THE OXFORD HANDBOOK OF

BIOETHICS

THE OXFORD HANDBOOK OF

BIOETHICS

Edited by

BONNIE STEINBOCK

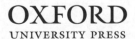

OXFORD
UNIVERSITY PRESS

Great Clarendon Street, Oxford OX2 6DP

Oxford University Press is a department of the University of Oxford.
It furthers the University's objective of excellence in research, scholarship,
and education by publishing worldwide in

Oxford New York

Auckland Cape Town Dar es Salaam Hong Kong Karachi
Kuala Lumpur Madrid Melbourne Mexico City Nairobi
New Delhi Shanghai Taipei Toronto

With offices in

Argentina Austria Brazil Chile Czech Republic France Greece
Guatemala Hungary Italy Japan Poland Portugal Singapore
South Korea Switzerland Thailand Turkey Ukraine Vietnam

Oxford is a registered trade mark of Oxford University Press
in the UK and in certain other countries

Published in the United States
by Oxford University Press Inc., New York

British Library Cataloguing in Publication Data

Data available

Library of Congress Cataloging in Publication Data

Data available

Typeset by Laserwords Private Limited, Chennai, India
Printed in Great Britain
on acid-free paper by
Biddles Ltd., King's Lynn, Norfolk

ISBN 978–0–19–927335–5

1 3 5 7 9 10 8 6 4 2

To Lindy Linder, my first cousin and first best friend

ACKNOWLEDGMENTS

THIS book is the brainchild of Peter Momtchiloff, who asked me to edit it many years ago, and refused to take 'no' for an answer. While I remain uncertain as to whether I owe him 'thanks' for this, I must acknowledge that the book would not have come into being, but for his persistence. I am grateful to all my contributors, especially those who actually handed in their work on time, or at least within a year of when they said they would get it in. (The delays led to John Arras suggesting that the contributors could be paid, not in cash or Oxford books, but death benefits, or possibly, assisted-living expenses.) I could not have finished this project without the painstaking work of Juliette Stevens. Juliette, you're wonderful. Thanks also to Darren Anderson for putting the manuscript on disk and putting together the index, saving me a lot of time and my sanity. Finally, I had the good fortune to have the best copy editor in the world: Laurien Berkeley. I am deeply grateful for her careful attention and unfailing good humor.

Contents

PART VI: GENETICS AND ENHANCEMENT

PART VII: RESEARCH ETHICS

PART VIII: PUBLIC AND GLOBAL HEALTH

Notes on the Contributors

Felicia Nimue Ackerman is Professor of Philosophy at Brown University. Her essays on bioethics have appeared in the *Hastings Center Report, Midwest Studies in Philosophy, Physician-Assisted Suicide: Expanding the Debate* (Routledge, 1998), *Ethical Issues in Modern Medicine* (McGraw-Hill, 2002), and elsewhere. Her short stories on bioethical themes have appeared in *Commentary, Mid-American Review, Prize Stories 1990: The O. Henry Awards* (Doubleday, 1990), *Clones and Clones: Facts and Fantasies About Human Cloning* (Norton, 1998), and elsewhere. She is writing *Bioethics Through Fiction*, a book of essays and short stories, forthcoming in the Rowman & Littlefield series *Explorations in Bioethics and the Medical Humanities*.

John D. Arras is Porterfield Professor of Biomedical Ethics and Professor of Philosophy at the University of Virginia, and a Fellow of the Hastings Center, Garrison, NY. His primary areas of interest currently include research ethics (with a focus on international trials), global justice and human rights, and methods of practical ethics. He consults regularly with the Centers for Disease Control and Prevention, Atlanta, Georgia, and the National Institutes of Health on ethical issues in research and public health practice.

Andrea Bonnicksen teaches courses in biomedical and biotechnology policy in the Department of Political Science at Northern Illinois University, where she is Presidential Research Professor. She is the author of three books, including *Crafting a Cloning Policy: From Dolly to Stem Cells* (Georgetown University Press, 2002). She is co-chair of the Ethics Committee of the American Society for Reproductive Medicine.

Allen Buchanan is James B. Duke Professor of Philosophy and Public Policy at Duke University. Buchanan's work is mainly in Bioethics and in Political Philosophy. His most recent books are *From Chance to Choice: Genetics and Justice* (co-authored with Dan W. Brock, Norman Daniels, and Daniel Wikler; Cambridge University Press, 2000) and *Justice, Legitimacy, and Self-Determination: Moral Foundations for International Law* (Oxford University Press, 2003).

James F. Childress is the John Allen Hollingsworth Professor of Ethics at the University of Virginia, where he teaches in the in the Department of Religious Studies and in the Schools of Law and Medicine, and directs the Institute for Practical Ethics and Public Life. He is the author of numerous articles and several books in bioethics, including (with Tom L. Beauchamp), *Principles of Biomedical Ethics*, (5th edn., Oxford University Press, 2001). He has served on a number of governmental bodies addressing bioethics and public policy, including the National Bioethics Advisory Commission 1996–2001.

John K. Davis is an Assistant Professor of Philosophy at the University of Tennessee, Knoxville. His research and teaching interests include bioethics, ethical theory, and philosophy of law. In addition to autonomy and end-of-life care, he is interested in the methodology and epistemology of applying ethics to cases.

Matthew DeCamp entered the Duke University Medical Scientist Training Program (MD/Ph.D.) in 2000 and is currently pursuing graduate work in the Department of Philosophy. His current research focuses on the relationship between intellectual property rules and global distributive justice in global health.

Gerald Dworkin is Professor in the Philosophy Department at the University of California at Davis. He is also an adjunct Professor in the School of Law. He is the author of many articles and books in moral, political, and legal philosophy. His most recent book (co-authored with Sissela Bok and R. G. Frey) is *Euthanasia and Physician-Assisted Suicide: For and Against* (Cambridge University Press, 1998).

Ezekiel J. Emanuel is the Chair of the Department of Clinical Bioethics at the Clinical Center of the National Institutes of Health. He is a Fellow of the Institute of Medicine, the Association of American Physicians, as well as the Hastings Center, Garrison, NY. He is author of *The Ends of Human Life: Medical Ethics in a Liberal Polity* (Harvard University Press, 1991) and *No Margin, No Mission: Health-Care Organizations and the Quest for Ethical Excellence* (Oxford University Press, 2003), and co-editor (with Robert A. Crouch, John D. Arras, Jonathan D. Moreno, and Christine Grady) of *Ethical and Regulatory Aspects of Clinical Research: Readings and Commentary* (Johns Hopkins University Press, 2003).

John Harris is Sir David Alliance Professor of Bioethics at the Institute of Medicine, Law, and Bioethics, University of Manchester. In 2001 he was the first philosopher to have been elected a Fellow of the Academy of Medical Sciences. He has been a member of the Human Genetics Commission since its foundation in 1999. The author or editor of fourteen books and over 150 papers, his recent books include *Bioethics* (Oxford University Press, 2001), *A Companion to Genetics: Philosophy and the Genetic Revolution*, co-edited with Justine Burley (Blackwell, 2002), and *On Cloning* (Routledge, 2004).

Søren Holm is Professorial Fellow in Bioethics at Cardiff Law School and Director of the Cardiff Centre for Ethics, Law, and Society. He is also adjunct Professor of Medical Ethics in the Section for Medical Ethics, University of Oslo. He has written on many subjects in bioethics and the philosophy of medicine, and his most recent publications have been on biobanking and on stem-cell research.

Louise Irving was formerly at the Institute of Medicine, Law, and Bioethics at the University of Manchester, where she was a research fellow on a three-year project, funded by the European Commission, which seeks to develop a legal and ethical framework for stem-cell research. She has written on the commodification of the human body, the relationship between analytic moral philosophy and bioethics, and issues of public health. Her main research interest is in the nature of freedom.

Bruce Jennings is Director of the Center for Humans and Nature, a private operating foundation that focuses on ethical issues in environmental and health policy, and Senior Consultant at the Hastings Center, Garrison, NY. He also teaches at the Yale University School of Public Health. He is author of numerous books and articles on ethical and social issues in health-care and public policy. He is co-author (with Willard Gaylin) of *The Perversion of Autonomy: The Uses of Coercion and Constraint in a Liberal Society* (2nd edn., Georgetown University Press, 2003). He is currently at work on a book on dementia, quality of life, and the ethics of long-term care.

Eric T. Juengst is Professor of Bioethics at the Case Western Reserve University School of Medicine, where he directs the Center for Genetic Research Ethics and Law. He has written widely on conceptual and ethical issues in genetics, and has served on the DNA Advisory Board of the FBI, the NIH National Advisory Council for Human Genome Research, the NIH Recombinant DNA Advisory Committee, the Ethics Committee of the American Society for Gene Therapy, and the National Academy of Sciences Committee on Human Genetic Diversity. He is an elected Fellow of the Hastings Center, Garrison, NY, and the Center for Genetics and Society, University of California, Los Angeles, and in 2006 was awarded the Golden Eurydice Prize for pioneering work integrating science and ethics from the European Commission's International Forum on Biophilosophy.

Jeffrey Kahn is the Maas Family Endowed Chair in Bioethics and Director of the Center for Bioethics at the University of Minnesota. He holds additional faculty appointments in the university's Medical School, School of Public Health, and Department of Philosophy. He has published over seventy-five articles in both the bioethics and medical literature, serves on numerous state and federal advisory panels, and speaks nationally and internationally on a range of bioethics topics. From 1998 to 2002 he also wrote the bi-weekly column 'Ethics Matters' on CNN.com.

Jason Karlawish is Associate Professor of Medicine, Fellow of the Center for Clinical Epidemiology and Biostatistics, and Senior Fellow of the Center for Bioethics and the Leonard Davis Institute of Health Economics at the University of Pennsylvania. He is the Associate Director of the Penn Memory Center and the Director of the Alzheimer's Disease Center's Education and Information Transfer Core, University of Pennsylvania. His research focuses on ethical issues in human subjects research and the care of persons with dementia.

Jeanette Kennett is Principal Research Fellow in the Centre for Applied Philosophy and Public Ethics, Australian National University, and School of Philosophy and Bioethics, Monash University. She is the author of *Agency and Responsibility* (Clarendon Press, 2001) and has published widely on philosophical and ethical issues related to moral responsibility, the self, and mental disorder.

Benjamin J. Krohmal is a fellow in the Department of Clinical Bioethics at the Clinical Center of the National Institutes of Health. His current focus is on research ethics and the ethics of health-care reform.

Alex John London is Associate Professor of Philosophy and an executive member of the Center for the Advancement of Applied Ethics and Political Philosophy at Carnegie Mellon University. The recipient of a New Directions Fellowship from the Andrew W. Mellon Foundation in 2005, he is also co-editor (with Bonnie Steinbock and John D. Arras) of *Ethical Issues in Modern Medicine* (6th edn., McGraw-Hill, 2003).

Florencia Luna is an Adjunct Researcher at CONICET (the National Scientific and Technological Research Council), Argentina. She is the Director of the Program of Bioethics at FLACSO (the Latin American University of Social Sciences) and co-director with Ruth Macklin of a research training grant of the National Institutes of Health in the United States. She was also the President of the International Association of Bioethics (2003–5). She is the author of *Bioethics and Vulnerability: A Latin American View* (Rodopi, 2006), and of *Ensayos de bioética: Reflexiones desde el Sur* (Fontamara, 2001), and co-editor (with Arleen L. F. Salles) of *Decisiones de vida y muerte* (Sudamericana, Buenos Aires, 1995) and (with Arleen L. F. Salles) *Bioetica* (Sudamericana, 1998).

Ruth Macklin is Professor of Bioethics at Albert Einstein College of Medicine in the Bronx, New York. She is the author or editor of twelve books and has published more than 200 articles in scholarly and professional journals. She is an elected member of the Institute of Medicine of the National Academies of Science, chairs the External Ethics Committee of the Centers for Disease Control and Prevention, Atlanta, Georgia, and serves as an adviser to the World Health Organization and the Joint United Nations Programme on HIV/AIDS. Her latest book is *Double Standards in Medical Research in Developing Countries* (Cambridge University Press, 2004).

Don Marquis is Professor of Philosophy at the University of Kansas. He teaches applied ethics and ethical theory.

Anna Mastroianni is Associate Professor at the School of Law and Institute for Public Health Genetics at the University of Washington. She holds additional faculty appointments in the University's School of Public Health and Community Medicine and Medical School. She has held a number of legal and federal policy positions in the United States and has served on several national advisory panels concerning issues of biomedicine and health policy. She has published numerous articles in the legal and bioethics literature, with specific interests in the legal, ethical, and policy issues related to human subjects research, public health, and the use of genetic technologies.

Dennis McKerlie is Associate Professor of Philosophy at the University of Calgary. He has published articles on egalitarianism, justice between age groups, and ancient philosophy.

Carolyn McLeod is Associate Professor of Philosophy at the University of Western Ontario. From 2004 to 2006 she was also a New Faculty Fellow in the Comparative Program on Health and Society at the Munk Centre for International Studies at the University of Toronto. She has published in bioethics and moral theory, on topics such as trust, autonomy, integrity, conscience, objectification, and commodification. Her book *Self-Trust and Reproductive Autonomy* (MIT Press, 2002), is part of the Basic Bioethics series of the MIT Press.

Jonathan D. Moreno is the Emily Davie and Joseph S. Kornfeld Professor and Director of the Center for Biomedical Ethics at the University of Virginia. He is an elected member of the Institute of Medicine and has served as senior staff to two presidential advisory committees and as a consultant to numerous public and private organizations. Among his books are *Undue Risk: Secret State Experiments on Humans* (Routledge, 2001) and *In the Wake of Terror: Medicine and Morals in a Time of Crisis* (MIT Press, 2003). His latest book is *Is There an Ethicist in the House? On the Cutting Edge of Bioethics* (Indiana University Press, 2005).

Ronald Munson is Professor of the Philosophy of Science and Medicine at the University of Missouri—St Louis. He has served as a bioethicist for the National Cancer Institute, the National Eye Institute, and the Veterans Administration, and is a member of the Human Studies Committee at Washington University School of Medicine. His books include *Reasoning in Medicine* (Johns Hopkins University Press, 1994), *Outcome Uncertain: Cases and Contexts in Bioethics* (Wadsworth, 2003), and *Raising the Dead: Organ Transplants, Ethics, and Society* (Oxford University Press, 2002). He is also the author of the novels *Nothing Human*, *Fan Mail*, and *Night Vision*.

Thomas H. Murray is President of the Hastings Center, Garrison, NY. He has written or edited many books including *The Worth of a Child* (University of California Press, 1996), *Cultures of Caregiving* (with C. Levine; Johns Hopkins University Press, 2004), *Genetic Ties and the Family* (with M. Rothstein, G. Kaebnick, and M. A. Majumder; Johns Hopkins University Press, 2005), *The*

Encyclopedia of Ethical, Legal, and Policy Issues in Biotechnology (with M. Mehlman; John Wiley, 2000), and *Feeling Good and Doing Better: Ethics and Nontherapeutic Drug Use* (Humana Press, 1984). He is Chair of the World Anti-Doping Agency's Ethical Issues Review Panel.

Alastair Norcross is Associate Professor of Philosophy at Rice University. His articles on ethical theory and applied ethics have appeared in such journals as *Philosophical Review, Journal of Philosophy, Philosophy and Public Affairs*, and *Social Theory and Practice*. He is co-editor, with Bonnie Steinbock, of *Killing and Letting Die* (2nd edn., Fordham, 1994).

Stephen G. Post is Professor in the Department of Bioethics, Case Western Reserve University School of Medicine, and was a Senior Research Scholar in the Becket Institute at St Hugh's College, University of Oxford. He is Editor-in-Chief of *The Encyclopedia of Bioethics* (3rd edn., Macmillan Reference, 2004). He is an elected member of the Medical and Scientific Advisory Panel of Alzheimer's Disease International, the recipient of a 'distinguished service' award from the Association's National Board (1998), and the author of *The Moral Challenge of Alzheimer Disease: Ethical Issues from Diagnosis to Dying* (2nd edn., Johns Hopkins University Press, 2000).

Julian Savulescu is the Uehiro Professor of Practical Ethics and Director of the Oxford Uehiro Centre for Practical Ethics at the University of Oxford, and Director of the Program on Ethics and the New Biosciences in the 21st Century School, University of Oxford. Qualified in medicine, bioethics, and analytic philosophy, he has published over 100 articles and is co-author (with R. A. Hope and Judith Hendrick) of the book *Medical Ethics and Law* (Churchill Livingstone, 2003).

Bonnie Steinbock is Professor of Philosophy at the University at Albany/SUNY. She is the author of *Life Before Birth: The Moral and Legal Status of Embryos and Fetuses* (Oxford University Press, 1992) and the editor of several books, including (with John Arras and Alex London) *Ethical Issues in Modern Medicine* (6th edn., McGraw-Hill, 2003).

Daniel P. Sulmasy, OFM is Sisters of Charity Chair in Ethics at St Vincent's Hospital Manhattan, and Professor of Medicine and Director of the Bioethics Institute of New York Medical College. He is Editor-in-Chief of the journal *Theoretical Medicine and Bioethics*. His latest books are *The Rebirth of the Clinic* and *A Balm for Gilead: Mediations on Spirituality and the Healing Arts* (both Georgetown University Press, 2006).

Stuart J. Youngner is the Susan E. Watson Professor of Bioethics and Chair of the Department of Bioethics at Case Western Reserve University School of Medicine. He has written and spoken extensively about definitions of death, organ and tissue transplantation, end-of-life decisions, and clinical ethics consultation.

INTRODUCTION

BONNIE STEINBOCK

THE aim of this *Handbook* is to provide an up-to-date picture of the state of the art in bioethics. It makes no attempt to cover every issue in the field—there are excellent encyclopedias that serve this purpose (Post 2004; Murray and Mehlman 2000). Instead, it is a selective representation of some of the most important issues in contemporary bioethics. The chapters are surveys in that they inform the reader of what has been happening recently in each area, through a discussion of the relevant literature. At the same time, they are not neutral, encyclopedia-like articles, but original essays that reflect the particular 'take' of their authors. They are not intended for undergraduates or general readers, but rather for those with some knowledge of the field (scholars and graduate students) who want an authoritative and stimulating account of bioethics today.

My task as editor was to get the best and most interesting individuals in the field as contributors. This might be interpreted as meaning the best-known or most prominent bioethicists, and certainly this *Handbook* includes some of the most respected names in bioethics, people who have shaped, and continue to shape, the field. However, I also wanted to include some who are not as well known because they are in the early stages of their careers. These 'up-and-comers' represent the next generation of bioethicists. In addition, the aim was to reflect the interdisciplinarity that is fundamental to bioethics. Therefore, the volume includes individuals not only from my own discipline (philosophy), but also from theology, medicine, law, political science, social science, and public health. Until recently, bioethics has been dominated by Americans. However, in recognition that bioethics is becoming increasingly international, a third of the contributors come from outside the United States. Equally importantly, the authors represent a diversity of opinions and viewpoints, sharpening and deepening the debate on a number of controversial issues.

A SHORT HISTORY OF BIOETHICS

Bioethics was preceded by medical ethics, which focused primarily on issues arising out of the physician–patient relationship. The ancient Hippocratic literature (which includes but is not limited to the Hippocratic Oath) enjoins doctors to use their knowledge and powers to benefit the sick, to heal and not to harm, to preserve life, and to keep in the strictest confidence information that ought not to be spread about (though precisely what must be kept confidential is not detailed). These basic values and principles remain an essential part of contemporary bioethics. However, after the Second World War it became clear that the old medical ethics was not sufficient to meet contemporary challenges.

Unprecedented advances in medicine, including the use of penicillin and immunizations against childhood diseases, have saved literally millions of lives. So have open heart surgery and cardiac catheterization, chronic hemodialysis, and organ donation. At the same time, many of the tools of modern medicine are very expensive, and thus out of the reach of many who might benefit from them. Medicine's success thus led to a debate about how to pay for health care. In most industrialized countries, the provision of health care is viewed as the responsibility of government, comparable to the obligation to provide public education. By contrast, in the United States many still regard payment for health care as an individual responsibility, or at least something that employers, not the state, should provide. Among those who agree that some kind of national health insurance is both fair and fiscally sound, a debate continues between egalitarians, who insist that no care should be provided unless it is available to all who need it, and those who favor a tiered health care system that allows some medical services to be distributed by the market. (This issue is thoroughly explored in Part II, Chapter 7, by Benjamin J. Krohmal and Ezekiel J. Emanuel.)

Medicine's successes in the post-war years raised another issue: the value of preserving life. Respirators were originally invented for people who were expected to recover and be able to breathe on their own. Within a short period of time they began to be used on people in persistent vegetative states, forcing medical professionals to ask whether this was an appropriate use of technology. Should people who are permanently and irreversibly unconscious be kept alive indefinitely? A similar issue resulted from the development of neonatal intensive care units (NICUs), which have saved the lives of many premature babies who would have died in earlier decades. Many of these babies go on to have normal, healthy lives, but many face a lifetime of severe disabilities and serious health complications.

Thus, NICUs raise the question: Ought life to be preserved regardless of the nature or quality of that life? And if there are times when life should not be preserved, who should be authorized to make these decisions?

During the 1960s these questions began to be debated at academic conferences and in scholarly journals, giving birth to the field of bioethics. In 1969 the Hastings Center in Garrison, NY, an independent, nonpartisan, and nonprofit bioethics research institute, was founded by Dan Callahan and Willard Gaylin to explore fundamental and emerging questions in health care, biotechnology, and the environment. Its journal, the *Hastings Center Report*, first appeared in June 1971. In July of that year the Kennedy Institute of Ethics at Georgetown University opened, with two research scholars: LeRoy Walters, who soon became its Director, and Warren Reich, who was the editor of the first edition of the *Encyclopedia of Bioethics*, published in 1978.

The term 'bioethics' was coined in the early 1970s by biologists who brought to the public's attention two pressing issues: the need to maintain the planet's ecology, on which all life depends, and the implications of advances in the life sciences toward manipulating human nature. In his book, *Bioethics: Bridge to the Future*, published in 1971, Van Rensselaer Potter focused on the growing human ability to change nature, including human nature, and the implications of this for our global future. This issue has been revisited in recent years in a growing literature on enhancement, genetic and otherwise, and is addressed from very different perspectives in Part VI Chapters 21 and 22, by Thomas Murray and Julian Savulescu respectively. Although the term 'bioethics' has referred almost exclusively to problems in biomedicine, in recent years the field has returned to 'the wider context provided by the life scientists of the early 1970s, including their environmental and public health concerns' (Post 2004, p. xi). (The relevance of public health for bioethics is covered in Part VIII, Chapter 28, by Jeffrey Kahn and Anna Mastroianni.)

While bioethics has been interdisciplinary since its inception, theology played a foundational role in its creation. It continues to have a profound influence today, as reflected in the careful analysis and defense of the rule of double effect by Daniel Sulmasy in Part I, Chapter 5. Three theologians in particular were instrumental in the birth of bioethics: Joseph Fletcher, an Episcopal minister; Paul Ramsey, a Methodist minister; and Richard McCormick, a Jesuit moral theologian. The theologians were soon joined by philosophers who rejected the emphasis in contemporary analytic ethics on meta-ethics, to the exclusion of normative ethics. Events in the 1960s—opposition to the war in Vietnam, the civil rights movement, and other social movements it spawned, such as the women's movement, the disability rights movement, and the gay and lesbian rights movement—played a role in the revitalization of normative ethics, and philosophical interest in applied ethics. Students began to demand that their courses were 'relevant', and professional philosophers also became interested in writing on the issues of the day. Philosophers now specialize in bioethics, but even philosophers not usually thought of as 'bioethicists', including Jonathan Bennett, Ronald Dworkin, Joel Feinberg, Jonathan Glover, Thomas Nagel, Onora O'Neill, Judith Thomson, and Bernard Williams, have made important contributions to the bioethics literature.

A new journal, *Philosophy and Public Affairs*, appeared in 1971, with lead articles on war and abortion. John Rawls's *A Theory of Justice* appeared the same year. The book had a huge impact on Anglo-American political philosophy, and indirectly on bioethics. As Jonsen (1998: 74) puts it, 'Rawls's thesis excited many moral philosophers, restored faith in a rational approach to ethics, provided a carefully articulated version of contractarianism, and bequeathed to some future bioethicists the basis for a theory of the allocation of medical resources.' The influence of Rawls can be seen in many of the chapters in this volume, especially in Parts I and II.

CENTRAL ISSUES IN BIOETHICS

At its inception, the central issues in bioethics were research with human subjects, genetics, organ transplantation, death and dying, and reproduction. As a glance at the table of contents reveals, these continue to be important issues today.

Methodology has been a central theoretical issue since the very beginning of bioethics. While some hoped that bioethics would generate a single correct normative theory, that idea has been given up by most practitioners. Indeed, bioethics reflects a wide range of theoretical approaches in normative ethics, including utilitarianism, deontology, natural law, contractarianism, virtue ethics, communitarianism, pragmatism, and feminist ethics (Steinbock et al. 2003). All of these approaches, and variations within these, are carefully enunciated by James Childress in Part I, Chapter 1. As Childress perhaps ruefully concludes, 'It is probably too much to expect consensus about the best possible method(s), all things considered—at most, we can take advantage of the strengths of each method and compensate for its special deficiencies.'

A related issue concerns the relationship between abstract principles and concrete particulars. An approach that has come to be known as 'principlism', famously advocated by Beauchamp and Childress in their classic text *Principles of Bioethics* (1979–2001), attempts to derive answers to bioethical dilemmas from the basic principles: autonomy, beneficence, and justice. Principlism has been criticized, as John Arras points out in Chapter 2, by casuists, feminists, partisans of narrative ethics, and pragmatists as 'too abstract, deductive, and "top down"'; as being 'insufficiently attentive to particulars, relationships, storytelling, and process'. In response, principlists have attempted to incorporate these insights into a principle-based approach, using Rawls's method of 'reflective equilibrium'. However, while this approach has considerable intuitive appeal, it is far from clear exactly how reflective equilibrium is to be interpreted or applied. Arras provides a clear and thorough analysis of the difficulties, ending on a moderately skeptical note about the value of method in moral inquiry. No method, he says, is a guarantor of truth, or even intersubjective agreement, but careful attention to the various approaches can improve practical reasoning and 'facilitate our quest for moral justification'.

In addition to methodological issues, theoretical issues in bioethics include certain concepts and principles. Of these, perhaps the most central is autonomy. The prominence of autonomy in biomedical ethics can be traced back to the Belmont Report (National Commission for the Protection of Human Subjects of Biomedical and Behavioral Research 1979), so called because it had its origins in a meeting held in February 1976 at Belmont House, a conference center of the Smithsonian Institution. Congress had instructed the Commission to identify the basic ethical principles that should underlie the conduct of biomedical and behavioral research involving human subjects. The Commission articulated three basic principles: respect for persons, beneficence, and justice. The articulation of these principles had a major impact on the development of bioethics, and indeed on virtually every chapter in this volume. These concepts found their way into the general literature of the field, and evolved from the principles underlying the conduct of research into the basic principles of bioethics. 'Respect for persons' became understood as 'respect for autonomy' or simply 'autonomy'. Yet while autonomy is unquestionably a central principle in bioethics, both its interpretation and its moral weight remain controversial, as Bruce Jennings illustrates in Chapter 3.

The issue of autonomy is considered from the perspective of moral psychology in Chapter 4, by Jeanette Kennett. While mental illness clearly can rob a person of the capacity for autonomous choice and action, it is also true that this has been exaggerated in the past by prejudice and stigmatization. What, then, is the correct attitude to take toward those suffering from mental illness? Kennett reminds us that 'agency comes in degrees, that autonomy is an achievement, and that respect for autonomy may require our active support for the agency of those in adverse circumstances', including mental illness. Acknowledging the difficulty of adopting 'the participant stance' toward those who are seriously mentally ill, Kennett argues that nevertheless we are morally required to adopt it, so far as possible.

Part II turns to issues of justice and policy. Like Arras in the preceding section, Søren Holm, a Danish philosopher and physician, starts with Rawls, although Holm is less interested in reflective equilibrium as a methodology, and more interested in the requirements of deliberative democracy. He notes that while policy making shares some of the values of ethical decision making (such as reasonableness, reciprocity, consistency, and integrity), it also incorporates features that may be anathema to philosophers, including political compromise, moratoria (waiting periods while scientific uncertainty is resolved), and the accommodation of minority positions. These political tools, Holm argues, are as important as philosophical reasoning for achieving 'peaceful public decision making in a context of fundamental moral disagreement'.

The next chapter, by Benjamin J. Krohmal and Ezekiel J. Emanuel, considers whether a just health care system must be strictly egalitarian (as in Canada and Norway), or whether a better approach allows for a tiered health care system, in which some people can pay for greater access to services than others with the same needs. After examining the arguments pro and con, the authors conclude that an egalitarian approach is unjust. Justice calls for a two-tier health care system with universal public coverage (as in Britain and Israel).

Another question of distributive justice arises because people have different needs for health care. For example, as people age, they are likely to need more and more expensive health care, including prescriptions, tests, and hospital stays. In Chapter 8 Dennis McKerlie, a Canadian philosopher, addresses this issue, asking, 'Are the elderly receiving less, or more, than their fair share of health resources and economic wealth?' An important part of the answer depends on how principles of justice are applied. McKerlie contrasts a 'complete lives' view, which focuses on people's lifetime expectations of receiving primary goods, with the prudential lifespan account, proposed by Norman Daniels and Ronald Dworkin, in which principles of justice have a temporal scope. He rejects both in favor of what he calls the 'life-stage view', which is more generous to the elderly than either the complete lives view or the prudential lifespan account, in large measure because they need help the most. The chapter ends with a thoughtful reflection on the effects of aging on individuals' abilities and values, and the implications this has both for respect for autonomy and for a just distribution of resources.

Part III addresses a set of issues turning around human bodies and parts of bodies. In Chapter 9 Ronald Munson outlines the history, economics, and ethics of organ transplantation, an issue that has been prominent in medical ethics since the first organ transplant in 1954. Most transplants are taken from dead donors, but many more lives could be saved if the number of living donors of kidneys and livers was increased. The risks to donors, however, are considerable, and the chance of coercion or undue influence is thought by some to undermine voluntariness and autonomy. However, Munson argues that paternalistically denying someone the opportunity to be a living donor is a greater threat to autonomy, especially since measures can be taken to protect voluntariness.

The next chapter, by Louise Irving and John Harris, on biobanking discusses the methods and purposes of tissue storage and collection. A major theme is the great importance of tissue collection to medical research, which at the same time raises issues of confidentiality, consent, stigmatization, and risk. While these need to be taken seriously, Irving and Harris argue that the ethical problems raised by biobanking are neither unique nor unresolvable.

Carolyn McLeod, in Chapter 11, addresses the issues of oocyte vending and commercial contract pregnancy from a feminist perspective. The commodification of women's reproductive capacity presents feminists with a classic double bind. Should a market in reproductive labor be viewed as degrading and rife with the potential for harm and exploitation of women? Or should the ability to sell one's labor (reproductive or otherwise) be viewed as empowering, and the denial of this right inconsistent with women's status as autonomous persons? McLeod does not resolve this issue, but suggests several ways in which the debate could be refined and clarified.

Part IV opens with an update on the problems with the definition and determination of death. Stuart J. Youngner illustrates the ways in which this is not only a scientific issue, but a matter of philosophy and policy as well. His chapter dovetails nicely with Munson's, on organ transplantation, since the possibility of transplanting organs from deceased donors has influenced, if not driven, the conceptual debates about death.

One of the challenges of the twenty-first century is the increase in lifespan, and the consequent increase in numbers of the very old, issues addressed by Stephen Post and Felicia Nimue Ackerman in Chapters 13 and 14. While both Post and Ackerman disagree with the natural law approach taken by, for example, Leon Kass, they disagree with each other about the value of extending life when this entails illness and deterioration.

John K. Davis returns, in Chapter 15, to the issue of autonomy in his discussion of advance directives (ADs). A number of writers have argued that ADs pose an insoluble problem. They express the values and preferences of the competent individuals who write them, but they go into effect only when the individuals are no longer competent. Once incompetent, they are likely to have very different interests than the interests they had when competent. They may no longer care about, or even be cognizant of, issues such as dignity and independence. Indeed, some would argue that the presently incompetent individual is so radically changed that he or she is not the same person as the individual who wrote the AD, and that therefore the writer of the AD does not have the moral authority to decide that lifesaving treatment should be withheld from the present incompetent person. Drawing a distinction between loss of capacity and loss of concern, Davis defends ADs against this particular criticism. Gerald Dworkin ends this part with a careful analysis of the arguments for and against physician-assisted death, and a defense of physician-assisted suicide, though not, for strategic reasons, euthanasia.

Part V concerns issues at the beginning of life, specifically the morality of abortion and embryonic stem cell research. In 1989 Don Marquis published a now classic article, 'Why Abortion Is Immoral', in which he argued that both pro-life and pro-choice approaches were seriously flawed. In their place, he offered a new approach, the future of value argument. It maintains that the best explanation for the wrongness of killing is that killing deprives us of our valuable futures. Because we were once fetuses, fetuses have the same futures of value that every one of us has, and therefore abortion is 'seriously presumptively wrong'. In this new chapter Marquis elaborates on the notion of having a future of value, and argues that this argument is superior to recent accounts of moral status provided by Mary Anne Warren and David Boonin.

My own contribution to the book concerns the moral status of extracorporeal embryos, and the implications this has for embryonic stem cell research (ESCR). The chapter builds on the interest view, which I elaborated in *Life Before Birth* (1992). I argue that very early embryos (blastocysts) have no moral *status*, because they lack interests of their own. This means that we cannot act in their interest or on their behalf; they cannot be harmed or benefited. Nevertheless, as developing forms of human life, they have moral *value*, and are entitled to respect. I distinguish between the respect owed to human embryos and Kantian respect for persons, and argue that the respect owed to embryos does not rule out using them merely as means to our ends. Instead, it requires that the ends served be morally important ones. Potentially valuable scientific research qualifies as morally important, and is therefore consistent with respect for human life.

In the last chapter in Part V Andrea Bonnicksen returns to an issue addressed in Part I by Søren Holm: policy making in pluralistic societies. In the United States ESCR is politically extremely divisive. There is no federal support for it, and hence no federal oversight. Yet several states (California, New Jersey, Massachusetts, Illinois) have passed legislation to allow and/or fund ESCR, including the cloning of human embryos. Moreover, several private laboratories are attempting to clone human embryos and derive stem cell lines, without, however, the kind of oversight and ethical reflection characteristic of the Human Fertilization and Embryology Authority in the United Kingdom. Bonnicksen suggests that a 'policy community', consisting of academics, policy analysts, interest group members, and others with shared interests, might be able to overcome the current stalemate, both within the United States and internationally, and address some of the pressing ethical concerns raised by therapeutic cloning.

In addition to the issue of enhancement previously mentioned, Part VI addresses issues in genomic medicine. In Chapter 20 Eric Juengst notes that while the interest in mapping the human genome was initially genealogical, interest soon developed in the possibility of tailoring diagnostic protocols, therapeutic interventions, and preventive measures to each patient's genetic profile. This would have profound implications not only for medicine, but also for public health (this is addressed in Part VIII, Chapter 28, by Jeffrey Kahn and Anna Mastroianni). At the same time, it has raised old questions about racism and discrimination, as well as new questions about the collective interests of groups being studied. In Chapter 23 Matthew DeCamp and Allen Buchanan focus specifically on the role pharmaceuticals play in genomic medicine. In addition to problems resulting from the reifying of race, pharmacogenomic technologies raise serious issues of distributive justice: who will get these new drugs, on what basis will decisions to produce them be made, and who will pay for them?

Part VII concerns the ethics of research on human subjects, a subject that has been at the heart of bioethics since its inception. For most of its history, medicine was primarily therapeutic. Experimentation was limited to trying new curative or palliative approaches on individual patients. As medicine became more of a science, physicians wanted to know if their treatments, standard and innovative, actually worked. To do this, one needed to perform experiments on people, not primarily to benefit them, but to learn things that might benefit others. This put physician–researchers into a double bind. In so far as they were acting as the patient's doctor, their aim was to benefit the patient. In so far as they were acting as scientific researchers, their aim was to perform a controlled experiment and get accurate results. Typically, this means assigning subjects randomly to the various arms of a clinical trial without regard to whether the standard treatment, the new treatment, or placebo would be in the patient–subject's best interest. It seems that physicians cannot satisfy both roles simultaneously.

As Alex London points out in the first chapter in Part VII, Charles Fried attempted to solve this dilemma through the notion of 'equipoise'. Physicians were justified in enrolling their patients in clinical trials only if they were uncertain about the relative therapeutic merits of various arms of the trial. However, as London notes, there is considerable uncertainty about how precisely to formulate the requirement of equipoise. After clarifying different versions of the equipoise requirement, and demonstrating their respective strengths and weaknesses, London proposes a novel approach to research ethics that better avoids the exploitation of research participants.

The problem of exploitation is central to the next three chapters as well. In Chapter 25 the physician Jason Karlawish examines the problem of research on individuals who, due to cognitive impairment, cannot give informed consent. Is it possible both to accomplish valuable research and also to protect vulnerable individuals? This issue is also addressed by Florencia Luna (and again in Part VIII in the chapter by Jeffrey Kahn and Anna Mastroianni) from the perspective of research on vulnerable populations, namely, individuals in developing countries. The problems of such research were brought into sharp relief in the late 1990s, when clinical trials were done in sub-Saharan Africa, Asia, and Latin America to find a more economical and effective treatment for preventing mother-to-baby transmission of HIV/AIDS. A proven treatment for preventing transmission existed, and was standard in the United States and other developed countries. However, it was not only expensive (far beyond the health care budgets of developing countries), but also burdensome to administer—perhaps even impossible in the conditions in most developing countries. To see if a less expensive, less burdensome regimen was effective, half the subjects in the trial were given the proposed regimen and half were given placebos. This was extremely controversial because normally a new treatment is tested against the proven treatment to determine if it is as effective.

This was not done in the so-called 'AIDS-African trials' because the proven regimen was beyond the economic reach of developing countries. The issue for them was not whether the new regimen was as effective as the proven regimen, but whether it was better than nothing (i.e. placebo). If it was not, there would be no point in using scarce health care dollars to provide it to HIV-infected pregnant women. This seemed reasonable, and yet such a protocol would never be approved in a developed country. Critics complained of introducing a double standard into international research—'a standard for industrialized countries that can provide the best existing therapies and another for poor countries with limited funding and a deficient healthcare system'. Exploitation of vulnerable populations is a real problem, but not one that can be solved with slogans, Luna argues. Obligations to research subjects during and after clinical trials must be considered, as well as the benefit to of individuals and communities who participate in research.

Part VII ends with a discussion of research on animals. Ever since Peter Singer's *Animal Liberation* appeared in 1975, there has been a lively debate about the moral status and treatment of animals. Although the treatment of human beings in research has at times been scandalous (with the experiments on Jews and others in Nazi concentration camps being the most heinous example), such treatment of non-human animals is pervasive. Animals are routinely killed, maimed, shocked, burned, and caused terrible pain, in the name of scientific and medical progress. In Chapter 27 Alastair Norcross examines various justifications for inflicting pain on non-human animals, and concludes that they are unsuccessful, and that this renders much animal experimentation morally unacceptable.

Part VIII explores some relatively new directions for bioethics: the turn to public and global health. On the one hand, public health seems at odds with bioethics because the focus in public health is the health of the population or community, whereas the focus in medicine is the health of the individual. Moreover, even as bioethics diverged from traditional medical ethics, it retained the principle of respect for individual autonomy, and correlative principles of confidentiality and privacy. On the other hand, there has been a kind of self-correction in the field of bioethics, away from an excessive individualism and toward engagement in questions of public health and global justice. In the first chapter in Part VIII Jeffrey Kahn and Anna Mastroianni discuss these issues, using as examples HIV/AIDS, resource allocation, and public health genomics.

In the next chapter Ruth Macklin explores the notion of 'globalization', and explains why in today's globalized world public health is global health. In part, this is because intercontinental travel makes the spread of disease so rapid, increasing the possibility of global pandemics. In addition, actions and policies carried out in one part of the world are likely to have significant, and often harmful, effects on people very far away. Thus, it becomes increasingly impossible to reject responsibility for those effects. Finally, the world's problems can only be solved by international cooperation.

In the last chapter Jonathan Moreno discusses the ethical problems raised by bioterrorism, including the tension between respecting civil liberties and protecting the public's health, triage in a bioterror attack, and the responsibilities of emergency health care professionals. Moreno's chapter is an excellent example of the way in which bioethics can draw on historical parallels even as it adapts in response to new developments and challenges. As science and medicine continue to advance, new issues are constantly being raised, for example, in neuroscience, bioengineering, and nanotechnology. Some of these emerging sciences and technologies may pose genuinely new questions for bioethics; others can be characterized as 'old wine in new bottles'. Controversy over this question (and others) is inevitable, as bioethicists identify and analyze new issues, thus framing the debates of the twenty-first century.

References

BEAUCHAMP, T., and CHILDRESS, J. (1979–2001), *Principles of Bioethics*, (1st–5th edns. New York: Oxford University Press).

JONSEN, A. R. (1998), *The Birth of Bioethics* (New York: Oxford University Press).

MARQUIS, D. (1989), 'Why Abortion Is Immoral', *Journal of Philosophy*, 89: 183–202.

MURRAY, T. A., and MEHLMAN, M. (eds.) (2000), *The Encyclopedia of Ethical, Legal and Policy Issues in Biotechnology* (New York: John Wiley).

NATIONAL COMMISSION FOR THE PROTECTION OF HUMAN SUBJECTS OF BIOMEDICAL AND BEHAVIORAL RESEARCH (1979), *The Belmont Report: Ethical Principles and Guidelines for the Protection of Human Subjects of Research* (Washington, DC: Government Printing Office).

POST, S. G. (ed.) (2004), *The Encyclopedia of Bioethics*, (3rd edn. New York: Macmillan).

POTTER, V. R. (1971), *Bioethics: Bridge to the Future* (Englewood Cliffs, NJ: Prentice-Hall).

SINGER, P. (1975), *Animal Liberation* (New York: Random House).

STEINBOCK, B. (1992), *Life Before Birth: The Moral and Legal Status of Embryos and Fetuses* (New York: Oxford University Press).

——— ARRAS, J. D., and LONDON, A. J. (2003), *Ethical Issues in Modern Medicine*, (6th edn. Boston: McGraw-Hill).

PART I

THEORETICAL AND METHODOLOGICAL ISSUES

CHAPTER 1

METHODS IN BIOETHICS

JAMES F. CHILDRESS

INTRODUCTION: QUESTIONS
ABOUT METHOD

In the preface to the first edition of his classic work *The Methods of Ethics*, Henry Sidgwick noted its focus on 'the different methods of obtaining reasoned convictions as to what ought to be done' (Sidgwick 1962, p. v). He defined a 'method of ethics' as 'any rational procedure by which we determine what individual human beings "ought"—or what it is "right" for them—to do, or to seek to realize by voluntary action' (Sidgwick 1962: 1). One major reason for the widespread interest in methods of doing bioethics is to determine how best to guide human action. Hence, assessments of different methods consider, in part, how well a bioethical theory, framework, or perspective guides action—other criteria include clarity, consistency, coherence, completeness, and comprehensiveness, as well as congruence with moral experience (Beauchamp and Childress 2001, ch. 8). But, even on Sidgwick's definition, there can be strong and weak conceptions of method. For instance, a method may illuminate an agent's choices without fully prescribing or determining what he or she should do. Indeed, a method may provide a complex rather than a tidy answer to the agent who asks, 'What should I (or we) do?'

Early bioethics, in the 1970s, was often viewed as a species of 'applied ethics': bioethics denoted the reflective activity of applying an ethical theory or ethical principles to the domains of the biological sciences, medicine, and health care.

The language of 'applied ethics' implies more action guidance from theories or principles than is usually available, and it has now been largely discarded in favor of the language of 'practical ethics', a phrase that Sidgwick (1998) also used. Not all methods for addressing practical moral problems entail applying, in a deductivist fashion, ethical theories, frameworks, or perspectives.

The philosopher R. M. Hare (1996), in examining 'the methods of bioethics' (the title of one of his articles), observes that the designation 'ethical or moral theories' covers different kinds of activities, as captured, for instance, in their broad and narrow meanings. On the narrow conception of ethical theory, the task is to examine the logic of moral reasoning, and representative theories, often called metaethics, including naturalism, intuitionism, subjectivism, emotivism, and prescriptivism. Hare (1996) believes that we have to start with these narrow theories, because they can make the greatest contributions to bioethics, but he focuses instead on normative theories, such as utilitarianism, virtue ethics, and ethics of care. I too will concentrate on normative ethical methods and theories rather than on metaethics, while recognizing that the line between them is not always clear.

Other broad uses of the term 'method' encompass a variety of descriptive approaches. Observing the wide range of methods used in scholarly inquiry about physician-assisted suicide, Daniel Sulmasy concludes that scholars who have employed such methods as history, law, theology, philosophy, quantitative methods, ethnographic methods, and so forth, are all 'properly called "medical ethicists", and their research is properly called "medical ethics"' (Sulmasy 2001: 259). However, this usage is too broad to be helpful. Although numerous methods of scholarly inquiry can and do make important contributions to medical ethics or bioethics, not all those contributions actually involve doing medical ethics or bioethics in the normative sense, and I will limit my attention to methods in normative bioethics. This restriction in no way denigrates other methods and their contributions—indeed, they are frequently illuminating, and often indispensable. Nevertheless, a scholarly inquiry into bioethics, or into some topic within bioethics, does not necessary translate into 'doing bioethics', however important it may be for 'doing bioethics'.

This chapter then will stay largely within boundaries of normative bioethics. It will examine major types of principle-based methods (consequentialist, deontological, and pluralistic principlist methods), case-based methods, virtue ethics, ethics of care, and communitarian perspectives, along with some critical points from feminist perspectives and from rule-based theories. One cautionary note is in order: most of these types of method, theory, or perspective encompass a number of approaches that involve some degree of family resemblance. Since it will be impossible to examine all of these approaches in detail, I will highlight some major themes and criticisms, discuss a few representative positions in more detail, and sketch a few of their implications for practical decision-making about physician-assisted suicide and active euthanasia, topics addressed by proponents of all these methods, theories, and perspectives.

PRINCIPLE-BASED METHODS

A principle-based method, some claim, dominates bioethics. This claim may be accurate when the whole range of principle-based positions is surveyed. However, principle-based methods encompass a wide and rich variety of more specific methods, all of which stress principles without necessarily sharing much more. Minimally, a bioethical method that is principle-based must hold that general moral action guides are central to moral reasoning in bioethics. It need not, however, reduce all moral reasoning to explicit principle-based reasoning. It may concede, for instance, that appeals to principles most often occur when there is uncertainty or conflict about the appropriate course of action.

Action guides are frequently distinguished into principles and rules. The most general action guides—for instance, utility or respect for autonomy—are usually labeled 'principles' while the more specific action guides—for instance, respect for confidentiality—are usually labeled 'rules'. Nevertheless, the terms 'principles' and 'rules' are frequently used interchangeably, and the lines between them are often unclear because they reflect different degrees of generality and specificity. I will later consider different interpretations of the relationship between principles and rules; for now I merely note that rules are often regarded as derivative from broader principles (Solomon 1978).

No single approach can be called *the* principles approach; hence, criticisms directed against one principle-based method may not apply to other such methods. For instance, criticisms aimed at a principle-based deontological theory may not apply to a principle-based consequentialist theory. Sometimes the language of 'principles' is mistakenly restricted to deontological theories, that is, theories holding that some inherent or intrinsic features of acts, such as truthfulness or lying, make them right or wrong. This restriction is misleading because consequentialist theories, which focus on the probable effects of actions, may also be principle-based. For example, utilitarianism, the most prominent contemporary consequentialist theory, appeals to the principle of utility in assessing acts or rules.

Consequentialist Principles

Most consequentialists focus on both the intended ends and anticipated effects of actions but consider those intended ends only in relation to the action's probable overall effects. Many, perhaps most, contemporary consequentialists are also utilitarians: the principle of utility provides the fundamental point of reference for their assessment of actions. This principle—in its simplest form, the requirement to produce the greatest good for the greatest number—presupposes some values for the evaluation of states of affairs that might result from different actions. Prominent values include pleasure, happiness, and individual preferences, but a variety of other values can be employed. Whatever the locus and range of values, consequentialists take different tracks, depending on whether they focus on the effects of particular actions (act-consequentialist methods) or on the effects of types of action and hence rules governing those types of action (rule-consequentialist methods).

Act-Consequentialist Methods

Contemporary act-consequentialists analyze the probable consequences of different courses of action and assess those actions according to their probable balance of good effects over bad effects. Many act-consequentialists are utilitarians. Act-utilitarians doing bioethics, such as the late Joseph Fletcher (1966) or Peter Singer (1993), apply the principle of utility directly to different possible acts in a situation to determine which would probably produce the greatest good for the greatest number; that act is then right and even obligatory. Act-utilitarians may face uncertainties about which course of action would satisfy the principle of utility, but they never face moral dilemmas created by conflicting principles.

No moral dilemmas arise because act-utilitarians recognize only one principle (utility) as binding and view other principles and rules as mere maxims or rules of thumb that may usefully summarize agents' experiences in the application of the principle of utility. Such principles or rules can help agents see the tendencies of different acts to produce good or bad consequences, but they lack prescriptive power. In short, the principle of utility binds, while other principles and rules, as generalizations based on past experience, only illuminate decisions. From the standpoint of the act-utilitarian, both rule-utilitarians and rule-deontologists are more alike than different: both make too much of principles and rules (other than utility) and too little of the consequences of particular acts. Such principles and rules create victims: people suffer bad consequences as a result of others' adherence to principles and rules (other than utility). It is not surprising then that act-utilitarians often support changes in laws, policies, and practices to allow agents to assist in suicide or to engage in voluntary active euthanasia because such actions can in some circumstances relieve patients' pain and suffering (Singer 1993).

Critics contend, among their other charges, that act-consequentialists, including act-utilitarians, fail to attend to the necessity of principles and rules to solve or at least to reduce problems of coordination, cooperation, and trust in human interactions. For example, G. J. Warnock (1971) considers the expectations that would be appropriate in a clinical encounter between an act-utilitarian physician and a patient. He notes that the patient could only expect the physician to attempt to cure him of his afflictions 'unless his [the physician's] assessment of the "general happiness" leads him to do otherwise' (Warnock 1971: 33). Asking the act-utilitarian physician

to declare his intentions truthfully or to promise to consider only the patient's welfare, in accord with the Hippocratic tradition, would not be helpful because all the
physician's declarations and promises would themselves be subject to utilitarian calculation. Trusting that the act-utilitarian physician would act only or even primarily
in the patient's best interest would be unwarranted because such a physician must
always, in every situation, attend to the greatest good of the greatest number. Such
problems of trust, coordination, and cooperation lead many utilitarians and other
consequentialists to focus on rules rather than only on particular acts.

Rule-Consequentialist Methods

Many rule-consequentialists, as already suggested, are utilitarians, but some have
a different and larger set of considerations than happiness, pleasure, or individual
preferences for evaluating the consequences of various actual and proposed moral
rules. Brad Hooker (2002) provides a major recent example of a well-developed rule-
consequentialist approach. He contends that the ethical assessment of acts should be
based on rules that can be justified impartially and that impartial justification occurs
if and only if the reasonably expected overall value of the general internalization of
those rules by the overwhelming majority is greater than the reasonably expected
overall value of any alternative rules. In short, we have impartially justified rules if
those public rules internalized by 'the overwhelming majority in each new generation' would have the greatest expected value and their implementation would be
cost-effective (including the costs of internalization) (Hooker 2002). This method
employs rules that are justified by their anticipated overall consequences if implemented.

Clearly this method presupposes a different moral psychology than the one we
find in act-consequentialism. Hooker contends that his version of rule-consequen-
tialism does not collapse into act-consequentialism because the moral agent aims
at justifiable rules rather than at overall maximization of the good— the rules are
designed to achieve that end. Furthermore, his moral psychology recognizes that
human agents are susceptible to both cognitive errors and affective distortions,
including impure motivations, and these points enter into his view of different rules
(Hooker 2002: 187).

Several questions arise. Questions about the relevant values plague consequentialist theories. Despite the apparent simplicity of consequentialism, the debates
about values are as serious as the debates about principles in deontological approaches. For Hooker (2002), the relevant value is objective well-being, and he
adds distributional patterns that assign some priority to the worst off. In addition,
questions arise about specification: What counts as an 'overwhelming majority'?
How do we choose between actual rules that function fairly well and possible rules
whose effects we may not be able to predict with great certainty? And what evidence
is required for determining the probable balance of expected value and disvalue of
possible rules?

One of Hooker's main examples concerns a rule that would permit euthanasia under certain conditions. Such a rule might appear to be prima facie warranted because it would respect autonomous choices and reduce suffering—both important consequences. Whether, however, it would be ethically justified overall depends on a reasonable prediction and assessment of its total impact if it were internalized by an 'overwhelming majority'.

Major concerns focus on whether allowing euthanasia would be accompanied by an unacceptably high level of intentional abuse and would erode communal inhibitions on killing the unconsenting innocent. Hooker recognizes that any answers to these questions must be at least 'partly speculative' (Hooker 2002: 186). The best judgment must be based not only on the prediction and assessment of probable outcomes of a permissive rule but also on an appreciation of the costs—in suffering and disrespect for autonomous choices—of current prohibitive rules (Hooker 2002: 187). In view of the facts of human psychology—susceptibility to both cognitive errors and affective distortions, including impure motivations—Hooker finds good reasons for imposing and enforcing 'tight restrictions on the use of euthanasia' (2002: 187). Then he concludes: 'With rigorously enforced restrictions, a rule allowing euthanasia, even active euthanasia, has (I believe) greater expected value than a complete ban' (2002: 187). In response to those who might suppose that empirical evidence from the experiment with euthanasia in the Netherlands would be helpful and perhaps even decisive, Hooker stresses the divergent interpretations and evaluations of that experiment, most of which reflect different ethical viewpoints (Hooker 2002: 187). (For a rule-utilitarian argument for not treating and even for 'active termination by anesthetic' of certain 'defective [*sic*] newborns', see Brandt 1992.)

Deontological Principles

Deontological approaches are usually contrasted with consequentialist ones. At a minimum, deontologists hold (1) that some features of actions other than or in addition to their consequences make those actions right or wrong, obligatory, or optional, and (2) that deontological considerations always, generally, or sometimes trump consequentialist considerations. Even if a bioethical theory recognized (1) but held that consequentialist considerations always triumph in a conflict, that theory would not be considered deontological.

While the label 'Kantian' is now often used rather than 'deontologist' for such positions, that common usage is more likely to distort than to illuminate. To be sure, Immanuel Kant and later interpreters of his ethical theory have greatly influenced modern bioethics, but the sources of deontological theories are broader, and few contemporary bioethical approaches are Kantian in a strict sense even if they draw on some Kantian language and themes, such as human dignity, autonomy, and respect for persons. Onora O'Neill (2002) is a distinguished exception. Indeed, deontologists in bioethics are as likely to draw on religious sources, texts, and traditions as on Kant and the Kantian tradition.

Some contemporary deontological approaches to bioethics are secular in nature, even if partially inspired by religious perspectives. For instance, Robert M. Veatch (1981, 1995), whose position I will discuss later as a pluralistic principle-based approach with a lexical or rank order, identifies several deontological principles (veracity, fidelity to promises, avoidance of killing, autonomy, and justice), which collectively take priority over consequentialist principles. Hence, he satisfies both conditions for a deontological theory. In addition, Kevin Wildes (2000) affirms deontological principles, based on natural law and reason, but he also notes the absence of the epistemological conditions for securing agreement on those principles in our pluralistic society.

In contemporary debates, two major deontological principles are often viewed as competitors: sanctity of life and respect for autonomy. They may point in different directions in debates about assisted suicide and active euthanasia. Defenders of a principle of sanctity of life usually oppose those acts and any moral, professional, or legal rules that would allow those acts, while defenders of respect for personal autonomy often (but by no means always) recognize the moral rights of individuals to choose suicide or euthanasia, and of others, including health care professionals, to assist them in committing suicide or to carry out the request for euthanasia. Hence, two prominent examples of deontological principles in contemporary bioethics appear on the side of libertarians—for example, the earlier Engelhardt (1986)—and on the side of religious thinkers with a commitment to the sanctity of life—for example, Pope John Paul II (1995) and Paul Ramsey (1970, 1978).

In the next section, on pluralistic principlism, I will examine the various moves that deontologists make. There I will explicate principle-based approaches that recognize at least one deontological principle and at least one consequentialist principle and then have to connect those principles to concrete cases through such maneuvers as application and deduction, specification, or balancing.

Principlist Approaches

Pluralistic Principlism

The term 'principlism' was coined by critics (Clouser and Gert 1990) to designate and disparage a particular principle-based approach to bioethics, especially the one associated with *Principles of Biomedical Ethics* by Tom L. Beauchamp and James F. Childress (1979–2001). Even though Clouser and Gert would oppose any principle-based framework, for reasons that will be clear later, their main target, designated 'principlism', is an ethical framework that employs several general and unranked principles that are all prima facie binding. A broader interpretation of principlism would encompass a wide variety of positions that appeal to moral principles, rules, and other guidelines, including some positions that rank principles and rules.

Many principle-based approaches incorporate consequentialist principles along with non-consequentialist ones without deriving one set from or reducing it to the other; for instance, a principle of utility may be included on equal footing with principles of respect for autonomy and justice. Such approaches can be called pluralistic. In this chapter, then, 'principlism' will refer to pluralistic principle-based positions that recognize both deontological and consequentialist principles and hence have to develop ways to address actual and potential conflicts within and between these two kinds of principles, particularly in moving from principles to cases in order to guide action.

Principlists differ greatly in the principles they affirm, how they justify those principles, and how they connect them to concrete cases. In *Principles of Biomedical Ethics* (5th edn., 2001, as well as earlier editions), Beauchamp and Childress identify four primary principles—respect for autonomy, non-maleficence, beneficence (including utility), and justice—and several derivative rules—veracity, fidelity, privacy, and confidentiality—along with various other rules, such as informed consent. Others have called this framework the 'four principles approach' (Gillon 1994; Gillon and Lloyd 1994). These principles and derivative rules are all prima facie binding; that is, they are binding other things being equal, but each can be outweighed in a particular context by another principle or rule. However, the principles' different weights cannot be assigned in advance; they can only be determined in particular contexts in addressing cases or policies.

In a similar vein, the influential National Commission for the Protection of Human Subjects of Biomedical and Behavioral Research (1978) identified three unranked, basic principles that should govern research involving human subjects: beneficence (which includes non-maleficence), respect for persons (which includes respect for autonomous choices and protection of persons who are non-autonomous), and justice—principles that still guide federally funded research in the United States (see also Childress et al. 2005).

As previously noted, Robert Veatch, in *A Theory of Medical Ethics* (1981) and subsequent works (e.g. 1995), offers a different list, but one that has substantial overlap with the above approaches: beneficence, contract-keeping, autonomy, honesty, avoiding killing, and justice. He also recognizes several moral rules, such as informed consent. The major difference between Veatch's principle-based method and the two already mentioned in this section is that he offers a rank order of his principles. (I will later examine Veatch's method of lexical ranking for resolving conflicts among these principles and rules.)

Rule-Based Critique

One major type of criticism of principlism holds that broad, general moral principles—of the sort associated with Beauchamp and Childress's work—are unnecessary because specific moral rules, such as non-deception, and moral ideals, such as going out of the way to help others, cover the whole moral terrain; that principles are too general and vague to guide action; and that, in the absence of a strong theory, it is not possible to resolve conflicts among principles (Clouser and Gert 1990). This critique, which can be described as a rule-based (or strong theory-based) approach, attacks any principle-based approach. Clouser and Gert write: 'for all practical and theoretical purposes, there are no moral principles', and 'Our quarrel is not so much with the content of the various "principles" as it is with the use of "principles" at all' (Clouser and Gert 1990: 235, 220). Nevertheless, they mainly target a pluralistic principlist approach that does not rank principles or provide a clear-cut decision procedure for resolving actual or potential conflicts.

Regarding the charge that moral principles are unnecessary and moral rules are sufficient, principlists could respond that they too recognize moral rules, often derived from their principles; for instance, rules of voluntary, informed consent can be derived from the principle of respect for persons or respect for autonomy. However, they doubt that all that is important in moral principles can be fully captured in specific rules, such as the ones proposed by Gert and colleagues: don't kill; don't cause pain; don't disable; don't deprive of freedom; don't deprive of pleasure; don't deceive; keep your promise; don't cheat; obey the law; and do your duty (Gert et al. 1997). These rules largely specify the harms that are to be avoided under the general requirement—what others might call a principle—of non-maleficence, but they do not adequately express what many principlists construe as obligations of respect for autonomy, beneficence, and justice.

Since space does not permit a full discussion, a single example must suffice. Elsewhere I have argued (Childress 1982) that neglect of a principle of respect for autonomy leads Gert and his colleagues to bizarre interpretations of particular cases, especially in their discussions of paternalism, as is evident in their reasoning about a particular case: Following a serious accident, a patient while still competent refuses a blood transfusion on religious grounds but then he falls unconscious and his physicians believe he will die unless he receives a transfusion. Gert and Charles Culver (1979) argue that the physician's provision of a blood transfusion under these circumstances would be paternalistic because, after the patient regains consciousness, it would lead to a violation of either the moral rule against deception or the moral rule against causing pain. If the physicians fail to tell the patient, they would violate the moral rule against deception; if they tell him, they would violate the moral rule against causing pain.

Gert and Culver are forced to take such a circuitous and problematic path of moral analysis precisely because they neglect the principle of respect for autonomy.

They fail to see that the reason the transfusion is paternalistic, and prima facie wrong, is that it violates the patient's autonomously expressed wishes and choices in order to provide a medical benefit (Childress 1982). As a result, the Gert–Culver analysis implies that if the patient dies without regaining consciousness, no paternalistic or wrongful act has been committed, because no moral rules have been violated.

The content of the moral rules proposed by Gert and colleagues does not adequately express the principle of respect for persons and their autonomy; such moral rules as 'do not deprive of freedom' will not cover all the critical cases involving self-determination. Nor will their subsequent expansion of this moral rule adequately address this problem; the later expansion appears in the interpretation added in parentheses after 'Do not deprive of freedom (includes freedom to act and from being acted on)' (Gert et al. 1996: 44). Although this expansion comes closer to addressing the problem created by the narrow rule, it does so only by building in enough to bring the rule closer to a principle, and clarity would be served by explicit recognition of a principle of respect for autonomy.

Regarding the charge that principles are too vague to guide action, principlists can respond that they too seek to specify their principles in rules that move closer to concrete action guidance. And they attempt to resolve conflicts in various ways, for instance, through lexical ordering, specification, and constrained balancing—all methods that will be examined in the next section on 'From Principles to Cases'. Even so, many principlists, especially those who seek 'reflective equilibrium' in a coherentist strategy, will not satisfy the Gert et al. requirement of a strong and unified theory: 'the value of using a single unified moral theory to deal with the ethical issues that arise in medicine and all other fields, is that it provides a single clear, coherent, and comprehensive decision procedure for arriving at answers' (Clouser and Gert 1990: 233; for an examination of reflective equilibrium, see Chapter 2, by John Arras, in this volume). For many principlists, including this one, that goal is unrealistic and efforts to realize it are misguided and ultimately distort morality and moral decision-making.

From Principles to Cases

Moral principles require interpretation because they are indeterminate. It is often unclear whether a case falls under a principle or rule; a single principle or rule may point in two different directions in the same situation; and there may be apparent or real conflicts among principles and rules—perhaps even dilemmas as well as interpersonal conflicts. Henry Richardson (1990) has identified three models of connection between principles and cases: (1) application, which involves the deductive application of principles and rules, (2) balancing, which depends on intuitive weighing, and (3) specification, which proceeds by 'qualitatively tailoring our norms to cases'. I will use these three models for analytic purposes (without considering and assessing Richardson's constructive argument). I will indicate how these models become even more illuminating when we consider two dimensions of moral principles (and rules): (*a*) their meaning, range, and scope of application (e.g. broad or narrow), and (*b*) their weight, strength, and stringency (e.g. absolute, prima facie, or suggestive).

These two dimensions are closely related rather than totally independent. For instance, if we interpret 'lying' as 'any intentionally false or deceptive statement', it is utterly implausible to defend an absolute rule against lying. However, if we understand 'lying' as 'deliberately deceiving someone who has a right to the truth'—another definition commonly offered for lying—it is not implausible to hold that a rule against lying, with this meaning, range, and scope, is absolute. But then all the important moral analysis in conflict cases would center on who has a right to the truth in particular circumstances.

Applying Principles

As I noted at the outset, bioethicists now generally eschew or at least criticize the language of application. This point holds for most principlists as well as for their critics, even though act-utilitarians may reasonably be viewed as applying the principle of utility. While there may be some genuine applications of principles to concrete cases, the language of application does not cover all or even the most significant connections between principles and particular judgments about cases. Not all such connections involve rational deduction of particular case judgments from general moral principles. On the one hand—as will be developed further in conjunction with casuistry—most principlists concede that particular case judgments are often made in relative independence of general moral principles. We often know what we ought to do without explicit reference to general moral principles even if we could articulate such principles if we were challenged to do so. On the other hand, principlists can and should recognize that judgments about particular cases can and sometimes should also lead us to modify our general moral principles.

The application framework can function effectively only where we can assume that (*a*) the principle's scope and range of applicability can be firmly established, (*b*) the principle's weight or strength can be established a priori, and (*c*) the principle will never come into conflict with other equally significant principles. In concrete cases, conflicts between moral principles—e.g. between benefiting patients and respecting their autonomous choices—generate moral perplexities that lead to adjustments in (*a*) or (*b*). In such situations, we often proceed by specifying or balancing the principles in conflict. Specifying principles is a way to try to reduce or eliminate the conflict; balancing principles is an effort to resolve the conflict through determining which principle outweighs the other in the circumstances.

Some bioethicists seek to resolve conflicts not by specifying or balancing moral principles but by arranging them in some a priori order. This represents yet another version of the application–deduction framework for connecting principles to concrete cases. For instance, a bioethical framework might hold that a rule against killing always outweighs a principle of beneficence or—in an example that combines specification with a rank order—that the principle of respect for autonomy always overrides the principle of beneficence when the only beneficiary is the competent person whose wishes, choices, or actions are at stake.

Much of Robert Veatch's work, including *A Theory of Medical Ethics* (1981), attempts to find a defensible lexical ordering of principles, which can provide a framework within which some balancing can occur. Focusing on what he considers to be the relatively neglected but critical task of resolving conflict among competing principles, he proposes a 'mixed strategy' (Veatch 1995). This 'mixed strategy' presupposes a sharp distinction and separation between consequentialist principles (beneficence and non-maleficence, which are consequence-maximizing) and non-consequentialist principles (veracity, fidelity to promises, avoidance of killing, autonomy, and justice). While moral agents can balance various consequentialist principles and various non-consequentialist principles, they cannot balance consequentialist principles against non-consequentialist ones. Instead, there is a lexical rank order: the balanced non-consequentialist principles are lexically ranked over the balanced consequentialist principles (Veatch 1995). Such an application–deduction framework is subject to the same challenges that confront other application–deduction frameworks: plausible counterexamples.

Specifying Principles

Specifying general moral principles is another way to connect them to particular cases. This process of specification presupposes a distinction between general and specific and between degrees of generality and specificity. However general our moral principles—for example, respect for personal autonomy or justice—we interpret them in part by formulating them more specifically or by delineating the types of cases that we believe fall under them. This process is inevitable because, as R. M. Hare observes, 'any attempt to give content to a principle involves specifying the cases that are to fall under it .... Any principle, then, which has content goes some way down the path of specificity' (Hare 1989: 59). Indeed, drawing on the distinction between principles and rules, it is plausible to view many rules in bioethics as specifications of broad principles so they can function as concrete action guides. For instance, rules of voluntary, informed consent specify the requirements of the principle of respect for persons and their autonomous choices.

Specifying ethical principles is often indispensable and valuable for action guidance, especially but not only in conflict situations. In face of apparent moral dilemmas, specification always merits a trial to see if the conflict can be avoided, eliminated, or reduced. How far the method of specification can be expected to succeed will depend in part on fundamental beliefs about the moral universe, including harmony and conflict within that universe. It is important to note that specification proceeds by restricting the range or scope of a principle's applicability, rather than by adjusting its weight or strength. However, one effect of narrowing a principle's range or scope of applicability may be to increase its weight or strength within that narrower range or scope.

A good example of specification appears in the way Roman Catholic moral theology has over time interpreted the Decalogue's prohibition of killing. This use of specification is complex because it is combined, as specification often is, with application and deduction and with absolutism: 'from the beginning, faced with the many and often tragic cases which occur in the life of individuals and society, Christian reflection has sought a fuller and deeper understanding of what God's commandment prohibits and prescribes' (John Paul II 1995, para. 55). Specification was undertaken in light of what the Church deemed to be fundamental and unchanging beliefs and values—human beings as created in God's image and God's sovereignty over human life. In this light, the Church determined the precept's meaning by restricting its range and scope of application in at least two ways: first, to innocent human life; second, to direct action. Hence, given the first restriction, killing in self-defense, warfare, and capital punishment could be justified. Given the second restriction, a few cases of indirect fetal death (e.g. in the case of ectopic pregnancy) and some cases of letting patients die could be justified.

Specification has been praised as a way to reduce the role of intuition in concrete decisions (Richardson 1990), but there is debate about how far it can actually succeed in doing so. Some critics suggest that balancing occurs in the very process of specification or at least that specification falls prey to the same problems that many see in balancing. As John Arras asks: 'what motivates and guides the modification and specification of abstract principles, what compels one to lard them with qualifying clauses, if not precisely the sort of countervailing values and principles encountered by the principlist [engaged in balancing]?' (Arras 1994: 997). Specification thus may be as arbitrary as intuitive balancing in cases of conflict, especially in the absence of controls over the interpretation of key moral categories, such as 'lying' or 'killing'.

Some specification, as noted earlier, is unavoidable as part of the process of giving concrete content to broad, abstract principles, and it enables principlists to avoid or rebut some of the charges leveled by the strong rule critics. Indeed, specification generates rules. In addition, in conflict situations, specification, as developed by Richardson (1990), and extended by David DeGrazia (1992) in 'specified principlism', is promising. Beauchamp and I have also featured this strategy in later editions of *Principles of Biomedical Ethics* (1994, 2001; for a critique, see Strong 2000, with a response by Beauchamp 2000). However, as suggested above, specification's overall value in connecting principles and particular judgments in situations of apparent conflict will depend in part on more fundamental beliefs about whether moral conflict, not only between people but also within the moral universe, is inevitable, since the goal of specification is to reduce if not eliminate those conflicts.

Balancing Principles

While specification addresses the meaning, range, and scope of principles, a second question also arises: How much weight, or what degree of stringency, do different principles have in relation to each other if they come into conflict?

If moral principles are more than merely suggestive, illuminative, or advisory, then it is important to determine just how binding they are in order to address any conflicts that emerge. Absolutism presents one extreme possibility: absolutists maintain that some moral principles and rules are absolutely binding whatever circumstances arise. But they face irresolvable moral dilemmas if they recognize more than one absolute principle and those principles come into conflict. As a result, absolutists often carefully specify the meaning, range, and scope of their principles in order to avoid such conflicts (see Ramsey 1968, 1970).

Another possibility—discussed above under application—is to try to establish a lexical or rank order that would itself be absolute. However, this approach too seems implausible in the face of counterexamples that appear to constitute legitimate exceptions: it is hard to establish an absolute priority for all cases. A single-principle approach could be absolutist, as act-utilitarianism is, but then it will be forced to view all other principles (and rules) as mere maxims or rules of thumb with illuminative but no prescriptive power.

Yet another approach—one often associated with principlism in its narrow sense—views moral principles as prima facie or presumptively binding, rather than as absolutely binding or lexically ordered (Beauchamp and Childress 2001). It thus balances various principles when they come into conflict in particular cases, if the process of specifying the principles does not eliminate the conflict. An act is morally right or obligatory in so far as it has the features that, according to the relevant principles, establish moral rightness or obligatoriness. For example, an act is right in so far as it is truthful, wrong in so far as it is a lie. However, a particular act, in particular circumstances, may have features that express some principles while contravening others; for instance, a truthful act may also be unjust or cause harm. In such a case, the agent must determine whether one principle or the other is weightier or stronger, a judgment that cannot be made on the basis of prior, abstract formulations.

In part to reduce (but not eliminate) the role of intuition, Beauchamp and Childress (2001) offer several conditions for restricting or constraining judgments about balancing conflicting prima facie moral principles. These conditions are:

1 Better reasons can be offered to act on the overriding norm than on the infringed norm...

2 The moral objective justifying the infringement must have a realistic prospect of achievement.

3 The infringement is necessary in that no morally preferable alternative actions can be substituted.

4 The infringement selected must be the least possible infringement commensurate with achieving the primary goal of the action.

5 The agent must seek to minimize any negative effects of the infringement.

6 The agent must act impartially in regard to all affected parties...

(Beauchamp and Childress 2001: 19–20)

These conditions or constraints express the logic of prima facie principles. Prima facie principles are weightier or stronger than mere maxims or rules of thumb, but lighter or weaker than absolute principles. They are morally binding other things being equal. Hence, in a case of conflict, infringing or overriding one prima facie principle in order to protect another prima facie principle requires attention to various circumstances, including the often overlooked or neglected conditions of necessity, or last resort, and least infringement. Nevertheless, according to its critics, this form of principlism still relies excessively on intuition, whatever procedures it introduces to reduce the role of intuition in the process of balancing its various principles and rules.

Instead of viewing application, balancing, and specification as three mutually exclusive models, it is better, I believe, to recognize that all three are important in parts of morality and for different situations or aspects of situations, as well as often intertwined and overlapping. Sometimes principles (and rules) can be applied, and sometimes they need to be specified, but at times conflicts may emerge that can only be resolved by (constrained) balancing. It is a substantive, and not merely a formal, moral debate as to which method works where and when.

CASE-BASED METHODS

The Gert–Clouser critique, as we have seen, faults principlism for failing to develop a rationalistic, unified theory with concrete directives for action (in the form of rules). According to this critique, principlism is insufficiently 'top-down' and deductivist. By contrast, proponents of case-based methods charge that principlism is too 'top-heavy' and 'top-down' because it fails to attend sufficiently to particular judgments about cases. Case-based methods involve a 'bottom-up', inductive approach to ethical justification. Casuistry, as one case-based approach, can be defined as 'a method for arriving at justifiable decisions about what to do in specific cases' (Strong 2000). There are several important case-based and casuistical methods (Brody 1988, 2003; Strong 2000; Kuczewski 1997), but I will concentrate on the casuistical approach offered by Albert Jonsen and Stephen Toulmin in their influential book *The Abuse of Casuistry* (1988), and in their various individually authored articles.

The Abuse of Casuistry claims, among other points, (1) that 'casuistry is unavoidable', (2a) that 'moral knowledge is essentially particular, [(2b)] so that sound resolutions of moral problems must always be rooted in a concrete understanding of specific cases and circumstances', and (3) that moral reasoning proceeds by paradigm cases (moral precedents) and analogical reasoning (Jonsen and Toulmin 1988: 330). The first point (1) is relatively uncontroversial. While the essential particularity of moral knowledge (2a) can be interpreted in several different ways, major qualifications are necessary on any interpretation; however, (2b) is defensible. Finally, while identifying an important feature of moral reasoning, the last claim (3) tends to exaggerate the role of this mode of reasoning to the neglect of principle-based reasoning.

In explicating and justifying claim (2a) about the essential particularity of moral knowledge, *The Abuse of Casuistry* vigorously resists what Toulmin had earlier called 'the tyranny of principles' (Toulmin 1981). This rhetoric is exaggerated, because, in fact, Jonsen and Toulmin have as their target not the inevitable tyranny of any and all principles but only the tyranny of certain conceptions of principles, that is, 'eternal, invariable principles, the practical implications of which can be free of exceptions or qualifications' (Jonsen and Toulmin 1988: 2). They contend that such principles lead to deadlocks and fruitless standoffs, among other problems. In short, this casuistry-based attack on tyrannical principle-based methods focuses on absolutist versions, rather than on versions that view principles and rules as prima facie binding and require specification, balancing, and other modes of interpretation in situations of decision.

This rhetoric is also overblown because Jonsen and Toulmin themselves do, in fact, recognize principles. At one point, they state that their aim is to argue for 'good casuistry', that is, casuistry 'which applies general rules to particular cases with discernment [in contrast to] bad casuistry, which does the same thing sloppily' (Jonsen and Toulmin 1988: 16). And elsewhere Toulmin (1981) concedes that principles have special relevance and importance in relations between strangers rather than intimates. If so, then one important question is how we can best characterize relations in research and also in medicine and health care—they are often relations between strangers rather than relations between intimates.

In view of their nod to principles, how should we understand and assess Jonsen and Toulmin's claims about the primacy or priority of particular judgments? On the one hand, such a claim might mean that particular judgments came first chronologically and gave rise to general judgments (principles). Even if that claim could be established—a difficult and perhaps impossible task—its implications may be quite limited for the ways we are now acculturated and reason ethically. We all participate in communities of moral discourse that embody and extend traditions of moral reflection. These traditions incorporate both general principles and particular case judgments, including paradigm cases, and these communities build both into their formal and informal moral instruction. Indeed, moral education is virtually unimaginable without general principles and rules as well as paradigm or precedent cases that help specify their content.

On the other hand, claims about the primacy of particular judgments could refer to logical or normative priority of case judgments over principles. However, the relation between particular judgments and general judgments (principles) is better viewed as dialectical, with neither fully and completely derived from the other and each potentially modifying the other. Where there are conflicts, adjustments may need to be made in either the particular or the general judgments (principles), but there is no justification for insisting that either one should always take priority. Indeed, what is sought is a kind of 'reflective equilibrium' within a coherentist strategy (see Arras 1991; Beauchamp and Childress 2001).

Suppose that, upon reflection, we make a judgment that an action in a particular set of circumstances is wrong, without regard to general moral principles. What are the implications of this particular judgment, if we take seriously both ethical consistency and universalizability, which entail treating similar cases in a similar way? If we have made a judgment about a case—that X is wrong or right—then, R. M. Hare notes, 'we have acquired a precept or principle which has application in all similar cases. We have, in some sense of that word, learnt something' (Hare 1989: 55–6). And if we learn something useful from reflection on a particular case, the principle we gain, Hare contends, must be somewhat general rather than having unlimited specificity. Since no two real cases are exactly alike, the results of reflection can be useful in the future only if we 'have isolated *certain broad features* of the cases we were thinking about—features which may recur in other cases' (Hare 1989: 56; italics added). To isolate these 'broad features' is to identify a principle or rule (for the principlist) and a paradigm or precedent case (for the casuist).

Casuists also make another important claim ((3) above) about their inductive method of moral reasoning and justification: Practical reasoning proceeds by analogy from paradigm cases, i.e. settled cases or precedents, to new or unsettled ones. Such reasoning is widespread in bioethics, among principlists as well as casuists. Hence, it is not surprising, for example, that much of the ethical debate about a controversial case of research involving human subjects will reason analogically in relation to the negative paradigm case of the Tuskegee syphilis study in which close to 400 African American men were left untreated for syphilis for decades so that researchers could study the history of untreated syphilis in the African American male. If a current case is relevantly similar to the Tuskegee case, then, on grounds of ethical consistency and universalizability, we are committed to judging the current case as wrong. Such an analogical mode of moral reasoning can and often will be illuminating.

The principlist could agree but could also argue that cases such as Tuskegee are paradigms or precedents for moral reasoning precisely because of the principles they embody—for instance, the Tuskegee syphilis study became a negative paradigm case because it violated fundamental principles of justice, respect for autonomy, beneficence, and non-maleficence. The differences between principles, on the one hand, and paradigms and precedents, on the other, appears to be minimal, especially because each identifies 'broad features' of types of cases. They usually differ in degree of generality or specificity—the paradigm or precedent case may have more details and greater specificity. However, to use a legal analogy, even with the rich, specific details of the case, it may still be necessary to identify the 'holding' in the case, and this will bring us closer to a principle or principles. Furthermore, some of the maxims that casuists see embedded in cases appear to function as mid-level principles or rules.

Other important—but often neglected—questions for casuists (and for others) concern cases and their descriptions: How are cases identified and labeled? How does the casuist determine what kinds of cases they are? These are necessary first steps in the process of taxonomic analysis. However, identifying and labeling cases often seems to be more implicit than explicit, more intuitive than reasoned, with insufficient attention to the process of 'evaluative description', which is perhaps the most adequate way to conceive case presentations. Narrative analysts who have turned their spotlight on bioethical cases, as mini-narratives, have directed our attention to the evaluative and other assumptions that often structure cases and lead to both classifications and conclusions that may not be adequately examined or warranted (Chambers 1999).

Consider two evaluative descriptions of cases, the first relatively uncontroversial and the second quite controversial. First, several years ago the *Journal of the American Medical Association* (*JAMA* 1988) reported a case under the title 'It's Over Debbie'. In this case, the authenticity of which has been questioned, a medical resident injects a terminally ill woman with enough morphine to end her life in response to her request, uttered in their first encounter, 'Let's get this over with'. The casuist Jonsen classifies this case as one of killing, hence bringing it under a taxonomy of cases of killing, governed by various maxims, and then reasons analogically in relation to paradigm cases in this taxonomy (Jonsen 1991). Jonsen's case description, classification, and analysis appear to be quite straightforward in this case, but conflicts can emerge about the evaluative descriptions of cases according to their type and classification, as is evident in the next example.

A few years ago a clinical case involving the disconnection of a ventilator maintaining the life of a patient with amyotrophic lateral sclerosis (Lou Gehrig's disease) was presented as an end-of-life case, in which the 'patient' decided to discontinue the ventilator. However, members of the audience, many of whom had themselves experienced long-term ventilator use, disputed this classification, viewing the case instead as a disability case in which the clinicians should have provided better care, fuller information, and more options to the 'consumer', particularly after the recent death of his spouse (Kaufert and Koch 2003). Interpreters contend that this conflict illustrates the importance of narrative analysis, which examines the assumptions and perspectives that operate in the description of cases: 'What to the clinicians was a textbook case of "end-of-life" decision making was, for their audience, a story in which a life was ended as a result of failures of information and assistance by the presenters themselves' (Kaufer and Koch 2003: 462).

At the very least, casuists (and others) need to pay more explicit attention to 'moral diagnosis' (Arras 1991) and hence to how they describe and frame cases. Of particular importance is the recognition and reduction of bias in 'describing, framing, selecting and comparing of cases and paradigms' (Kopelman 1994: 21). Bias reduction strategies, at a minimum, should include richer, fuller descriptions of cases, and the incorporation of a wide range of possible descriptions.

Case-based and casuistical methods lack a clear way to identify relevant features of cases, in part because they lack content. According to some critics, casuistry is 'a method without content. It is a tool of thought that displays the fundamental importance of case-comparison and analogy in moral thinking, but it lacks initial moral premises' (Beauchamp and Childress 2001: 395). Or, stated differently, it is 'more a method than a doctrine, more an engine of thought than a moral compass' (Arras 1998: 112). Hence, the engine's direction depends on the values—individual, professional, communal, etc.—casuists bring to bear on the case. If, of course, casuists were to identify the maxims in an array of cases, e.g. on killing, they would perhaps then have a framework of mid-level principles or rules that could be critically examined and employed in describing cases and recommending actions—but then it would be even harder to distinguish casuists from principlists.

General principles may also provide ways to criticize practices that are not available in case-to-case analysis. This point may hold even if the principles themselves are discerned in practices, rather than established by an ethical theory. John Arras (1991) worries that, in the taxonomic approach of moving from actual case to actual case, the casuist may be limited to what practitioners and others present for ethical analysis and assessment because of felt problems or dilemmas. However, general principles may help us identify other cases that should be on the moral agenda because of some 'broad features', and they may direct our attention to real problems and dilemmas that have not yet been experienced as such. In addition, principles, such as justice, may help us identify and correct the distortions that our social structures, policies, and practices create in our perception of cases and our analogical reasoning.

The contrasts between principle-based and case-based methods or between generalist and particularist approaches may be less significant and less illuminating if these methods gravitate more and more toward the middle as they mature (Sumner and Boyle 1996). Indeed, most debates about these methods and positions already tend to feature caricatures rather than real opponents. One question is whether these methods become virtually identical or whether they are complementary. Even though casuists and principlists—in their best moments—attend to both principles and cases and seek rigorous and imaginative ways to relate them—for example, dialectically—the methods are better understood as complementary than, as Mark Kuczewski (1998: 521) claims, 'largely the same method'.

VIRTUE ETHICS

A modern alternative to principle-based (and rule-based) approaches appears in virtue ethics, which draws on ancient philosophical resources, especially Aristotle. In a sense, as Michael Slote (1997: 233) observes, virtue ethics has awakened from 'a long slumber', but, in view of its extended dormancy, it is, practically speaking, 'the new kid on the block' compared to consequentialist and deontological approaches. It (re)emerged as a critique of the inadequacies of various principle-based approaches, but has now morphed into a distinctive, constructive alternative.

(Re)emerging as a critique, virtue ethics has routinely been characterized as a corrective. According to proponents of virtue ethics, principle-based as well as case-based methods—which from the standpoint of virtue ethics are more similar than different—tend to neglect moral character, discernment, motivation, emotions, etc. By contrast, virtue ethics attends to the agent rather than the act; to character rather than conduct; to what sort of persons we should become rather than what sorts of actions we should perform; and so forth. While partially illuminating the different positions, such characterizations and contrasts also inevitably oversimplify and distort them.

Principle-based approaches—as well as casuistical approaches—usually recognize the importance of the virtues. While the list of specific virtues will vary from theory to theory and method to method, they all presuppose certain conceptions and kinds of virtues, as established traits of character, including motivation to act according to certain principles and rules or to act on casuistical judgments. Nevertheless, it is fair to say that neither principle-based nor case-based approaches have adequately attended to the virtues they presuppose for their own successful operation.

Principle-based approaches tend to identify (at least some of) the relevant virtues by their correspondence to different principles—e.g. the virtue of benevolence corresponds to the principle of beneficence—or by their value for morality as a whole—e.g. courage (see Beauchamp and Childress 2001). From this standpoint, the virtues, as motivational structures and dispositions, are important because they enable agents to adhere to moral principles. As William Frankena put it, 'principles without virtues are impotent' (Frankena 1973: 36). There is thus little dispute that the virtues are important and even indispensable in ethics and in bioethics.

However, for principled and casuistical approaches, the virtues are important and indispensable in a secondary, derivative way—to provide motivation to realize what is already known independently through principle-based or case-based judgments.

For principle-based and case-based methods, then, the virtues have no independent cognitive or normative significance for human action. Virtues do not guide action but, instead, motivate action. Indeed, emphasizing that virtues do not direct action, Frankena holds that 'virtues without principles are blind' (Frankena 1973: 36). In a similar vein, R. M. Hare claims: 'It looks as if any ethics of virtue would have to borrow extensively from an ethics of principle in order even to tell us what virtue consists in' (Hare 1996: 22). Given these points, it might be unclear just what virtue ethics can contribute to bioethics other than calling attention to neglected virtues as indispensable motivational resources for principle-based and case-based methods.

One problem is that conceptions of the virtues as dispositions to act, in a one-to-one correspondence with independent principles and rules, reduce each of the virtues to what Hursthouse (2003) calls a 'single track disposition'. However, such a reductionist conception distorts the virtues. For instance, the virtue of honesty cannot be reduced to a 'single track disposition to do honest actions, or even honest actions for certain reasons'—instead, it is 'multi-track' because it denotes a 'complex mindset', consisting, in addition to honest actions, of other actions, such as disapproving of others' dishonesty, along with various associated emotions, attitudes, perceptions, sensibilities, and the like (Hursthouse 2003). One important implication is that not even a wide range of agent X's acts of honesty can warrant the judgment that X is honest, in part because X's reasons (motives) are crucial to the judgment but also because honesty is a 'multi-track disposition' that may be embodied and expressed in degrees.

While one set of action-guiding virtues—variously called practical wisdom, prudence, or discernment—functions in part through the interpretation and application of principles, it too is more complex. As Alisa Carse rightly argues, 'recognizing that a general principle or rule is relevant to the situation at hand, and knowing how it is fittingly to be acted upon requires a capacity for discernment that is distinct from, and presupposed by, the application of principles themselves' (Carse 1991: 11). She further observes that discerning responses are not always principle-driven or the result of principled deliberation; rather they may involve sensitivity to other people through a sympathetic attunement to their needs and concerns. Principle-based approaches need not and should not deny these points: principles do not exhaust the moral life and its decisions, and even when principles are relevant they must be discerningly interpreted and employed in the situation.

Proponents of virtue ethics contend that virtues provide more action guidance than other theorists often recognize. A major misconception that pervades much of the contemporary debate about ethical theory and method, according to Rosalind Hursthouse, a virtue ethicist herself, is that 'virtue ethics does not, and cannot, provide action guidance, the way utilitarianism and deontology do' (Hursthouse 2003). Against this misconception, she argues that

virtue ethics provides a specification of 'right actions'—as 'what a virtuous agent would, characteristically, do in the circumstances'—and such a specification can be regarded as generating a number of moral rules or principles (contrary to the usual claim that virtue ethics does not come up with rules or principles). Each virtue generates an instruction—'Do what is honest', 'Do what is charitable'; and each vice a prohibition—'Do not . . . do what is dishonest, uncharitable'.   (Hursthouse 2001: 17)

Despite such points about virtue ethics' capacity for action guidance, critics still often view an examination of the virtues as a subject better suited for the novelist than for the ethicist, because they are so numerous, unspecifiable, and potentially in conflict without some way to arrange and order them. Hence, beyond claims that virtues lack independent action-guiding content, questions arise about whether the virtues can guide action because of their limited specifiability. As Justin Oakley observes, 'a virtue ethics criterion of rightness is less precisely specifiable and less easily applicable' than some other approaches (Oakley 1998: 94). The very nature of the virtues, according to Robert Louden, means that we can reasonably expect 'a very limited amount of advice on moral quandaries . . . from the virtue-oriented approach. We ought, of course, to do what the virtuous person would do, but it is not always easy to fathom what the hypothetical moral exemplar would do were he in our shoes' (Louden 1984: 229).

In response to concerns about whether virtue ethics can guide decisions in conflict situations, Hursthouse argues that the goal should not be 'to provide a decision procedure which any reasonably clever adolescent could apply [without moral wisdom or discernment]' (Hursthouse 2001: 18). This is part of her—and virtue ethics'—rejection of the idea that ethics is 'codifiable'. She also distinguishes 'resolvable dilemmas', or hard cases, from 'irresolvable and tragic dilemmas', noting that the virtue ethicist may try to specify the virtues and to distinguish merely apparent from real dilemmas—a task that presupposes moral wisdom and discernment (Hursthouse 2001). (As Hursthouse recognizes, some forms of principlism also distinguish the apparent from the real by further specifying principles to avoid or reduce the apparent conflict.) Sometimes, however, irresolvable and tragic dilemmas remain. Even though action guidance is impossible in such situations, virtue ethics can depict how the agent should respond, that is, with appropriate attitudes and emotions, such as distress and guilt.

One critique of virtue ethics, leveled by a variety of principlists, is that good or virtuous people can act wrongly and do bad things (Hare 1996; Oakley 1998). Neither a settled motivational structure nor guidance from the virtues themselves, including prudence, may be sufficient to preclude wrong actions. Indeed, even if an agent's motivation is virtuous, certain dominant virtues may lead him or her to act wrongly. For example, a caregiver's virtue of benevolence may lead her to find active euthanasia acceptable for a particular patient, even though that patient is not able to speak competently for himself.

Virtue ethicists could respond that the virtues need to be considered as an integrated whole, as a unity, and that a virtuous person has discernment to draw appropriate lines. Furthermore, unless virtue ethics reduces all general standards of action to virtue standards—a move that is unnecessary and indefensible—then, as previously noted, virtue ethics can incorporate other principles of action guidance.

Even though many theories have grounded the moral virtues in conceptions of human flourishing or fulfillment, those conceptions have floundered in the wake of the collapse of teleological notions of science and the prevalence of diverse conceptions of the good life. As a result, some virtue ethicists have resorted to traditions of particular communities—such as religious communities—which may embody a unified conception of human flourishing that can warrant a set of virtues.

A promising alternative in bioethics grounds the virtues in particular professional traditions, such as medicine and nursing. In contrast to general ethics, Edmund Pellegrino argues that 'professional ethics offers the possibility of some agreement on a telos—i.e. an end and a good', which, in the case of the relationship between the health care professional and the patient, would be the good of the patient (Pellegrino 1995: 266). From the clinical relationship with its telos of healing, Pellegrino develops a list of virtues: fidelity to trust and promise, benevolence, effacement of self-interest, compassion and caring, intellectual honesty, justice, and prudence. According to Pellegrino, this list, while not exhaustive, identifies the virtues 'most essential to the healing purposes of the clinical encounters' (Pellegrino 1995: 268). In short, 'they are "entailed" by the end of the healing relationship; that is, they are required if the end is to be attained' (Pellegrino 1995: 268). These different virtues are mutually reinforcing—compromising one would compromise the others—such that no priority order is possible.

Questions still arise about whether this list of virtues is sufficiently comprehensive. Critics note the absence of a virtue that would correspond to respect for patients' autonomous choices and wonder whether Pellegrino's virtue-based framework thus allows and supports excessive professional paternalism. In addition, the professional relationships and traditions, on which Pellegrino builds, have suffered, in recent decades, from widespread consumerism in market-driven interactions. Hence, it is unclear whether they can engender and sustain the virtues Pellegrino affirms.

Virtue-based methods would approach questions about euthanasia in part by drawing out the implications of character and specific virtues in light of the telos that the particular method recognizes. For example, focusing on the telos of human flourishing, Philippa Foot examines the moral possibility of various kinds of euthanasia (passive or active and voluntary or non-voluntary) from the standpoint of the virtues, contending that charity as the virtue of attachment to the good of others can support euthanasia while justice sometimes opposes and sometimes allows it (e.g. justice opposes non-voluntary active euthanasia, may accept non-voluntary passive euthanasia, and supports active voluntary euthanasia) (Foot 1977: 106). However, in considering changes in legal and professional rules, Foot's argument differs little from many rule-consequentialist arguments, in stressing the importance of keeping a 'psychological barrier' and the dangers of abuse as well as the alteration of social expectations about care of the sick and elderly (Foot 1977). By contrast, Pellegrino (1998) totally rejects active euthanasia, at least by physicians, because it is opposed to specific professional virtues in clinical relationships aimed at healing.

ETHICS OF CARE

Another approach that also seeks to provide an alternative to principle-based methods is an ethic of care or caring. It is similar in many respects to virtue ethics, with care or caring viewed as a specific virtue. After decades of research into human moral development, some psychologists noticed that principle-based approaches tend to echo male voices about male experiences, while neglecting women's voices and experiences. They further observed that theories of moral development were based exclusively on male models. In her pioneering research along these lines, Carol Gilligan (1982) reported that women tend to concentrate on narratives, contexts, and relationships of care. By contrast, males tend to emphasize what Gilligan calls an ethic of justice, involving tiers of general moral principles and employing a logic of hierarchical justification. (These tendencies do not mark gender exclusivity—men may take a care perspective and women a justice perspective.) From a care perspective, the moral agent is relational and interdependent with others rather than an independent decider who applies abstract, general principles—even autonomy is often construed as 'relational autonomy' (Mackenzie and Stoljar 2000).

Beyond studies of moral development, philosophers have highlighted a variety of features of a care perspective. Viewing an ethic of care as 'a way of understanding one's moral role, of looking at moral issues and coming to an accommodation in moral situations', the philosopher Rita Manning finds in it five central ideas: moral attention, sympathetic understanding, relationship awareness, accommodation, and response (Manning 1998: 98). Another central theme is 'appropriate trust', which Annette Baier (1985, 1994) emphasizes.

Given the focus on care as a moral sentiment and response in particular relationships, and its similarities to virtue ethics, it is not surprising that 'care as a standard does not prescribe specific actions in the way an ethic of rules or decision procedures strives or claims to do' (Blum 2001: 186). Methodologically, as Alisa Carse observes, ' "care" reasoning is concrete and contextual rather than abstract; it is sometimes principle-guided, rather than always principle-driven, and it involves sympathy and compassion rather than dispassion' (Carse 1991: 17). In so far as the ethics of care is contextual, it overlaps with casuistry.

However, turning from principles to context, including relationships, still leaves open difficult questions about setting priorities when responsibilities to concrete others in particular relationships come into conflict with each other or with responsibilities to stakeholders outside those particular relationships. In many cases, moral agents have to determine, at least in part through principles and rules, how much weight to give to different relationships. For example, a physician may have to determine whether to breach confidentiality in order to warn a stranger of a patient's threatened violence.

An ethic of care appears to be best suited for intimate relations, including some in health care. However, it must also address the stranger, the person outside specific relationships. Indeed, a major challenge to an ethic of care focuses on its particularity and its partiality. The question is whether care, in many of its formulations, is too partial and parochial, without pressures generated by a more principled approach. For instance, care in particular relationships may need to be limited in strength or weight even as care is expanded in scope—i.e. rendered more general and universal—perhaps under a principle of beneficence (or virtue of benevolence) or a principle or virtue of justice. As Gilligan (1982) recognizes, care and principles (which she characterizes in terms of 'justice') are generally complementary rather than opposed.

Even though much of the interest in and early work on an ethic of care emerged from feminist contexts, many feminists challenge such an ethic, especially if taken by itself without further attention to principles. Certainly principles of justice, particularly in the form of equality and impartiality, as well as respect for personal autonomy, strongly support often neglected women's rights. In addition, some feminists distinguish a feminist approach to ethics from a feminine approach, associating an ethic of care with the latter. For example, some feminists, who take seriously the oppression of women, are suspicious of a feminine ethic of care that originates and operates under oppression (and thus lacks independent standing) and that may actually perpetuate oppression. Such an ethic may foster further oppression through the liberal division of private and public spheres, with care being deemed appropriate in the private sphere but not in the public sphere, and with women being viewed as the primary bearers of caring—for instance, in the care of elderly family members (Sherwin 1992). For others, the care perspective is potentially transformative, since the personal and the interpersonal are also publicly and politically significant. One possible formulation is 'just care' (see Manning 1998: 103–4 on care and justice).

Just as a virtue ethic, an ethic of care can lead in different directions in debates about physician-assisted suicide or active euthanasia. At the very least, it would give priority to long-standing relationships in which care has been evident—for instance, it would tend to find Dr Timothy Quill's assistance to his patient Diane in her suicide much more acceptable than Dr Jack Kevorkian's assistance in the suicide of persons whom he barely knew and had not cared for (Quill 1991). Still the appropriate, fitting, responsible response in such situations will depend greatly on what is built into the notion of care and its limits.

In the final analysis, the care perspective offers an important corrective to some principle-based approaches by attending to context, narrative, relationships, emotion, compassion, and the like. At a minimum, principle-based approaches must attend to—and, if necessary, be reformulated in light of—the whole range of human moral experience, including women's experiences of caring as well as of oppression. Fidelity to moral experience is one important criterion for any acceptable ethical theory, perspective, or method.

COMMUNITARIAN PERSPECTIVES

Communitarianism, another family of approaches to ethics—a somewhat loosely related family because of the variety of meanings of community—has often criticized principle-based approaches to bioethics, whether deontological, consequentialist, or pluralist. Some communitarians charge that principlism is a foundationalist approach that neglects the role of community and tradition in moral reflection. However, principlists are not necessarily foundationalists in the theoretical sense. Some principle- and rule-based approaches appeal to at least a thin sense of community in notions of 'common morality' (Gert 1989; Gert et al. 1997; Beauchamp and Childress 2001). And some principlists argue further that communities and traditions regularly embody and convey moral principles, just as they transmit settled judgments about cases and seek to engender certain traits of character. Some communitarians have stressed shared, deep, thick communal values that can engender, support, and sustain both casuistical practices as well as virtuous persons (Kuczewski 1997, 2001). One difficulty in thinking from a communitarian perspective, as these points suggest, is determining the relevant community, e.g. whether a whole society or a particular community within that society.

Communitarianism may be primarily important as a perspective on ethical problems rather than as a way to resolve them. Most communitarians would agree with Daniel Callahan that 'the first set of questions to be raised about any ethical problem should focus on its social meaning, implications, and context, even in those cases which seem to affect individuals only' (Callahan 2003: 287). With its ecological bent, the point of communitarianism in Callahan's sense is to offer 'a way of thinking about ethical problems, not to provide any formulas or rigid criteria for dealing with them' (Callahan 2003: 288). It presupposes both analytical skills (rationality, imagination, insight) and personal virtues. It often seeks deliberative methods for the community, however defined, to develop and express its values (Emanuel 1992). In addition, communitarians often criticize principle-based approaches for their tendency to 'block substantive ethical inquiry' (Callahan 2003: 288).

The debate about principles has been caught in the larger and tangled web of debate about individualism versus communitarianism. Communitarians charge that individualistic interpretations of bioethical principles have dominated moral discourse and now need to be corrected. Even though some defenders of principle-based approaches are individualists—for example, deontologists who concentrate on respect for autonomy and liberty or utilitarians who simply sum up the effects of actions on individuals' interests—many principlists also recognize that moral agents are social and that communal values are very important. Furthermore, communitarians need not reject principles—though they may ground, interpret, and weight them differently than individualists and may propose additional principles, for instance, what some bioethicists call a principle of community or respect for community.

At the first meeting of the National Bioethics Advisory Commission in October 1996, Ezekiel Emanuel, then a member, contended that the three Belmont principles (respect for persons, beneficence, and justice), developed by a predecessor national body (the National Commission for the Protection of Human Subjects), and related guidelines for research involving human subjects do not adequately address *community*. Such a challenge could mean, among other possibilities, that we should add community as a fourth principle to the Belmont list—the approach that Emanuel recommends—or that we should interpret all these principles through the lens of relationships and community. According to Emanuel and Weijer (2005), an independent principle is needed in order adequately to recognize that communities have moral status, values, and interests (such as avoidance of communal stigmatization) that merit protection—beyond the sum of individual values and interests—and to describe and address the conflict between individual and communal interests. However, communitarians are rarely clear about how such conflicts are to be resolved, particularly in view of the different kinds of community involved.

An alternative way to correct the putative individualism of principlism is through a richer interpretation, or reinterpretation, of ethical principles through the lens of relationships and community. After all, the question for principles is not only their content, or their weight, but also their scope, as is indicated by the rubric Raanan Gillon (1994) has used for Beauchamp and Childress's principles—'four principles plus scope'. Among other things, scope can include such matters as moral status—for instance, of communities as well as embryos and the environment.

Reinterpreted through the lens of relationships and community, appeals to the principle of respect for persons, or respect for autonomy, would consider persons not merely as isolated individuals, who consent or refuse to consent, but also as members of communities. Individuals are embedded, to varying degrees, in their communities with various traditions, beliefs, values, and practices, and respect for cultural values is important. However, it is not possible or justifiable to determine an individual's wishes and choices by reading them off community traditions, beliefs, values, and practices, and it is not ethically acceptable to subordinate the individual's autonomy to the community's will without satisfying stringent justificatory conditions. Similar points can be made about other basic bioethical principles: each one can be interpreted through the lens of relationships and community. For instance, researchers should recognize that some communities can be harmed in genetics research—for example, through stigmatization—in violation of the principles of beneficence and non-maleficence, and that the principle of justice may require involving such communities to participate in the design of genetics research involving their members.

CONCLUSIONS

Significant conflicts remain about which bioethical method, if any, provides the best guidance for decisions and actions in clinical and policy settings. From the standpoint of action guidance, as well as other criteria, each method has significant problems, and yet each method is also helpful in some respects, particularly in identifying relevant features of agents, actions, ends, consequences, contexts, and relationships that merit attention in deciding and acting. Furthermore, several methods overlap with each other, or converge, or supplement each other. It is probably too much to expect consensus about the best possible method(s), all things considered—at most, we can take advantage of the strengths of each method and compensate for its special deficiencies.

REFERENCES

ARRAS, J. D. (1991), 'Getting Down to Cases: The Revival of Casuistry in Bioethics', *Journal of Medicine and Philosophy*, 16: 29–51.

—— (1994), 'Principles and Particularity: The Role of Cases in Bioethics', *Indiana Law Journal*, 69: 983–1014.

—— (1998), 'A Case Approach', in H. Kuhse and P. Singer (eds.), *A Companion to Bioethics* (Oxford: Blackwell), 106–14.

BAIER, A. C. (1985), *Postures of the Mind: Essays on Mind and Morals* (Minneapolis: University of Minnesota Press).

—— (1994), *Moral Prejudices: Essays on Ethics* (Cambridge, Mass.: Harvard University Press).

BEAUCHAMP, T. L. (2000), 'Response to Strong on Principlism and Casuistry', *Journal of Medicine and Philosophy*, 25: 342–7.

___ and CHILDRESS, J. F. (1979–2001), *Principles of Biomedical Ethics*, (1st–5th edns. New York: Oxford University Press).

BLUM, L. (2001), 'Care', in L. C. Becker and C. B. Becker (eds.), *Encyclopedia of Ethics*, (2nd edn. New York: Routledge), 185–7.

BRANDT, R. B. (1992), 'Public Policy and Life and Death Decisions Regarding Defective Newborns', in Brandt, *Morality, Utilitarianism, and Rights* (Cambridge: Cambridge University Press), 354–69.

BRODY, B. (1988), *Life and Death Decision Making* (New York: Oxford University Press).

___ (2003), *Taking Issue: Pluralism and Casuistry in Bioethics* (Washington, DC: Georgetown University Press).

CALLAHAN, D. (2003), 'Principlism and Communitarianism', *Journal of Medical Ethics*, 29: 287–91.

CARSE, A. L. (1991), 'The "Voice of Care": Implications for Bioethical Education', *Journal of Medicine and Philosophy*, 16: 5–28.

CHAMBERS, T. (1999), *The Fiction of Bioethics: Cases as Literary Texts* (New York: Routledge).

CHILDRESS, J. F. (1982), *Who Should Decide? Paternalism in Health Care* (New York: Oxford University Press).

___ MESLIN, E. M., and SHAPIRO, H. T. (eds.) (2005), *Belmont Revisited: Ethical Principles for Research with Human Subjects* (Washington, DC: Georgetown University Press).

CLOUSER, K. D., and GERT, B. (1990), 'A Critique of Principlism', *Journal of Medicine and Philosophy*, 15: 219–36.

DEGRAZIA, D. (1992), 'Moving Forward in Bioethical Theory: Theories, Cases, and Specified Principlism', *Journal of Medicine and Philosophy*, 17: 511–39.

DUBOSE, E. R., HAMEL, R., and O'CONNELL, L. J. (eds.) (1994), *A Matter of Principles? Ferment in U.S. Bioethics* (Valley Forge, Pa.: Trinity Press International).

EMANUEL, E. J. (1992), *The Ends of Human Life: Medical Ethics in a Liberal Polity* (Cambridge, Mass.: Harvard University Press).

___ and WEIJER, C. (2005), 'Protecting Communities in Research: From a New Principle to Rational Protections', in Childress et al. (2005: 165–83).

ENGELHARDT, H. T. (1986), *Foundations of Bioethics* (New York: Oxford University Press).

FLETCHER, J. (1966), *Situation Ethics: The New Morality* (Philadelphia: Westminster Press).

FOOT, P. (1977), 'Euthanasia', *Philosophy and Public Affairs*, 6: 85–112.

FRANKENA, W. K. (1973), *Ethics*, (2nd edn. Englewood Cliffs, NJ: Prentice-Hall).

GERT, B. (1989), *Morality: A New Justification of the Moral Rules* (New York: Oxford University Press).

___ and CULVER, C. (1979), 'The Justification of Paternalism', *Ethics*, 89: 199–210.

___ et al. (1996), *Morality and the New Genetics* (Sudbury, Mass.: Jones and Bartlett).

___ CLOUSER, K. D., and CULVER, C. (1997), *Bioethics: A Return to Fundamentals* (New York: Oxford University Press).

GILLIGAN, C. (1982), *In a Different Voice: Psychological Theory and Women's Development* (Cambridge, Mass.: Harvard University Press).

GILLON, R. (1994), 'Medical Ethics: Four Principles Plus Attention to Scope', *British Medical Journal*, 309: 184–8.

___ (ed.) and LLOYD, A. (asst. ed.) (1994), *Principles of Health Care Ethics* (Chichester: John Wiley).

HARE, R. M. (1989), 'Principles', in Hare, *Essays in Ethical Theory* (Oxford: Clarendon Press), 49–65.

—— (1996), 'The Methods of Bioethics: Some Defective Proposals', in L. W. Sumner and J. Boyle (eds.), *Philosophical Perspectives on Bioethics* (Toronto: University of Toronto Press), 18–36.

HOOKER, B. (2002), *Ideal Code, Real World: A Rule-Consequentialist Theory of Morality* (Oxford: Oxford University Press).

HURSTHOUSE, R. (2001), *On Virtue Ethics* (Oxford: Oxford University Press).

—— (2003), 'Virtue Ethics', in E. N. Zalta (ed.), *The Stanford Encyclopedia of Philosophy* (Fall 2003), <http://plato.stanford.edu/archives/fall2003/entries/ethics-virtue/>, accessed 8 Oct. 2005.

JANSEN, L. A. (2003), 'The Virtues in Their Place: Virtue Ethics in Medicine', *Theoretical Medicine*, 21: 261–76.

JOHN PAUL II, POPE (1995), *Evangelium vitae* (The Vatican).

JONSEN, A. R. (1991), 'Casuistry as Methodology in Clinical Ethics', *Theoretical Medicine*, 12/4: 295–307.

—— and TOULMIN, S. (1988), *The Abuse of Casuistry* (Berkeley: University of California Press).

JAMA (1988), 'It's Over, Debbie', 259/2: 272.

KAUFERT, J. K., and KOCH, T. (2003), 'Disability or End-of-Life: Competing Narratives in Bioethics', *Theoretical Medicine*, 24: 459–69.

KOPELMAN, L. M. (1994), 'Case Method and Casuistry: The Problem of Bias', *Theoretical Medicine*, 15: 21–37.

KUCZEWSKI, M. G. (1997), *Fragmentation and Consensus: Communitarian and Casuist Bioethics* (Washington: Georgetown University Press).

—— (1998), 'Casuistry and Principlism: The Convergence of Method in Biomedical Ethics', *Theoretical Medicine and Bioethics*, 19: 504–24.

—— (2001), 'The Epistemology of Communitarian Bioethics: Traditions in the Public Debates', *Theoretical Medicine*, 22: 135–50.

LOUDEN, R. (1984), 'On Some Vices of Virtue Ethics', *American Philosophical Quarterly*, 21: 227–36.

MACKENZIE, C., and STOLJAR, N. (eds.) (2000), *Relational Autonomy: Feminist Perspectives on Autonomy, Agency, and the Social Self* (New York: Oxford University Press).

MANNING, R. C. (1998), 'A Care Approach', in H. Kuhse and P. Singer (eds.), *A Companion to Bioethics* (Oxford: Blackwell), 98–105.

NATIONAL COMMISSION FOR THE PROTECTION OF HUMAN SUBJECTS OF BIOMEDICAL AND BEHAVIORAL RESEARCH (1978), *The Belmont Report: Ethical Guidelines for the Protection of Human Subjects of Research*, DHEW publication no. (OS) 78–00 (Washington, DC: Department of Health Education and Welfare).

OAKLEY, J. (1998), 'A Virtue Ethics Approach', in H. Kuhse and P. Singer (eds.), *A Companion to Bioethics* (Oxford: Blackwell), 86–97.

O'NEILL, O. (2002), *Autonomy and Trust in Bioethics* (Cambridge: Cambridge University Press).

PELLEGRINO, E. D. (1995), 'Toward a Virtue-Based Normative Ethics for the Health Professions', *Kennedy Institute of Ethics Journal*, 5/3: 253–77.

_____ (1998), 'The False Promise of Beneficent Killing in Regulating How We Die', in L. Emanuel (ed.), *Regulating How We Die* (Cambridge, Mass.: Harvard University Press), 71–91.

QUILL, T. (1991), 'Death and Dignity: A Case of Individualized Decision Making', *New England Journal of Medicine*, 324: 691–4.

RAMSEY, P. (1968), 'The Case of the Curious Exception', in G. Outka and P. Ramsey (eds.), *Norm and Context in Christian Ethics* (New York: Charles Scribner's).

_____ (1970), *The Patient as Person* (New Haven: Yale University Press).

_____ (1978), *Ethic at the Edges of Life* (New Haven: Yale University Press).

RICHARDSON, H. S. (1990), 'Specifying Norms as a Way to Resolve Concrete Ethical Problems', *Philosophy and Public Affairs*, 19: 279–20.

_____ (2000), 'Specifying, Balancing, and Interpreting Bioethical Principles', *Journal of Medicine and Philosophy*, 25: 285–307.

SHERWIN, S. (1992), *No Longer Patient: Feminist Ethics and Health Care* (Philadelphia: Temple University Press).

SIDGWICK, H. (1962), *The Methods of Ethics* (London: Macmillan).

_____ (1998), *Practical Ethics: A Collection of Addresses and Essays* (New York: Oxford University Press).

SINGER, P. (1993), *Practical Ethics*, (2nd edn. Cambridge: Cambridge University Press).

SLOTE, M. (1997), 'Virtue Ethics', in M. W. Baron, P. Pettit, and M. Slote, *Three Methods of Ethics* (Oxford: Blackwell), 175–238.

SOLOMON, W. D. (1978), 'Rules and Principles', in W. T. Reich (ed.), *Encyclopedia of Bioethics*, i (New York: Free Press), 407–13.

STRONG, C. (2000), 'Specified Principlism: What Is It, and Does It Really Resolve Cases Better Than Casuistry?', *Journal of Medicine and Philosophy*, 25: 324–41.

SULMASY, D. P. (2001), 'Research in Medical Ethics: Physician-Assisted Suicide and Euthanasia', in J. Sugarman and D. P. Sulmasy OFM (eds.), *Methods in Medical Ethics* (Washington, DC: Georgetown University Press), 247–66.

SUMNER, L. W., and BOYLE, J. (1996), 'Introduction', in Sumner and Boyle (eds.), *Philosophical Perspectives on Bioethics* (Toronto: University of Toronto Press), 18–36.

TOULMIN, S. (1981), 'The Tyranny of Principles', *Hastings Center Report*, 11/6: 31–9.

VEATCH, R. M. (1981), *A Theory of Medical Ethics* (New York: Basic Books).

_____ (1995), 'Resolving Conflicts Among Principles: Ranking, Balancing, and Specifying', *Kennedy Institute of Ethics Journal*, 5/3: 199–218.

_____ (2005), 'Ranking, Balancing, or Simultaneity', in Childress et al. (2005: 184–204).

WARNOCK, G. J. (1971), *The Object of Morality* (London: Methuen).

WILDES, K. W. (2000), *Moral Acquaintances: Methodology in Bioethics* (Notre Dame, Ind.: University of Notre Dame Press).

CHAPTER 2

THE WAY WE REASON NOW: REFLECTIVE EQUILIBRIUM IN BIOETHICS

JOHN D. ARRAS

In the world of bioethics, the air is abuzz with reflective equilibrium. Not too long ago, this same air echoed the din of clashing moral methodologies. Casuists,[1] feminists,[2] narrativists,[3] and pragmatists[4] had been collectively engaged in a tag

This chapter is dedicated to the memory of John Fletcher. Many thanks to Alex London and Bonnie Steinbock for helpful discussion along the way.

[1] Casuistry in bioethics has been championed by Albert Jonsen and Stephen Toulmin as an alternative methodology to principlism, one that supposedly works from the 'bottom up' by means of analogical case analyses, much like the common law, rather than 'top down' by means of moral theories and theoretically derived principles. (See Jonsen and Toulmin 1988; Arras 1991.)

[2] Feminist criticism in bioethics has focused primarily on gender-related power imbalances in the health care system. As contributors to the debate over method in bioethics, feminist critics of principlism have lamented the latter's alleged overemphasis on abstract principle and neglect of personal relations, the emotions, and power in the analysis of moral problems. Many feminists are also moral particularists, and thus have much in common with casuists and narrativists. (See e.g. Wolf 1995.)

[3] Narrative ethics, like casuistry, gives pride of place to the particularities of persons and social contexts as these are articulated within personal narratives. The emphasis here is on the trajectory of the 'patient's story', rather than on the abstractions of theory and principles. (See Arras 1997.)

[4] Bioethical pragmatists embrace the rejection of epistemological and ethical foundationalism that they find in traditional pragmatists like John Dewey and William James. They view ethical principles as

team debunking exercise at the expense of the embattled defenders of principlism, the heretofore dominant method in the field of practical ethics (Beauchamp and Childress 1979–2001). These methodological malcontents shared a common core of grievances: Principlism was too abstract, deductive, and 'top down'; it was insufficiently attentive to particulars, relationships, storytelling, and process. Each claimant to the throne adamantly pressed its case for methodological supremacy in bioethics. In response, the avatars of principlism, Tom Beauchamp and James Childress, politely thanked all their critics for making so many truly helpful suggestions, assuring them that they would each be respectfully subsumed into principlism's evolving grand synthesis. Each hostile critique would, however, first have to be shorn of its excesses before being assigned its very own section in the next edition of *Principles of Biomedical Ethics*. Thus, to the casuists, Beauchamp and Childress granted that principles not only ruled over case judgments but were actually derived from particular intuitions in a dialectic between 'top down' and 'bottom up'. To the feminists, they conceded the importance of relationships and the need to address inequality and domination in the relations between the sexes. To the partisans of narrative ethics, they affirmed the importance of narrative detail for the successful deployment and specification of principles. And, finally, to the pragmatists, they admitted the flexible, tool-like nature of principles, and the indispensability of good judgment in their application (Arras 2002).

Central to this project of principlist assimilation was the notion of reflective equilibrium (henceforth, RE), a method of doing moral and political philosophy originally developed by the great political philosopher John Rawls (1971, 1975). According to Rawls, the project of justifying ethical beliefs ideally involves the attempt to bring our most confident ethical judgments, our ethical principles, and our background social, psychological, and philosophical theories into a state of harmony or equilibrium. Our most confident moral judgments or intuitions (e.g. 'Slavery is wrong') provide a touchstone for the adequacy of our principles; any moral principle that justified slavery would be either reformulated or rejected. Meanwhile, principles invested with a great deal of confidence could be used to reject some conflicting intuitions while extending our ability to judge confidently in less familiar moral settings. We thus zip back and forth, nipping an intuitive judgment here, tucking a principle there, building up or reformulating a theory in the background, until all the disparate elements of our moral assessments are brought into a more or less steady state of harmonious equilibrium. According to this view, moral justification must be sought, not in secure, incorrigible foundations outside of our processes of reflection, but rather in the coherence of all the flotsam and jetsam of our moral life.

flexible tools that evolve over time in the service of social problem solving, rather than as absolute dos and don'ts; and they tend to emphasize the importance of democratic process as well as the substance of ethical judgments. (See McGee 2003.) It should go without saying that all of these brief vignettes in nn. 1–4 are hopelessly oversimplified.

Although Rawls limited the deployment of RE to the theoretical construction of his social contract theory, applied ethicists in many fields have more recently taken up this method as a vehicle for solving practical moral problems in their respective disciplines. (See e.g. Benjamin 2002; Nussbaum 1992; Daniels 1996; van der Burg and van Willigenburg 1998.) Although this more practical deployment of RE might raise eyebrows among those philosophers who view ethical theory and practical ethics as existing on two entirely different planes, it has made perfect sense for the growing number of practical ethicists who regard their work as existing on a continuum with that of theorists in normative ethics. It has, in fact, become something of a commonplace for philosophers straddling the theoretical and practical domains to remark that their modes of thinking and justification are pretty much identical in both areas, even if the role of abstraction is obviously greater in the domain of theory construction (Beauchamp 1984; Brock 1995). Although there is no doubt much to be said on behalf of this claimed continuity between practical and theoretical ethics, it remains to be seen whether RE, at least in its most expansive contemporary manifestations, can serve the theorist and practical ethicist equally well. As I explain below, I have my doubts on this score.

One of the many attractions of RE as a method in practical ethics has been its ability to appeal to just about every faction in the method wars. It is agreeably flexible, non-dogmatic, and non-foundationalist in claiming that there are no incorrigible elements of morality on which everything else must be grounded and from which all justification flows. It enforces an appealing egalitarianism with regard to all the various elements of our belief systems, including our beliefs about particular cases, moral principles, and background theories. Within the method of RE, there are no privileged beliefs. Every belief is fair game for pruning in the service of more strongly held beliefs of the same or other kinds. Thus, casuists are happy to hear that intuitive case judgments are crucially important in moral justification; principlists are pleased with the robust role of moral principles; and high-flying philosophers and social theorists are relieved to hear that there's even a place for background theorizing about the nature of persons and society. It was thus no great surprise, then, when Beauchamp and Childress, confronting that unruly mob of rival methodologists gesticulating from the other side of the moat, hoisted the unifying flag of RE, declaring it to be henceforth *the* method of principlism in bioethics (4th edn., 1994). All our methodological differences would henceforth merely be matters of emphasis. We would all just be fellow bozos on Neurath's boat—out at sea, unable to reach dry dock where foundational work could be done, we patch, mend, and stitch our moral bark with the disparate materials at hand.[5] As Mark Kuczewski observed at the time, 'Who could ask for anything more?' (1997).

---

[5] 'We are like sailors who on the open sea must reconstruct their ship but are never able to start afresh from the bottom. Where a beam is taken away a new one must at once be put there, and for this the rest of the ship is used as support. In this way, by using the old beams and driftwood the ship can be shaped entirely anew, but only by gradual reconstruction' (Neurath 1966).

Indeed, who could ask for more than this? As a philosopher, however, my job is to make life more difficult for people, so I will proceed to ask some hard questions about the method of RE in practical ethics. I do this not simply to make trouble, but rather because this method raises some very difficult and troubling questions which I shall explore below. I do so with some trepidation, however, because I have previously recommended a modest version of this very method (Arras 2003), and I am hard-pressed to identify a better way of justifying our judgments of right and wrong in practical ethics. I begin, then, with some preliminary remarks about the general features and basic varieties of RE in moral reflection. I shall then consider a couple of preliminary doubts about this method. One claims that the most plausible interpretation of RE is so comprehensive that it risks paralyzing our thinking, while the other claims that this same version of RE is insufficiently determinate in practical contexts and will thus fail to be sufficiently action-guiding. I then proceed to explicate the sense in which RE qualifies as a coherence theory of justification, and I consider several objections to RE that flow from its reliance on the putative connection between coherence and moral justification. I will then bring this chapter to a close with some reflections on the very idea of method in ethics—that is, on what we might realistically expect of methodology as a vehicle to advance justification and truth in the domain of practical ethics.

STANDARD FEATURES OF REFLECTIVE EQUILIBRIUM

Considered Judgments and Principles in RE

In his first paper devoted to a 'decision procedure' in ethics, Rawls elaborated an interesting picture of the relationship between moral principles and the intuitive or 'considered' judgments out of which they develop (1951). We begin, says Rawls, with a notion of 'competent moral judges'—i.e. people who are intelligent, impartial, reasonable, well informed, imaginative, empathetic, and so on. Now, let us assume, first, that these judges are capable of filtering out their less plausible moral judgments. They are on guard against operating under conditions that usually yield bad or untrustworthy decisions—i.e. they are not judging in haste, under a cloud of intense emotions, driven by their own self-interest, and so on. Let us then suppose that these competent judges confront a wide spectrum of moral situations or cases and deliver judgments based not upon some sort of sophisticated theory or set of principles, but rather, assuming there to be such, simply upon their direct, unmediated, most reliable intuitions of right and wrong. Later on, in *A Theory of Justice*, Rawls calls these responses 'considered moral judgments'—i.e. those moral judgments in which we have the most confidence (1971: 47/1999: 42). Although

Rawls, as always, is loath to cite concrete examples here, the paradigm cases might be examples of free speech, religious liberty, and racial equality. Putting it mildly, a competent moral judge would look unfavorably upon both the goals and methods of the Spanish Inquisition. Forcing all people to abandon their own visions of the good and the nature of the universe at the altar of Catholic orthodoxy—and to do so by threatening the rack, thumbscrew, or burning pyre—would definitely strike our competent moral judges as being morally out of bounds. So the initial 'data' of moral reflection are these intuitive judgments of competent judges directed at various cases. A good bioethical example of this would be our intuitive negative responses to the infamous Tuskegee syphilis study, in which US government researchers charted the doleful effects of untreated syphilis in black sharecroppers over a period of forty years.

The next step in the method is to develop moral principles that 'match', 'explicate', 'accord with', 'fit', or 'account for' the body of intuitions amassed by competent moral judges. Thus, a principle of religious freedom might explicate the fact that various competent moral judges would intuitively condemn the torture and burning of heretics and similar behaviors. Rawls likens this process to the inductive scientific method, whereby inquirers assemble a set of observation statements or data points, and then attempt to formulate a principle or mathematical function that best makes sense of them. According to this interpretation of RE, moral principles are hypotheses advanced to make sense of the set of considered moral judgments of competent judges. Principles 'explain' moral judgments if we could deduce exactly the same judgments just from the principles and relevant facts alone, without the benefit of any moral intuitions or sentiments. In short, moral principles are supposed to yield conclusions in particular cases that would match our considered judgments. If our suggested principles mesh perfectly with our considered judgments, then we are in equilibrium; if they don't fit, then we have to amend either our particular moral judgments or our principles, depending upon which element of our moral system merits the most confidence.

In addition to their explanatory function sketched above, moral principles also have normative functions within the framework of RE. First, principles that have been forged over time in the crucible of RE can help us recognize and reject mistaken moral judgments; second, Rawls asserts that principles should help us resolve moral perplexities posed by conflicting intuitions in difficult cases. Deploying a set of firmly held principles can assist us in extending the reach of our convictions, even in those situations where we initially lack confidence in our judgments.

A number of questions arise with regard to this initial Rawlsian sketch of RE. First, it is reasonable to ask whether our considered judgments about cases really present themselves in isolation from more 'theoretical' considerations in the way that Rawls initially suggested they might (1951). I suspect, with Brian Barry, that most such intuitive judgments about cases already harbor the germ of some sort of larger, quasi-theoretical reflection. For example, our repulsion at the burning of heretics or at the withholding of proven treatment from syphilitic black sharecroppers is not some sort of brute 'datum', but is rather most likely a reaction already suffused with the 'quasi-theoretical' judgment that the Inquisition and Tuskegee violated, *inter alia*, important moral norms mandating equality among human beings (Barry 1989: 264; Arras 1991).

Conversely, it is equally problematic to assert that moral principles can be relied upon to yield, exclusively on the basis of the relevant facts, the very same conclusions reached by confidently uttered case judgments. Just as case judgments are infused with quasi-theoretical elements, so principles, in order to actually reach practical conclusions in concrete circumstances, must be supplemented with all sorts of judgments, intuitions, and analogous comparisons with other cases. Although we might be able to 'derive' or 'deduce' correct practical conclusions from principles in clear-cut cases of moral evil like the Tuskegee experiment, we cannot do so in hard cases involving conflicting principles or difficult problems of interpretation—that is, in precisely those cases that provide the grist for most bioethical reasoning.

A second problem with Rawls's initial formulation of RE is his claim that moral principles should be understood as hypotheses developed to explain or match whatever deeply felt intuitions we happen to have (Barry 1989: 263). At the least, proponents of RE need to explain how moral intuitions can play the same justificatory role as observation statements in the physical sciences, each one providing its own particular kind of basic 'datum' for further theorizing. (I shall say more about this issue later on.) Even some of the most zealous defenders of RE have abandoned this suggested analogy between observation statements in science and considered moral judgments (Daniels 1979). More plausible recent expositions of RE simply acknowledge the existence of most of our commonsensical moral principles—e.g. keep promises, respect autonomous choices—and then attempt to show what is valuable and important about the norms they articulate and to state the best reasons why it is wrong to violate them (Scanlon 1992). In other words, instead of deploying RE to discover new principles, these theorists harness RE for the more modest but still crucially important task of becoming more reflective about the meaning, functions, and justifications of whatever moral principles we happen to endorse. Sometimes the process of RE will reveal that we have misunderstood the values protected by a principle, and this will have implications for what the principle is now taken to sanction. More rarely, this process may reveal that we have simply given up entirely on the reasons behind a principle ('Shield your patients from troubling diagnoses'), and at that point we jettison the principle.

Finally, and most importantly, it is unclear how RE, as explicated so far, has any serious normative bite. At best, such a bouncing-back-and-forth between considered judgments and derivative principles will yield a fully rounded inventory of our collected moral intuitions, but the justification of those very intuitions remains unsettled. It is a commonplace that people often feel supremely confident in their most basic moral judgments, but it is unsettling, to say the least, to acknowledge that some of those very judgments have in the past affirmed the naturalness of slavery, the necessity of burning heretics at the stake, and the unsuitability of atheists and women for public office. Construed narrowly to encompass only particular judgments and the principles that explain them, RE offers an easy target to critics, who claim that it is hopelessly parochial and conservative (Hare 1975; Singer 1974; Kagan 1998). This suspicion of moral intuitions is nicely captured by James Griffin, who observes that 'It is especially in ethics that intuitions have risen so far above their epistemological station' (Griffin 1996: 5). In order to meet this challenge, the partisans of RE reach for a distinction between 'narrow' and 'wide' versions of the method.

Narrow versus Wide RE

The version of RE that we have considered so far is called 'narrow reflective equilibrium' (henceforth NRE); it can help us identify our most confidently held moral judgments and the principles that best explain them, but it apparently lacks the resources to actually *justify* those intuitions and matching principles. To do that, RE must expand its inventory of moral considerations and widen its scope. Towards this end, Rawls and Norman Daniels have developed an alternative account of RE that they call 'wide reflective equilibrium' (henceforth WRE; see Rawls 1975; Daniels 1979: 258). In addition to considered judgments and principles, then, WRE encompasses a wide variety of theoretical considerations, including (1) alternative 'moral conceptions' (e.g. utilitarianism, perfectionism, Kantian ethics) and their respective philosophical warrants; (2) theories of moral personhood; (3) theories of procedural justice; (4) theories of moral development; and (5) empirical theories bearing on the nature of society and social relations. In spite of the evident shortcomings of our considered moral judgments with regard to the problem of justification, the partisans of WRE contend that we have no other choice but to embrace them. Crucially, however, they contend that these judgments are only 'provisional fixed points' that must be scrutinized from every possible angle. The above theoretical considerations are imported into RE in order to provide just that kind of critical scrutiny. Importantly, Daniels insists that these background theories are not dependent upon our moral intuitions in the same way that our principles are, so they can, he argues, be counted upon to provide independent justification for the deliverances of RE (1979: 260).

WRE thus provides us with a highly complex and multi-layered approach to moral justification. Considered judgments, principles, and background theoretical considerations incorporate as many moral and empirical beliefs as possible, and allow us to test each of these elements or strata against all of the others. Crucially, as mentioned before, no single element or stratum of this dynamic mix of beliefs is considered to be foundational or immune to criticism. We shuttle back and forth from judgments, to principles, to theories, and back again—always adjusting, pruning, and seeking coherence among the widest possible set of relevant beliefs. WRE is thus both a coherentist and non-foundationalist approach to moral justification.

WRE and Methods of Bioethics

It's time to pause in our exposition and draw out some important initial implications of WRE for our methodological debates in bioethics. Remember, Beauchamp and Childress have explicitly embraced WRE as the official methodology of principlism. (In their fourth edition they write, 'we have agreed with Rawls that justification is "a matter of the mutual support of many considerations, of everything fitting together into one coherent whole"' (1994: 23). One important question is whether this move is consistent with their long-standing advocacy of principlism as a distinct methodology. As I understand it, principlism has traditionally emphasized the centrality of moral principles in bioethical reflection. As the very title of their oft-revised book implies, for Beauchamp and Childress bioethical reasoning is ultimately about the identification, justification, specification, weighing, and balancing of moral principles against one another in the context of specific cases. As Beauchamp once remarked, principles provide the 'spine of ethical analysis' (personal communication). Now, it may well have been a commendable move for these distinguished partisans of principlism to endorse WRE and thereby usher in the peaceable methodological kingdom, but it is difficult to comprehend how they could do so while still giving pride of place to principles in moral analysis. We must recall in this connection that WRE doesn't play favorites with regard to the various *kinds* of beliefs, whether they are about cases, principles, or background theories. No single stratum or cluster of moral considerations is privileged. All that matters as we go about our business of adjusting, pruning, and rendering our beliefs coherent is the *strength* of particular beliefs, our degree of commitment to them, rather than the objects of belief or the level of their concreteness (Scanlon 1992: 14; DePaul 1993: 157). Thus, our beliefs about principles are always subject to revision at the bidding of more strongly held beliefs about particular case judgments or background theories of the person, due process, or society. If this is the case, then principlism seems to have effectively placated and silenced its critics at the cost of its own methodological distinctiveness. Were brevity and aesthetics not factors to consider, the title of their next edition should read: *Considered Case Judgments, Principles, and Background Theories in Bioethics: How They Can All Be Brought into Coherence Within the Ambit of Reflective Equilibrium.* Principles no longer deserve top, let alone exclusive, billing.

What's true for principlism is also true for each of the other rival methodologies in bioethics. Just to take one additional example, casuistry can also be taken up into the larger synthesis of WRE, but only at the cost of sacrificing its distinctiveness. According to Albert Jonsen and Stephen Toulmin (1988), the prime movers of casuistry as a rival method to principlism, the primary locus of moral justification and certitude is the paradigm case. Modeling their vision of ethics on the common law, these authors assert that moral knowledge results from the slow accretion of cases and our efforts to distill principles out of them. According to Toulmin (1981), moral principles are just so many afterthoughts trailing behind our intuitive responses to paradigm cases. If we are looking for normativity, we will find it, asserts Toulmin, in the paradigm case—not in principles distilled *post hoc*, and certainly not in abstract ethical theories. Thus, just as principlism gave pride of place to moral principles (the 'spine' of ethical inquiry), casuistry locates the 'real action' in ethical reflection at the level of the paradigm case. In so far as both of these rival methodologies favor one level of moral belief over others, they both must be shorn of such favoritism before being allowed to play their respective roles in our search for wide reflective equilibrium.

The take-home message here is that if WRE is taken to be the preferred method in moral philosophy and bioethics, then both principlism and casuistry as traditionally understood must be rejected as partial and incomplete moments in a grander, all-encompassing methodological synthesis. As Hegel would put it, both methods are *aufgehoben*—that is, they are shorn of whatever is partial, fragmentary, or one-sided about them, while their remaining valuable features are preserved and elevated within a more comprehensive synthesis.

Again, who could ask for anything more? The beauty of WRE is that it makes room for *all* beliefs that might potentially contribute to a richer synthesis. As Michael DePaul (1993: 107 ff.) notes, WRE is the only fully *rational* method of moral inquiry. Whatever its faults or limitations might be, WRE is uniquely capable of leading the moral inquirer to accept a rational system of beliefs through a set of rational steps. Alternatives to WRE cannot make this claim. Take, for instance, R. M. Hare's project of grounding ethics on a foundation of meta-ethical propositions bearing on the meaning of moral terms like 'good' and 'right' (1963). According to Hare, moral intuitions and considered moral judgments are far too untrustworthy to help guide moral reflection in a process like RE. ('Garbage in, garbage out.') He therefore urges us to submit all of our moral beliefs, including beliefs about moral intuitions and moral principles, before the tribunal of epistemic principles and background theories. DePaul asserts that Hare's proposed method is irrational in so far as it would require us to subordinate or jettison our strongly held moral beliefs about cases and principles even if we think, on due reflection, that they are more likely to be true than any theory of moral language that Hare or others might concoct. This, DePaul concludes, cannot be a rational move (1993: 124). The same thing could be said about a method like casuistry that submits background theories and moral principles to the tribunal of paradigm cases. Even if someone were suddenly to come to believe that a moral or political theory (e.g.

Marxism) was more likely to be true than any other item in their inventory of beliefs, the casuist would require her to give up her theory if it conflicted with her pre-existing moral intuitions about paradigm cases, *even if the born-again Marxist now views those intuitions (e.g. those relating to private property) to be the products of false consciousness.*

The intuitive attractiveness of WRE, then, rests upon its inclusiveness. If you don't like the way the process of RE is going, if you think that it currently overlooks some crucial pieces of the moral picture—such as a different moral outlook or a background theory of social stability—then WRE simply asks you to toss it into the mix alongside all our other beliefs. Who could ask for a more accommodating method of moral reflection?

Preliminary Doubts About Wide Reflective Equilibrium

Notwithstanding the inclusiveness and intuitive attractiveness of WRE, there are difficulties and objections that must be squarely confronted. Although I think that the most philosophically interesting and important challenges to WRE relate to its embrace of coherence as the engine of moral justification, I shall begin with worries focused on the scope and action-guiding potential of this method.

WRE is too Comprehensive

Although the inclusiveness of WRE initially strikes us as a major advantage over foundationalist theories, it is also a source of pragmatic concerns about the method's practicability. Consider the length and breadth of WRE's welcome mat for the ingredients of moral reflection. Judgments about cases, moral principles, competing moral outlooks (i.e. moral theories), the accompanying philosophical arguments for those rival outlooks, theories of the role of morality in society, theories of moral personhood, notions of procedural justice, general social theories, and theories of moral development all have a role to play in the working out of RE. If we wish to know whether any particular proposition is morally justified, we have to subject it to the competing pushes and pulls of this entire network of beliefs. The daunting nature of such a mission comes to light when we consider just one ingredient of this overall process of justification, namely, those competing moral conceptions and their accompanying philosophical justifications. Suppose we wish to ascertain whether our views on cloning are morally justified. The method of WRE would demand, *inter alia*, that we at some point consider the rival claims of all the live options in moral theory—e.g. utilitarianism, Kantian theories of autonomy, Thomistic perfectionism, feminism, Aristotelian virtue theory—assess their competing arguments, and embrace the one moral conception that best coheres with the rest of our moral intuitions and background theories. This, of course, could well constitute the life's work of a professor of moral philosophy, but it is not all that would be required. We would then have to perform similar work on competing theories of the person, of social organization, and of the role of morality in society. Once all this work (and more) was done, we would need to see how all of our disparate beliefs and theories fit together, making sure to nip and tuck those that conflicted with those beliefs and theories in which we had the greatest confidence. In contrast with casuistry, which views justification as a relatively simple and straightforward matter of bringing our judgments within the gravitational pull of paradigm cases, this picture of justification in WRE is daunting in the extreme. It truly seems like a job not for ordinary mortals, but rather for Ronald Dworkin's legendary but fictional judge Hercules.[6]

This problem of over-inclusiveness need not necessarily be a huge problem for the moral theorist. Rawls (1971: 49–50/1999: 43), for example, concedes that 'it is doubtful whether one can ever reach this state'. He contents himself, however, with the thought that the theorist can at least canvass some of the most salient options in moral theory, if not all such options, and still regard WRE as a regulative ideal towards which the theorist should strive. It is less clear, however, whether the practical ethicist has this same luxury. Once we transcend narrow RE to encompass standard moral theories and their philosophical justifications—not to mention all those other background moral, political, and empirical theories—the ordinary working stiff bioethicist is likely to find WRE to be a hopelessly cumbersome method of moral justification. If she is to make any progress at all, she will no doubt have to bracket many beliefs and theories that would normally play integral roles in an ideal process of RE. Indeed, it would not be surprising if Reflective Equilibrium for Working Bioethicists, Version 1.0 were to bear a striking resemblance to narrow RE in the majority of cases.

WRE is too Indeterminate

A closely related problem concerns a disconcerting lack of precise guidance in coming to terms with all those competing moral outlooks and their corresponding supportive arguments. Exactly how is the process of analysis and comparison

---

[6] Hercules is portrayed by Dworkin as an idealized omniscient judge who decides hard cases by forging legal principles that best 'fit' all the legal precedents, best mesh with our legal history and institutions, and are most compellingly justified by our best moral and political theories of justice and equality. Dworkin realizes that fallible human judges cannot conceivably work their way through all these steps, but he asserts that this would be the ideal process of legal justification (Dworkin 1977: 197).

supposed to proceed? Rawls and Daniels say precious little about this. Even Rawls's attempt in *A Theory of Justice* to vindicate his famous two principles of justice against the claims of various versions of utilitarianism has run into a barrage of cogent criticisms. The same worry obviously haunts the project of choosing among rival social theories or theories of the person. What criteria should we use to select one such theory over others? How should the reasoning go? Here again, WRE appears to be more a rather massive effort of hand waving than a precise road map to moral justification (Raz 1982: 309). Given the inherent vagueness in the charge to review all these various objects of belief, to vindicate some but not others, and to bring all of the remaining beliefs into the broadest possible circle of coherence, it appears highly unlikely that WRE will eventually yield definite action-guiding results.

The combined effect of these two related criticisms of WRE—i.e. that this method is both too comprehensive and too indeterminate—is to suggest a distinction between an ideal method of justification and a more rough-and-ready decision procedure that might helpfully guide our thinking in practical contexts.[7] WRE might well serve as a regulative ideal of moral justification for theorists, especially if we were given more information about how the various moral conceptions and background theories should be evaluated and compared; but it is hard to imagine a more cumbersome or less action-guiding program for practical moral decision making. The omniscient but unfortunately fictional judge Hercules might be able to manage all those justificatory hoops, but ordinary mortals will have to settle for much less.

WRE and the Limits of Coherence

As we have seen, WRE rejects foundationalism in ethics, the view that a certain favored set of beliefs—e.g. meta-ethical propositions, human nature, paradigm cases, moral theory, certain key intuitions, or the Bible—constitutes the incorrigible bedrock of moral reflection from which all other beliefs must flow. Within foundationalist moral systems, beliefs are justified by being 'derived from' or 'based upon' those more fundamental or foundational beliefs. Within WRE, by contrast, beliefs are justified—i.e. they acquire the greatest measure or warrant or support—by being brought into coherence with the widest possible set of other beliefs we hold. As Rawls (1971: 21/1999: 19) puts it, the justification of moral principles 'is a matter of the mutual support of many considerations, of everything

---

[7] Alex London has cogently developed this theme in a series of articles on method in practical ethics. Rather than viewing the various proposed methods of bioethics as routes to justified true beliefs, he views them as helpful procedures for ensuring that non-ideal agents deliberating under real-world circumstances have the best chance to decide an issue on the merits (London 2000).

fitting together into one coherent view'. RE is, thus, a particular version of the 'coherence theory' of moral justification, which has applications not just in ethics but also in the theory of knowledge generally (Pollock 1986). While much of the attraction of WRE derives from its repudiation of foundationalism, its embrace of coherence theory is viewed by some as deeply problematic. In this section I shall try to sketch, albeit all too briefly, the most salient of these doubts and worries and to assess their significance for the viability of WRE as a bioethical method.

What Kind of Coherence Justifies?

If beliefs are justified by being brought into coherence with other beliefs, we first have to determine exactly what we mean by 'coherence'. There are several different interpretations of coherence, and it matters which one we select because they have very different implications for the project of moral justification. We might, for example, interpret coherence to mean the consistency of each element in the overall belief system, including both moral and empirical beliefs, vis-à-vis all the other elements. Although this gloss on coherence would no doubt be somewhat helpful, allowing us to ferret out contradictions among our various beliefs, it's hard to see how mere consistency with other beliefs can serve to justify any particular belief.

A more robust notion of coherence can be found in commentaries on the natural sciences, where the justificatory power of coherence is bolstered by two special features. First, coherence in the natural sciences is buttressed by observation statements that provide the data for theory building. True, even in the natural sciences some observations might be ignored if they happen to conflict with an especially powerful theory, so science, like RE, takes a holistic approach to justification. Still, most of us think that the observation statements in physics are on a much firmer epistemological footing than the considered moral judgments of various people, especially when we note that these sources of considered judgments may reflect major and irreconcilable cultural, religious, and class differences. Second, the kind of coherence available in science features not just mutually consistent beliefs, but also mutually supporting beliefs or 'credibility transfers' that can reliably raise the level of the whole set of beliefs (Griffin 1996: 16). Assuming that the same natural world is the subject matter of all the sciences, beliefs developed in one zone of inquiry will have the effect of supporting similar beliefs developed in others. The upshot of this cross-cutting system of mutual support among scientific beliefs is that coherence in science exhibits a certain 'bootstrapping' effect that appears to be lacking in the moral domain. We appear, then, to confront a dilemma: If we construe coherence weakly to mean consistency with our other moral beliefs and known facts, then just about any live option in moral philosophy will pass the test of coherence, and we won't have a test that will allow us to choose between such live options. Alternatively, if we construe coherence to entail the sort of bootstrapping and credibility transfers that we encounter in scientific webs of belief, then we would indeed have a conception of coherence with legs, one that offered real justificatory power. Unfortunately, however, it is highly doubtful that the sort of relationships connecting our considered judgments, moral principles, and background theories can rise to this level. Certainly, various relationships can be discerned among these disparate elements of RE; but it is highly uncertain, to say the least, whether they can bestow the sort of heightened credibility on display in mutually supportive scientific beliefs.

Can Coherence Teach Us What and How to Prune?

According to Daniels (1979: 258), the method of WRE is an attempt to generate coherence in an ordered triple of sets of beliefs encompassing (*a*) considered moral judgments, (*b*) a set of moral principles, and (*c*) the set of relevant background theories. We thus attempt to bring our beliefs at one distinct level (e.g. considered judgments) into harmony with our beliefs at the other levels (e.g. moral principles or background theories). If we encounter a disparity between any two of these disparate elements of our moral system, then RE calls for a movement to and fro, pruning a bit here, tucking a bit there, until the discrepancies are ironed out and harmony among our beliefs is restored. But now a question arises: Assuming the appearance of a conflict between two different elements of our moral system—e.g. between a considered judgment and a given moral principle—*which one* should be pruned? As D. W. Haslett (1987) observes, coherence considerations by themselves are not enough to enable us to decide between any two conflicting elements within the ambit of RE. While coherence can indeed direct us to prune either the judgment or the principle, it cannot tell us *which one* should be sacrificed in its name. Given any two sets of considered judgments and matching principles, there could, then, be *innumerable* different wide reflective equilibria corresponding to different (arbitrary) choices for nipping and tucking.

Haslett's objection gives us an additional reason to demand more from coherence than mere consistency. If that is all coherence means, then Haslett has indeed delivered a crushing blow to the claims of RE. The defenders of RE can respond, however, that coherence encompasses not just the bare-bones notion of consistency, but also such important relations as providing the 'best fit' or 'strongest mutual support'. While this gloss on coherence could be helpful in pointing our pruning shears in the right direction, it generates problems of its own. As Bo Petersson (1998) points out, the larger the network of intersecting elements in RE, the more disparate their contents and varieties of interdependence, the more difficult it will be to assign a definite meaning to such notions as 'maximal coherence' and 'strongest mutual support'. In WRE we have a vast network of considered judgments, moral principles, and both moral and empirical background theories. The way in which empirical background theories may support various moral theories, for example, may differ significantly from the way in which considered judgments support moral principles. How are we to determine the relevance and strength of these different kinds of support in coming to an all-things-considered judgment about 'maximal coherence'? For this purpose should the number of supportive relations count for more than their 'strength'? Since WRE contains such a huge mix of disparate elements and differing kinds of supporting relationships—e.g. exhibiting logical entailment, inductive support, or mere consistency—the notion of degrees of coherence implied by this alternative approach turns out to be yet another exercise in hand waving. If we cannot clearly ascertain which particular arrangement of all these disparate elements is the 'most coherent', then the method of WRE will fail to provide a useful guide to either theory construction or practical ethics.

Will the Coherence Approach Yield Convergence?

It's hard to think of a better method than RE to help each of us organize, systematize, and smooth out inconsistencies within our respective inventories of moral beliefs. Indeed, most discussions of RE stipulate that it is a method to be used by each individual inquirer to achieve moral justification of his or her own beliefs. What happens, however, when we abandon this first-person perspective and consider the reflective equilibria of other people in society? Will the widespread use of WRE tend to foster convergence of belief with regard to individual cases, moral principles, and background theories?

This is an important question because it goes to the heart of the whole rationale for employing a *method* of moral reasoning in the first place. In most fields of inquiry, the promise of method, as opposed to mere ad hoc, episodic ruminations, is that it will reliably guide us to discover correct results. At its most rigorous, the notion of method works as a kind of procedural guarantee that anyone who submits to its discipline, going through all the prescribed steps, will come out at the other end with an intersubjectively verifiable truth. A more realistic expectation for method in bioethics is that following its dictates will at least increase our chances of converging upon the truth. I will come back later in this chapter to the very notion of method in ethics, but for now I want to focus on the claims of WRE to facilitate convergence around proposed solutions to bioethical problems.

One indicator of intersubjective reliability is the ability of a method to produce a confluence of opinion or belief among those who use it. Although mere consensus is obviously no guarantee of moral truth—witness the Third Reich, which was remarkably successful in achieving consensus—it's hard to imagine a method of thought being reliable in the required sense unless it can produce convergence of belief among those who deploy it. It is thus an important question whether WRE can be counted upon to effect this sort of convergence with regard to moral beliefs.

Interestingly, Rawls (1971: 50/1999: 44) never committed himself on this question, and apparently for good reason. A moment's reflection on the matter should make it rather painfully obvious that in a liberal, pluralistic democratic society, different groups of people will enter WRE with very different considered moral judgments. Although such judgments are not sacrosanct and incorrigible within WRE, they do exert a significant influence upon the moral principles we eventually embrace and the sorts of background theories we are willing to accept. Thus, we should expect fundamentalist Christians from the Midwestern United States to start with dramatically different considered judgments from those of Jewish leftists living on the upper west side of Manhattan; and we should, moreover, expect both of these types to differ fundamentally with the considered moral judgments of Shi'ite clerics in Baghdad or Shining Path Marxist revolutionaries in Peru. It is reasonable to expect, then, that the members of all four of these demographics will end up in very different *moral* places once they have gone through the required motions of WRE in their own heads. Clearly, their considered judgments will not all be mutually exclusive; they will share a good deal with regard to nearly universal values bearing on truthfulness, respect for property (except those Marxists and anarchists who equate property with theft!), and the avoidance of gratuitous cruelty. They will, nevertheless, tend to differ on such key bioethical issues as the fair distribution of health care, the permissibility of artificial reproductive technologies, and the enhancement of human nature through biomedical technology. In short, then, the method of WRE can ideally yield justification to those individuals who engage in the process, but it cannot be counted upon to yield convergence with regard to typical front-burner issues in bioethics; and if it can't yield convergence among different sorts of people in a pluralist society, then it cannot be considered to be a reliable method of arriving at moral truth. There may well be no other method of moral inquiry that could possibly achieve this kind of convergence and reliability; the moral world may simply be too fragmented for that. Even Rawls's staunchest defenders have admitted that WRE cannot achieve intersubjective consensus within the context of pluralistic societies, at least with regard to those controversies that implicate divergent visions of the good beyond the 'overlapping consensus' on basic principles of justice. As Daniels (1996: 144–75) now puts it, it was a 'philosopher's dream' to imagine that the kind of philosophical reflection driving WRE could bring about convergence within pluralistic societies, and he has therefore turned to other methods of justifying practical moral solutions within such societies, such as the political procedures of 'deliberative democracy' (Daniels and Sabin 2002). Along with Rawls, Daniels still believes that RE can generate an overlapping consensus on the core principles governing the basic structure of a liberal democratic society, but he now contends that we must seek the resolution of controversies arising beyond the basic structure, where most bioethical problems lurk, in a *political process* bounded by the norms of basic justice.

This is in many ways a salutary move. One problem with the method of RE as developed so far is that it tends to focus on the solitary theorist and her struggle to achieve coherence among all of her disparate beliefs. Notwithstanding the importance of this project, it tends to neglect the social dimension of reasoning in an area like bioethics. More often than not, we *reason together* in bioethics in the context of hospital ethics committees, governmental ethics commissions, and collaborative group projects. In contexts like these, it is important not simply to align our respective beliefs in reflective equilibrium, but also to justify them to other free and equal citizens within a process of inquiry governed by democratic norms.

Local versus Global Coherence?

According to the partisans of WRE, we should seek coherence among the *widest possible* set of moral and non-moral beliefs. But how far and wide can we expect this set to extend into the entire domain of morality? What, in other words, is possible? On one view, morality can be properly regarded as a *unified system* of beliefs, principles, and theories. Any inconsistencies between disparate regions of the 'moral world' should, from this angle, be ultimately remediable. On this reading, the sort of coherence we seek in moral reflection is ultimately *global*. This is a very ambitious thesis. Just how ambitious it is can be gauged by reflecting for a moment on the sort of phenomenon morality is. For those of us who don't believe that morality is given to us by God, helpfully inscribed on extremely durable stone tablets, or by nature in such a way that the solutions to our disputes in practical ethics can be 'read off' the nature of humans and society, morality will present itself to us as a historically and culturally conditioned achievement. Different considered judgments and moral principles developed in different historical settings exist side by side in contemporary cosmopolitan societies, and these differences may well prevent morality from being viewed as a coherent whole. If the domain of law can be aptly characterized by one of our most distinguished theorists as a 'higgledy-piggledy assemblage of the remains of contradictory past political ambitions and beliefs' (Raz 1994: 296), then, a fortiori, the same could be said of morality (Nagel 1991; Scanlon 1992; Brock 1995). This does not mean that achieving coherence isn't a desirable thing, for it clearly is; it does mean, however, that the sort of coherence that we can realistically seek among our moral beliefs is most likely local rather than global. As Raz (1994: 317) nicely puts it, we should expect to find 'pockets of coherence' rather than vast unified expanses of it. Thus, the principles developed to govern the physician–patient relationship may be inadequate or counterproductive in other domains of the moral life, such as public health, environmental ethics, or assessing our obligations to the distant needy in other lands (Scheffler 2001).

What's So Great About Coherence?

I wrap up this excursion into coherence theory and RE with some brief remarks about the epistemological value of coherence. This topic runs very deep, so I can only scratch the surface here. This is the problem: Once we abandon foundationalist approaches to justification in ethics, we are apparently left with coherence as the only remaining source of justifiability. Yet coherence, on the face of it, seems an unlikely candidate for this role. The first thing to notice is that coherence per se is not necessarily a compelling virtue of moral outlooks. It's quite possible for someone to inhabit a seamlessly unified moral world-view and yet fail to be justified in his moral judgments.[8] Consider the case of Rush, a hypothetical teenager of middling intellectual gifts, sub-acute moral perception, and an embarrassingly bad complexion, who immerses himself in the world of right-wing politics in order to provide himself with 'an identity'. All day long, he tunes into the rants of right-wing ideologues on talk radio, reads and rereads their screeds in pamphlets and books, and avidly participates in their website chat rooms. Rush emerges from this ideological bath feeling much better about himself as a committed Republican, free-marketeer, political libertarian, and a sworn enemy of the welfare state, which he decries as a haven for losers and a drain on the energies of virtuous, wealthy entrepreneurs. What shall we say about Rush's world-view and his dismissal of the poor as a bunch of pathetic losers? Clearly, Rush's moral universe is exceedingly coherent. His moral, political, economic, and even artistic views all hang together quite nicely now, and his judgments about events and policy flow spontaneously from that coherent world-view. Still, many of us, even many conservatives, would probably say that Rush's moral and policy judgments are anything but morally justified. They would perhaps point to Rush's lack of intelligence, his lack of experience in the real world, and the urgency of his need for self-validation as factors vitiating the trustworthiness of his confident denunciations of the poor. Even if he has reached, within his own mind, a state of reflective equilibrium, most of us would deny that this equilibrium justifies anything about Rush's judgments. We would, for starters, recommend that he broaden his experience of the world, perhaps by joining Habitat for Humanity or the Peace Corps, and enlarge his reading list to include (at least) Charles Dickens, Victor Hugo, John Steinbeck, Frantz Fanon, and Martin Luther King. Once he has exposed himself to such potentially transformative texts and experiences, he might well abandon his former beliefs; but even if he continues to embrace some version of political conservatism, his former beliefs will have been tested and transformed in the crucible of conflicting evidence. At least compared to his earlier beliefs, Rush's new beliefs will be more justified for having emerged from that crucible, even if his old web of belief was entirely coherent. This is where

---

[8] The same reservations about coherence surface with regard to particular moral theories. One of the most coherent moral outlooks, by far, is the theory of act utilitarianism, yet this theory is regularly assailed by its many critics as overly simplistic and tolerant of immoral results.

Daniels's exhortation for us to achieve coherence among the 'widest possible' set of beliefs becomes absolutely crucial.

Here's another case. Consider Sophia, a hypothetical young woman—a smart, well-educated, widely read, well-traveled, progressive, and deeply thoughtful early twentieth-century amateur eugenicist who advocates sterilization of the 'unfit'. Like Rush, Sophia inhabits an extremely coherent moral viewpoint. All the disparate elements of her inventory of belief—including the Bible, as she has learned to interpret it; 'common sense'; the then-ascendant social Darwinist theory of political economy; and, of course, then-current theories of genetics—tell her the same thing: namely, that the white race is superior, that it is under siege, and that sterilizing the 'unfit' represents the quintessence of social responsibility. In contrast to our response to Rush, it's harder to say that Sophia is intellectually dim, sheltered, badly educated, or psychologically deformed. She is, in the opinion of her contemporaries, a very serious, thoughtful, and politically progressive person.[9] Still, most of us would say that, in retrospect, her beliefs about sterilization were wrong and destructive, primarily because they were based upon background scientific and social theories that we now know to be empirically false. Were we to use time travel miraculously to inject our contemporary knowledge of genetics into her constellation of beliefs, Sophia would have to prune many of her considered judgments and background theories right down to their stumps.

Here we need to make an important distinction between justifying moral theories or positions on controversial issues, on the one hand, and, on the other, asking whether a given agent is justified in believing some proposition. With regard to this latter question, we can ask, as we did in Rush's case, whether a given agent is 'justified' in making the claims that he does. Perhaps he really isn't epistemologically 'entitled' to make various claims because he is lazy or uninformed. Although important in its own right, this latter question is not within the original purview of the method of RE, which is concerned with the marks or criteria that are most likely to indicate the presence of a true belief. More specifically, the method of WRE claims that any given belief is most likely to be true if (and only if) that belief can be shown to belong to a maximally coherent set of other beliefs.[10]

The case of Sophia shows us, then, that even when we abstract from the question of whether *a particular agent* is epistemologically entitled to believe a proposition, we can still raise questions about the truth of beliefs that happen to meet the coherence criterion of justification. Thus, even supposing that Sophia had subjected her belief in eugenic sterilization to the test of maximal coherence, and even if that belief had passed the test in 1920, we would now say that it was wrong, both because it was based upon what we now know to be junk science, but also because we now place a

---

[9] I don't mean to suggest here that enlightened opinion at that time was unanimously in favor of eugenic sterilization. There were eloquent dissenters, such as G. K. Chesterton, but they were unfortunately in the minority (Chesterton 1927).

[10] I thank Alex London for helpful discussion on this point.

much higher value upon individual autonomy and bodily integrity than people did back then.

Our reflections on these two hypothetical individuals yield the following preliminary conclusions. First, any given agent's state of reflective equilibrium can fail to justify various elements of his moral outlook and practice if that agent is sufficiently obtuse, inexperienced, unimaginative, callous, or otherwise psychologically warped. So when Daniels defines WRE as the search for the 'widest possible' network of coherent beliefs, we have to ask whether we should develop an objective or subjective gloss on 'widest possible'. A subjective gloss, as might be rendered by Rush at the nadir of his immersion in right-wing ideology, would appear to be a wholly inadequate basis of moral justification. Second, someone can possess all the requisite 'epistemic virtues'—i.e. intelligence, open-mindedness, zeal in the pursuit of truth, etc.—and yet still be wrong about some very important moral issues, such as eugenic sterilization. So even if we grant that, in cases like Sophia's, WRE can yield maximal coherence, we have to acknowledge that this is not the same thing as actually yielding moral truth. So even if we insist on a more objective gloss on the notion of the 'widest possible' network of beliefs in Daniels's definition of WRE—a gloss that would include reference to all those beliefs that a reasonable person would have to consider in her quest for WRE—this would mark a big improvement, but would still tend to underscore the important difference between the weak sense of moral justification provided by RE and moral truth. Another way to put this is to say that while any true moral belief is likely to pass the test of WRE, merely passing this test does not guarantee that any particular belief will, in fact, be true.

The second major problem with coherence theories of moral justification is summed up in what I'll call the 'circularity objection'. According to this objection, RE yields results as reliable (or unreliable) as the considered moral judgments that get the ball rolling. As we have already seen, if we limit ourselves to the relatively narrow ambit of NRE, the problem is obvious: considered moral judgments give rise to moral principles that 'explicate' or 'fit' them, yet why should we credit the moral bona fides of those considered judgments? If we cannot give a satisfactory answer to this question, we will be highly motivated to adopt WRE as our method, since it promises to advance both moral and empirical background theories to test the adequacy of our considered judgments and our principles derived from them. Now, it won't do us much good at this juncture if the background theories deployed in WRE turn out to owe their credibility to the same considered moral judgments that gave rise to our moral principles. That would obviously amount to question begging. So defenders of WRE must contend that the background theories they endorse, both moral and empirical, do not owe their existence or credibility to the same set of considered moral judgments that animate NRE. They must, that is, demonstrate that the considered moral judgments that ultimately give rise to various morally saturated background theories (e.g. theories of the person, of the role of morality in society, etc.) are somehow independent of those that shaped the moral principles in NRE. Daniels calls this the 'independence constraint' (1979: 260).

This is a plausible defense of WRE, and Daniels carefully works it out with his usual blend of scholarly precision and philosophical sophistication. There is, however, one remaining problem. Supposing that the background theories we use to discipline both our considered moral judgments and our principles all satisfy the independence constraint; suppose, in other words, that whatever moral judgments go into the development of those theories are drawn from a different set than those that go into the development of our moral principles. This would solve the circularity problem, but it remains something of a mystery how it is that the stock of our considered or 'pretheoretical' moral judgments could be compartmentalized in this way (Haslett 1987). One would naturally think that *all* of our considered moral judgments would be pretty much cut from the same cloth of moral sensibility. If they are, then the circularity objection re-emerges. But if they aren't, if some of our considered moral judgments can morph into background theories capable of criticizing the considered judgments that animate NRE, then we would have to explain how we are capable of generating two conflicting sets of considered moral judgments within the structure of the same moral personality, only one of which falls under the purview of NRE. It's unclear, to me at least, how this can be done. It's also unclear why this second set of considered judgments, lurking in the background until the stage of theory formation in RE, would have any greater degree of epistemic warrant than the first set that went into the formation of NRE. The fact that, as incorporated into morally informed background theories, this latter set of judgments might be used to criticize the first set does not establish that they actually provide firmer moral footing. The fact that they are different does not necessarily make them more trustworthy.

CONCLUSIONS

At the end of this long rumination on method in bioethics, we can draw together our conclusions. First, we can say that RE deserves its status as a *regulative ideal* for achieving ethical justification, but only on certain conditions. We are justified in our actions and beliefs to the extent that we have maximal confidence in them, and there appears to be no better way of achieving such confidence than by testing those beliefs against the widest possible set of other beliefs, including those that conflict with the belief in question. In this connection, RE is clearly a powerful engine of rationality and consistency, which afford it a good measure of critical edge. On the other hand, we have seen that mere confidence in our beliefs is not enough, and that this confidence must be sufficiently warranted. It's not enough, in other words, merely to achieve coherence among the beliefs that we happen to have on hand, no matter what our degree of intelligence, our level of empathy, and moral perspicacity, and no matter what efforts we have made to enhance the quality and credibility of those beliefs. An insensitive, provincial, and intellectually lazy dullard, like our hypothetical friend Rush, may have a coherent set of beliefs in which he is supremely confident, but most of us would (correctly) see this not as a justification of those beliefs, but rather as evidence of his intellectual and moral inadequacy. We can thus conclude that RE may be a necessary condition of moral justification, but coherence alone is not sufficient.

Second, we have seen that even warranted confidence in a coherent system of beliefs, such as that possessed by our other hypothetical friend Sophia—i.e. confidence *earned* through the diligent application of intelligence and moral perception to the thorough testing of all the various strata in our system of belief—we have seen that even this kind of moral justification is not enough to guarantee moral truth or credibility. Sophia was well brought up, smart, and progressive, and conscientiously tested her beliefs against the best that contemporary religion, genetics, and social science had to offer. Although many of us might perhaps still fault her for a lack of empathy for the victims of involuntary sterilization, she could make a strong case that her belief system was justified (because maximally coherent) even though its scientific bases were later shown to be manifestly false. So even though the process of RE at its very best can promise ethical justification as a regulative ideal, we should not mistake this for a promise of ethical truth.

Our third conclusion has been that *wide* RE is an unattainable ideal, especially in practical contexts, and that both its requirements (e.g. the critical evaluation of all live options in moral and social theory) and its putatively global scope will have to be significantly scaled back before this method can achieve traction in an area like bioethics. If we take seriously the suggestion developed above that the most we are likely to get is local, rather than global, coherence, then WRE, at least in its most ambitious global form, is not even a necessary condition for moral justification.

Finally, our fourth conclusion is that even if WRE, properly hedged with the conditions stipulated in conclusion 1, can serve as a regulative ideal of ethical justification, we should not expect it to deliver intersubjective convergence around particular moral judgments bearing on actions and policies. As we have seen, the fact of ethical, cultural, and religious pluralism within contemporary cosmopolitan societies will insure a broad multiplicity of reflective equilibria bearing on bioethical questions. Each of these differing sets of belief in equilibrium will be shaped by differing respective visions of the good belonging to the agents in question. So even though we can reasonably expect WRE to have some salutary potential for rendering our beliefs more justifiable, and even though WRE practiced on the societal level might occasionally be helpful in bringing the disparate members of society together on some issues, we should not expect this method to deliver intersubjective agreement on most bioethical controversies.

SOME FINAL THOUGHTS ON METHOD

Similar deflationary thoughts loom over the very notion of *method* in moral inquiry. As we have seen, the unspoken assumption behind appeals to method in various disciplines and practices is that following all the prescribed steps will at least make it more likely that we will reach correct results. At its most daring, some might say presumptuous, this assumption amounts to the claim that just about anybody can reach the correct result, just so long as he or she adheres to the proper method. In the domain of morality this would mean that no matter who employs it, the method of RE can be counted upon to lead the enquirer to moral justification and truth. The focus here is on purifying, as far as possible, our initial considered judgments, and then systematizing all the disparate elements of our moral and empirical inventories. As DePaul (1993: 181) observes, this project fits within a very intellectualist or even scientistic picture of moral philosophy.

Now, the main point that I want to make in closing is that if the project of RE actually harbors the above assumption about the power of method, then we should abandon that assumption. It is highly unlikely that method can live up to this billing anywhere else than in mathematics and the physical sciences, if even there. If we continue to speak of *method* in the area of moral philosophy and practical ethics, we will have to lower our expectations considerably. In this domain, while it is certainly important to try to get the various sectors of our moral world to fit together into as coherent a whole as possible, it is equally if not more important, as Nussbaum (1992) urges, to try to improve our capacity for making sensitive and discriminating moral judgments. As DePaul (1993: 174) puts it, tweaking what he takes to be the intellectualist–scientistic pretensions of RE, we need to spend equal if not more amounts of time attempting to refine the measuring instrument itself—i.e. our own sensibility as moral agents. Thus, he suggests that we need to focus more on developing the inquirer's capacity for making discriminating moral judgments, rather than merely tidying up and systematizing whatever judgments this capacity happens to crank out. If DePaul is right about this, then our efforts to achieve RE would need to be supplemented, as I have suggested above in conclusion 1, by traditional Aristotelian concerns about character formation and training in virtue. And within the story of RE's development, we would have to dust off and rehabilitate Rawls's initial emphasis, dropped from later versions of the method, on the important role of 'competent moral judges' in this scheme (Rawls 1951). Were we to go this route, then the cultivation of good judgment would share center stage with the cultivation of consistency and coherence; and formative works of art, such as novels and films, would assume much greater importance both in moral education and in our quest to improve the output and reliability of RE.

What, then, can or should we expect of method in the domain of practical ethics? While this is surely the subject of another paper, a few modest propositions can be advanced here. First, if method is to play a role in our work, it cannot be the role that Descartes (1637/1967) envisioned for it in 'first philosophy', or metaphysics. That is, we should not conceive of method as something we should first have to learn before we go off and start arguing about cloning, justice in health care, and randomized clinical trials in Africa. It is highly unlikely that there are any sure-fire steps that, once mastered, will lead us to correct results.

Second, we need to distinguish between an idealized method of justification like WRE and helpful suggestions for 'going forward' in ethical analysis and argument (London 2000). As we have seen, in order to head off charges of circularity and insularity, NRE had to morph into WRE; but WRE turned out to be hopelessly clunky and complex as a recipe for moral justification. Not only do we have to make sure that our considered judgments and moral principles are in equilibrium, but we also have to consider all the available 'moral outlooks' and their respective philosophical defences, as well as all those background theories—a morning's work before breakfast for Hercules, perhaps, but a crippling justificatory burden for us mortals. So if we are going to extend the function of RE from contractualist theory building à la Rawls to practical ethics, we will have to direct those pruning shears to WRE itself. In the vast majority of cases (but not in all, to be sure), it will probably turn out that NRE, for all its limitations, will be a tolerably helpful methodological tool. Such an approach would, I suspect, be more or less extensionally equivalent to the more sophisticated varieties of casuistry that envision a dialectical relationship between case judgments, moral principles, and background institutions (Jonsen 1995; Kuczewski 1997).

Finally, just as we should not view method in bioethics as a foolproof guarantor of justification—no matter how callow or unperceptive the moral agent might be—neither should we view it as a complete waste of time in our search for answers. Anyone who has seriously studied the methodological reflections of principlists, casuists, feminists, narrativists, and pragmatists realizes that each of these disparate approaches to thinking about morality points us in helpful directions. It is important to know, for example, about the processes of specifying, weighing, and balancing competing principles; about reasoning by analogy from paradigm cases; about the effects of power and domination on moral relationships; about the importance of narrative for comprehending the rich texture of practical situations; and, finally, about the flexible, tool-like character of moral principles and the importance of deliberative processes for bioethics. These are all important lessons that will surely improve our practical reasoning and facilitate our quest for moral justification, even if they won't guarantee truth.

REFERENCES

ARRAS, J. D. (1991), 'Getting Down to Cases: The Revival of Casuistry in Bioethics', *Journal of Medicine and Philosophy*, 16/1: 29–51.

ARRAS, J. D. (1997), 'Nice Story, But So What? Narrative and Justification in Ethics', in H. Nelson (ed.), *Stories and Their Limits: Narrative Approaches to Bioethics* (New York: Routledge), 65–88.

—— (2002), 'Pragmatism and Bioethics: Been There, Done That', *Journal of Social Philosophy and Policy*, 19/2: 29–58.

—— (2003), 'The Owl and the Caduceus: Does Bioethics Need Philosophy?', in F. G. Miller, J. M. Humber, and J. C. Fletcher (eds.), *The Nature and Prospect of Bioethics* (Totowa, NJ: Humana Press), 1–42.

BARRY, B. (1989), *Theories of Justice* (Berkeley: University of California Press).

BEAUCHAMP, T. L. (1984), 'On Eliminating the Distinction Between Applied Ethics and Ethical Theory', *Monist*, 67/4: 514–31.

—— and CHILDRESS, J. (1979–2001), *Principles of Biomedical Ethics* (New York: Oxford University Press; 1st edn., 1979; 2nd and 3rd edns., 1983; 4th edn., 1994; 5th edn., 2001).

BENJAMIN, M. (2002), *Philosophy and This Actual World: An Introduction to Practical Philosophical Inquiry* (Totowa, NJ: Rowman & Littlefield).

BROCK, D. (1995), 'Public Moral Discourse', in R. E. Bulger, E. M. Bobby, and Harvey V. Fineberg (eds.), *Society's Choices: Social and Ethical Decision Making in Biomedicine* (Washington, DC: National Academy Press), 215–40.

CHESTERTON, G. K. (1927), *Eugenics and Other Evils* (New York: Dodd, Mead).

DANIELS, N. (1979), 'Wide Reflective Equilibrium and Theory Acceptance in Ethics', *Journal of Philosophy*, 76: 256–82.

—— (1996), *Justice and Justification: Reflective Equilibrium in Theory and Practice* (Cambridge: Cambridge University Press).

—— and SABIN, J. E. (2002), *Setting Limits Fairly: Can We Learn to Share Medical Resources?* (New York: Oxford University Press).

DePAUL, M. (1993), *Balance and Refinement: Beyond Coherence Methods of Moral Inquiry* (London: Routledge).

DESCARTES, R. (1637/1967), 'Discourse on Method', in *The Philosophical Works of Descartes*, i, ed. E. S. Haldane and G. R. T. Ross (Cambridge: Cambridge University Press), 79–130.

DWORKIN, R. (1977), 'Hard Cases', in Dworkin, *Taking Rights Seriously* (Cambridge, Mass.: Harvard University Press), 81–130.

GRIFFIN, J. (1996), *Value Judgement: Improving Our Ethical Beliefs* (Oxford: Clarendon Press).

HARE, R. M. (1963), *Freedom and Reason* (Oxford: Oxford University Press).

—— (1975), 'Rawls' Theory of Justice', in N. Daniels (ed.), *Reading Rawls* (New York: Basic Books), 82–107.

HASLETT, D. W. (1987), 'What Is Wrong With Reflective Equilibria?', *Philosophical Quarterly*, 37/148: 305–11.

JONSEN, A. R. (1995), 'Casuistry: An Alternative or Complement to Principles?', *Kennedy Institute of Ethics Journal*, 5: 237–51.

—— and TOULMIN, S. (1988), *The Abuse of Casuistry: A History of Moral Reasoning* (Berkeley: University of California Press).

KAGAN, S. (1998), *Normative Ethics* (Boulder, Col.: Westview Press), 11–16.

KUCZEWSKI, M. (1997), 'Bioethics' Consensus on Method: Who Could Ask for Anything More?', in H. L. Nelson (ed.), *Stories and Their Limits: Narrative Approaches to Bioethics* (New York: Routledge), 134–48.

LONDON, A. J. (2000), 'Amenable to Reason: Aristotle's Rhetoric and the Moral Psychology of Practical Ethics', *Kennedy Institute of Ethics Journal*, 10/4: 287–305.

McGEE, G. (ed.) (2003), *Pragmatic Bioethics*, (2nd edn. Cambridge, Mass.: MIT Press).

NAGEL, T. (1991), 'The Fragmentation of Value', in Nagel, *Mortal Questions* (Cambridge: Cambridge University Press), 128–41.

NEURATH, O. (1966), 'Protocol Sentences', trans. G. Schick, in A. J. Ayer (ed.), *Logical Positivism* (New York: Free Press), 199–208.

NUSSBAUM, M. (1992), 'Perceptive Equilibrium: Literary Theory and Ethical Theory', in Nussbaum, *Love's Knowledge: Essays in Philosophy and Literature* (New York: Oxford University Press), 168–94.

PETERSSON, B. (1998), 'Wide Reflective Equilibrium and the Justification of Moral Theory', in van der Burg and van Willigenburg (1998: 130–3).

POLLOCK, J. L. (1986), *Contemporary Theories of Knowledge* (Totowa, NJ: Rowman & Littlefield).

RAWLS, J. (1951), 'Outline of a Decision Procedure for Ethics', repr. in S. Freeman (ed.), *John Rawls: Collected Papers* (Cambridge, Mass.: Harvard University Press, 1999), 1–19.

_____ (1971/1999), *A Theory of Justice* (Cambridge, Mass.: Harvard University Press; rev. edn., 1999).

_____ (1975), 'The Independence of Moral Theory', in *John Rawls: Collected Papers*, ed. S. Freeman (Cambridge, Mass.: Harvard University Press, 1999), 286–302.

RAZ, J. (1982), 'The Claims of Reflective Equilibrium', *Inquiry*, 25/3: 307–30.

_____ (1994), 'The Relevance of Coherence', *Ethics in the Public Domain: Essays in the Morality of Law and Politics* (Oxford: Clarendon Press), 277–325.

SCANLON, T. M. (1992), 'The Aims and Authority of Moral Theory', *Oxford Journal of Legal Studies*, 12/1: 1–23.

SCHEFFLER, S. (2001), 'Individual Responsibility in a Global Age', in Scheffler, *Boundaries and Allegiances: Problems of Justice and Responsibility in Liberal Thought* (New York: Oxford University Press), 32–47.

SINGER, P. (1974), 'Sidgwick and Reflective Equilibrium', *Monist*, 58/3: 490–517.

TOULMIN, S. (1981), 'The Tyranny of Principles', *Hastings Center Report*, 11/6: 31–9.

VAN DER BURG, W., and VAN WILLIGENBURG, T. (eds.) (1998), *Reflective Equilibrium: Essays in Honor of Robert Heeger* (Dordrecht: Kluwer Academic Publishers).

WOLF, S. (ed.) (1995), *Feminism and Bioethics: Beyond Reproduction* (New York: Oxford University Press).

CHAPTER 3

···

AUTONOMY

···

BRUCE JENNINGS

INTRODUCTION

···

No single concept has been more important in the contemporary development of bioethics, and the revival of medical ethics, than the concept of autonomy, and none better reflects both the philosophical and the political currents shaping the field. In this chapter I propose to consider autonomy in three of its facets and functions: first, as a concept in ethical theory; second, as a concept in applied ethics; and finally, as what might be called an ideological concept—that is, one that both draws from and reinforces non-philosophical interests at work in the profession of medicine, biomedical science and technology, and the broader liberal individualistic culture of Anglophone countries, particularly the United States, where a bioethical discourse centred on autonomy has flourished.

Two theses stand behind this discussion. First, there is a significant difference between the meaning and history of the concept of autonomy in moral philosophy (and political theory) and its appropriation in the normative and applied work of bioethics. This difference is often overlooked, and the deployment of autonomy in bioethics has usually been presented as the straightforward 'application' of a philosophically grounded concept and principle to particular cases or decision-making situations. In fact, the relationship between the meaning of autonomy in bioethics and its status in deontological or rights-based theory—particularly its most natural homes, contractarian and libertarian liberalism—is highly selective and tenuous. This is best illustrated, I believe, by contrasting *autonomy* as Kant understood it with *liberty* as it has been understood by John Stuart Mill and more recently Isaiah Berlin. Indeed, to talk about 'autonomy' in bioethics is something of a misnomer and a category mistake; the concept that is actually much more influential in bioethics is a version of Millian 'liberty', the version that Berlin dubbed 'negative liberty'. Bioethicists by and large have been suspicious of 'positive liberty', as Berlin himself was, and which is closely akin to Kantian or rationalistic autonomy. Modern bioethics has largely rejected the theoretical tradition and legacy of autonomy not so much by explicit critique as by rendering it invisible. This is done when the term 'autonomy' is used to mean and to do the ethical work of negative liberty.

My second thesis is that this conceptual displacement has occurred in bioethics partly owing to the sociology of the field and partly owing to the conditions that have been required of it to gain intellectual legitimacy (and thereby some measure of power and influence) in professional and policy domains.

AUTONOMY'S INFLUENCE IN BIOETHICS

I

Beginning with the Belmont Report of the National Commission on Ethical Issues in Human Subject Research (or perhaps even earlier, with Telford Taylor's resounding statement at the Nuremberg Doctors' Trial), the concept of autonomy (sometimes referred to as 'self-determination' or 'respect for persons') has played a central role in the modern field of bioethics. This centrality was reinforced by the tremendous influence of the seminal work of Tom Beauchamp and James Childress *The Principles of Biomedical Ethics*, first published in 1979, which has since become the standard work in the field and has gone through four significant revisions and expansions. There the principle of autonomy is presented as a middle-range principle, not dependent upon any single more general or abstract ethical theory and compatible with many. It stands alongside the other principles in the Beauchamp and Childress edifice—beneficence, non-maleficence, and justice—as a *primus inter pares*.

In soon-to-follow agenda-setting documents for the field, such as the influential reports of the President's Commission for the Study of Ethical Problems in Medicine and Biomedical and Behavioral Research in the early 1980s, the principle of self-determination again took a leading role in the analysis and recommendations made about everything from whistle blowing to genetic testing to health care access to decisions to forgo life-sustaining treatment. Before long autonomy-centred work in bioethics was beginning to appear in other countries beside the United States, in the Canadian Law Reform Commission, in the Waller Commission in Australia, in the work of the noted Australian philosopher Max Charlesworth (1993), and in the United Kingdom with the work of Raanan Gillon (1986), to name only a few.

This is not the proper place to rehearse all the countless ways and occasions in which the concept of autonomy has been pressed into service in bioethics. By the late 1960s and early 1970s it was an idea whose time had come. Let four areas of debate in bioethics provide brief examples to indicate the power of autonomy (or, more precisely, various conceptions of autonomy, for there are several) in bioethics. These are abortion, medically assisted reproduction, genetic counselling, and decisions to forgo life-sustaining medical treatment.

II

One thinks first of the evolution of the abortion debate during these years, particularly polarizing in the United States, and culminating in the landmark decision of the US Supreme Court *Roe* v. *Wade*, in which the woman's autonomous control of her own body and her own pregnancy became the central tenet. Autonomy was clearly central for those who did not ascribe moral significance to the early embryo and fetus. But even more interesting and indicative of the moral force of the concept of autonomy was an argument put forward by Judith Jarvis Thomson (1971), who was willing to grant even personhood status to the fetus and yet still argued that the pregnant woman's autonomy overrode any moral claims of fetal persons. As the pro-choice or pro-abortion line of argument developed, the question of the morally right choice came to be subsumed under the question of who had the moral right to choose. Some, like Daniel Callahan (1970), would argue that the law should not interfere with a woman's autonomy by prohibiting abortion, but that from a moral point of view there should be good reasons, some account beyond appeal to the woman's subjective will alone, for terminating a pregnancy; good reasons, that is, for cashing in one's autonomy.

In general, I think it is fair to say that Thomson's position prevailed over Callahan's position, but in so far as they both appealed to moral reasons (other than the autonomous right to choose) to justify a particular choice, neither of these positions gave the concept of autonomy the strength that it acquired in the more popular, less philosophical debate. The abortion controversy became so polarized and so bitter that asking for moral reasons for autonomous choice or action was rejected by the pro-choice side of the debate as a covert means of taking autonomy and power away from women. Being autonomous came to mean not being second-guessed by anybody or anything about one's choices or the use that one makes of one's freedom.

Closely related was the larger issue of medically assisted reproduction and reproductive autonomy. New technologies and drugs to overcome infertility, such as *in vitro* fertilization (IVf) grew in efficacy and popularity in the 1980s. Autonomous control of one's gametes—for donation, stimulation, implantation, and cryo-preservation—was the dominant orientation of bioethics, as various early restrictions were set aside that would make IVF and related technology accessible only to married heterosexual couples, or only to those couples who could demonstrate good health and good character and potential to be good parents and to provide well for the child. Concerns about the unknown effects on the child, psychological effects, social stigma, even possible genetic damage caused by the procedure itself were all set aside as so much idle speculation, and, in any case, were not considered sufficiently weighty to override the moral importance of protecting autonomy and choice for infertile men and women (Robertson 1994).

In the new field of genetic counselling, dealing as it did with a sordid history of racism, discrimination, and eugenics, the concept of respecting autonomy was the foundation upon which the doctrine of non-directive counselling was built. That same orientation and issue quickly moved over into the field of reproductive counselling as well.

The ideal of 'non-directive' behaviour by the counsellor raises a number of interesting problems in relation to the concept of autonomy. In essence, this doctrine limits the counsellor's role to providing clear, understandable factual information about test results, treatment options, and the like. Counselling should never discuss which course of action may be more reasonable, wise, prudent, or ethically appropriate. Even non-binding advice on such matters is regarded, not as helpful additional information, but rather as intrusive, even coercive, influence by a professional authority figure. As such it interferes with, instead of assisting or promoting, the client's exercise of autonomy. This makes sense when autonomy is conceived as being the independent exercise of individual will or choice, but it seems odd and overly restrictive if autonomy requires some degree of reason and is subject to some norms of cogency and correctness (perhaps norms built into the very concept of reason itself).

Here many of the difficult issues related to the concept of autonomy become apparent. If we stress the notion of reason and rational choice, how tightly do the norms of reason constrain action? Is there one right and reasonable decision to be made in each situation, and are only those who embrace the 'right' choice truly autonomous? On the other hand, if we stress the notion of liberty and independent choice, does the value of autonomy then preclude all other ethical judgements concerning actions (including perhaps the agent's own reflexive judgements)? Does it set up an internal conceptual conflict between autonomy and all other ethical values? Kant, for example, held that to be autonomous was to be rational in the sense of adopting principles that met certain conceptual tests, such as universality. John Stuart Mill held that diversity and experiments in ways of life were important and that what is the right way to live for one person may not be the right way for another. Finally, a century later Isaiah Berlin developed this side of Mill's thought even further and eloquently articulated a defence of liberty and ethical pluralism that was quite far removed from Kant. Often, in bioethics, as is illustrated by the doctrine of non-directive counselling, the term 'autonomy' more closely resembles Berlin's liberty than Kant's reason.

Finally, in the so-called right to die area, the concept of autonomy plays a central role in the notion that persons have the right to forgo life-extending treatment, even when they have lost decision-making capacity and another person must exercise that autonomy right on their behalf. Until the 1990s the boundaries of autonomy in end-of-life medical care had been drawn by the active–passive or killing–letting die distinction. The national grassroots efforts to legalize assisted suicide (in Oregon and briefly in the Northern Territory of Australia) and even active euthanasia by lethal injection (in the Netherlands) pushed the domain of autonomy further than the court cases and laws on the right to refuse treatment. Few official documents pertaining to bioethics are more influenced by the ethical concept of autonomy than the majority ruling of the US Ninth Federal District Court (covering the states of California, Oregon, and Washington) striking down the state laws criminalizing physician-assisted suicide in those jurisdictions (*Compassion in Dying* v. *Washington* 1996).

III

Further testimony to the influence of autonomy in bioethics is the fact that autonomy is facing a backlash. Patients do not always want to be the partners of their doctors in making health care decisions, argues Carl Schneider in *The Practice of Autonomy* (1998). Feminist bioethicists and others have tried to blunt the radical individualism that use of the concept of autonomy so often seems to imply. Such arguments can be found in work by George Agich, *Autonomy and Long Term Care* (1993), in the important collection *Relational Autonomy*, edited by Catriona Mackenzie and Natalie Stoljar (2000), and in my own work with Willard Gaylin, *The Perversion of Autonomy* (Gaylin and Jennings 2003).

Another notable work in this vein is Onora O'Neill's book *Autonomy and Trust in Bioethics* (2002: 75), where she argues:

The claims of individual autonomy, in particular of patient autonomy and reproductive autonomy, have been endlessly rehearsed in bioethics in recent decades. By
themselves . . . conceptions of individual autonomy cannot provide a sufficient and convincing starting point for bioethics, or even for medical ethics. They may encourage
ethically questionable forms of individualism and self-expression and may heighten rather
than reduce public mistrust in medicine, science and biotechnology. At most individual
autonomy, understood merely as an inflated term for informed consent requirements, can
play a minor part within a wider account of ethical standards.

O'Neill holds that the concept of autonomy that bioethics has appropriated bears little resemblance to Kant's understanding and use of this concept, and she offers a counter-reading of Kant, stressing the role of practical reason in his ethics and the fundamental importance, in the ethical life, of the social fabric of mutual and institutional trust.

AUTONOMY: A COMPLEX CONCEPT

I

Let us turn now to matters of definition and the place of autonomy in ethical theory outside bioethics.

The word 'autonomy' comes from the Greek *autos* (meaning 'self') and *nomos* (meaning 'rule', 'governance', or 'law'). Literally, therefore, 'autonomy' means 'the state of being self-governed or self-sovereign'; living autonomously means living by a law that you impose on yourself. In other words, autonomy is the right to live your own life in your own way.

Beauchamp and Childress (1994: 121) state that autonomy is the 'personal rule of the self that is free from both controlling interference by others and from personal limitations that prevent meaningful choice.... The autonomous individual freely acts in accordance with a self-chosen plan.' Numerous social and political philosophers express the same general idea. 'To regard himself as autonomous', says Thomas Scanlon (1972: 215), 'a person must see himself as sovereign in deciding what to believe and in weighing competing reasons for action.' For his part, Robert Paul Wolff (1970: 14) places autonomy in the context of a struggle among human wills for control:

As Kant argued, moral autonomy is a submission to laws that one has made for oneself. The autonomous man, insofar as he is autonomous, is not subject to the will of another. The autonomous ... man may do what another tells him, but not because he has been told to do it .... By accepting as final the commands of the others, he forfeits his autonomy.

Other philosophers and psychologists, such as R. S. Peters and Lawrence Kohlberg, say that autonomy requires a deliberate self-consciousness about obedience to rules. They place it at the pinnacle of moral development. 'Children finally pass to the level of autonomy', Peters writes (1972: 130), 'when they appreciate that rules are alterable, that they can be criticized and should be accepted or rejected on a basis of reciprocity and fairness. The emergence of rational reflection about rules ... central to the Kantian conception of autonomy, is the main feature of the final level of moral development.' Kohlberg (1981) also pictures the best moral agent as standing judgementally above the existing rules, laws, traditions, habits, and norms of his society, and choosing with rational detachment which rules to follow and which to disregard. Autonomy is a catalyst for moral growth and social enlightenment. It is a sign of moral adulthood in the individual; only autonomous persons are truly grown-up, regardless of their age. Kant (1963) likewise saw autonomy as a sign of the enlightenment and maturity of mankind.

Lawrence Haworth, author of one of the few book-length studies of the concept of autonomy, defines autonomy as having what he calls 'critical competence'. He writes: 'Having critical *competence* a person is first of all active and his activity succeeds in giving effect to his intentions. Having *critical* competence, the active person is sensitive to the results of his own deliberation; his activity is guided by purposes he has thought through and found reasons of his own for pursuing' (1986: 46).

These philosophical views of autonomy are widely shared in intellectual circles. Perhaps they are summed up most succinctly, if not most grammatically, by the philosopher Joel Feinberg: 'I am autonomous if I rule me, and no one else rules I' (1972: 161).

II

I rule me, myself. It is important to note that autonomy is not a single idea but a cluster of closely related, overlapping ideas. And it is not only a philosophical or theoretical construct. The idea, if not the actual term, is part and parcel of contemporary culture and everyday self-consciousness in the West. One of the things that has distinguished bioethics from academic philosophy is that each has a different audience. If one wishes to address a lay audience or a professional audience that is not widely read in philosophy, then one both must use the concept of autonomy, if one is to be appealing and understood, and must only use it in certain ways. This is why O'Neill's attempt to reconstruct and make more robust the concept of autonomy, whatever its appeal to other professional philosophers, is quite difficult within the context of bioethics, at least within American bioethics. Similarly, her attempt to concentrate attention elsewhere in our ethical understanding of medicine, to focus on the crucial concept of trust, for example, will also be difficult to achieve. The fact is that in the broader audience to which bioethics must appeal, the need to mean much more than 'informed consent requirements' when one appeals to autonomy is not apparent. Nor is this audience likely to agree on which forms of individualism and self-expression are ethically questionable. Again, at least in the American context, individualism, self-expression, and autonomy are closely conjoined and enormously appealing.

AUTONOMY AND THE CULTURAL CONTEXT OF BIOETHICS

I

The idea of autonomy in contemporary culture and society has been the focus of important studies by leading social theorists and social scientists. How far back one should trace this is debatable (Tocqueville?), but the groundwork for modern work on autonomy in American sociology was already established in the influential work of David Riesman *et al.*, *The Lonely Crowd* (1950).[1] A generation later, an implied critique of autonomy can be found in what the historian Christopher Lasch (1978) called the 'culture of narcissism'. It has affinities as well with what the philosopher Charles Taylor (1991) has referred to as the 'ethics of authenticity'. Robert Bellah and his colleagues (1985) called it 'expressive individualism'. Finally, at the heart of what I am concerned with under the heading of autonomy is a notion that the sociologist Alan Wolfe (2001) has called 'moral freedom'. He defines his subject in the following way:

The old adage that America is a free country has, at last, come true, for Americans have come to accept the relevance of individual freedom, not only in their economic and political life, but in their moral life as well. The defining characteristic of the moral philosophy of the Americans can therefore be described as the principle of moral freedom. Moral freedom means that individuals should determine for themselves what it means to lead a good and virtuous life. Contemporary Americans find answers to the perennial questions asked by theologians and moral philosophers, not by conforming to strictures handed down by God or nature, but by considering who they are, what others require, and what consequences follow from acting one way rather than another. Some of our respondents adopt moral freedom as a creative challenge... they find themselves quite comfortable with the idea that a good society is one that allows each individual maximum scope for making his or her own moral choices. (2001: 195)

Wolfe goes on to argue that the widespread (but by no means universal) embrace of moral freedom amounts to a cultural revolution in America:

never have so many people been so free of moral constraint as contemporary Americans. Most people, throughout most of the world, have lived under conditions in which their morality was defined for them. Now, for the first time in human history, significant numbers of individuals believe that people should play a role in defining their own morality as they contemplate their proper relationship to God, to one another, and to themselves. (2001: 199)

Many social commentators have been critical of the autonomy orientation of contemporary culture. These writers usually direct their criticism of the culture of autonomy along one of two lines. One such line, developed by the theologian Stanley Hauerwas (1974), is that autonomy is morally flabby because it is little more than an ethic of selfishness and self-indulgence. In a similar expression of the same kind of criticism the sociologist Daniel Bell (1976) decried what he called the dominant 'hedonism' behind the cultural transformations begun in the late 1960s.

The second line of criticism of the general cultural emphasis on individual autonomy is that the widespread deference accorded to autonomy today in the

---

[1] Riesman employs the term 'autonomous self' to designate an alternative character type that avoids the respective weaknesses of the 'inner-directed' and the 'other-directed' personalities. A useful sampling of social commentary on individualism and what we today would probably refer to as autonomy can be found in Bellah *et al.* (1987).

law and in secular morality threatens to undermine the moral order itself. A spate of books published in the last few years has developed variations on this theme, including Robert Hughes (1993) and Jean Bethke Elshtain (1995).

These books have in common a sense of disorder, albeit a disorder still just short of normlessness or anomie. Claims to rights and demands for dignity and respect, no matter how well deserved, are overloading the system. This sense of disorder and the need to respond aggressively to it are captured in the very titles or subtitles of many of these works: the 'fraying of America' (Hughes's subtitle), 'on trial', 'defence', 'death', and 'suffocating America'. In other works, America is being 'de-moralized' (Himmelfarb 1995) or 'disunited' (Schlesinger 1992).

II

Many of these recent criticisms of the effects of the concept of autonomy in our moral discourse and in our social lives cast an overly broad net. Rather than subjecting autonomy to a more careful conceptual analysis, they tend to use the term (or the concept) as a lightning rod for many different social complaints and criticisms.

To be sure, autonomy has been very influential in the broader moral culture as it has been in the field of bioethics. What is most needed now, however, is not a broad-brush critique but a more careful sifting of meanings and inconsistencies in the way the term is used. I have already mentioned the distinction between autonomy understood as the exercise of reason and autonomy understood as the exercise of liberty, and I will return to that distinction below. First, though, let us consider the broad and general meaning of autonomy further.

Autonomy is not an ethic of selfishness, nor is self-indulgence the same as rational self-fulfilment. Autonomy means freedom from outside restraint and the freedom to live one's own life in one's own way. To be autonomous is to live by your own law, or only by laws that you have embraced and accepted as your own. It is to be self-sovereign. It is to be the author of your life, your self, and your actions. Nothing in these notions necessitates selfishness or egoism. Self-determining conduct need not be exclusively self-serving. Being the author of your own life says nothing per se about the moral content of that life.

As an ethic, autonomy means living according to your own values and principles, as these are refined in the light of informed, rational deliberation and settled conviction. This ethic is a far cry from an anything-goes, do-your-own-thing morality. There is no obvious reason why an autonomous person cannot identify with principles of justice and moral virtue that are founded on reason. Not only is autonomy compatible with just and altruistic ideals, it seems to go naturally with them. The free and secure person is a more open and charitable person. It is insecurity about one's worth that often breeds defensiveness and hostility.

While autonomy is not an ideal of selfishness or disorderly self-indulgence, it is individualistic. It can be—according to most philosophers it *has* to be—based on rational will rather than licence; but it is the self's reason, not that of a community or a higher authority. Autonomy's mood is always possessive. It speaks in the first-person singular rather than the first-person plural. It is a vision of free *Is*, not free *Wes*.

In order to illuminate the special role of autonomy in modern culture, Joel Feinberg (1980), a leading proponent of autonomy and civil liberties, has asked what would be missing if we lived in a society that did not understand the concepts of autonomy and rights. He imagined a prosperous and benevolent society, not a tyranny or a despotism. He imagined a society in which individuals possessed all the other virtues and lived by the Ten Commandments and the Golden Rule. Even in such a good and happy society, Feinberg said, something essential to morality and humanity would be lacking. Individuals would not be able to make claims on each other for dignity and respect.

Autonomy allows one person to demand respect from another as a matter of right. Not to ask meekly for respect as a matter of goodwill, friendship, or charity, but to *demand* it. Proudly. And not necessarily on the basis of some accomplishment, but just because one is a person, an adult human being, a first-class member of the moral community. It is through the concepts of autonomy and rights that we gain our sense of identity as moral persons and free agents worthy of the respect of others.

Self-sovereignty in the moral realm; the right to live your own life in your own way so long as you do others no harm; being true to yourself above all—these notions are at the core of individualism, authenticity, moral freedom, and autonomy, if not as all professional philosophers would define them, then at least as many ordinary people define them in their own social and self-consciousness.

III

In sum, there are several key tenets that give autonomy its extraordinary moral power and appeal. They can be stated as follows. One tenet is *moral individualism*, the belief that the human individual is the centre of the moral universe, the subject of ultimate worth to whose well-being all other things that may be said to have moral value must finally contribute. Another is what might be called *moral constructivism*, the notion that the basic features of society are ultimately products of human choice and artifice, and as such the social world is a human world, a world fashioned not by God or nature but by the amazingly plastic, adaptive human will.

The final root idea underlying autonomy is the doctrine of *moral voluntarism* or *consent*. The moral life of the individual is made up of relationships, commitments, and obligations that the individual has freely chosen, not those into which she was born or that were imposed upon her. Rather, autonomy means living in accordance with rules that one gives to oneself. If an autonomous person does her duty, it is because she has freely and rationally chosen to do so. Autonomy gives an inward turn to moral duty, obligation, or responsibility, grounding them not in nature or history but in the domain of will and rational choice.

OBJECTIVE AUTONOMY (REASON)
AND SUBJECTIVE AUTONOMY (LIBERTY)
IN BIOETHICS

I

There are, of course, a number of ways in which the concept of autonomy can be used in ethical theory. It can be a good or goal to be obtained in some type of consequentialist theory, but such traits or aspects of human flourishing are usually differentiating concepts, something that only a few can obtain by special effort or circumstance, while autonomy is more commonly taken to be a universal potentiality, a common property or constitutive feature of our humanness as such. If a given individual does not possess autonomy it is rarely taken to be the result of failed effort and more often taken to be the result of some extrinsic condition, oppression, coercion, ignorance, or mental illness, for example. Thus autonomy is often used in deontological or contractarian type theories to designate a condition of mind and agency that adheres to individuals as a matter of right. The right to be allowed to be autonomous is an individual right or moral claim that can be made against others who might interfere with that condition and who thereby have a correlative obligation of non-interference with the autonomy of the other. Whether this is a negative obligation of forbearance only, or also a positive obligation of assistance, is a nice question.

For our purposes here the most important set of theoretical questions about the concept of autonomy concerns the issue of how and on what basis autonomy imposes any moral restrictions on the will of the autonomous person. This has to do with the difference between what might be called an objective understanding of autonomy versus a subjective one. *Alternatively, as I would prefer to formulate it, the question has to do with the relative emphasis one gives to reason or to liberty in one's understanding of autonomy.* This difference marks out the two principal pathways within the liberal tradition that the concept of autonomy has followed. The first may be seen in Locke and Rousseau, but certainly finds its most sophisticated philosophical expression in the ethical writings of Kant. The second can be seen as a course charted by John Stuart Mill in *On Liberty* and pushed even further a century later by Isaiah Berlin in his famous essay 'Two Concepts of Liberty'.

II

Kant was more concerned with duty than with freedom.[2] Autonomy is obedience to self-imposed law, but not just any law or indeed any aspect of the self. Autonomy is obedience to the moral law or categorical imperative as it is discerned by the self exercising reason. Autonomy is objective because reason and the moral law it discerns are objective. Moreover, Kant was primarily concerned with universalism and the formal preconditions for something to be a universal and rational moral law or principle. Mill was a naturalist and was more concerned with individual choice and action in a context of political and social constraint. Reason is not a formal and universal kind of knowing for Mill and it does not establish the formal preconditions for either autonomy or right. Reason is a faculty for determining conduct and for the choice of means to protect and preserve interests and desires, particularly those compatible with cooperative and mutually beneficial life with others similarly motivated and inclined.

Hence, with Mill one finds a version of subjectivity introduced into the notion of autonomy (a term that Mill rarely used) because each person is the most reasonable custodian and definer of his or her own interests and objectives. If the power to determine those interests is exercised over one by others, especially by officials of the state, one is deprived of liberty (autonomy) and one is hampered in the development of intelligence, skill, and self-reliance that Mill considered to be some of the hallmarks of human flourishing. On this account of autonomy there is no independent standard of moral knowledge or reason to determine if one use of freedom is inherently superior to another; the individual should decide as a matter of right, and if individuals are permitted by social and political arrangements to have this liberty, the society as a whole will prosper and the arrangement will be justified from a utilitarian point of view.

In this line of thinking, reason as a universal standard of right gives way to liberty as the exercise of judgement and choice by each individual person. Moral law and duty as bridles on natural desires and preferences give way to freedom as a claim-right to be asserted by the individual against others. Autonomy moves from being the basis of obligation to being the object of obligation.

One obvious question arises at this point. If there is no universally rational or objective basis for distinguishing qualitatively among the choices individuals make or the way each uses liberty, on what basis can any limits to the exercise of individual liberty be set? Mill's own attempt to answer this question is sketched in the following famous passage from *On Liberty* (1956: 13):

the sole end for which mankind are warranted, individually or collectively, in interfering with the liberty of action of any of their number is self-protection. . . . the only purpose for which power can be rightfully exercised over any member of a civilized community,

---

[2] In the following discussion I have relied heavily on Schneewind (1998) and Wolff (1970).

against his will, is to prevent harm to others. His own good, either physical or moral, is not sufficient warrant. He cannot rightfully be compelled to do or forbear because it will be better for him to do so, because it will make him happier, because, in the opinions of others, to do so would be wise or even right. These are good reasons for remonstrating with him, or reasoning with, or persuading him, or entreating him, but not for compelling him or visiting him with any evil in case he do otherwise. To justify that, the conduct from which it is desired to deter him must be calculated to produce evil to someone else. The only part of the conduct of anyone for which he is amenable to society is that which concerns others. In the part which merely concerns himself, his independence is, of right, absolute. Over himself, over his own body and mind, the individual is sovereign.

This shifts the question from the definition of reasonable, rightful choice to the definition of harm and to discriminations among various kinds and degrees of harm. It is not obvious that this latter is an easier concept with which to deal, but harm does have a certain solidity, a naturalistic and tangible quality that the concept of reason seems to lack. Nonetheless, problems abound. Define harm too expansively, and autonomy shrinks. How serious does harm have to be? Is it only serious physical harm or injury, or do psychological damage, pain, and suffering count as well? What is the gradation between harm, offence, annoyance, and inconvenience? Where should we draw the line?

Generally speaking, the species of harm that has most preoccupied bioethics is precisely the denial of autonomy or negative liberty of the other. Closely related, and of special importance in medicine, is the right to privacy and bodily integrity, in a word, informed consent. The autonomy or liberty limiting harms that are most prominent in bioethics are those things that encroach on my private space, those things that I don't invite in, whether it be an experimental drug, a life-saving surgery, or the implantation of an artificial nutrition and hydration tube that serves to prolong my dying from an underlying incurable disease.

III

There are some limitations on voluntary transactions imposed on grounds of moral standards, to be sure. But they are coming fully into the literature of bioethics only rather slowly, and they tend to come in the area of health policy and questions of the allocation of scarce resources. For example, the insurance system now confounds John Stuart Mill's distinction between other-regarding and purely self-regarding behaviour. Corporations will soon begin to take a greater interest in the health-related behaviours and characteristics of their employees—diet, exercise, smoking, genetic make-up—in order to hold down their insurance costs. This interest poses a substantial threat to the privacy and autonomy of large numbers of individuals in the coming years. But for those bioethicists inclined to justify it, it will be justified, as autonomy as negative liberty holds that all abridgements of freedom must be, on the basis of protecting the rights of healthy, well-behaved, and genetically well-endowed employees against the costly profligacy and self-abuse of those who get sick and drive up health care costs. Not because the choices of the profligate are inherently objectionable, but because their social effects cause harm to others.

Nonetheless, it is difficult, when discussing morality, especially within the domain of will, autonomy, and freedom, not to hold out some kind of interpersonal ideal, some notion of what counts as a higher kind of life and a better kind of choice. The tension between objective autonomy and subjective autonomy lingers even today in bioethics, although I believe that it is fair to say that the subjective conception of autonomy, which stresses liberty over reason, holds sway, subject pretty much only to those side constraints that Mill and his liberal successors have placed on it, such as the harm principle, justice, equity, and fairness. This is why it is helpful to consider Berlin as a kind of missing step as we move from Mill to modern bioethics.

One rarely acknowledged source that anticipates, if it did not directly influence, an important intellectual trend in bioethics is the key distinction between negative and positive liberty that was coined and first suggested by Berlin in his 'Two Concepts of Liberty'.

Negative liberty has to do with establishing a zone of privacy and non-interference around each person, a zone within which the person can exercise his own faculties and pursue his own life in his own way. Berlin (1969: 127) explains the concept this way:

The defence of liberty consists in the 'negative' goal of warding off interference. To threaten a man with persecution unless he submits to a life in which he exercises no choices of his goals; to block before him every door but one, no matter how noble the prospect upon which it opens, or how benevolent the motives of those who arrange this, is to sin against the truth that he is a man, a being with a life of his own to live.

Autonomy understood as negative liberty appeals to metaphors of space. It wants elbow room, a place of one's own. It is the single-family dwelling of ethics. Negative liberty requires fences and boundaries for protection against outside intruders. It rests on a conflict-ridden and antagonistic picture of social existence, in which each individual struggles with everyone else to control his own patch of ground. Negative liberty does not appeal to Napoleons or Don Juans. It appeals to ordinary folks who simply wish not to be dominated, who wish to be left alone.

Autonomy is also linked to liberty in another sense, through what Berlin and others have called *positive liberty*. Positive liberty is very close to self-mastery and detached judgement. Berlin (1969: 131) explicates it this way:

The 'positive' sense of the word 'liberty' derives from the wish on the part of the individual to be his own master. I wish my life and decisions to depend on myself, not on external forces of whatever kind. I wish to be the instrument of my own, not of other men's, acts of will. I wish to be a subject, not an object; to be moved by reasons, by conscious purposes, which are my own, not by causes which affect me, as it were, from outside. I wish to be somebody, not nobody; a doer—deciding, not being decided for, self-directed and not acted upon by external nature or by other men as if I were a thing, or an animal, or a slave incapable of playing a human role, that is, of conceiving goals and policies of my own and realizing them.

One is free in the positive sense when one's reason, one's higher self, is in charge of one's conduct. Negative liberty is the absence of control by others; positive liberty is more like self-control. Berlin is suspicious of positive liberty, which at least once he calls 'autonomy', as a manifestation of a dangerous objectivist, universalist conception of the fully human person and the fully human life. In the name of attaining this ideal, individuals have been asked, or required, to subordinate their ordinary freedoms and interests to Causes, with a capital C. Totalitarian ideologies of the mid-twentieth century talk of reforming and improving 'human nature'. This is the dark side that Berlin sees not only in various romantic and irrationalist bodies of thought, but in the legacy of Kantian rationalism itself. Autonomy and authenticity are dangerous elements in the Enlightenment. Better to stay on the more solid, mundane ground of ordinary interests and negative liberty.

IV

While acknowledging this danger in autonomy as positive liberty, I would still maintain that some vital elements of both moral philosophy and bioethics are missing without it, and that autonomy understood as negative liberty alone is too thin. The missing element in negative liberty has mainly to do with moral duties beyond rights, with relationality, a reaching out to establish modes of solidarity, mutual assistance, and care. These values, I argue, are constitutive of an autonomous form of life and human flourishing not simply instrumental to some self-directed project that contingently one happens not to be able to pursue alone.

The world of autonomy as negative liberty is a world of absences and omissions. As such, it is a clean, well-lighted place. One of autonomy's best emblems is the revolutionary-era flag in America that shows a coiled snake and the motto 'Don't Tread on Me'. The world of positive liberty is a messier space, filled with shadows. It is a much more human space. In it people do things to and with one another. They cannot get by simply by steering clear. 'Don't tread on me' gives way to 'Help me up'.

AUTONOMY AND THE SUCCESS OF BIOETHICS

One of the primary things to be observed by a review of the concept of autonomy in bioethics is a kind of conceptual displacement. This, at I noted at the outset, has occurred in bioethics partly owing to (*a*) the sociology of the field and partly to (b) the conditions that have been required of it to gain intellectual legitimacy, and thereby some measure of power and influence, in professional and policy domains.

The sociological factor to which I refer is the growing distance in the field between those who practice moral philosophy and political theory in academic settings and the rather insular literature in bioethics that purports to address its theoretical, conceptual, and philosophical underpinnings. William F. May (1980) once quipped that the relationship of the applied ethicist to the moral philosopher was as one who draws and carries water from wells they have not dug. Today that requires amendment. Applied ethicists are digging their own wells and carrying ideas from them to share with professional practitioners in medicine, science, and other fields. However, the new wells are not so deep nor their water always pure. That is perhaps unfair and too harsh. Another way of saying it is that the conditions under which theorizing takes place in bioethics have changed and are different from what they are in philosophy and cognate disciplines. To be in a bioethics centre in a medical school is not the same as being in a philosophy department in a school of arts and sciences. Thirty-five years ago bioethics was made up mainly of individuals who were at home in both places; today few move easily between them.

The problem of legitimacy in bioethics arises from the necessity for the field to make a transition from its origins in movements that arose in opposition to mainstream medicine, health care, and biomedical science to an established consulting discipline that has gained access to both clinical and policy settings. These movements of the late 1960s and early 1970s voiced concerns about obstetric practices and women's health generally, consumer rights, health care access for the elderly, children, and the poor, and advocacy for persons living with disabilities, and for those mistreated in certain types of medical research, such as the syphilis study conducted around Tuskegee, Alabama, by the United States Public Health Service. An important part of gaining this type of respectability and acceptance, while at the same time avoiding a total and abject co-optation, was to build an ethical stance around a concept such as autonomy that effectively straddled the powerful forces of libertarian individualism in the broader political and moral culture while redirecting the use of the expertise and authority of medicine without fundamentally challenging or undermining that authority. The concept of autonomy, understood as it has been in bioethics as negative liberty, has been well suited to this task. The practice of medicine in the service of respect for the rights, dignity, and personhood of the patient replaces medicine in the service of beneficent paternalism. But in this shift medicine retains its power based on scientific expertise, cultural influence, control over access to medical technology and treatment modalities, and considerable (albeit somewhat attenuated of late by the fiscal crises of universal insurance systems or by the commercial interests of managed care systems in the United States) leverage over the allocation of resources, conditions of practice, lobbying power, and the like.

CONCLUSION

The component ideas of autonomy—individual rights, freedom of choice, privacy, independence, freedom from outside interference—are vested with great moral legitimacy. They express deeply felt aspirations and worthy ideals. At the same time, other principles that remind us of our social natures and our interdependence as human beings—community, citizenship, authority, obligation, responsibility, reciprocity, tradition, rules, limits—are also ideas of potent resonance. They are the words of civilization and moral order; they are the elements of an essential vision of the human good. In fact, we perceive them as indispensable, since they are firmly rooted in our psychological natures. These ideas derive from the fact that the human identity is shaped by—and the human good is lived within and through—social roles (such as being a parent), relationships (such as providing care), and institutional structures (such as the family and civic and religious groups).

No moral discourse is truly adequate to the richness of human moral experience if it lacks either vocabulary—the vocabulary of autonomy or that of relationality and mutuality. It is critical that we retain what is of enduring value in the language of liberty and autonomy, but it is no less critical that we sustain the language of responsibilities and relationships. If there is a danger inherent in bioethics today—and I am convinced that there is—it comes from an excessive emphasis on autonomy and too little appreciation of human interdependence and mutual responsibility.

REFERENCES

AGICH, G. J. (1993), *Autonomy and Long Term Care* (New York: Oxford University Press).

BEAUCHAMP, T., and CHILDRESS, J. (1994), *Principles of Biomedical Ethics* (4th edn. New York: Oxford University Press).

BELL, D. (1976), *The Cultural Contradictions of Capitalism* (New York: Basic Books).

BELLAH, R. N., MADSEN, R., SULLIVAN, W. M., SWIDLER, A., and TIPTON, S. M. (1985), *Habits of the Heart: Individualism and Commitment in American Life* (Berkeley: University of California Press).

———— ———— ———— ———— ———— (eds.) (1987), *Individualism and Commitment in American Life: Readings on the Themes of Habits of the Heart* (New York: Harper and Row).

BERLIN, I. (1969), 'Two Concepts of Liberty', in Berlin, *Four Essays on Liberty* (New York: Oxford University Press), 118–72.

CALLAHAN, D. (1970), *Abortion: Law, Choice, and Morality* (New York: Macmillan).

CHARLESWORTH, M. (1993), *Bioethics in a Liberal Society* (Cambridge: Cambridge University Press).

Compassion in Dying v. *Washington* (1996), 79 F. 3d 790 (9th Cir.)

ELSHTAIN, J. B. (1995), *Democracy on Trial* (New York: Basic Books).

FEINBERG, J. (1972), 'The Idea of a Free Man', in R. F. Dearden, *Education and the Development of Reason* (London: Routledge & Kegan Paul).

_____ (1980), 'The Nature and Value of Rights', in J. Feinberg, *Rights, Justice, and the Bounds of Liberty* (Princeton: Princeton University Press), 143–58.

GAYLIN, W., and JENNINGS, B. (2003), *The Perversion of Autonomy: Coercion and Constraint in a Liberal Society* (2nd edn. Washington, DC: Georgetown University Press).

GILLON, R. (1986), *Philosophical Medical Ethics* (New York: John Wiley).

HAUERWAS, S. (1974), *Vision and Virtue* (Notre Dame, Ind.: Fides).

HAWORTH, L. (1986), *Autonomy* (New Haven: Yale University Press).

HIMMELFARB, G. (1995), *The De-Moralization of Society: From Victorian Virtues to Modern Values* (New York: Alfred A. Knopf).

HUGHES, R. (1993), *Culture of Complaint: The Fraying of America* (New York: Oxford University Press).

KANT, I. (1963), 'What Is Enlightenment?', in L. W. Beck (ed.), *On History* (Indianapolis: Bobbs-Merrill), 3–10.

KOHLBERG, L. (1981), *Essays on Moral Development*, i: *The Philosophy of Moral Development* (New York: Harper and Row).

LASCH, C. (1978), *The Culture of Narcissism: American Life in an Age of Diminishing Expectations* (New York: W. W. Norton).

MACKENZIE, C., and STOLJAR, N. (eds.) (2000), *Relational Autonomy: Feminist Perspectives on Autonomy, Agency, and the Social Self* (New York: Oxford University Press).

MAY, W. F. (1980), 'Professional Ethics: Setting, Terrain, and Teacher', in D. Callahan and S. Bok (eds.), *Ethics Teaching in Higher Education* (New York: Plenum Press), 205–41.

MILL, J. S. (1956), *On Liberty* (Indianapolis: Bobbs-Merrill).

Olmstead v. *United States* (1928), U.S. 438, 478.

O'NEILL, O. (2002), *Autonomy and Trust in Bioethics* (Cambridge: Cambridge University Press).

PETERS, R. S. (1972), 'Freedom and the Development of the Free Man', in R. F. Dearden (ed.), *Education and the Development of Reason* (London: Routledge & Kegan Paul).

RIESMAN, D., with GLAZER, N., and DENNY, R. (1950), *The Lonely Crowd: A Study of the Changing American Character* (New Haven: Yale University Press).

ROBERTSON, J. A. (1994), *Children of Choice* (Princeton: Princeton University Press).

SCANLON, T. M. (1972), 'A Theory of Freedom of Expression', *Philosophy and Public Affairs*, 1: 204–26.

SCHLESINGER, A. M., Jr. (1992), *The Disuniting of America* (New York: W. W. Norton).

SCHNEEWIND, J. B. (1998), *The Invention of Autonomy: A History of Modern Moral Philosophy* (Cambridge: Cambridge University Press).

SCHNEIDER, C. (1998), *The Practice of Autonomy: Patients, Doctors, and Medical Decisions* (New York: Oxford University Press).

TAYLOR, C. (1991), *The Ethics of Authenticity* (Cambridge, Mass.: Harvard University Press).

THOMSON, J. J. (1971), 'A Defence of Abortion', *Philosophy and Public Affairs*, 1/1 (Fall), 47–66; repr. in M. Cohen, T. Nagel, and T. Scanlon (eds.), *The Rights and Wrongs of Abortion* (Princeton: Princeton University Press, 1974), 3–22.

WOLFE, A. (2001), *Moral Freedom: The Search for Virtue in a World of Choice* (New York: W. W. Norton).

WOLFF, R. P. (1970), *In Defense of Anarchism* (New York: Harper and Row).

CHAPTER 4

MENTAL DISORDER, MORAL AGENCY, AND THE SELF

JEANETTE KENNETT

INTRODUCTION

LET me begin by quoting from Ann Deveson's account of life with her son Jonathan, who suffered from chronic schizophrenia:

At the end of the afternoon I was driving through North Adelaide when I spotted [Jonathan] walking along the middle of the road. He waved at me to stop. He asked me for a milkshake so we went into a cafe, and talked for a few minutes before he began glowering at me, and muttering. The tension of the past few weeks . . . was bound to erupt sometime. It erupted over me.

One minute Jonathan was blowing into his chocolate malted. The next he had thrown the milkshake into my face, followed by the pepper and salt, upturned the table, and chucked a chair at me. People gasped, the waiter came running and Jonathan shot off, out the door and up the street.

I would like to thank Dean Cocking, Steve Matthews, François Schroeter, Janna Thompson, and audiences at the universities of Melbourne, Edinburgh, and Glasgow, the Australian Catholic University, and the Australian National University for helpful comments on earlier versions of this chapter.

I shook the milk off me and tried to rub the pepper out of my eyes, which made it worse. The waiter hovered, hoping for an explanation. I couldn't think of one that wouldn't take half an hour so I paid the bill and left.

Brenda and Margaret [workers] thought I should charge Jonathan with assault. They said I had to set limits. The idea appalled me. But I did feel angry: angry with Jonathan for hurting me, angry with the system for not helping him, angry with the illness. The hardest anger to deal with was the anger with Jonathan, because of its paradox. Can you be angry with someone if it is their illness that makes them so destructive? But I *was* angry, so angry that I felt like thumping anyone and everyone, so angry that I had to belt my rage out on some cushions, and even then I could not assuage it because I felt so powerless.   (Deveson 1998: 82)

Here and at other points in Deveson's narrative we see a wide variety of responses to Jonathan and the manifestations of his illness, from blaming, excusing, pity, anger, and resentment, to a detached managerial approach, to withdrawal altogether from interaction. Two connected questions are raised here. What happens to the person who is the subject of such attitudes, and what should our moral responses be towards those who suffer serious mental disorders? Or, to put it in terms of a central debate in moral philosophy, how does mental disorder affect the agency, responsibility, and the moral standing of the affected person? In the philosophical debate, the more general question, as I first put it, of what happens to the person whose responsibility is of such theoretical interest is left almost untouched. Yet, a full understanding of the impact of mental illness on agency and responsibility must also examine the impact of mental illness on the self-conception[1] of people with mental illness, and on their interpersonal relations, for these are intimately connected with the exercise of their agency and their capacities for autonomy.

A person suffering a mental illness or disorder may differ dramatically from his or her previous well self. Family and close friends who knew the person before the onset of illness tend to regard the illness as obscuring their loved one's true self and see the goal of treatment as the restoration of that self. 'He is not really like this,' they will say with increasing desperation. Treatment teams and others, who have no acquaintance with the person when well, respond to what they see in front of them and do sometimes make harmful judgments of character based on the person's presentation when ill. 'He knows exactly what he is doing', 'He's just being manipulative', 'There's no excuse for that kind of language', and so forth. One mother I know took to carrying around a scrapbook filled with photos, letters, school reports, and testimonials recording her son's academic and sporting prowess, his popularity, and his deep moral concerns prior to the onset of schizophrenia. She kept this record to try to show treating teams what they could not or would not see for themselves,

---

[1] When I talk about self-conception I mean it in the most everyday sense: that is, how we see ourselves, our history, character, personality, relations with others, and so forth, and how we project ourselves into the future. It encompasses both self-esteem and personal narrative.

to try to ensure that her son was not seen either as a collection of symptoms or as straightforwardly difficult and bad: uncooperative, rude, aggressive, and dirty.[2]

The identity of those who suffer from mental illness, their character, and their capacities, can thus become contested by those surrounding them. But what happens to the person at the centre of this contest? I think that at least in a very common subset of cases—those where the mental illness is chronic or cyclical with onset during late adolescence—the central project we all have of constructing and maintaining our identity is profoundly undermined. This is in part because of the disunifying effect of such illnesses on one's agency; it is in part because certain identity-constituting relationships, such as our friendships and other close voluntary reciprocal relationships, may be largely unavailable when in the grip of the illness; and it is in part because those family and patient–client relationships left over provide an impoverished and perhaps even a stultifying environment for self understanding and self-creation. The person's self-conception and agency is, over time, affected by his illness, both directly and indirectly, to the point where we may well conclude that there is no univocal answer to the question. 'Is it him or is it his illness?'

When we ask this question we are partly interested in issues surrounding the person's capacities for autonomy and responsibility. For example, we might want to know whether it would be appropriate to charge Jonathan with assault and punish him, or conversely to subject him to involuntary treatment. But we are also, and in everyday circumstances, perhaps *primarily* interested in establishing what kinds of interpersonal dealings and relations are possible with the person. Is he always like this? When can we rely on what Jonathan tells us? Do we have special obligations towards him? Would we be able to take him to the theatre or the football or a family gathering? Or should we keep him at arm's length? Some philosophers have held that the capacities necessary for responsible agency and the capacities required for decent reciprocal relationships are two sides of the same coin. In what follows, I try to show how they are related but argue that there is a strong moral case for drawing a distinction between our assessment of someone's present capacity for autonomous choice and action and our preparedness to engage in reciprocal relations with him or her.

AUTONOMY AND RESPONSIBILITY

> I would prefer jail or halfway house to nuttery. I will always tell the truth because I have metal in my brain. (Jonathan, quoted in Deveson 1998: 157)

---

[2] Here and at other places in the text I am grateful to members of the Bridging the Gaps Forum, a parent support and advocacy group in Melbourne, for sharing their experiences and insights with me.

[Jonathan] said jail was heavy, but hospital was humiliating.

(Deveson 1998: 164)

As Jennifer Radden (2002) notes, questions of autonomy have been held to be especially important in psychiatric ethics as well as more broadly in moral philosophy. The assessments we make of each other's capacities for autonomous choice and action have significant moral and practical implications. For those suffering mental illnesses and disorders it may, at the limit, mark the difference between forced treatment on the one hand, and imprisonment on the other. But well before we reach the criminal justice system we find a polarization in community and professional attitudes to sufferers, each of which risks injustice. Radden (2002: 399) puts the problem this way:

This inquiry is a delicate one. Stigmatizing attitudes towards mental disorder have undeniably exaggerated the extent to which the mentally ill are imperfectly rational and autonomous agents, and modern day efforts to extend the presumption of autonomy . . . have gone some way towards undoing the ill-effects of such prejudicial attitudes. Nonetheless, it must be possible to acknowledge and avoid the wrongs associated with the cruel and discriminatory attitudes of the past without resorting to a misapplication of the autonomy model. Unwarrantedly attributing capabilities to the psychiatric patient when such capabilities are at least temporarily compromised involves its own inhumanity and injustice.

The task is indeed a difficult and delicate one, and part of the project of this chapter is to draw out why this is so. In this part of the chapter, I outline the capacities necessary to autonomy and their relation to responsibility as it has been traditionally conceived. I then consider a more fundamental condition of effective agency, unity of agency, which is disrupted in many cases of mental disorder but which is largely ignored in standard accounts of responsibility. I then examine the ways in which the exercise of our agency can be affected in and through our interactions and relations with others, and the disruptions caused by mental disorder to these relations, before returning to questions of responsibility and moral standing.

Autonomous Agency and Reflective Self-Control

What capacities do agents need in order to act autonomously and be held responsible for their actions? To what extent are people suffering mental illness impaired in these capacities? At one extreme of the spectrum Thomas Szasz (in The Myth of Mental Illness, 1961/1974, and in many places since) famously urges the view that the odd behaviour of those conventionally regarded as mentally ill is chosen as a way of dealing with 'problems in living' and that any form of compulsory treatment is a brutal measure of social control. If such persons commit crimes, they should be punished according to law. Anything else is dishonest and disrespectful.[3] He argues

---

[3] Szasz says in a recent piece, 'I do not deny that there are in our society, poor, homeless, lonely people who talk to themselves. However I do disagree . . . that this phenomenon is evidence that these

that 'insane behaviour, no less than sane, is goal directed and motivated' (Szasz: 113, cited in Moore 1975/1982). Szasz apparently believes that the mere capacity for intentional action is decisive evidence of the autonomy of the actor. This is a very thin account of the conditions of autonomous agency and one that is not shared by many moral philosophers. For, on such an account, young children and even dogs would count as autonomous and so as morally and legally responsible for their actions.[4]

R. Jay Wallace, in adopting a broadly Kantian account of agency, notes that

to be an accountable agent—an agent who is subject to moral requirements, and who may be appropriately held responsible for failing to comply with such requirements—it is not enough merely to be subject to desires and capable of acting to promote the ends set by such desires. Moral agency requires, in addition, the capacity to step back from one's given desires and to assess the ends they incline one to pursue in the light of moral principles. (Wallace 1994. 13)

Wallace articulates a widely shared view in insisting that free autonomous agents must possess the powers of 'reflective self-control'.[5] What are these? First, the person must possess moral concepts and have the capacity to recognize and apply moral reasons appropriately in their practical deliberation. Second, they must have the capacity to control their behaviour in accordance with these reasons. These capacities are not all or nothing. They come in degrees, and so responsibility, too, comes in degrees. While most persons with psychiatric illnesses or disorders will have acquired ordinary moral concepts (psychopaths are arguably the exception), disordered thinking, delusions, hallucinations, clinically depressed or elevated mood, and so forth may reduce or remove their capacity to recognize, or to weigh appropriately, relevant moral considerations and to judge accordingly.[6] Further,

persons suffer from a mental-brain disease . . . and that ostensibly compassionate–therapeutic attitude towards such individuals justifies our depriving them of their liberty (when they are innocent of crime), and of excusing them of responsibility for crime (when they are guilty of it)' (Szasz 1998: 205). I take it that by 'guilt' here he means only that they performed the action proscribed by the law.

[4] Unfortunately the incidence of mental illness and other psychiatric disorders in our prison populations suggests that the view expressed by Szasz—that mentally disordered persons are rightly held responsible for their offences—is not uncommon. A recent *New York Times* report puts the figure at about 20 per cent of the prison population ('Study Finds Hundreds of Thousands of Inmates Mentally Ill', 22 Oct. 2003). This is a time when it is increasingly difficult to mount a successful insanity defense in the United States even for defendants who are clearly severely impaired. Among philosophers, though, there is fairly consistent support for the idea that people with mental illnesses are not, or not fully, responsible for those actions symptomatic of their illness. Discussion here has tended to focus on the case of schizophrenia. See Christian Perring (2002).

[5] The idea that autonomous agency centrally involves the capacity to stand back from and evaluate one's first-order desires is widely shared by philosophers of both a Humean and a Kantian cast. See e.g. Bratman (2000); Kennett (2001); Korsgaard (1996); Watson (1982); Frankfurt (1971); Velleman (1997).

[6] For an argument that mentally ill defendants usually do know both what they are doing and that it is wrong, see Schopp (1991). Schopp argues that, nevertheless, such individuals may be substantially

these conditions may impair the ill person's capacity to exercise control over their actions in accordance with the moral considerations they do accept. Deveson writes movingly of finding desperate notes written by Jonathan to himself, perhaps as reminders or injunctions: 'Don't hurt Anne'. But such attempts to control his future actions were always vulnerable to defeat by his symptoms. On standard accounts Jonathan cannot count as an autonomous, responsible agent. *He*, at least, ought not be blamed for many of his actions. But even where we can make such a clear determination on responsibility for particular harmful actions, it does not determine in full what our attitude should be towards Jonathan or how he should be treated. For that we need to acquire a more substantial understanding of the losses the illness imposes on Jonathan himself.

Unified Agency and Self-Authorship

David Velleman has remarked that the philosophy of autonomy and the philosophy of personal identity seem to intersect at something called 'the self'.[7] My discussion here is located at this intersection: at the interrelation between effective agency and self-conception. Christine Korsgaard (1988: 101), in providing a Kantian account of personal identity, argues that a person is 'both active and passive, both an agent and a subject of experiences'. She argues that effective agency requires unity both at a time, in order that we may eliminate conflict among our motives and do one thing rather than another, and over time, since many of the things we do form part of longer-term projects and make sense in the light of these projects and life plans. And she says that in pursuing these long-term projects and commitments '*we both presuppose and construct a continuity of identity and of agency*' (1988: 113; my emphasis). What does this mean? We do not simply act, as Michael Bratman (2000: 40) points out, from moment to moment. We conceive of ourselves as agents who persist over time, and so we commit ourselves to future directed plans, which we intend should structure and coordinate our more particular decisions and activities. But we can only do so if we can be confident that our future directed decisions will be *effective*, that we are able to 'determine today what gets done by us tomorrow' (Velleman 1997: 45). If we don't have this ability we lack autonomy here and now. For, as Korsgaard says: 'to the extent that you regulate your choices by identifying yourself as the one who is implementing something like a particular plan of life, you need to identify with your future in order be *what you are even now*' (1988: 113–14).

Velleman argues that we achieve diachronic autonomy because the plans we adopt now provide reasons for us into the future, reasons we will then buy into

impaired in their capacities of rational choice. They may have, for example, delusional beliefs of such force that they cannot reason properly about their actions. For further discussion of issues surrounding criminal responsibility and mental impairment, see Kennett and Matthews (2004).

[7] Formerly on his website.

but might not otherwise have had. We identify these plans and commitments as our own and implementing them thus usually makes the best sense of our life stories (Velleman 1997: 45–8; 2000). Hence it would seem that autonomous agency depends upon significantly unified agency. Unity is fundamental to the capacity to make, shape, and revise plans *and* to carry them out: to engagement in those long-term projects and commitments, such as an education, a career, a marriage, or a friendship, which are the sources of our deepest satisfactions. Unity is an essential condition of both the capacity for competent deliberation and the capacity for self-control over time that standard accounts of moral agency and responsibility insist upon. In short, it underwrites our authorship of our lives. While not all aspects of the self, or even, I would argue, all valuable aspects of the self, are subject to agential control, agency is surely central to the self and is a condition of access to a wide variety of important normative goods.

Of course unity of one's agency does not, on its own, ensure a good life. *Successful* self-authorship relies on the possession of a variety of fairly sophisticated skills that fall under the rubric of either competent deliberation or self-control. There is the rational requirement of getting one's projects to cohere, there are means–end managerial skills; there are value judgments about the quality of different projects; there are prioritization skills; and importantly, predictive imagination—'If I take that job, then I'll turn into that kind of person, can I imagine myself as being like that, is that the way I want to be . . . ?', and so on.

A view of the self as author allows for rational revision of plans in the light of changed circumstances or new information, and so allows for personal development and change over time. Indeed we may have projects that quite explicitly aim at changing our very characters, and so at changing the way we may come to view ourselves, and our projects, in the future. One of my projects may be to write a cookbook, another may be to learn to service my car. Yet another may be to develop a greater sensitivity to the suffering of others and a less judgmental attitude to their misfortunes. If I am successful in this latter character-building project, I may come to see new reasons for action in the future; these lead me to take on new projects, and so by incremental steps I become very different from how I am now. Nevertheless, I retain authorship of the overall process and identify with each stage of it.

But now consider what happens when we undergo dramatic changes—not in our external circumstances, but in ourselves—which we have not chosen. What if we find we can no longer rely, in the normal way, on our future selves being appropriately affected by our present plans and decisions? What if our projects, large and small, were at constant risk of derailment? What if even those traits and dispositions which we might think of as fundamental to our characters—openness, generosity, efficiency, and so forth—were in danger of being masked or reversed? Then it would seem that we would lack authorial control over our lives, and our identity, our self-conception, as well as our autonomy would be gravely undermined. In cases of serious, recurrent, or chronic mental illness I suggest that this is what happens. The onset of illness is like a grenade or a series of grenades exploding in one's path. The impact of the repeated failure of one's plans and one's hopes for the future must damage one's self-conception and autonomy in ways that extend beyond the more obvious and direct disabling of the capacities for rational reflection and self-control. As Korsgaard says, we need to see ourselves as agents of our future, we need to identify with our future, to be what we are even now. If mental illness changes a person's view of their future, and of their ability to shape their future, it changes them now.

Agnetti and Young (1993: 69) argue that, for patients (and their families) with a long-standing psychiatric disorder:

life seems like it has always been dominated by the illness and always will be. The past is seen as the same as the present and the future offers nothing new. . . . If the temporal dimension is lost in one's view of the world, then the possibility of hope, growth and change is also lost . . . events stand still and individual action is paralysed.[8]

Repeated experiences of illness, of hospital, of (perhaps coercive) treatment, of failed plans, of other ill people, and of the reactions of others to one's illness, must *all* over time profoundly affect the way the agent sees themselves and influence the ways in which they can project themselves into the future. This is vividly illustrated in Jay Watts and Stephen Priebe's (2002: 447) study of users of assertive community treatment services:

Most of the participants described the psychiatric system and the labelling of diagnosis as an attack on their identity. For example: 'I get sick, I get cracked up, and this is my life. I can't keep fighting against it and trying to be someone else . . . I had people that could depend on me. I liked independence . . . To lead, and I am not in a position to lead no more.'

Though people with chronic mental illnesses still wish for the same goods as everyone else, and may hold much the same values as they did prior to illness, a loss of confidence in their power to see through valued plans and projects may mean that they are given up, and the person lives an impoverished life dominated by short-term considerations. They may come to see themselves quite generally as subjects, rather than agents, of their experiences.

There is much more to be said, and much more precisely, than there is room for here, about how the various symptoms of the various illnesses might affect or impair one's authorial capacities as well as about the possibilities of regaining authorship of one's life in a way that integrates and organizes one's experience of illness. I leave further exploration of that to the reader.[9] Here I want to focus on one

---

[8]   There is also evidence that treating teams are vulnerable to this paralyzing sense of timelessness when dealing with patients or clients with chronic psychiatric conditions. For discussion of this and of ways in which treating teams can 'restart the clock' for their clients, see Young (1994).

[9]   But see Wells (2003); Kennett and Matthews (2003); Phillips (2003); Radden (2003); Velleman (2005).

particularly central way in which one's sense of self, and opportunities for effective agency, may be affected when one suffers a mental illness, which has especially strong moral implications for those with social, professional, and institutional contact with persons suffering mental disorders or illnesses.

RECIPROCAL INTERACTION
AND THE VISIBILITY OF THE SELF

Successful negotiation of the social environment is a condition of success for almost all of our activities and projects, from going shopping to holding down a job. Further, our most central and long-term commitments may be to loving reciprocal relationships. Talking in terms of an individual person's projects and capacities, as I have until now, may suggest that to the extent to which persons have authorship at all, we are *sole* authors of our identity and life story. But of course, as social beings, as agents whose actions impact on others and who regularly need the cooperation of others in order to complete action, we are not. Other people contribute very significantly to how we see ourselves, and so to the selves that we become. How do these social interactions and relationships proceed? How do they make their contribution to the self-building and maintenance project? And how does this enhance or impair our agency and autonomy?

Nathaniel Branden (1993: 67), in an essay entitled 'Love and Psychological Visibility', argues that it is to a large degree through our interactions with others that we become visible to ourselves. He begins by analyzing the pleasure he gets from playing with his dog:

The key to understanding my pleasurable reaction . . . was in the self-awareness that came from the nature of the feedback she was providing. From the moment I began to 'box' she responded in a playful manner . . . Were I to push or jab at an inanimate object, it would react in a purely mechanical way; it would not be responding to *me*; there would be no possibility of its grasping the meaning of my actions, of apprehending my intentions, and of guiding its behaviour accordingly . . . The effect of Mutnik's behaviour was to make me feel *seen*, to make me feel *psychologically visible* . . . And as part of the same process, I was experiencing a greater degree of visibility to *myself*; I was making contact with a playfulness . . . which . . . I generally kept severely contained, so the interaction also contained elements of *self-discovery* . . .

Branden argues that this experience of visibility to oneself and others is a product of all positive human interaction that reaches its pinnacle in romantic love. He further claims that to do the job of providing visibility, the interaction must be both positive and appropriately responsive to the other and to what is conveyed by the other. Let's look at some of those interactions.

RECIPROCITY, INTERPRETATION, AND THE REACTIVE ATTITUDES

As social beings we must, necessarily, engage in a wide variety of transactions and interactions with others. Social life is shot through with interpretive practices. Grasping each other's meaning, recognizing each other's intentions, guiding our actions accordingly to coordinate with each other, these all involve a degree of interpretation of the other. The interpretation is largely *implicit*. For the most part we don't think about the particular messages we give to others: we are skilled at mind reading, at picking up behavioural cues and responding to them appropriately, and many social situations and transactions are governed by rules, roles, or conventions that we have internalized. All social transactions, from getting a haircut, to asking for directions, to having dinner with friends, require a degree of mutual responsiveness and interpretation of the other for success. In these transactions with other our default stance, our natural stance, is what Peter Strawson (1982: 62) has called the participant stance. Within this stance we are exposed to the reactive attitudes of, for example, 'gratitude, resentment, forgiveness, love, and hurt feelings'. My attitude to you will depend crucially on my picture of your motivations towards me. As Strawson (1982: 63) remarks: 'If someone treads on my hand accidentally, while trying to help me, the pain may be no less acute than if he treads on it in contemptuous disregard of my existence . . . but I shall generally feel in the second case a kind and degree of resentment that I shall not feel in the first.' Strawson claims that just in being prone to these kinds of reactive attitudes we manifest *respect* for each other. In taking up the participant stance, he says, we signal that we regard those with whom we engage as fit for ordinary adult human relationships. So successful social interactions should provide, at least, a basic visibility and affirmation of the self as social participant with rightful expectations of mutual goodwill. Often enough they do more. We might receive more specific feedback on how we're doing and on how we're seen, for example a compliment on our good service, thanks for some basic assistance like helping someone pick up the contents of a spilled trolley, or we might share a moment's camaraderie with a stranger at a football match. Such interactions involve positive reactive attitudes and provide positive reinforcement to the self. They allow us to proceed with confidence. But now consider those of the negative variety.

Whether we stand to the other as friend, lover, colleague, customer, or patient, we expect and indeed demand that their actions where we are concerned reflect good rather than ill will. That we make this demand, and that the attitudes of others matter to us, is evident in our reactions when our ordinary expectations are disappointed. The rudeness of a shop assistant, the brusque dismissiveness of a doctor, each occasions hurt feelings and a degree of resentment that may bear little relation to any actual disadvantage we suffer. The shop assistant rolls her eyes at my clumsiness with my purse, ignores my attempts at pleasantries, and displays obvious impatience in answering my queries, but she wraps my purchases efficiently and gives the correct change. The injury here is in the attitude not the action. Attitudes of contempt or indifference are in themselves injurious; attitudes of goodwill and esteem, in themselves, confer a benefit on the recipient. But what is the nature of the injury? I suggest that it is, at least in part, an injury to our conception and presentation of ourselves. When we lose control of how we *appear* to others, when our self-presentation misfires, we will typically experience some anxiety about who we *are*. I am trying to be pleasant and cooperative but am coming across as fussy and incompetent. Maybe I *am* fussy and incompetent. Or maybe she is just rude. In the case of one-off interactions such as with the shop assistant where there is a failure of reciprocity and interpretive charity there is no chance to negotiate or revise the interpretation as there may be in longer-term relationships. I am stuck with the dissonance between the way I thought I was and the picture I gained in seeing myself through her eyes. (Of course I may come to believe that her interpretation of me is correct and I will then modify my view of myself and maybe make an effort to change in order to avoid the negative feedback.) In cases of the worst kind I cannot see myself at all through the other's eyes. I am simply invisible to them. This is frequently the experience of members of minority or oppressed groups in interactions with members of dominant groups. In these cases the default assumption of mutual goodwill and respect doesn't even get off the ground. The effect of such invisibility and exclusion from social interaction on the agent's sense of efficacy, and on their capacity to act, is particularly severe.

FAILED RECIPROCITY AND FRAGILE IDENTITY

> I started hearing voices, I started talking to myself, she couldn't take it any more, the relationship broke up . . . and I ended up on my own.
>
> (quoted in Watts and Priebe 2002: 445)

In cases where the agent suffers a mental illness, the kinds of social misfirings I've described above happen more often. Though most people with a mental illness manage well enough with most public social interactions, going to the corner shop, catching public transport, etc., the features of their illnesses can often create the conditions for things to go wrong. Depressed or anxious persons may seek to make *themselves* invisible, others go the opposite way; their lack of judgment or social disinhibition leads them to press too much personal information on strangers, resulting in withdrawal. Other oddities in behaviour and presentation, for example, talking too loudly or standing too close, can also lead to avoidance. Sufferers may have difficulty seeing themselves through others' eyes and so may not make the appropriate modifications to their behaviour: alternatively they may be too ready to adopt a negative self-evaluation on the basis of others' reactions to them. Thus these experiences will fail to provide visibility of the right kind and may feed back in a negative way to the agents' conception of themselves.

Of course these kinds of public social interactions are not of a deep, extended, or intimate nature and so they would not normally provide, contribute to, or *challenge* a deep view of the self. Our close and intimate relationships do, on the other hand, contribute very significantly to the way we see ourselves and to the selves that we become. The more stable, positive, and sensitive interpretations offered in the context of our intimate relationships can counter and resolve dissonant experiences in the public social sphere. The reassurance and affirmation we receive there strengthen and protect the self. Unfortunately these relations too are often weakened or unavailable to the agent suffering a mental disorder, since many such people are impaired precisely in the responsiveness and attentiveness to others needed to form and maintain them.

Since Aristotle it has been accepted that friendship is a central human good and an important source of self-knowledge. In addition it provides a means to self-growth and development. Let's examine how. In close friendships we engage in the broad interpretive practices outlined above of grasping each other's meaning, recognizing intentions, coordinating actions. But, ideally at least, these will be more finely tuned and attentive in friendship. One's close friend will be better able than acquaintances or strangers to read one's mood, and friends, as I've claimed elsewhere, are especially receptive to responding to each other's wishes and coordinating their activities in accordance with each other's suggestions.[10] So I might notice, where others would not, a slight stiffening in my friend's demeanour when she is cornered by someone she dislikes but doesn't wish to be rude to at a social gathering, and will move to rescue her from the situation. If she then says 'Let's get out of here', I will take that as sufficient reason to leave. My responses to her are highly particularized and thus provide a high degree of visibility and affirmation of self.

Beyond this particularized *implicit* interpretation of her I also, as her close friend, offer *explicit* interpretations that contribute in a deeper way to her understanding of who she is. I may, for example, point out, after rescuing her, that she quite generally exhibits discomfort with men of a certain status and that perhaps this is colouring her view of the individual who cornered her. I may say that he's not so bad, that she may have misread his intentions, or I may affirm her own assessment of the situation. Assuming that what I say is, as Branden insists, appropriately responsive, she is likely to take it on board and this will help shape and develop

---

[10] The account of friendship given here draws upon that developed in Dean Cocking and Jeanette Kennett (1998, 2000). See also Dean Cocking and Steve Matthews (2000). The example below originated in a talk given by Dean Cocking, 'Intimacy and Privacy Online', at the Australian National University in 2002.

her view, not just of the situation, but also of herself. Mutual deep interpretation is a central and defining activity of close friendship without which much of its intimacy would be lost. Within friendship we receive and accept input and feedback that importantly contributes to our self-building project, and affirmation, which is vital to its maintenance. This, what we might call, *drawing* of each other, further enhances the relationship between us: there is a positive and dynamic feedback loop.

Such interpretations may not be taken on board at all, and certainly not in the same way, if made in the context of a different relationship, say by one's mother or even by one's therapist. The point is that in close friendship we are especially receptive to such interpretations and so friendship provides an important arena for self-development and the acquisition of self-knowledge that may not be replaceable. Aristotle (*MM* 1213^{a}10–26) says: 'If, then, it is pleasant to know oneself, and it is not possible to know this without having someone else for a friend, the self-sufficing man will require friendship in order to know himself.' There is here, as John Cooper (1980) says, recognition 'of the social bases of a secure self-concept and of the role intimacy plays in providing the means to it'. This supposed necessary base of a secure self-concept is placed at risk when one party develops a chronic mental illness.

The nature of the difficulty that, for example, delusional individuals must face in establishing and maintaining close friendships is obvious when we look at the role reciprocal interpretation plays in friendship. Delusional individuals often have beliefs about themselves and others that are bizarre and resistant to revision. A lack of response or a highly inappropriate response to the interpretations offered by another will constitute a barrier to friendship. Conversely the ill person is often not well placed to offer the kinds of interpretations of others that the *other* can integrate into *their* self-conception. So an important mutual activity of friendship that contributes to the intimacy between friends, as well as to self-knowledge and self-development, may be less available to those suffering delusions. More generally the mere presence and expression of the delusion can disturb the friendship since this may lead to wariness on the part of the friend with respect even to non-delusional communication. Other psychiatric conditions will also affect one's fitness here. For example, deep depression, paranoia, or wild mood swings may so bias interpretations that they are unacceptable to the recipient.

Even the apparently less demanding broad interpretive activities of grasping the other's meaning and anticipating their intentions, forming joint intentions, and coordinating activities can be more difficult for people with serious mental illnesses. The presence of delusions or obsessions, for example, may dictate activities or routines that cannot be altered and which others cannot understand or share; or the illness may affect the agent's motivation and planning capacities such that they cannot reliably take part in joint activities, even in the absence of positive symptoms. Poor or absent motivation is well recognized as one of the negative symptoms of schizophrenia. Further, the loss of confidence in one's future that comes from repeated interruption of one's projects does, as we have seen, affect how the agent thinks of themselves in the present and so affects the way they proceed in relationships as in other matters.

The loss of friendships and other close relationships leads to social isolation and contributes to the social invisibility of the ill person, and it is well known that such isolation has a significant detrimental effect. As Watts and Priebe (2002: 446) point out, the literature on chronic illnesses shows that 'the overwhelming implications of illness on identity is mitigated by intervention from significant others'. But this mitigation was largely unavailable to the psychiatric patients in their study, many of whom had lost significant others 'early in their psychiatric career'. Without the stabilizing influences that good relations with others provide, psychological function deteriorates further.[11] A vicious loop can develop as the feedback from others becomes increasingly impoverished, negative, and defensive, or somewhat artificial and paternalistic, as in many professional encounters.[12] It is hard to construct a rich positive sense of self as we become increasingly invisible to others, as they refuse eye contact, turn away at our approach, end conversations abruptly, and show less and less interest in what we say and do.

The argument to this point suggests that the consequences of impaired social interaction and the loss of deep interaction on self-concept and the development and exercise of one's agential capacities can be severe. What it does not support is the idea of a neat division between the person and the symptoms of their illness that we can use in allocations of responsibility, since the illness can affect the person via its effects on their plans, projects, expectations, and relationships even during periods of quiescence. The person they would have become if they had not become ill is an increasingly distant fiction, and the self they are now is constructed out of experiences of illness and of remission, and of their own responses to these experiences and others' responses to them. It is not identical either to a set of symptoms or to the self prior to illness.

If the illness now forms part of the person and has shaped their identity, we cannot dismiss it or glide over it in our moral evaluation of the person. Our responses to the person must also be responses to their illness. However, if we accept the claim that in our relations with others we can become, invited, welcomed, or not, part authors of that person's self-conception and life story, we need carefully to consider the responsibility that is thus placed on us, particularly in our dealings

---

[11] Indeed impaired adolescent friendship patterns are a significant predictor of a sustained delusional outcome in persons with schizoaffective disorder (Coryell, Keller, et al. 1990).

[12] Watts and Priebe outline the therapeutic experiences of their subjects as follows: 'the approach focused on medication . . . Relationships were seen as impersonal and paternalistic because of short appointment times and frequent turnover of staff' (2002: 448). They quote one subject, Mr B: 'When you are on the ward, you get staff that think it's a prison or something. And that you've done something and they try and boss you around. Control you, control you' (2002: 446).

with those whose identity and agency is already fragile. Given the undermining effects of social failure and withdrawal by others on the self, it may seem obvious that in both professional and personal contexts we should not withdraw, as people often do, from those suffering a mental illness. Simple beneficence dictates that we should actively seek to maintain engagement with the other even where their capacity to reciprocate appropriately is impaired. But there is a problem with this simple conclusion. For mental illness is widely (and properly) seen as exculpatory, and in several influential writings it is argued that reciprocal relations and the presumption of responsibility are not separable.

FAILED RECIPROCITY AND THE OBJECTIVE STANCE

The consequences of the mentally ill agent's impaired capacity for interpersonal relations and social interaction have deep and troubling implications not only for the development and maintenance of the self and the exercise of agency, but also for the ill person's *moral* standing in the community. As we have seen, to the extent that we find someone's actions odd or unintelligible and unmodified by our reactions to them, to the extent to which they seem incapable of understanding or taking an interest in our interests, or of responding to us as we are, we may decide that our interaction with them is insufficiently rewarding and withdraw from it. Peter Strawson (1982: 66) takes a position at the opposite end of the spectrum to Szasz in suggesting that in the case of the severely mentally ill, the participant reactive attitudes are altogether out of place. When faced with such individuals we move, and *should* move, to the *objective* stance. Here is his description of this stance:[13]

To adopt the objective attitude to another human being is to see him, perhaps, as an object of social policy; as a subject for what, in a wide range of sense, might be called treatment; as something certainly to be taken into account, perhaps precautionary account of; to be managed, handled, cured or trained; perhaps simply to be avoided. . . . The objective attitude may be emotionally toned in many ways, but not in all ways: it may include repulsion or fear, it may include pity or love, though not all kinds of love. But it cannot include the range of reactive feelings and attitudes which belong to involvement or participation with others in inter-personal human relationships; it cannot include resentment, gratitude, forgiveness, anger, or the sort of love which adults can sometimes be said to feel reciprocally for each other. If your attitude towards someone is wholly objective, then though you may fight with

---

[13] The following passage may present Strawson's view as rather more black and white than it is. Strawson does acknowledge that we may move between the two stances particularly in the case of children. I argue below that there is a distinction between a fitting objectivity of judgment that may inform aspects of our relations with others, including professional relations, and the objective stance as described by Strawson.

him, you cannot quarrel with him, and though you may talk to him, even negotiate with him, you cannot reason with him. You can at most pretend to quarrel, or to reason, with him.

Seeing some one then, as warped or deranged or compulsive in behaviour . . . tends, at least to some extent, to set him apart from normal participant reactive attitudes on the part of one who sees him, tends to promote, at least in the civilized, objective attitudes.

Though the objective attitude, so described, sounds anything but civilized, we may find ourselves moving towards it, in both personal and professional contexts, for the reasons I have given. Disappointed reciprocity and failures of interpretation can lead to feelings of frustration and impotence. Then the objective stance may indeed act as a refuge from the strains of involvement. But further argument is needed to support Strawson's implied suggestion that we *should*, normatively speaking, adopt the objective stance when dealing with people suffering severe mental illness. If reciprocal relations are, as Strawson suggests, the ordinary basis even for respect and goodwill, then we would expect to find, what we largely do find, that mentally ill persons are treated with less respect and less goodwill than other adult members of the community including by some members of the helping professions. It does not seem right or desirable that one's moral entitlements should depend so heavily upon one's social competence. So what can be said in favour of Strawson's position?

For Strawson, resentment is arguably the most central of the reactive attitudes, so I will focus on that. Let's consider the kinds of consideration that allowably modify or remove resentment and the disposition to blame in circumstances where one would normally expect it to be operative; that is, in circumstances where one has suffered some injury or offence at the hands of the other. Strawson suggests that the considerations fall into two kinds, which, following Wallace (1994), I shall call excuses and exemptions.

Excuses do not call into question those capacities of the agent that seem essential for engagement with others and for making and responding to the demand for goodwill and respect. They do not invite us 'to view the agent as one in respect of whom these attitudes are in any way inappropriate' (Strawson 1982: 64). Excuses draw our attention to the fact that, for example, the action was performed inadvertently or on the basis of misinformation, or that it was coerced or accidental. 'I couldn't help it', 'I didn't know', 'I was pushed', 'The accelerator jammed'. Resentment is inappropriate here, since the agent's actions do not signal any lack of goodwill, and the suspension of interpersonal attitudes is also inappropriate, since there is no indication that the agent is unfit for social life. The agent is seen as in general accountable for her actions, but the presence of an excusing condition indicates that the agent did not, on this occasion, *do* anything deserving of blame.

Exemptions, on the other hand, do invite the suspension of some or all of the reactive attitudes. It is admitted that the agent did do something wrong, but it is suggested that this agent, in particular, is not accountable for it on this occasion. Strawson believes that there are two subgroups to the exemptions. The first points to a temporary lack of accountability—e.g. 'He's been under a very great strain lately.' The second suggests a more thoroughgoing lack of accountability. Strawson gives the following examples: 'He's only a child', 'He's a hopeless schizophrenic', 'His mind has been systematically perverted', 'That's purely compulsive behaviour on his part'. These pleas, Strawson claims, do invite the suspension of our ordinary reactive attitudes. The second subgroup, in particular, invites us to see the agent as 'psychologically abnormal—or as morally underdeveloped', as 'incapacitated for normal human relationships'. He argues that when we see someone in such a light, 'all our reactive attitudes tend to be profoundly modified' (1982: 66). It is apparent that Strawson places mental illness in the class of type-2 exemptions rather than excuses and sees the presence of serious mental illness as a reason to suspend or 'profoundly modify' our reactive attitudes, rather than to see them as undeserved in just this instance. He argues that 'the participant attitude, and the personal reactive attitudes in general, tend to give place and, it is judged by the civilized, should give place, to objective attitudes, just in so far as the agent is seen as excluded from ordinary human relationships by deep-rooted psychological abnormality' (1982: 67).

Strawson believes that holding people responsible for what they do, praising or blaming them, or even excusing them on some occasion for their actions, is something we can *only* do in so far as we, actually or vicariously, occupy the participant stance with regard to them. Gary Watson (1987: 257) points out that, for Strawson, the reactive attitudes 'are constitutive of moral responsibility; to regard oneself or another as responsible just is the proneness to react to them in these kinds of ways under certain conditions'. We find a similar position put forward by Christine Korsgaard (1992: 305) in her paper 'Creating the Kingdom of Ends: Reciprocity and Responsibility in Personal Relations'. There she argues that to hold someone responsible 'is to adopt an attitude towards him rather than to have a belief about him or about the conditions under which he acts'. It is, effectively, to enter a certain kind of relationship with the other: a relationship of reciprocity. Reciprocity, she claims, involves acting in concert with another, sharing ends and sharing reasons with each other. You will only enter into such a relationship on the expectation that the other will deal with reasons rationally as you would. 'In this sense' she argues, 'reciprocity requires that you hold the other responsible' (1992: 311). She says:

If my friend fails me in a serious way, and I do not blame her, shrugging it off as I would the misdemeanours of a child or a pet, then I was not holding her responsible after all and probably I was holding myself back.... Blame is important...as an expression of the tenacity of disappointed respect. At its best it declares to its object a greater faith than she has in herself. Yet it is still not central. The willingness to take a chance on some form of reciprocity is the essence of holding someone responsible.... In everyday personal interaction, we cannot get on without the concept of responsibility. (1992: 311–12)

Both Strawson and Korsgaard see fitness for reciprocal relations, rather than the possession of the capacities mentioned earlier, for deliberative judgment and self-control, as primary to an account of responsibility. It appears that for them there is a conceptual connection between the reactive attitudes, to which reciprocal relations expose us, and holding people responsible for what they do. And they do not detach this from according the other moral standing and respect.

So there is a two-step argument in defense of Strawson's seemingly unpalatable suggestion. The first step is to point out the person's impaired capacity for reciprocal relations, and to say that in such cases the participant stance is, in truth, *unavailable*. We delude ourselves if we think it is; the reactive attitudes simply misfire. Deveson's anger, understandable though it is, lacks a proper object when directed at ill Jonathan. She might as well be angry with her car for failing to start. She might as well try to set limits for her car as for Jonathan, for all the good it would do in getting either of them to shape up. Second, if we agree with Strawson and Korsgaard that it is actual or vicarious engagement in or fitness for reciprocal relationships that grounds attributions of responsibility, the reactive attitudes of resentment and so forth to which engagement exposes us are simply *unfair* to the mentally ill. To the extent that they cannot share our reasons and ends and coordinate their activities with ours, they don't deserve to be the subject of such harmful attitudes as resentment. Such attitudes may also get in the way of our helping them and managing their behaviour. We can do this much better if we can remain calm and detached in the face of odd or 'challenging' behaviour.

However, if we move all the way to the objective stance, if we treat persons as things 'to be managed, handled, cured or trained', we make them socially invisible and so, as I have argued, to a significant extent, invisible to themselves. The person is visible merely as a threat, a nuisance, an embarrassment. Their already fragile agency is further frustrated and undermined by the lack of recognition, support, and positive feedback. It looks as though whichever stance we adopt will be damaging. People with psychiatric conditions too often walk a thin line between being the recipients of undeserved blame and resentment on the one hand, and exclusion from the participant stance and so from social life on the other.

RECIPROCITY AND RESPONSIBILITY

We have arrived back at the dilemma outlined by Radden at the beginning of this chapter. It is a very real one and desperately hard to resolve in practice, as Deveson's account of life with Jonathan makes clear. However, I think Strawson's solution rests on a mistake. First, it is not clear that there is the strong conceptual connection claimed by Strawson and Korsgaard between occupying the participant stance with respect to another and attributions of responsible agency. So it is not clear that adopting the participant stance will be unfair to the mentally ill. Second, the participant stance is elastic; it encompasses a wide variety of reciprocal interactions that are commonly adapted to take account of the particular capacities and characteristics of those with whom we engage. It is unlikely that in any but the most extreme cases the participant stance would be wholly unavailable to us.

It seems clear in both Strawson's and Korsgaard's accounts that judgments of responsibility made from within the participant stance must presuppose the existence and importance of just those capacities for deliberation, planning, and self-control over time that I earlier described as belonging to autonomous agency. Indeed it is precisely the presence, impairment, or absence of these capacities that Strawson implicitly, and sometimes explicitly, draws upon in distinguishing the varieties of excusing conditions from each other and from those that exempt one from blame and modify or remove resentment. Resentment serves, often, to alert us to the violation of an other-regarding reason. But we may only fairly hold people responsible for such violations if they have both the capacity to recognize the reason and the capacity to conform their conduct to it. Though those capacities are for the most part developed and supported through our relations with others, they are nonetheless conceptually distinct from these relationships. Further, we can make judgments about those capacities and about the degree of responsibility to be borne by the agent without entering, actually or vicariously, into a relationship with them and exposing ourselves to the participant reactive attitudes.

According to what Korsgaard calls the theoretical conception of responsibility, which is the conception familiar in philosophical and legal discussions, a person is responsible for her actions just in case she possesses certain characteristics or capacities essential for responsible agency and is in a condition to exercise those capacities in the circumstances (or to determine the condition she is in). It will be a matter of fact, though perhaps difficult to determine, whether or not the person has those capacities. Korsgaard (1992: 313) believes that this is not the model we adopt in our practical interactions with others. On the practical construal that she favours, she argues that holding someone responsible 'is adopting an attitude towards her, or, much better, placing yourself in a relationship with her'. On this conception, facts about the agent's condition at the time of action *guide* decisions about responsibility but do not determine them. She says:

I do not believe there is a stable relationship between the voluntariness of an action or attitude and the appropriateness of holding someone responsible for it. If a bad action is found to have been involuntary in some straightforward sense we will withdraw blame; we may also do this if a person is under severe emotional stress. But there is neither need nor reason to reduce the second kind of excusing condition to the first and say that people under severe emotional stress *cannot* control themselves. We do not need to understand a form of debilitation as a form of impossibility in order to make allowances for it; we only need to know what it is like.   (1992: 313)

Korsgaard is right, I think, to point out that judgments of an agent's responsibility made within relationships—from within the participant stance—are not, and should not be, strictly forensic. But though the facts about the agent's capacities may need to be put in their place, they still have a central place. Given that even judgments of responsibility made from within the participant stance are highly (and properly) dependent on our assessment of the person's capacities for reflective self-control, it seems that perhaps Korsgaard, at least, is claiming, not that responsible agency and reciprocal relations are conceptually inseparable, but that the capacities that constitute us as responsible agents are *prerequisites* for decent reciprocal relations. She says: 'in everyday personal interaction we cannot get on without the concept of responsibility'. Is this right?

Korsgaard (and Strawson too, to some extent) presents a model for relations between persons, one requiring responsive and responsible agency. The model is one of perfect reciprocity, described in Kantian terms as a sharing of reasons and ends.[14] Now, the relationship Korsgaard uses to illustrate this model is close friendship. But close friendship is not an appropriate model to govern all our relations with others, requiring, as we have seen, a very high degree of equality and responsiveness across domains. This sets the bar for reciprocity too high. While one might need to qualify as an autonomous agent to be a fit subject for the reactive attitude of resentment, it is not at all obvious that full autonomy is needed to fit one for the many other participant reactive attitudes, or must be present to ground the moral demand for respect and goodwill. (It is not even clear that it is necessary to every case where there is a sharing of ends—for example, the end of recovery or a normal life.) This puts the cart before the horse. We are born into the participant stance. We engage in reciprocal exchanges long before we become autonomous agents; indeed it is entirely plausible that such exchanges are essential to the development and maintenance of our agency. Admission to the participant stance cannot and should not depend on the equal capacity of the parties. Annette Baier (1995: 28–9) points out:

we begin as helpless children, at almost every point in our lives we deal with both the more and the less helpless . . . equality of power and interdependency, between two persons or groups, is rare . . . The recognition of the importance for all parties of relations between those who are and cannot but be unequal, and of their effect on personality formation and so on other relationships, goes along with a recognition of the fact that not all morally important relationships are freely chosen.

---

[14] The description also recalls Aristotle's description of virtuous friendship.

IMPERFECT RECIPROCITY
AND THE GROUNDS OF RESPECT

Let's go back, briefly, to Mutnik. Here is an example of an (admittedly primitive) reciprocal social interaction that is not subject to the demand that the other deal with reasons as I would—and yet does provide the psychological visibility and affirmation that is so important to the development or maintenance of a positive sense of self. And there are many other examples of exchanges of affection, shared amusement, sadness, and so forth where this demand is similarly absent, highly domain-specific, or beside the point of the interaction. A father and his young son may share their enjoyment of the slapstick comedy of the Three Stooges without there being any requirement on the son that he be able to appreciate any more sophisticated humor and without the fact that he cannot leading to any diminution of the respect and goodwill owed to him quite generally by his father. Similarly, the person whose spouse develops Alzheimers may come to accept and find value in a changing relationship worked around and respecting those aspects of the self—the values, memories, habits, and emotions—that remain.[15]

These and the earlier examples of interactions between friends serve to highlight the fact that what is valuable in our relations with each other, and our moral standing within those relations, is not given wholly by the features that make us accountable agents. I can value your clumsiness, your ill-fated attempts to hide your fear of spiders, your warmth, your laugh, the way you look at me. These sorts of valuings are part and parcel of relationships and help structure the kinds of communication that go on in them and the conditions under which the particular reactive attitudes arise. Impairments in agency and social responsiveness such as occur in many mental disorders also structure what is possible in interpersonal interactions; they may place restrictions on its scope and depth, they may require the modification of some, though not all, of the reactive attitudes. It is commonly the case, though, in relationships that we adjust our responses and expectations in the light of facts about the other, their sensitivities, temperament, etc., and we do this without abandoning the participant stance. A survivor of the Changi prisoner of war camp may be utterly rigid in his views of all things Japanese and perhaps understandably so. If I say 'Don't talk to Granddad about Japanese art. You'll only get him going', I am taking an objective view of this feature of Granddad and of the situation, but I need not thereby depart from the participant stance. I may in fact be showing a highly particularized concern and respect for him.

The 'sort of love' that adults have with their unimpaired close friends or partners may be out of reach for some people suffering mental illness or disorder, and this, I have argued, can be a great misfortune, but it would be a mistake to think of such

---

[15] See Agnieszka Jaworska's perceptive discussion in Jaworska (1999).

high-level, wide-ranging mutual responsiveness as providing a description or a norm for interpersonal relations in general. We are neither forced nor normatively required to move to the objective stance in our dealings with the mentally ill, since not all social interactions must presuppose full autonomous agency and since we can establish or maintain areas of reciprocity with persons whose agency and social responsiveness is underdeveloped, impaired, or intermittent. However, given that it can be difficult to remain in the participant stance without falling prey to misplaced resentment or other harmful reactive attitudes, we might wonder whether anything *obliges* us to remain, or to try to remain, there, and to pursue engagement when our ordinary expectations of reciprocity and reason sharing are disappointed.

Here I believe that the best argument (though perhaps not the whole argument) is to be found within a Kantian perspective. I've argued that a wholesale shift to the objective stance denies the mentally ill person psychological visibility and so further depletes or undermines their picture of themselves and their efficacy as agents. It fails to acknowledge or to support their stake in constructing a unified autonomous self and in regaining authorship of their actions and lives. In moving to the objective stance we deny or ignore the agency of the other. That is what it is to treat someone as 'an object of social policy... to be understood and controlled in the most desirable fashion' (Strawson 1982: 66). Now, as beings with the goal of autonomy—as beings constitutively concerned with discovering and acting for reasons—Kant believed that persons had intrinsic worth and dignity and as such were never to be used merely as means. To treat a person as an object is clearly to mistreat them. The demand for respect and goodwill in our dealings with each other is, in the first place, the demand that we approach each other from within the participant stance. It is minimally the demand that we do not ignore or undermine each other's agency. For many latter-day Kantians it is more. They recognize that agency comes in degrees, that autonomy is an achievement, and that respect for autonomy may require our active support for the agency of those in adverse circumstances. Mental illness is such an adverse circumstance. In especially severe cases we may not have any great reason for optimism about the prospects of the ill person regaining control of their lives and achieving the goods conditional upon unified agency; even in less severe cases we may not always be sure to what extent the person's actions are symptoms of her illness rather than manifestations of her (albeit impaired) agency, and so we may not be sure that our responses are appropriate. But our uncertainty does not counter the moral reason to adopt as far as possible the participant stance and to adapt it in response to the capacities of the ill person. The demand for goodwill from each other is a powerful moral demand and one that mentally ill people are as entitled to make as mentally well people. In the professional context and the broader social context as well as in more personal contexts it is a demand for patience and charity of interpretation of the other's words and actions particularly as they reflect on the person's character. It is the demand that we remain receptive to, and promote, opportunities for engagement;

for shared activities and shared goals. Where mental illness plays a causal role in cases where an agent causes injury or offence this should inhibit blame, though maybe not always, but it need not inhibit the participant reactive attitudes more generally. Given the importance of social relations in building, supporting, and strengthening agency, and so in securing access to central human goods, the default stance in both personal and professional dealings with those suffering a mental illness or disorder, as with anyone else, must be the participant stance.

REFERENCES

AGNETTI, G., and YOUNG, J. (1993), 'Chronicity and the Experience of Timelessness: An Intervention Model', *Family Systems Medicine*, 11/1: 67–81.

ARISTOTLE, (1984), *Magna Moralia*, ed. J. Barnes, in *The Complete Works of Aristotle: The Revised Oxford Translation*, ii, Bollingen Series (Princeton: Princeton University Press), 1868–1921.

BAIER, A. (1994), 'The Need for More Than Justice', in Baier, *Moral Prejudices: Essays on Ethics* (Cambridge, Mass.: Harvard University Press, 1995), 18–32; first pub. in *Canadian Journal of Philosophy*, suppl. vol. 13: 197–220.

BRANDEN, N. (1993), 'Love and Psychological Visibility', in N. K. Badhwar (ed.), *Friendship: A Philosophical Reader* (Ithaca, NY: Cornell University Press), 65–73.

BRATMAN, M. (2000), 'Reflection, Planning, and Temporally Extended Agency', *Philosophical Review*, 109: 35–61.

COCKING, D., and KENNETT, J. (1998), 'Friendship and the Self', *Ethics*, 108/3: 502–27.

_____ (2000), 'Friendship and Moral Danger', *Journal of Philosophy*, 97/5: 278–96.

_____ and MATTHEWS, S. (2000), 'Unreal Friends', *Ethics and Information Technology*, 2: 223–31.

COOPER, J. (1980), 'Aristotle on Friendship', in A. Rorty (ed.), *Essays on Aristotle's Ethics* (Berkeley: University of California Press), 301–40.

CORYELL, W., KELLER, M., LAVORI, P., and ENDICOTT, J. (1990), 'Affective Syndromes, Psychotic Features and Prognosis. II: Mania', *Archives of General Psychiatry*, 47/7: 658–62.

DEVESON, A. (1998), *Tell Me I'm Here* (Ringwood, Vic; Harmondsworth: Penguin).

FRANKFURT, H. G. (1971), 'Freedom of the Will and the Concept of a Person', *Journal of Philosophy*, 68: 5–20.

GARETY, P. A., and FREEMAN, D. (1999), 'Cognitive Approaches to Delusions: A Critical Review of Theories and Evidence', *British Journal of Clinical Psychology*, 38: 113–54.

JAWORSKA, A. (1999), 'Respecting the Margins of Agency: Alzheimer's Patients and the Capacity to Value', *Philosophy and Public Affairs*, 28/2: 105–38.

KENNETT, J. (2001), *Agency and Responsibility* (Oxford: Clarendon Press).

_____ and MATTHEWS, S. (2003), 'The Unity and Disunity of Agency', *Philosophy, Psychiatry, Psychology*, 10/4: 305–12.

_____ (eds.) (2004), *International Journal of Law and Psychiatry*, 27/5, special issue: *Responsibility and Mental Impairment*.

KORSGAARD, C. (1988), 'Personal Identity and the Unity of Agency: A Kantian Response to Parfit', *Philosophy and Public Affairs*, 18: 101–32.

_____ (1992), 'Creating the Kingdom of Ends: Reciprocity and Responsibility in Personal Relations', in J. E. Tomberlin (ed.), *Philosophical Perspectives*, vi: *Ethics* (Atascadero, Calif.: Ridgeview), 305–32.

_____ (1996), *The Sources of Normativity* (Cambridge: Cambridge University Press).

MOORE, M. S. (1975/1982), 'Some Myths About Mental Illness', *Archives of General Psychiatry*, 32: 1483–97; repr. in R. B. Edwards (ed.), *Insanity, Rational Autonomy and Mental Health Care* (New York: Prometheus Books, 1982), 33–49.

PERRING, C. (2002), 'Mental Illness', in Edward N. Zalta (ed.), *The Stanford Encyclopedia of Philosophy (Summer 2002 Edition)*, <http://plato.Stanford.edu/archives.sum2002/entries/mental-illness/>.

PHILLIPS, P. (2003), 'Psychopathology and the Narrative Self', *Philosophy, Psychiatry, Psychology*, 10/4: 313–28.

RADDEN, J. (2002), 'Psychiatric Ethics', *Bioethics*, 16/5: 397–411.

_____ (2003), 'Learning from Disunity', *Philosophy, Psychiatry, Psychology*, 10/4: 357–60.

SCHOPP, R. F (1991), *Automatism, Insanity, and the Psychology of Criminal Responsibility* (Cambridge: Cambridge University Press).

STRAWSON, P. F. (1982), 'Freedom and Resentment', in G. Watson (ed.), *Free Will* (Oxford: Oxford University Press, 1982), 59–80; first pub. in *Proceedings of the British Academy*, 48 (1962), 1–25.

SWEENEY, P. D., ANDERSON, K., and BAILEY, S. (1986), 'Attributional Style in Depression: A Meta-Analytic Review', *Journal of Personality and Social Psychology*, 50/5: 974–91.

SZASZ, T. (1961/1974), *The Myth of Mental Illness* (New York: Harper and Row).

_____ (1998), 'Commentary on "Aristotle's Function Argument and the Concept of Mental Illness"', *Philosophy, Psychiatry & Psychology*, 5/3: 203–7.

VELLEMAN, J. D. (1997), 'Deciding How to Decide', in G. Cullity and B. Gaut (eds.), *Ethics and Practical Reason* (Oxford: Clarendon Press), 29–52.

_____ (2000), 'Well-Being and Time', in Velleman, *The Possibility of Practical Reason* (Oxford: Clarendon Press), 56–84.

_____ (2005), 'The Self as Narrator', in J. Christman and J. Anderson (eds.), *Autonomy and the Challenges to Liberalism* (Cambridge: Cambridge University Press), 56–76.

WALLACE, R. J. (1994), *Responsibility and the Moral Sentiments* (Cambridge, Mass.: Harvard University Press).

WATSON, G. (1982), 'Free Agency', in Watson (ed.), *Free Will* (Oxford: Oxford University Press), 96–110.

_____ (1987), 'Responsibility and the Limits of Evil: Variations on a Strawsonian Theme', in F. Schoeman (ed.), *Responsibility, Character, and the Emotions: New Essays in Moral Psychology* (Cambridge: Cambridge University Press), 256–86.

WATTS, J., and PRIEBE, S. (2002), 'A Phenomenological Account of User's Experiences of Assertive Community Treatment', *Bioethics*, 16/5: 439–54.

WELLS, L. A. (2003), 'Discontinuity in Personal Narrative: Some Perspectives of Patients', *Philosophy, Psychiatry and Psychology*, 10: 297–303.

YOUNG, J. (1994), 'The Loss of Time in Chronic Systems: An Intervention Model for Working with Longer Term Conditions', *Australian and New Zealand Journal of Family Therapy*, 15/2: 73–80.

CHAPTER 5

....

'REINVENTING' THE RULE OF DOUBLE EFFECT

....

DANIEL P. SULMASY

THE Rule of Double Effect has played an important role in bioethics, especially during the last fifty years. Its major application in bioethics has been in providing physicians who are opposed to euthanasia with a moral justification for using opioid analgesics in treating the pain of patients whose death might thereby be hastened. It has also prominently been applied to certain obstetric cases. The scope of application of double effect is actually much broader than medical ethics, extending to cover such topics as strategic bombing in warfare. This chapter, while general in theory, will concentrate on its applications in medical ethics.

The Rule of Double Effect has been heatedly debated in the literatures of philosophy, theology, and bioethics. Some have tried to derive all of morality from it (Knauer 1979). Some have pronounced it a dead idea, riddled with confusions and inconsistencies (Davis 1984; Quill et al. 1997). Some have felt that it contains some kernel of truth and have either tried to revise it radically in order to preserve that truth (Quinn 1989) or have suggested that whatever kernel of truth it contains must be defended in some other form of moral analysis (McIntyre 2001; Foot 1978). Still others have defended it in a more or less traditional formulation (Boyle 1980).

Even the name given to the notion of double effect has proven controversial. Some have called it a Dogma; some a Doctrine. Some have called it a Principle; others a

Rule. Following Beauchamp and Childress,[1] I will call it the Rule of Double Effect. It seems to me that it is best to label it a rule since it is not sufficiently fundamental to any ethical theory to be called a principle. Rather, it seems to be a meta-rule used in deciding about certain types of case in which more fundamental rules appear to clash. Calling it a dogma or a doctrine has the potential to obscure debate by suggesting theological and/or legal overtones, or by suggesting a prominence that may be unwarranted.

While many philosophers have dismissed it as an anachronism, the persistence of the debate about double effect suggests that the idea has some staying power. In this chapter, I will propose a substantial reformulation of the requirements of the Rule of Double Effect (RDE), making use of recent developments in the philosophy of mind and taking seriously the critiques of those who quite simply have found many suggested applications of the RDE to be incredible. One should understand that by 'reformulation' I will not simply be defending the traditional form of the RDE. But one should also understand that I will not be completely revising it. My intention is to show how the rule itself is fundamentally sound, both morally and conceptually, but that the conditions governing the rational application of the RDE, particularly with respect to the intention–foresight distinction, must be substantially tightened if that soundness is to be preserved.

The Traditional Formulation
of the RDE

Most commentators turn to Mangan (1949) for an authoritative historical account of the RDE and its traditional formulation. While I agree with Mangan that the historical discussion and evolution of the RDE finds its beginning in Aquinas' discussion of killing in self-defense, Aquinas himself never articulated the RDE or anything that looked much like the rule as it is known today. Properly speaking, the RDE emerged after centuries of reflection on Aquinas' discussion of self-defense and its application to an ever widening circle of cases.[2] As will become clear from what I argue below, I do not think the RDE actually works as a justification for using lethal force in cases of self-defense.[3] Aquinas' justification of killing in self-defense

[1] Beginning with the fourth edition of their very widely used textbook, Tom L. Beauchamp and James F. Childress (1994: 206) changed from calling it a 'principle' to a 'rule'.

[2] The first clear formulation of the RDE that approximates its present form does not come until Jean-Pierre Gury in the 19th century (see Kaczor 1998).

[3] Thomas A. Cavanaugh (1997) thinks that Aquinas would not permit the use of force that one knew would be lethal, while Joseph M. Boyle (1978) thinks Aquinas would permit this. Cavanaugh seems correct about Aquinas' logic, while Boyle seems correct about what Aquinas thought he was proving. That such confusions have never been resolved suggests the need for a fresh approach.

would fall outside the narrow constraints of the intention–foresight distinction that I articulate below. Nonetheless, part of the genius of Aquinas was to articulate enough ideas that an RDE eventually emerged. And that RDE, I believe, can be rendered in a manner that is conceptually and morally sound.

The traditional formulation, according to Mangan, is as follows. A person may licitly perform an action that he foresees will produce a good and a bad effect provided that four conditions are verified at one and the same time:

1. that the action in itself from its very object be good or at least indifferent;
2. that the good effect and not the evil effect be intended;
3. that the good effect not be produced by the evil effect;
4. that there be a proportionately grave reason for permitting the evil effect.

The classical case in medical ethics to which the RDE has been applied has been the use of morphine to treat the pain of dying patients. Applying the RDE to morphine injections, one notes that (1) they are at least morally indifferent actions; (2) one may presume that the physician only intends to relieve the patient's pain and not to hasten the patient's death; (3) the cessation of respiration and subsequent death of the patient are not the means by which morphine relieves pain; and (4) given serious pain and imminent death, there seems to be a proportionately grave reason for permitting the risk of hastening death. Therefore, even a scrupulously conscientious physician who is morally opposed to euthanasia may licitly perform the action of injecting the morphine according to the RDE.

Nonetheless, the RDE has raised serious controversies in the literatures of medical ethics and philosophy. I will argue that much of this discussion has been hampered by two significant errors that have made it difficult to evaluate this discussion.

Two Significant Errors

Two significant errors have plagued the last fifty years of debate about the RDE. These errors have resulted in many fruitless efforts to defend and to refute the rule. I intend to discuss these errors briefly. Following this discussion, I will present a 'reinvented' version of the RDE—a version that I will argue is philosophically sound and morally credible.

Lack of Appreciation of Developments in the Philosophy of Mind

The first significant error that has plagued recent debates about the RDE is one that has afflicted both its opponents and its proponents, although the impact of this error has been greater for opponents. The error is this: contemporary discussions of the RDE have largely ignored important developments in action theory and have been written as if moral philosophy and philosophy of mind were parallel universes that never communicate or influence each other. An important example in this regard is the treatment of the RDE by Beauchamp and Childress. They write that 'the distinction between what is intended and merely foreseen in a planned action is not viable', and cite John Searle in support of this position.[4] However, in citing Searle, the authors appear to misinterpret him.[5] In the passage they cite, Searle is actually making a distinction between different kinds of unintended consequences of actions. He is not discussing the distinction between the intended and the foreseen. Searle actually fully and explicitly defends the distinction between the intended and the foreseen in his later book *Intentionality*, stating, 'A common confusion is to suppose that if someone knows that something will be a consequence of his action then he intends that consequence' (1983: 103). That bioethicists simply insist (without philosophical argument) that there is no distinction between the intended and the foreseen, and pay so little attention to recent developments in philosophical action theory, seems a serious lapse in scholarly rigor.

In this chapter I will offer an explanation and defense of the distinction between the intended and the foreseen based on the work of John Searle (1983), Michael Bratman (1987), and Alan Donagan (1987). This will lead me to a reformulation of the requirements for the rational application of the RDE that will address some of the worries expressed by opponents of the RDE. I fully realize that this approach will never satisfy those who simply hold that intentions never matter in the moral evaluation of human acts, or who insist that contemporary theories of human action are all mistaken. But the burden of proof would seem to be upon those who raise such objections to show how contemporary scholars in philosophy of mind are all wrong about the distinction between the intended and the foreseen, or admit that the distinction is valid but supply moral arguments about why it is nonetheless morally irrelevant.

Historical Misapplications of the RDE Now Function as Paradigm Cases

A second significant error has been committed by proponents of the RDE. In the early twentieth century they misapplied the rule in a way that has subsequently stretched the distinction between the intended and the foreseen beyond the point

---

[4] See Beauchamp and Childress (2001: 131 and n. 44).

[5] See Searle (1980: 65). Searle's concern in this passage is with the unintended aspects of actions that seem to count as relevant aspects of the action (such as Oedipus' marrying his mother) and the unintended aspects of the action that seem so far removed from the core of what the agent is doing and thinking that they cannot be considered parts of the action at all (such as Oedipus' causing some neurons in his brain to fire and say, 'I do').

of credibility.[6] This may have solved certain moral problems from the perspective of Catholic theology in the short run, but in the long run it has proven disastrous to the defense of the RDE in the wider world.[7] I would argue that the mistake was the application of the RDE to the cases of tubal ectopic pregnancy and the cancerous gravid uterus. Both proponents and opponents seem to accept the traditional view that these are typical applications of the RDE (even paradigmatic instances of its use), and have conducted their debates accordingly. But if these cases represent a misapplication of the RDE, then the moral and conceptual soundness of this rule does not rise and fall with discussions of these cases.

In hindsight, it seems that the RDE was applied to these cases by Catholic medical moralists in an attempt to justify their intuitive belief that life-saving operations upon women who carried tubal ectopic pregnancies or were pregnant while suffering from cancer of the uterus were morally justifiable and distinct from the ethics of abortion. Since Catholic teaching in opposition to abortion has been absolute, and the theological climate of the day was not very open to innovation, I suspect that the only principle to which these Catholic moralists felt they could appeal in order to justify this procedure was the RDE. Unfortunately, however, this application of the RDE has rendered the whole notion (which I will contend is basically sound) incredible to many observers both inside and outside the Catholic faith. In extending the RDE to cover these cases, they have jeopardized the intellectual standing of this important moral rule with respect to cases in which it does readily apply.

Once one gives up on the idea that the RDE applies to these cases, however, the task of defending it becomes much easier. In 'reinventing' the RDE, I will formulate the conditions for the rational application of this rule in such a way that the cases of ectopic pregnancy and the cancerous gravid uterus are excluded. I believe that surgical interventions for these conditions can be justified, morally and conceptually, on grounds other than the RDE that do not require an acceptance of the moral permissibility of abortion. Explaining fully how this is so is beyond the scope of this chapter.

For the duration of this chapter I will proceed as follows: First, I will present my 'reinvented' set of requirements for the correct application of the RDE. Second, I will present the underlying action theory that corrects the first significant error and supports and explains my reformulation of the distinction between the intended and the foreseen in the RDE. Third, I will apply this reinvented RDE to the cases of morphine and ectopic pregnancy to show how this corrects the second significant

---

[6] This complex and fascinating history is detailed by David F. Kelly (1979: 274–309). The morality of hysterectomy in the cancerous gravid uterus case was justified under double effect at the very beginning of the 20th century. After decades of debate, the doctoral dissertation of an American Jesuit named Bouscaren, by applying the rule of double effect, finally won acceptance within the Church for surgery for ectopic pregnancies in 1933.

[7] See, for instance, relatively early attacks by Williams (1957: 200–5) and Glover (1977: 86–91).

error. Fourth, I will consider some major objections and suggest how I think the arguments that I have presented can move the debate about the RDE forward constructively.

A Reformulation of the Rule of Double Effect

If one encounters a conflict between a specific duty to do good and one's general duty to avoid evil, and

1. this conflict arises from one intentional act with at least two foreseeable effects;
2. the act itself is either morally good or morally neutral;
3. the conflict of duties arises because intentionally bringing about one effect is morally good while intentionally bringing about another effect is morally bad;
4. all other reasonable means of achieving the good effect with less risk of causing the bad effect have been exhausted;[8]
5. the good and bad effects are not foreseen as coming about by way of intervening agents;[9]
6. one's prior intention is to act in such a way that one's intention in acting is to bring about the good effect while the foreseen bad effect is not part of one's intention in acting;
7. one is sincere and rational in one's report of one's complex prior intention, such that, at the very least:
   (a) the intended act itself is not an alternative definite description of the bad effect;
   (b) the good effect is not an alternative definite description of the bad effect;
   (c) the bad effect is not wholly spatiotemporally contained within the intended act itself;
   (d) the bad effect is not wholly spatiotemporally contained within the good effect;
   (e) the intended act does not entail the bad effect logically;
   (f) the good effect does not entail the bad effect logically;
   (g) the bad effect is not one's further intention in so acting;
   (h) the bad effect is not an empirically necessary causal condition for the good effect;
   (i) one does not intend the good effect by way of the bad effect;

---

[8] Space precludes me from defending each of the amendments I am making to the classical formulation of the RDE. For a discussion of Requirement 4, see Sulmasy (2000).

[9] If there are intervening agents, the proper moral category for analysis is cooperation or complicity, not double effect. See Sulmasy and Pellegrino (1999).

8. and the act is undertaken with due proportionality, which is to say:
   (a) the good effect is proportionate to the bad effect;
   (b) the means under consideration are proportionate to the expected effects,[10]

then one is morally *responsible* for having undertaken the act with due diligence, in accordance with this rule, and in this sense one is morally *responsible* for all of the good effects and bad effects of the act one has undertaken intentionally. But one is not morally *culpable* for having brought about the bad effect of the act.[11]

THE ACTION THEORY UNDERLYING THIS REFORMULATION OF THE RDE

The first point to establish is that intentions matter in the moral evaluation of human acts. This is, of course, denied by utilitarians and other consequentialists, who discount the moral significance of agency and look only to consequences. The importance of intention is sometimes discounted by those who worry about the public verifiability of intentions and prefer to limit the moral evaluation of human acts to the observable aspects. Some will accept the moral relevance of intention, but reduce it to a character trait: something that is good in so far as it produces morally good actions or morally good results.

But it seems plain to the common person that intentions matter in the moral evaluation of acts. One learns from childhood that one is far more deserving of blame for what one has intentionally brought about than for what one has not intentionally brought about. Judges and juries expend great energy in distinguishing between manslaughter, homicide, and the degrees of murder based upon complex evaluations of the intentions of the defendant. Intentions are the backbone of the agency that is *in* moral acts. Moral acts do not merely happen. They happen because agents make them happen. And agents make their acts happen through intentions. To discount the importance of intentions in the moral evaluation of human acts is

---

[10] This requirement is infrequently noted. Not only must the outcomes be proportionately balanced, the means used must 'fit' the end intended. For example, normally one would not be justified in using an expensive, toxic, intravenously administered drug such as amphotericin B to treat athlete's foot. See Kaczor (1998: 310–12).

[11] This is another very important point often lost on critics of the RDE, but perhaps because it is rarely made explicit by proponents. The RDE does not abolish moral responsibility. There is a distinction between what one does intentionally and what one intentionally does. The former simply refers to an act that one freely undertakes. The latter refers to what one aims at accomplishing in so acting. A physician who administers morphine to a dying patient does so intentionally, and is morally responsible for the act and all of its outcomes. This means that she should not do so without engaging in some form of double effect reasoning, so that she is acting responsibly. But this does not mean that she is intentionally aiming at making the patient dead. If she did, she would be morally culpable. See Bratman (1987: 124–5).

to discount the central feature that makes these happenings *moral* happenings in the first place.

This is not to say that it is easy to explain what an intention is, or easy to know what an agent's intentions actually are in any given act. But for moral philosophers to give up on ever doing so because it is too hard would be analogous to medical students giving up on molecular biology because it is too hard. Nearly half a century ago moral philosophers were challenged by Elizabeth Anscombe (1958) to take up the questions of philosophical moral psychology. Few have done so. Even fewer bioethicists have done so.

Bioethicists have sometimes dismissed the importance of intention in the moral evaluation of clinical acts because they claim that intention is an unclear or philosophically underdeveloped notion.[12] And yet, exciting work in the philosophy of mind has emerged over the past few decades, full of rich insights that can contribute importantly to ongoing work in moral philosophy and in bioethics. This work undergirds the reinvention of the RDE that I am proposing, especially with respect to the task of making the distinction between the intended and the foreseen clearer and more rigorous.

Definitions

The reformulation of the RDE that I have offered uses a number of technical terms from the philosophy of mind that may not be familiar to readers of the bioethics literature. I will therefore provide some useful definitions:

Definition 1: Acts. Donagan holds that the voluntary doings of agents constitute the class of things that are known as acts, and that acts are 'a species of event' (1987: 19). Acts are voluntary human doings that can be explained by their doers' propositional attitudes (Donagan 1987: 23).

Definition 2: Propositional attitudes. A propositional attitude is a cognitive relationship between a person and a proposition (Wagner 1995). Examples include Joan's believing, hoping, desiring, being disappointed, or being surprised that her mother has been cured of cancer.

Definition 3: Events. An event is a spatiotemporal occurrence. Events are changes or persistences in states of continuing objects. Ontologically, 'events are genuine individuals', not states of affairs (Donagan 1987: 38–9). They are represented linguistically, as other individuals are, by individual names or definite descriptions, not by sentences (Donagan 1987: 19).

Definition 4: Intentions. An intention is an irreducibly simple attitude, ascribable to an agent, that takes as its object a proposition about an event that the agent himself chooses to bring about under a definite description. If the event occurs in the way the agent has chosen, this attitude will explain the event.

---

[12] See e.g. Kuhse (1987: 24) and Brock (1993: 172–5).

Definition 5: Conditions of fulfillment. Searle (1983: 14) notes that as propositions have truth conditions, so intentions have conditions of fulfillment. If an event comes about in the way the agent intends it, the agent's intention has been fulfilled.

Definition 6: Prior intentions. To have a prior intention means that an agent has consciously chosen to bring about an event (i.e. an end) in advance of an act. When fully *mature*, this prior intention also includes a choice of a means of bringing about the intended end. When *complex*, this prior intention includes all those (generally multiple) cause and effect relationships that are part of the agent's plan.

Definition 7: Intention in acting. To have an intention in acting means that an agent has acted or is acting, and that one can ascribe to the agent's act the choice of a complete act—both an end and a means of achieving that end.

Definition 8: Further intention. To have a further intention means that the agent intends to act upon a complex prior intention that includes not only the immediately intended event, but also some further event that the agent has chosen as part of her plan.

Intentional Causation

Causation is itself a vexatious philosophical topic. For the purposes of this chapter, however, all that is required is an intuitive grasp of what is meant by causation. The theory of intention that I present should be compatible with almost any theory of causation one would choose to believe.

Agents act in the world. Acts are, as defined above, those events that take place in the world that are explained by the intentions of agents. Agents *cause* events in the world by way of their intentions. Precisely how this comes about is beyond the scope of this chapter, but it is a great marvel that the events we call acts are causally explained by way of the intentions of agents.

Yet one can be more precise. Acts are causally explained by the propositional content of intentional choices that must refer to some agent's intention in acting (Searle 1983: 85 ff.; Donagan 1987: 88). Acts are events that are explained when the conditions of fulfillment of the intention of an agent are realized by way of the agent himself or herself carrying out that intention. There is a necessary self-referentiality to one's intentional causation. Thus, not everything that happens after an agent acts can be explained as having been intentionally caused. While an agent may have caused events other than the condition of fulfillment of her intention, properly speaking, these other events are not part of the agent's act. Ethically speaking, events that are not properly part of the agent's act are evaluated differently from those that are.

For example, suppose that Tim should intend to write Diane a prescription for 2 grams of secobarbital so that she could commit suicide, and were to have told her that this was his intention. Suppose that he were to have written a prescription for Debbie for 2 grams of secobarbital, but had not yet written the prescription for Diane. Now, suppose further that Diane were to have shown up at Tim's office, seen the prescription for secobarbital written for Debbie, thought it was for her, had it filled, consumed all the pills, and died. It would be true that Tim's intention caused Diane to die, but it would not be true that Diane's death could be explained as having been intentionally caused by Tim. Her death did not come about by way of Tim's acting upon the full propositional content of his actual intention. If the district attorney were to investigate him as the agent of Diane's death, he would need only to show that the prescription that Diane filled was written for Debbie, and the charges would be dropped.

Agents need no theory of causation in order to act, but agents grasp the causal potential of their intentions. The plans that agents make often involve complex causal paths. As I shall explain in greater detail below, if an agent has formed a complex prior intention that includes further intentions as part of a plan, the conditions of fulfillment of that complex prior intention include all of the events that are foreseen as causally required in order to fulfill the furthest intention in that plan. As I will explain in greater detail later in this chapter, this is why conditions (g), (h), and (i) of Requirement 7 of the Reformulated RDE are so important. They address the agent's intended causal chain, not merely the agent's intended results.

For example, if Jack intends that Janet should die by way of her pushing a button that causes a programmed series of injections of drugs that will first cause her to be sedated, then cause her to be paralyzed, then cause her heart to stop beating, and thus cause her death, the condition of fulfillment of Jack's intention is that Janet's death should come about by way of his having that complex prior intention—a complex prior intention that includes all of the causally necessary conditions for her dying in just this way.

The Irreducibility of Intention

Knowing something about what one means by intentional causation still does not ensure that one has adequately understood what an intention is. Understanding intention as a propositional attitude raises questions about the relationship between intention and other propositional attitudes. It became common in the twentieth century, under the influence of positivism and behaviorism, for many philosophers to hold that intentions were reducible to beliefs, desires, or some combination of these other propositional attitudes. Against this, Aristotle (1985: 1111^b12) wrote that, 'Those who say decision is appetite or emotion or wish or some sort of belief would seem to be wrong.' Contemporary philosophy of action now holds that Aristotle was correct.

Donagan takes an Aristotelian position and argues that the propositional attitude of intention *cannot* be reduced to any other propositional attitude. And he and others have amassed a significant array of arguments to make it clear that while certain beliefs and desires might be relevant to an intention, no combination of belief and desire is sufficient to account for an intention.

While intentional acts require a whole nexus of background beliefs, intention cannot be reduced to belief alone. There are several reasons for this. First, beliefs alone, as Brand (1984: 94–7) points out, cannot initiate acts the way intentions can. For example, Tim's belief that he will write a prescription for a lethal dose of secobarbital for Diane is not sufficient for him to act on that belief, nor would it be sufficient to explain his so acting if he were to write such a prescription. No matter how strong his belief, the act will not take place unless Tim is moved to do so, and a belief is not a being-moved-to-act.

Second, Searle (1983: 3) simply points out that the 'direction of fit' differs in intention and belief. Belief has a 'mind to world direction of fit'. That is, the truth conditions for beliefs involve the conforming of the believer's mind to the world. On the other hand, intention has a 'world to mind direction of fit'. The conditions of satisfaction of intentions involve the world coming into conformity with the agent's mind. Given this fundamental asymmetry between intentions and beliefs, it is hard to see how one could be reduced to the other (Searle 1983: 9–10).

Finally, it does not seem necessary for an agent to believe that the intended outcome of an intentional act will be accomplished by the act. It would seem that one can very strongly intend what one believes one will not accomplish, and there is nothing illogical about this. One can intend what one does not believe will happen. For example, one could intend to withstand torture even if one were to believe that the overwhelming likelihood were that one would eventually crack (Gustafsen 1986: 68). Similarly, a doctor could intend to save a patient's life and act accordingly even if she were to believe that this would be, to a reasonable degree of medical certitude, impossible. One can intend to do either what one believes one will accomplish or what one believes one will not accomplish.

Intentions Are Not Desires

Neither can intentions be reduced to desires (Anscombe 1969: 5–6). It is certainly true that desires have the same direction of fit as intentions, directed towards the conforming of the world to the mind of the agent, and this may have led certain thinkers to try to account for intention solely on the basis of desire. But having the same direction of fit does not mean that desire and intention are the same. Desire is neither necessary nor sufficient for intention (Brand 1984: 122–3).

First, equating intention with desire makes accounting for the problem of wayward causal chains an insoluble problem (Gustafsen 1986: 44). The fact that something an agent desires actually comes to pass in no way implies that its occurrence was intentional. Suppose that Tim desired to give Diane the knowledge and the means to commit suicide. Suppose that he had discussed this with his postdoctoral fellow, a young and enthusiastic general internist. Suppose that, while Tim was off giving a lecture about assisted suicide, Tim's postdoctoral fellow were then to write a prescription for an overdose of secobarbital and were then to give it to Diane along with instructions on how to use it. If Diane were then to take the overdose, would one say that her death was intentional on the part of Tim simply because he desired it? Hardly. And if that is the case, how could one say that what happens intentionally is what one desires to happen and actually comes about?

Second, it seems clear that one can easily intend what one does not desire, and that one can desire what one does not intend (Brand 1984: 122–3). My desire to eat ice cream does not mean that I intend to eat ice cream. At the moment, I have a strong desire to eat ice cream. I enjoy it very much. But I do not intend to eat ice cream. In the short run it would ruin my appetite for dinner. In the long run it would contribute to the ruin of my arteries by clogging them with cholesterol-rich atherosclerotic plaques. And because I think it would be noble to set a good example for my patients (whom I instruct to refrain from eating ice cream), I overrule my desire for ice cream and do not intend to eat it. Similarly, I often intentionally do what I do not desire to do. I frequently do not desire to stay at the office and see patients who show up late and happen to be very sick and in need of immediate medical attention. This is particularly true when my colleague who is supposed to be on call for such emergencies can't be reached and I have had to stay late and have missed supper the two previous nights in a row and the patient who has shown up late but very sick has not followed my instructions and has a habit of showing up late and I have a tennis court reserved and love to play tennis. Despite my desires to the contrary, I act intentionally in staying with the patient and providing the necessary care. Intention cannot be reduced to desire alone.

A frequent response to such arguments is to say that there is no such thing as an intention contrary to desire. On this theory, one really *always* does what one desires the most in any given situation. In the example given above, it can be argued, the desire to eat ice cream is simply not as strong as the desire to enjoy dinner or to maintain cardiovascular health or not to appear hypocritical to my patients. In the other example, it might be said (charitably) that my desire to help patients or (less charitably) my fear of a malpractice suit are my predominant desires and that I simply desire these more than playing tennis.

But this argument can be dispensed with on several grounds. First, one must note that this begs the question in a serious way. If one has presumed that there is no such thing as an undesired intentional act, one simply reinterprets every other kind of explanation of an act as a disguised desire.

Second, as Bratman (1987: 19) points out, even the postulation of such a predominant desire 'does not guarantee that my desire will control my conduct' the way that it seems an intention would. For example, Tim may begin an office visit with Diane feeling as if he can offer her no more help except by giving her the knowledge and the means to commit suicide and may have a predominant desire to do just that: to help her commit suicide. But this does not mean that he has *settled* upon giving her the means and the knowledge, nor has he settled on a plan for doing so (like a prescription for secobarbital). He still might not be sure that he will do so. He might also have a desire to make a breakthrough in the quality of medical care by launching a national campaign for assisted suicide and might see this case as a possible test case for his idea. But he might see his acts as constrained by certain principles. Tim might think that he would not assist Diane in suicide if she had relapsed in either her alcoholism or her depression, and so might not have formed an intention to write the lethal prescription and give the lethal instructions before talking to her, even though he might be quite desirous of doing so. This is *not* to say, of course, that intentions could not be formed on a provisional basis and later reconsidered. Bratman (1987: 5) is only arguing that intentions can constrain behavior even in the face of a dominant desire.

Third, most of the examples of a conflict between desire and intention involve the concepts of duty and external coercion. As Brand (1984: 123) points out, in these conflict situations it is simply not the case that doing one's duty or giving in to external pressures is equivalent to desiring what one does not desire. Brand gives the example of Richard Nixon resigning as President. Nixon could not truly be said to have resigned because he desired not to be impeached more than he desired to remain in office. Nixon's predominant desire, one supposes, was to remain in office more than anything else. Yet his resignation was an intentional act.

Or suppose that I desire that my patient should die. Suppose she has widespread metastatic cancer of the breast, is suffering great pain that is mostly, but not completely, relieved by medication, but that this incomplete pain relief had to come at the price of being sleepy most of the time. I might very well desire that she should die quickly, thinking that this would be for the best. I might even pray for her quick death. I might come to consider her death my predominant desire. But it seems clear that, even though I might strongly desire that she die, this does not mean that I intend that she should die. This desire would make my decision morally difficult, to be sure. If I were to believe that I had a duty not to practice euthanasia or assisted suicide, I would need to act against my desires. But I can do that. Intentions can override desires. And one can take this as evidence that desires are not intentions.

To see why the reduction of intention to desire is so conceptually problematic, it might help to examine the problem of the 'package deal'. Most choices made in cases of conflict can be regarded as choices of 'package deals'. On the theory that intention can be reduced to a predominant desire, one would be forced to say that the choice of such a package deal implies that, on the whole, this 'package' is what the agent most desires. Consider again the case above regarding the physician who gets stuck late in the office caring for an acutely needy patient. On the theory that intentions can be reduced to predominant desires, one would say that the agent's intention represents a desire that the event (staying late to care for the sick and not playing tennis) should occur. But this would not seem to be the case, as can be seen when one examines the implications of this hypothesis carefully.

There are three different ways by which desires for individual events can be related to the desire for the conjunction of these individual events: conjunctions of desires can be aggregative, complementary, or antagonistic.[13] Desires for things that are valued for themselves individually (such as a desire for chocolate and a desire for a Nobel Prize) are aggregative. Those that are complementary (such as gin and tonic) are desired in conjunction, but not necessarily separately. Those that are antagonistic (such as a Hawaiian shirt and a tuxedo) may be desired individually, but not in conjunction. When desires are aggregative, these desires distribute, logically, over the conjunction, so that if one desires (A and B), one would desire A and one would desire B.

Take an example of a tragic choice like Sophie's (Styron 1979). Sophie chooses that (child A live and child B die)—tragically. But her desires cannot account for this choice. On the presumption that Sophie desires equally that each child individually should live, the most that the predominant desire theory could say would be that she desires ((that child A live and child B die) or (that child B live and child A die)) more than she desires that (child A die and child B die). But the disjunction is not a choice. If her desire for each child is truly equal, no amount of desire can result in a choice of which child should live and which should die. The predominant desire theory thus reduces to a Buridan case.[14] Her predominant desire does not specify a choice.

Further, her desire is that both children should live, and this desire is clearly aggregative: each child is valued for its own sake. But if that is the case, and one believes that her choice (that child A live and child B die) is simply explicable as her dominant desire, without any need to invoke intention as a distinct propositional attitude over and above her desires, it would follow (by the logical rule of the distribution of aggregative desire over conjunctions) that Sophie would, other things being equal, desire that child A otherwise should live and also desire that child B otherwise should die. And that is certainly not the case if we presume that she loves both equally. Nor could one suggest that Sophie desires the death of child B to the extent that this helps to fulfill her predominant desire that child A should live. She desires nothing of the sort. Nor does her choice (her fully determinate intention) prove that she desires that child A live more than she desires that child B live. Such accounts conflict violently with our deepest intuitions.

---

[13] The first term is borrowed from economic theory. 'A complement is a good which tends to be purchased when another good is purchased since it "complements" the first' (Pearse 1992: 73). The rest of the analysis is based on permutations of this principle.

[14] In a famous case, attributed to Jean Buridan but not found in his writings as they are known to us today, an ass starves to death because it is unable to choose between two equally attractive and equidistant bales of hay.

Choice requires something that desire alone cannot supply—namely, intention. The nature of tragic choice and the moral life requires that intentions not be reduced to desires.

Intentions, by contrast, do not logically distribute over conjunctions of events. To intend (A and B) does not imply that one otherwise intends A and otherwise intends B. Sophie's choice of this conjunction does not imply, logically, that Sophie, other things being equal, otherwise intends that child A should live and otherwise intends that child B should die, any more than my choice to stay in the office and not play tennis implies that, other things being equal, I otherwise would intend to stay in the office and otherwise would not intend to play tennis.

Intention cannot be reduced to desire because intention involves a commitment of some sort—a choice. And choices are often hard. They sometimes involve doing what one does not desire. A choice is, as Donagan (1987: 51) would put it, a fully determinate intention.

In addition, it seems simply implausible that doing one's duty should *always* be doing what one most desires, even for a saint. If a duty is a real duty, it would seem that it should be capable of constraining desire. And this would cast further doubt on the notion that intention can be reduced to desire.

Further, as both Searle (1983: 103) and Brand (1984: 124) point out, desires can be contradictory while intentions cannot. For instance, Jack can desire that he should euthanize Thomas and also desire that he not transgress the law by doing so. But presuming that he is fully informed about the law and understands that euthanizing Thomas would break the law of the State of Michigan as it stood in September 1998, then he cannot intend to euthanize Thomas in the State of Michigan in September 1998 without intending to break the law.

Brand (1984: 124) also points out that desires admit of degrees, while intentions do not. For instance, one can say of Tim that he greatly desires to help Diane commit suicide, but it makes no sense to say that he greatly intends to help her commit suicide. Intention requires, as Davidson (1980: 101) once put it, an all-out judgment. Intentions do not admit of degrees the way desires can. Intentions are not reducible to desires.

The Belief–Desire Model is Inadequate

The most sophisticated model proposed by those who are not convinced that intentions actually exist is the belief–desire model. Such a model suggests that a combination of belief and desire accounts for intention. A good example of this approach is given by Faden and Beauchamp (1986: 242–8). By their account, a surgeon who desires to operate on a patient, believing that it is possible to operate and believing that it is possible that he will scar the patient, intends to operate on the patient and intends to scar the patient. While I suspect most surgeons would find it perplexing to be told that they intend to scar their patients, for Faden and Beauchamp, nothing more need be said.

But no such combination of beliefs and desires will accomplish what neither belief nor desire alone could do—account completely for intention. There are several reasons for this.

First, Searle argues that while intentional states may involve belief and desire, intentionality is not reducible to belief and desire. For example, to be annoyed that p, to be remorseful that p, and to be sad that p all imply the belief that p and the desire that not-p. But annoyance, remorse, and sadness are not the same. Likewise, the fact that intentions might involve belief or desire does not imply that intention can be reduced to belief and desire (Searle 1983: 35–6). Second, the arguments made above point out that desire is not merely insufficient, it is in fact unnecessary to account for intention. If belief is insufficient and desire is unnecessary, then no combination of belief and desire will be both necessary and sufficient to account for intention.

Third, as Aquinas pointed out long ago (Aquinas 1964: I-II q. 13 a. 6 ad 3), human agents are not paralyzed by equal choices. When one is faced with choices that are equally desirable or undesirable and one believes that both choices are available and can be achieved with equivalent effort and equivalent satisfaction of one's desire, one is still able to choose between the two courses of action. Intentional choice is something over and above belief and desire.

Bratman (1987: 11 ff.) makes the same point by discussing a set of problems known as Buridan cases (see note 14). If one sits before two equally desirable boxes of cornflakes believing that eating either will satisfy one's desires equally, and believing that one will satisfy one's desire by eating cornflakes and believing that it is equally likely that either box could be obtained with equal convenience and equal success, has one thereby formed an intention? Does one thereby intend to eat either box of cornflakes? Both boxes of cornflakes? It hardly seems so. Belief and desire do not add up to intention.

It is important to note that the foregoing does not mean that one cannot simultaneously desire and intend that the same event should come about, or that one cannot simultaneously believe and intend the same event, or that one cannot simultaneously desire, believe, and intend the same event. Nor should the foregoing be taken as an argument that only intentions matter in morality, and that beliefs and desires do not matter or that consequences do not matter. On the contrary, moral agents can have multiple propositional attitudes towards the events they bring about intentionally, and a robust philosophical moral psychology will have something to say about all of these propositional attitudes. Intention is important, but morality is not limited to intentions. All I have tried to establish is that intentions cannot be reduced to desires and beliefs and that intentions have a special importance in the evaluation of the acts human beings undertake.

Intentions Are Not Motives

Neither should intentions to be confused with motives. A criminal investigation of homicide provides a good example of the difference between intention and motive. When the police look for a motive for a fatal knifing, or for a suspect with a possible motive, they have often already assumed that the act was intentional. They generally presume, that is, that the stabbing was the ascribable condition of fulfillment for the suspect's intention in acting, and they often believe that the death of the victim by way of the suspect himself stabbing her was the condition of fulfillment of the suspect's mature complex prior intention. When searching for a motive, however, they want to know what could have initiated or led someone to perform such an intentional act. As Davidson (1980: 105) puts it, a motive is a reason for intending. Gustafsen (1986: 181–2) agrees, pointing out that motives *start* intentions.

However, ordinary language sometimes confuses motives with what I have called further intentions. Anscombe (1969: 20–1) distinguishes backward-looking motives from forward-looking motives. She means by a backward-looking motive that the main ground of the motive is something that happened in the past, or is happening now. By contrast, the main ground of a forward-looking motive is something that has yet to take place. It is forward-looking motives that are most easily confused with intentions.

As an example of a backward-looking motive, one might be seeking to understand the motive for a person's suicide. If the person's motive were to 'get even' with those who had failed to show adequate concern for her suffering—to cause them suffering in return by making them feel guilty—it would be a backward-looking motive. Revenge is something that gets started by something in the past. One can look forward to the day of revenge. And the revenge would be present in the suicide, but it would have started because of past events. The memory of past hurts to the person committing suicide and a desire to respond by returning the hurt would be the complex state of affairs that constitutes the motive.

By contrast, a person might commit suicide to prevent some undesired future state of affairs. This would be a forward-looking motive. For example, Janet might fear that as a carrier of the ϵ-4 allele of Apolipoprotein E, she is at such high risk for Alzheimer's disease that at the first signs of memory loss she would rather commit suicide than face further dementia. If this were her motive for committing suicide, it would be forward-looking.

While ordinary language can be sloppy in this regard (especially regarding forward-looking motives) a motive is not some further desired event. Death is what Janet intends, but death is not her motive. Her motive might be fear, or embarrassment, or some other psychological state regarding her future. Anscombe also names admiration, spite, and friendship as forward-looking motives, but these attitudes or states of affairs are not events that could function as the objects of genuine intentions. A motive is a psychological state of affairs that helps to explain how an agent comes to have an intention. Properly speaking, the propositional content of an intention must refer to an event. Intentions and motives are not the same.

Event Identity

Thus far, I have explained what intentions are and how they differ from beliefs, desires, and motives. However, merely establishing that intentions are not reducible to beliefs and desires does not suffice for establishing a plausible distinction between the foreseen and the intended. Certain beliefs must necessarily be ascribable to the agents that undertake acts. Those beliefs must be coherent and plausible if the description of the agent's intentional state is to be coherent and plausible. Intentions, by definition, explain the events brought about by agency. So, while intention cannot be reduced to beliefs, incoherence or implausibility in an agent's beliefs about the events that she brings about can render her explanation of those events as having come about under a particular intentional description incoherent or implausible.

Critical to any proposed account of the distinction between the intended and the foreseen are beliefs regarding descriptions of events. Especially crucial is the question of whether two or more particular descriptions describe the same event or different events. With this in mind, I will propose a definition of event identity. This definition is modified somewhat from Myles Brand's work. I will suggest that, formally,

> *Definition 9: Event identity.* If 'x' and 'y' are descriptions that pick out events, then if x and y occupy the exact same spatiotemporal coordinates, 'x' and 'y' pick out the same event.

This means, for instance, that if x is an event (described, say, as 'Oedipus marries Jocasta') and y is an event (described, say, as 'Oedipus marries his mother') and both of these events occupy the same spatiotemporal coordinates, then they are the same event. 'x' and 'y' may be two true definite descriptions, but both descriptions pick out the same event.

Conditions of Plausibility and Coherence: Distinguishing the Intended from the Foreseen

Armed with the philosophy of action I have just outlined, I can now specify a set of conditions that will permit one to test whether any particular report of a distinction between the intended and the foreseen is plausible and coherent. This, I believe, has always been the purpose of the causation requirement of the classical formulation of the RDE (Requirement 3 in Mangan's formulation). In fact, if one is rational and sincere, the requirement that the unintended bad effect not cause the intended good effect adds *nothing* to the classical requirement that one must foresee but not intend the bad effect. Thus, I suspect that the purpose of the causation requirement in the classical formulation of the RDE has been to render plausible and coherent reports about what is foreseen but not intended, so that one would not deceive oneself or others in reporting on one's beliefs and intentions.

However, one may question whether the causal requirement is sufficient to quell doubts about the rationality and sincerity of reports about what someone claims to foresee but not to intend. I believe that exclusive reliance upon this 'test' has led to significant errors in the application of the RDE. There are quite a number of other ways in which one can, in reporting on what one believes and what one intends, be insincere or irrational. The purpose of Requirement 7 of my 'reinvented' RDE is to expand the set of tests for the coherence and plausibility of reports about what is foreseen but not intended. The correct application of this requirement of the Reformulated RDE must treat the object of an intention as a proposition regarding an event. Events, as I have discussed, are best understood as particulars. As particulars, events will have logical implications and alternative true definite descriptions, and will have the potential to cause other events.

Double effect cases are typically quite complex. Often, when an agent forms a prior intention to bring about some event, there are many different implications, alternative true definite descriptions, and cause and effect relationships connected to that event. Accordingly, one must consider, at the very least, the following three types of scenario, each specifying a different set of relationships between intention and causation: linear causal chains, causal forks, and alternative causal routes:

Scenario I: Linear Causal Chains

(*p* causes *r*) & (*r* causes *q*)

$$p \longrightarrow r \longrightarrow q$$

e.g. I intend to drink alcohol (*p*) in order to relax (*r*), but I do not intend that this experience should make me an alcoholic (*q*).

Scenario II: Causal Forks

(*p* causes *q*) & (*p* causes *r*)

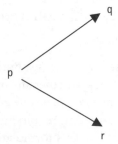

e.g. I intend to prescribe penicillin (p), in order to cure strep throat (r), but I do not intend to cause an anaphylactic reaction (q).

Scenario III: Alternative Causal Routes

(p causes q)& (p causes r) & (q causes r)

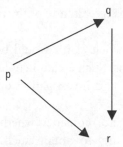

e.g. I intend to perform a bone marrow transplant (p) in order to treat leukemia (r), but not intending to cause high-grade graft v. host disease (q), even though high grade graft v. host disease also has a profound anti-leukemic effect (r).[15]

Having described these causal scenarios, I can now set forth the list of conditions I propose for plausibly and coherently maintaining that one foresees but does not intend a particular upshot of one's intentional act. I will set these forth without argument, since it seems to me that once one understands what is meant by intention and event identity, these conditions are self-evidently true.

CONDITIONS FOR RATIONALLY DISTINGUISHING BETWEEN INTENDED AND FORESEEN EVENTS

If an Agent (S) believes that the causal situation is such that it can be illustrated by any of the Scenarios (I–III), it is plausible and coherent for S to maintain that he or she foresees two results (q and r) from a chosen means of acting (p), but only intends r, given the following conditions:

(C1) p and q are not alternative true definite descriptions of the same event;

(C2) q and r are not alternative true definite descriptions of the same event;

(C3) q is not wholly spatiotemporally contained within p;

(C4) q is not wholly spatiotemporally contained within r;

(C5) p does not logically entail q;

---

[15] Currently, clinicians are actually aiming at (intending) mild graft v. host disease (GVHD) because of its anti-leukemic effect, but no one aims at high grade GVHD.

(C6) r does not logically entail q;

(C7) q is not S's further intention;

(C8) q is not an empirically necessary causal condition for r;

(C9) S does not intend r by way of q.

If conditions C1 through C9 are met, it would be coherent and plausible to claim to intend r, but not q, by means of p, in any of the three scenarios, as the examples amply demonstrate.

This is not to say that any such claim would be a true and sincere report of the agent's intentions and plans. Such a claim could be rebutted. But that rebuttal would require further inquiry and investigation of the facts and reported beliefs and intentions of the agent.

Further, this analysis does not consider whether the agent actually has the requisite knowledge (or the duty to obtain such knowledge) in order to have true and correct beliefs about these events and their casual relations and logical implications. Some ignorance is culpable, and some excuses. For example, it matters whether one thinks that Oedipus had a responsibility to know that Jocasta was his mother.

In addition, it must be noted emphatically that having a plausible and coherent report of what one foresees but does not intend is not sufficient to justify the act from a moral point of view. It is necessary that the agent also satisfy the other requirements of the Reformulated RDE.

Finally, while these conditions are proposed as necessary, I am making no claim that they exhaust all the conditions for rendering a coherent and plausible account of a complex prior intention in which it is claimed that at least one effect of an act is foreseen but not intended. This analysis only presents a first defense of a tightened set of conditions for the coherence and plausibility of distinguishing between the foreseen and the intended.

This analysis requires some further explication. First, one should note that each of these conditions corresponds to a matching condition under Requirement 7 of the Reformulated Rule of Double Effect, as it was laid out above. This more formal rendering of these conditions makes use of the technical vocabulary in philosophy of mind that I have presented.

Second, this set of conditions can be viewed as a significant amplification of the third requirement of the classical RDE. I believe that the major purpose of this classical 'causal' requirement (that the purportedly unintended bad effect cannot be the cause of the intended good effect) was to provide a check on the sincerity of the agent—to provide at least one condition for a report on beliefs and intentions that was coherent and plausible. However, this was simply insufficient. There are other ways to be incoherent and implausible in one's reports on what one foresees but does not intend. Thus, the purpose of these conditions is to 'tighten the rules' by setting up further tests for the coherence and plausibility of such reports.

It will doubtless prove helpful to the reader if I describe these conditions in words and give examples. In words, p is the Agent's (S's) intended means—the act itself. q is the purportedly foreseen but unintended causal result of p, and r is the intended causal result of p. Condition 1 states that the purportedly unintended result (q) cannot be an alternative true definite description of the intended means (p). Condition 2 states that the purportedly unintended result (q) cannot be an alternative true definite description of the intended result (r). Condition 3 states that the purportedly unintended result (q) cannot be an event that is completely subsumed within a wider event that constitutes the intended means (p). Condition 4 states that the purportedly unintended result (q) cannot be wholly spatiotemporally contained within a wider event that constitutes the intended result (r). Condition 5 states that the purportedly unintended result (q) cannot be logically implied by the intended means (p). Condition 6 states that the purportedly unintended result (q) cannot be logically implied by the intended outcome (r). Condition 7 states that the purportedly unintended result (q) cannot be, in fact, the agent's actual further intention. Condition 8 states that the purportedly unintended result (q) cannot be an empirically necessary causal condition for the intended result (r). And Condition 9 states that it cannot be the case that the agent actually intends the intended result (r) by way of the purportedly unintended result (q).

Intention and Foresight: Electroconvulsive Therapy

As an example, consider a physician who is contemplating the use of electroconvulsive therapy (ECT) for a patient suffering from a severe manic state, in the setting of bipolar affective disorder, refractory to medical treatment.

According to C1, it would not be coherent and plausible for the physician to claim to use ECT as his means (p) of treating mania (r), and also claim that he did not intend to subject the patient to electro-shock psychotherapy (q), since these are two alternative definite descriptions of the same procedure.

According to C2, it would not be coherent and plausible for the physician to claim to use ECT as his means of treating mania (p), intending as a result of ECT to produce a seizure (r), but not intending to produce an epileptic fit (q), since 'seizure' and 'eplileptic fit' pick out the same event.

According to C3, it would not be coherent and plausible for the physician to claim that if, in the course of ECT, he were to draw the patient's blood (p) as a means of monitoring the patient's drug levels, he only intended thereby to measure lithium levels (r), but did not intend to remove any red blood cells (q), because the removal of red blood cells (q) is an event wholly spatiotemporally contained within the event he intends as his means—namely, the drawing of the patient's blood (p).

According to C4, it would not be coherent and plausible for the physician to claim to use electrical current as his means (p) of achieving his intended aim of producing a seizure sufficient to cause motor movement of a non-paralyzed limb (r), while not intending to cause synchronous electrical discharges in the patient's brain (q), since the event of synchronous electrical discharges in the brain (q) is an event wholly contained within the wider event that he intends as his aim—namely, a seizure (p).

According to C5, it would not be coherent and plausible for the physician to claim to use a ten-treatment course of ECT as his means (p) of treating mania, but claim that he did not intend to give a multi-treatment course (q), since a ten-treatment course (p) logically implies a multi-treatment course (q).

According to C6, it would not be coherent and plausible for the physician to claim to be using ECT as his means (p) of treating mania, intending the complete remission of the manic episode (r), but not intending to end the patient's decreased sleep requirement (q), because a decreased sleep requirement (q) is a defining characteristic of mania, and the complete remission of mania (r) logically entails ending the decreased sleep requirement.

According to C7, it would not be coherent and plausible for the physician to claim to use ECT as his means (p), intending only to produce seizures (r), but not intending to cause memory loss (q), if it were the case that (for some nefarious motive) his actual further intention were to produce permanent memory loss in the patient (q) by means of ECT.

According to C8, it would not be coherent and plausible for the physician to claim to use ECT as a means (p) of bringing the patient's mania into remission (r), but not to cause any ongoing electrochemical changes in the brain of the patient (q), when the production of ongoing electrochemical changes in the brain of the patient (q) is an empirically necessary causal condition for the remission of the patient's mania (r).

According to C9, it would not be coherent and plausible for the physician to claim to use ECT as a means (p) of bringing about a remission of mania (r) but not to intend to cause seizures (q), when the physician's plan was to produce ten seizures of approximately one minute's duration each over the course of two weeks (q) as a way of bringing about the relief of the patient's mania (r).

However, it would be coherent and plausible for the physician to claim to intend to perform ECT (p) as a means of relieving mania (r), while foreseeing but not intending permanent memory loss (q), under Scenario II (Causal Forks). It would also be plausible and coherent to make this claim under Scenario III (Alternative Causal Routes).[16] The Alternative Causal Routes Scenario is especially interesting to consider in discussing ECT because it was once thought (although the view is now largely discredited) that the relief of psychiatric symptoms through ECT was at least in part caused by memory loss. Even were this to be true, it would still not be

[16] Since the relief of mania (r) does not cause memory loss (q), Casual Scenario I (Causal Chains) would not seem to apply here.

implausible or incoherent to claim to intend to relieve the mania without causing memory loss (unless memory loss were known to be an empirically necessary causal condition for the relief of psychiatric symptoms by ECT).

The RDE and the Concept of a Side-Effect

The distinction between the intended and the foreseen is of critical importance to any account of the practice of medicine. In fact, it is the structural basis of the concept of a side-effect. Side-effects (such as memory loss) are not merely unwanted. They are *unintended*, even if foreseen.

To see why this is so, consider the fact that, occasionally, side-effects are foreseen, unintended, and yet desirable. For example, consider the case of a depressed and anxious patient who smokes, has difficulty sleeping, and has a chronic seizure disorder. Suppose the patient's anxiety and depression have not responded to fluoxetine (Prozac). The clinician might then face a choice between bupropion and nortriptyline as the next drug to try. She quickly realizes that bupropion has a side-effect (unintended and very undesirable) of lowering the seizure threshold, and so chooses nortriptyline. In this case she intends to treat the anxiety and depression and to avoid seizures. The clinician might note that it would have been nice if she would have been able to use bupropion since it would also have helped the patient to quit smoking. Yet she is also aware that notriptyline is a second-line drug for smoking cessation (Hughes et al. 2003). In this case smoking cessation is foreseen as a potential beneficial and desirable side-effect, but it is not intended, since if it were the intention of the treatment, bupropion would have been the first choice. If, two weeks later, the patient returns and has quit smoking in addition to having improved anxiety and depression, the clinician and the patient would both have achieved a desirable, but unintended, side-effect. It would be coherent and plausible for a physician to say, 'I did not choose to prescribe bupropion with the intention in so acting of causing the patient to quit smoking, even though I was able to foresee that this unintended effect was possible, and I am glad that it has happened'.

APPLICATION TO CASES

The foregoing discussion of the RDE, as I have reformulated it, is significant for the debate about the place of the RDE in the philosophy of medicine and in medical ethics. The additional conditions I have proposed for judging the plausibility and coherence of a claim that a particular upshot of a proposed act is foreseen but not intended results in a reclassification of controversial cases that should affect this debate in important ways. Cases that have been used routinely by opponents of the RDE to show that the distinction between the foreseen and the intended makes no sense could no longer be used to discredit the RDE because these are not examples of its correct application. However, if the RDE were no longer a legitimate justification for the acts described in these cases, proponents of the RDE would either be required to consider these cases immoral or be forced to find some other means of showing that these acts are justifiable. While space limitations will not permit a full discussion of the implications of this reformulation of the RDE for many contested cases, an examination of its application to the tubal ectopic pregnancy case and the morphine case will readily illustrate the clinical and ethical implications of the Reformulated RDE.

The Tubal Ectopic Pregnancy Case

Those who are morally opposed to abortion, but would defend the permissibility of surgery for tubal ectopic pregnancy as an application of the RDE, must assume that the intention of the operator is not to abort the fetus but to remove the diseased Fallopian tube. They suggest that one can hold that direct abortion is morally wrong in all circumstances yet claim that in operating under such conditions, foreseeing but not intending the death of the fetus, the abortion is indirect and therefore morally permissible (Griese 1987: 268–71). Is this a coherent claim according to the above analysis?

Initially it would *not* seem that the case could be made that the removal of the diseased tube and the abortion of the fetus are two distinct events. Many would suggest that since the removal of the fetus and the removal of the tube require the same motor movements and occupy the same space and occur at exactly the same time, these two descriptions pick out the same event and are therefore nothing more than alternative definite descriptions of that event. If so, it would be incoherent, according to my analysis, to claim that one foresaw but did not intend the abortion of the fetus.

However, the proponent of the applicability of the RDE to this case could respond that the fetus is contained *within* the Fallopian tube and is therefore, in fact, spatially distinct from the tube. Such a person might suggest that this justifies the intention–foresight distinction in this case. But one must question whether this claim is plausible. Suppose the proponent were to argue that this case involved a Causal Forks Scenario (Scenario II). The event of the operation (p) causes one good effect (r, the intended removal of the diseased tube), and also causes one bad effect (q, the unintended removal of the fetus). However, it would seem that this claim would be implausible because Condition 2 of Requirement 7 would still be violated. It would still seem that 'q' and 'r' pick out the same event. The diseased tube is diseased because it contains a fetus. The fact that it contains a fetus *is* what is wrong with it. Granted, the fetus and the tube are spatially distinct things. But the only good event one could suggest that one hoped to achieve in such a case would be the removal of a *diseased* tube. In the case of tubal ectopic pregnancy, 'the removal of the fetus' and 'the removal of the diseased tube' seem to pick out the same event. So, even if one were to claim to foresee but not intend the removal of the fetus while intending the removal of the tube, it does not seem *plausible* to suggest that one intends the removal of a diseased tube but not the removal of the fetus. In other words, this is not a Causal Forks scenario.

Further, even if one were to grant the (implausible) suggestion that 'the removal of the diseased tube' and 'the removal of the fetus' pick out different events, one would still be left to contend with the question of whether this procedure violates Condition 4. It seems that the event of removing the fetus is wholly spatiotemporally contained within the event of removing the diseased tube. No part of the event of removing the fetus would be spatiotemporally outside the event of removing the diseased tube unless one were to perform a salpingotomy (i.e. an incision in the tube) and were simply to remove the fetus from the tube. But then it would clearly be a directly intended abortion and the RDE could not apply. So, even if one were to grant that this construal of the act would survive scrutiny according to Condition 2, it would not survive scrutiny according to Condition 4.

In fact, with methotrexate treatment, one may now remove the disorder from the tube without damaging the tube (Lipscomb *et al.* 1999). This may be safer for the mother since it is a medical, not a surgical, technique. Therefore, those who hold that the RDE justifies the surgery for tubal ectopic pregnancy are now in the awkward position of either (1) recommending the possibly more dangerous surgical procedure to the mother, or (2) claiming that the aim of intervention with methotrexate is to remove the diseased trophoblastic tissue that connects the fetus to the wall of the Fallopian tube, not to remove the fetus (Clark 2000). It should be clear that the latter construal would not stand up to scrutiny according to the conditions I have delineated for distinguishing the foreseen from the intended any more than for the surgical case. Many traditional defenders of the application of the RDE to the tubal ectopic pregnancy case have concluded that it is implausible and incoherent to claim that one intends only to remove the trophoblastic tissue, not to cause an abortion. Yet they fail to see that it is equally implausible and incoherent to say that one is merely removing a diseased tube, not the fetus inside it. This has led some to recommend the more invasive, expensive, and dangerous surgical approach, which is an awkward position to defend. It therefore seems better to give up on the idea that it is the RDE that justifies treatment in cases of tubal ectopic pregnancy, no matter what treatment modality one uses.

An alternative move for the proponent of the application of the RDE might be to suggest that the tubal ectopic pregnancy case falls under the broad rubric of a type III scenario, not a type II scenario. It might be argued that what is intended (p) is better described more narrowly as the removal of the tube, rather than broadly as the performing of an operation for tubal ectopic pregnancy. The good one intends by this means is the health of the mother (r). The bad one foresees but does not intend is the removal of the fetus (q). One might also acknowledge fully that the event of the removal of the fetus (q) is an alternative causal route to the event of the health of the mother (r), but not the route one intends. But is this a coherent and plausible claim?

The answer would again be no because it violates Condition 8 of Requirement 7 of the Reformulated RDE. The event of the removal of the fetus is a necessary causal condition for the event of the health of the mother. With current surgical techniques, the fetus cannot be left inside the mother to develop normally.[17] And given current surgical techniques, if one *did* leave the fetus floating freely inside the abdominal cavity, or even partially attached to the abdominal wall, it would still constitute a grave threat to the life of the mother and the likely result would be two deaths instead of one. So, under a Scenario III interpretation, a plan to keep the fetus inside the mother would be inconsistent with one's stated good intentions—to save the life of the mother. And this would seem quite irrational. Therefore, an attempt to argue that one foresees but does not intend the death of the fetus in operations for ectopic pregnancies is implausible and incoherent.

A proponent might at this point concede that the removal of the fetus is within the scope of the intention, and offer one final move. The proponent might try to redescribe the act as the removal of the tube and the fetus, with the specific intention in acting of saving the life of the mother, while foreseeing but not intending the death of the fetus. However, this leads to a even more serious conundrum, for if this argument were acceptable for the ectopic pregnancy case, it would be acceptable for many, many other cases. Every act of abortion could thereby be justified by the same sort of act redescription: intending only to remove the fetus, not intending to kill it. One must bear in mind that the proponent of the use of the RDE to justify surgery for tubal ectopic pregnancies was initially led to use this argument because of opposition to abortion. It would be devastating to concede that the argument justifying the application of the RDE to the tubal ectopic pregnancy case could also justify abortion on demand.

Operations for tubal ectopic pregnancies would therefore appear to be cases of killing the fetus.[18] If such operations are justifiable, as almost everyone would agree that they are, and one is otherwise morally opposed to abortion, such operations must be justified some another way than by invoking the RDE. Space limitations (in an already very long chapter) do not allow a full discussion of the alternative.[19]

[17] This is true at the present level of technology. However, if progress ever allowed physicians to do so safely, then one would presumably be morally impelled to reimplant the conceptus elsewhere (such as in the uterus) and there would be no point to saying that one did not intend the death of the fetus because it would be an avoidable event, and would violate Requirement 4 of the Reformulated RDE.

[18] For a more complete definition of killing, see Sulmasy (1998).

[19] For a more extensive discussion, see Sulmasy (1995).

But briefly stated, rather than its traditional formulation, the moral rule prohibiting killing, as I see it, ought best to be formulated as follows.

Prohibited Killing

Acting on individual authority, one may never make the death of a human being the condition of fulfillment of one's intention in acting, except in forced choice situations in which one *cannot* act intentionally without making the death of a human being the condition of fulfillment of one's intention in acting. Classically, these are cases of self-defense or rescue, where self-defense and rescue are narrowly defined to include only direct, serious threats of death (and no lesser harms). In such cases, the threatened person (or the rescuer of the threatened person) is permitted to use lethal force against the attacker provided all other means have been exhausted, the threat is truly imminent, and it is truly direct (i.e. the attacker is the agent of the threat, not some other party such as a hired assassin or a subordinate ordered to kill). In these cases, one is not culpable for acting directly against human life, since one cannot act without taking human life. One is *not* acting against the *value* of life in such forced choice situations, because no choice is available except one that involves taking life. One either kills or is killed. In these cases, one may employ other considerations (such as number of lives involved, role responsibilities, or the like) in choosing one life or the other.

In removing a tubal ectopic pregnancy, one is killing, but since one is doing so to rescue the mother from a serious imminent threat of death, caused by the fetus, despite its innocence, with no intervening agents, this is an allowable exception. When either one or the other must die (or, more specifically in such cases, either one dies or both die), one is allowed to choose, by action or omission, who will survive and who will die. Thus, vigorous defenders of the value of human life can justify surgery or methotrexate in cases such as tubal ectopic pregnancy without diminishing their allegiance to a principle of equal respect for the value of each human life, prenatal or postnatal. But they also ought not invoke the RDE in such an incoherent way that the significance of this important moral rule is jeopardized.

The Morphine Case

In contrast to the way in which my Reformulated RDE excludes the tubal ectopic pregnancy cases from its ambit, the Reformulated RDE continues to justify its application in most traditional cases. To illustrate this, I will 'walk through' its application to the morphine case.

In the morphine case, proponents of the RDE suggest that in giving powerful opioid analgesics such as morphine to dying patients, one intends only pain relief, not the hastening of death that one knows can occur through respiratory depression. According to my Reformulated RDE, such a combination of intentions is coherent, plausible, and morally justifiable.

Although in such a case it might not seem immediately obvious, there *are*, in fact, two separable events, distinct in time and space: pain relief (intended) and respiratory depression (unintended). To see why these really are two distinct events, making the application of the RDE plausible, it is perhaps best to think about this case on a molecular level. The analgesic and respiratory depressant effects of morphine occur by the binding of morphine molecules at different subtypes of morphine receptors, populating different locations in the nervous system. The chemistry for each effect has a different time course (kinetics). Morphine achieves pain relief via μ_1 receptors and respiratory depression via μ_2 receptors. These molecular differences are manifested in the response of the patient to the drug. Pain relief occurs at lower doses and more rapidly than respiratory depression. Thus, while the effects are scattered throughout the body, conceptually this is still a Causal Forks Scenario (type II). So the claim that one intended pain relief and not respiratory depression is plausible and coherent.

However, since the event of death is also a potential cause of the event of pain relief, the skeptic might suggest that this could be construed as a type III scenario—an Alternative Causal Routes Scenario. Accordingly, one must ask whether the morphine case, so construed, would meet the conditions of Requirement 7 of the Reformulated RDE. I argue that even under this construal, the distinction between the foreseen and the intended would be plausible and coherent. 'Death' and 'administering morphine' do not pick out the same event. And neither do 'analgesia' and 'death' pick out the same event. The intention to administer morphine does not logically imply intending the death of the patient. Intending analgesia does not logically imply intending the death of the patient. The event of the death of the patient is certainly not a necessary causal condition for the event of pain relief. If it is not the doctor's further intention that the patient should die, and it is not the case that he intends analgesia by way of the patient's death, then the claim is at least plausible and coherent, and meets all of the conditions of Requirement 7 of the Reformulated RDE.

For the morphine case to be permitted, however, the remaining requirements of the Reformulated RDE must be met. This analysis turns out to be quite straightforward. A physician morally opposed to euthanasia has a conflict between a duty to relieve suffering and a duty not to kill (i.e. not to act with the specific intention in acting that a human being should die by way of that act except in cases of self-defense or rescue). In such cases, she may administer the morphine with the following provisos:

(1) the administration of morphine is one intentional act with the two foreseeable effects of pain relief and respiratory depression;

(2) injecting morphine is at least morally neutral;

(3) relieving pain is morally good and killing is morally bad;

(4) other means of pain relief such as non-steroidal anti-inflammatory drugs are no longer effective;

(5) no intervening agents are involved;

(6) she has the intention in acting of relieving pain and not depressing respirations and thereby hastening death;

(7) it is plausible and coherent for her to make this claim (as demonstrated by the above analysis), so one cannot rule out that she is sincere and rational in her report on her intentions;

(8) there is due proportionality, such as when the patient's death is inevitable and the pain is great, so that fears of hastening the patient's death seem overwhelmingly small when proportionately compared to the benefits of pain relief.

The act is then morally justified according to the RDE.

While space considerations prohibit analyzing more cases, the upshot is that under the Reformulated RDE, the tubal ectopic pregnancy, the cancerous gravid uterus, and the case of using lethal force in self-defense, all fall out of double effect analysis. Cases such as morphine for the dying, and almost any other clinical case that could be described as a treatment with a side-effect, fall within the scope of the Reformulated RDE.

CONSIDERATION OF POSSIBLE OBJECTIONS

This is a considerable reworking of the RDE, and I can anticipate that objections will be raised. Here I consider seven objections, and will leave discussion of other potential objections to the thoughtful analysis of colleagues.

First, some might wonder if the RDE has been rendered superfluous. If a case such as the tubal ectopic pregnancy case must be justified by some other moral rule, perhaps the moral rule about killing that I offered is sufficient, and the RDE unnecessary. Those who have suspected that the RDE is merely correlated with other moral intuitions that actually do all the necessary moral work might be tempted to think this way. However, this is not the case.

A rule justifying killing only in self-defense or rescue would not cover the morphine case. The morphine case involves only one life, not a forced choice between at least two. So a rule that justifies direct killing only in cases of self-defense or rescue would not apply.

Nor would it do to recast the morphine case as the 'rescue' of the person who is dying. While clever, such a move would implicate one in an untenable dualism, claiming that the person was being threatened by some 'other person' (perhaps the person's own body). And, clearly, the threat would not be a threat of death, but a threat of pain.

Similarly, the new rule prohibiting killing would not apply to a whole range of cases in which death is a side-effect, such as bone marrow transplantation for leukemia, in which the foreseeable risk of death is high, but not intended, but there is no 'other party' threatening death. Even cases such as the strategic bomber case would also still require the RDE, since the threat of harm posed to the bomber, her comrades, and her nation by the armaments factory (the intended target) would presumably not be imminent, and the schoolchildren next door (the unintended target) are not themselves the source of any threat. So, the RDE would be far from superfluous under my proposed reformulation.

Second, some might object that this reformulation is too complicated. Surely, with so many conditions and qualifications, one might suggest, there must be something suspicious about this theory. My argument against this is to remind readers that the purpose of ethical theory is to explain and justify morality. This is different from being a moral person or, more specifically, a moral clinician, and different from acting in a morally upright manner. If I am correct that the RDE is the theory that explains the concept of a side-effect, then clinicians act according to the RDE almost reflexively every day. Explaining what one means by a side-effect in a rigorous philosophical manner is a far more complex matter than having a common-sense working notion of a side-effect in clinical practice. One resorts to theoretical analysis if someone challenges the meaning of a common-sense notion such as the notion of a side-effect, or if someone objects to the application or plausibility of a moral rule such as the RDE with respect to a particularly difficult case.

Similar considerations apply to all sciences. Human bodies work according to the laws of biochemistry. One need not know all the theories of biochemistry in order to be a good doctor. But in exceptional cases one resorts to biochemistry to meet a particular clinical challenge or one explores biochemistry as a basic science in order to explain better what is common. No medical student would object to being taught about topoisomerases or enzyme kinetics 'because it is too hard'. It is puzzling that anyone seriously interested in medical ethics would feel entitled to complain that medical ethics 'is too hard'. This brings to mind Bernard Williams's (Williams and Smart 1973: 149) critique of utilitarianism as having, in its reduction of all of morality to the simplicity of consequences, 'too few thoughts and feelings to match the world as it really is'. If explaining biochemistry is complex, it seems reasonable to expect that the moral life of the human beings who arise out of these biochemical processes would be at least as complex.

A third anticipated objection is that this is all a religious theory that has no place in secular philosophical analysis. This objection is often repeated, or at least intimated, in the bioethics literature. However, it is also a puzzling objection. The RDE is a substantial topic of philosophical discourse. Nothing in my argument depends upon acceptance of any scripture, the teaching of any church, pope, or bishop, or the dogma of any religion. That it has its origin with the writings of a saint is no argument that it is an inherently religious notion, any more than one can argue legitimately that all theoretical defenses of the immorality of adultery are inherently religious simply because one of the Ten Commandments prohibits adultery. It is a form of the *ad hominem* fallacy to attempt to detract from an argument merely by citing what one considers its (arguably!) suspect source.

In fact, a fourth anticipated objection is actually an additional counterargument to the third. Adherents to the traditional Roman Catholic formulation of the RDE might well object that the reformulation I am proposing is too radical a break with the Catholic tradition on double effect. I have suggested that the intention–foresight distinction, as it originated in the writings of St Thomas Aquinas, was misapplied from the beginning. While this might worry some Catholics, it also ought to suggest that the origins of the idea (whether Catholic or not) are irrelevant to my analysis and therefore no objection to it.

I *do* think that the idea of the intention–foresight distinction is of critical importance, and that we can credit Aquinas with first presenting it, even if I do not agree that it applies to the case to which he first applied it. I think this distinction remains crucial to Catholic moral thinking, and that contemporary philosophy of mind helps to clarify and support it. But if the RDE has been misapplied in Catholic thinking, that mistake needs to be corrected *within Catholicism* as well as in philosophy. And I hope that Catholic proponents of the RDE will be able to see how my analysis strengthens their own defense of this important moral rule.

A fifth anticipated objection is a variation on the fourth. Proponents of the RDE might accuse me of having so radically reformulated it that, in a parody of a phrase associated with the Vietnam War (and the phrase itself is a dark parody of sorts), 'I had to destroy the RDE in order to save it'. There is no question that I have significantly restricted the use of the RDE by tightening the conditions for its rational application. But rendering a moral rule more rational can hardly be considered its destruction. Other attempts to reformulate this rule have changed its structure and moral tenor considerably more than mine. My reformulation simply makes the traditional formulation more stringent. If, as I believe is true, most of the objections to the RDE are raised by those who have found untenable the applications of the RDE that I also find untenable, then the proper metaphor is not that I have engaged in scorched earth warfare but that I have instead been pruning the vine. By pruning away branches of the RDE that are already dead, it is my hope that I will actually have breathed new life into this important moral rule and that, in its proper application, it will blossom.

A sixth anticipated objection is that the RDE, with its emphasis on intention, is not morally relevant. It is true, as I stated at the beginning of this chapter, that if one does not believe that intentions matter in the moral evaluation of human acts, the RDE will make no sense. Many, like Bennett, are skeptical about whether intentions actually exist. But these critics often, like Bennett, beg the question in a very serious way. Bennett (1995: 194) states, 'What a person intends in ϕ ing is defined, therefore, by which of her consequential beliefs explain her ϕ ing and by which of her desires do so.' Notice that he says 'consequential beliefs' and not 'consequences'. If he defines intentions in terms of beliefs and/or desires, it is simply vacuous for him to argue that intentions can be reduced to beliefs and/or desires. In yet another curious example of one of the two major mistakes I have tried to correct in this chapter, namely that of paying insufficient attention to developments in philosophy of mind, Bennett cites Searle, but then proceeds to ignore everything Searle has to say about why intentions cannot be reduced to beliefs or desires. Bennett offers no reply to any of the arguments to the contrary noted above, such as Buridan cases, wayward causal chains, or the differences in the logical properties of beliefs, desires, and intentions. He also makes no mention of self-referential causation. Therefore, nothing he says should cast any doubt on the theory of intention I have presented.

Still, to accept the RDE, even if one concedes that intentions exist, one must be convinced that intentions mark a moral difference that cannot be accounted for purely by consequences. Space does not permit a full discussion here, but intentions make acts human and give acts a moral structure that must be evaluated if acts are to be evaluated as human and moral. At least two simple, initial lines of argument are available against the consequentialist alternative. First, one can point out that anyone who would dismiss the moral importance of *how* medical events come about, basing moral judgments solely upon the consequences, faces a monumental task. She must show that a formidable history of collective moral judgment has been ill-considered. Physicians, the US Supreme Court, and most plain persons continue to hold a belief that there is a moral difference between injecting 150 mEq of potassium chloride into the right ventricle of a dying patient and giving that same patient an injection of a dose of morphine sufficient to relieve the patient's pain, and acting with that intention (*Washington* v. *Glucksberg* 1997; *Vacco* v. *Quill* 1997). The consequences of these two acts may be the same. I have argued elsewhere that the basis of the judgment that these acts are different depends upon intentions (Sulmasy 1998). It will not suffice, in the face of all that I have outlined about contemporary work in philosophy of action, simply to insist that intentions do not exist or to 'prove', via question-begging arguments, that everyone who believes these cases are morally different is misguided.

One can also offer counterexamples. I will offer a variation on one first proposed by Philippa Foot (1978). Suppose a physician were to have a limited supply of a life-saving drug and were suddenly to face five patients who needed it. Four of these patients would be highly likely to survive with a dose equivalent to $^1/_5$ of the supply of the drug, while the fifth would be likely to survive only if given the total dose. If one were to give each patient a dose equivalent to $^1/_5$ of the supply, foreseeing but not intending the death of the patient who needed a higher dose, one would fulfill all of the conditions of the Reformulated RDE and the act would be morally permissible. However, suppose one were to face a situation in which there were no drug supply, but the drug could be made by sacrificing one of the five, grinding him up, and making a life-saving serum out of him—enough to save the other four. This plan would not meet the conditions of the Reformulated RDE, since it would violate Requirements 7(h) and 7(i). One could not plausibly and coherently claim that one did not intend the death of the individual sacrificed to make the serum. Only the crassest of utilitarians would see these cases as morally equivalent—always making the best of a bad lot. What marks the moral difference that people of reason and goodwill sense here is not the net outcome (which is exactly the same in both cases). The difference can be ascribed to the fact that in the latter case the death was intended as part of the doctor's plan, while the death in the former case was foreseen but not intended.

Space limitations will not permit me to take up this debate in greater detail than I already have. Suffice it to say that the RDE matters in morality to the extent that intentions matter in morality.

Seventh, some objections might be based upon particular moral judgments about the cases that I discussed. For example, some might hold that euthanasia is not immoral, and therefore hold that killing a dying patient is not bad, and therefore conclude that the RDE does not apply to the morphine case. However, this sort of objection is not an argument against the RDE itself. Discussion would need to shift to arguments for and against the morality of acting with the specific intention in acting of making a human being dead by way of one's act in order to relieve that person's suffering. Even so, such a critic might not object to the role of intentions in morality in general and thus be persuaded by my reformulation of the RDE with respect to its application to cases in which it could be granted that the unintended side-effect actually would be bad, such as the foreseeable and uncontroversial badness of the hair loss that often accompanies cancer chemotherapy.

CONCLUSION

I have presented a reformulation of the RDE that addresses what I consider two fundamental mistakes: the failure of ethicists (particularly bioethicists) to consider developments in the philosophy of mind in relation to the RDE and the misapplication of the RDE to a class of cases that has proven contentious. Critical to this reformulation of the RDE has been the introduction of various notions from philosophy of mind in order to tighten the conditions under which one can be considered plausible and coherent in a claim to foresee a certain bad outcome while not intending it. This reformulation precludes the cases that have seemed most incredible to critics, thereby lessening their objections. This reformulation also forces proponents of the RDE to reconsider the basis by which they can justify the acts that they mistakenly have thought to be justified by the RDE.

Elizabeth Anscombe (1970) once observed that the denial of the RDE 'has been the corruption of non-Catholic thought, and its abuse the corruption of Catholic thought'. It is my hope that this chapter has helped to expurgate a little bit of that corruption.

REFERENCES

ANSCOMBE, G. E. M. (1958), 'Modern Moral Philosophy', *Philosophy*, 33: 1–19.

——— (1969), *Intention* (2nd edn. Ithaca, NY: Cornell University Press).

——— (1970), 'War and Murder', in R. A. Wasserstrom (ed.), *War and Morality* (Belmont, Calif.: Wadsworth), 42–53.

AQUINAS, T. (1964), *Summa Theologiae*, ed. T. Gilby (New York: McGraw-Hill).

ARISTOTLE (1985), *Nicomachean Ethics*, trans. T. Irwin (Indianapolis: Hackett).

BEAUCHAMP, T. L., and CHILDRESS, J. F. (1994), *Principles of Biomedical Ethics* (4th edn. New York: Oxford University Press).

——— (2001), *Principles of Biomedical Ethics*, (5th edn. New York: Oxford University Press).

BENNETT, J. (1995), *The Act Itself* (New York: Oxford University Press).

BOYLE, J. M. (1978), '*Praeter intentionem* in Aquinas', *The Thomist*, 42: 649–65.

——— (1980), 'Toward Understanding the Principle of Double Effect', *Ethics*, 90: 527–38.

BRAND, M. (1984), *Intending and Acting* (Cambridge, Mass.: MIT Press).

BRATMAN, M. (1987), *Intention, Plans, and Practical Reason* (Cambridge, Mass.: Harvard University Press).

BROCK, D. W. (1993), *Life and Death: Philosophical Essays in Biomedical Ethics* (New York: Cambridge University Press).

CAVANAUGH, T. A. (1997), 'Aquinas' Account of Double Effect', *The Thomist*, 6: 107–21.

CLARK, P. A., SJ (2000), 'Methotrexate and Tubal Pregnancies: Direct or Indirect Abortion?', *Linacre Quarterly*, 67 (Feb.), 7–24.

DAVIDSON, D. (1980), *Essays on Actions and Events* (Oxford: Clarendon Press).

DAVIS, N. (1984), 'The Doctrine of Double Effect: Problems of Interpretation', *Philosophical Quarterly*, 65: 107–23.

DONAGAN, A. (1987), *Choice: The Essential Element in Human Action* (London: Routledge & Kegan Paul).

FADEN, R., and BEAUCHAMP, T. (1986), *A History and Theory of Informed Consent* (New York: Oxford University Press).

FOOT, P. (1978), 'The Problem of Abortion and the Doctrine of Double Effect', in Foot, *Virtues and Vices and Other Essays in Moral Philosophy* (Berkeley: University of California Press), 19–32.

GLOVER, J. (1977), *Causing Death and Saving Lives* (New York: Penguin).

GRIESE, O. N. (1987), *Catholic Identity in Health Care: Principles and Practice* (Braintree, Mass.: The Pope John Center).

GUSTAFSEN, D. (1986), *Intention and Agency*, Philosophical Studies Series in Philosophy, 33 (Dordrecht: D. Reidel).

HUGHES, J. R., STEAD, L. F., and LANCASTER, T. (2003), 'Antidepressants for Smoking Cessation', *Cochrane Database of Systematic Reviews*, 2, CD000031.

KACZOR, C. (1998), 'Double-Effect Reasoning from Jean Pierre Gury to Peter Knauer', *Theological Studies*, 59: 297–316.

KELLY, D. F. (1979), *The Emergence of Roman Catholic Medical Ethics in North America* (New York: Edwin Mellen).

KNAUER, P. (1979), 'The Hermeneutical Function of the Principle of Double Effect', in C. E. Curran and R. A. McCormick (eds.), *Readings in Moral Theology*, i: *Moral Norms and the Catholic Tradition* (New York: Paulist Press), 1–39.

KUHSE, H. (1987), *The Sanctity of Life Doctrine in Medicine: A Critique* (Oxford: Clarendon Press).

LIPSCOMB, G. H., McCORD, M. L., STOVALL, T. G., HUFF, G., PORTERA, S. G., and LING, F. W. (1999), 'Predictors of Success of Methotrexate Treatment in Women with Tubal Ectopic Pregnancies', *New England Journal of Medicine*, 341: 1974–8.

McINTYRE, A. (2001), 'Doing Away With Double Effect', *Ethics*, 111: 219–55.

MANGAN, J. T., SJ (1949), 'An Historical Analysis of the Principle of Double Effect', *Theological Studies*, 10: 41–61.

PEARSE, D. W. (ed.) (1992), *The MIT Dictionary of Modern Economics* (4th edn. Cambridge, Mass.: MIT Press).

QUILL, T. E., DRESSER, R., and BROCK, D. W. (1997), 'The Rule of Double Effect: A Critique of Its Use in End-of-Life Decision Making', *New England Journal of Medicine*, 337: 1768–71.

QUINN, W. (1989), 'Actions, Intentions, and Consequences: The Doctrine of Double Effect', *Philosophy and Public Affairs*, 18: 334–51.

SEARLE, J. (1980), 'The Intentionality of Intention and Action', *Cognitive Science*, 4: 47–70.

——— (1983), *Intentionality: An Essay in the Philosophy of Mind* (New York: Cambridge University Press).

STYRON, W. (1979), *Sophie's Choice* (New York: Random House).

SULMASY, D. P., OFM (1995), 'Killing and Allowing to Die', Ph.D. thesis, Georgetown University.

——— (1998), 'Killing and Allowing to Die: Another Look', *Journal of Law, Medicine, and Ethics*, 26: 55–64.

——— (2000), 'Double Effect: Intention Is the Solution, Not the Problem', *Journal of Law, Medicine, and Ethics*, 28: 26–9.

——— and PELLEGRINO, E. D. (1999), 'The Rule of Double Effect: Clearing Up the Double Talk', *Archives of Internal Medicine*, 159: 545–50.

Vacco v. *Quill*, 117 S. Ct. 2293 (1997).

WAGNER, S. J. (1995), 'Proposition', in R. Audi (ed.), *The Cambridge Dictionary of Philosophy* (Cambridge: Cambridge University Press), 658–9.

Washington v. *Glucksberg*, 117 S. Ct. 2258 (1997).

WILLIAMS, B., and SMART, J. J. C. (1973), *Utilitarianism: For and Against* (Cambridge: Cambridge University Press).

WILLIAMS, G. (1957), *The Sanctity of Life and the Criminal Law* (New York: Knopf).

PART II

JUSTICE AND POLICY

CHAPTER 6

....

POLICY-MAKING
IN PLURALISTIC
SOCIETIES

....

SØREN HOLM

Now, the serious problem is this. A modern democratic society is characterized not simply by a pluralism of comprehensive religious, philosophical, and moral doctrines but by a pluralism of incompatible yet *reasonable* comprehensive doctrines. No one of these doctrines is affirmed by citizens generally. Nor should one expect that in the foreseeable future one of them, or some other reasonable doctrine, will ever be affirmed by all, or nearly all, citizens. Political liberalism assumes that, for political purposes, a plurality of reasonable, yet incompatible, comprehensive doctrines is the normal result of the exercise of human reason within the framework of the free institutions of a constitutional democratic regime (Rawls 1996, p. xviii; my emphasis).

Bioethics is not only concerned with analysing the actions of individual moral agents; it also analyses policy decisions and thereby has an interface with political philosophy. Bioethicists often give unsolicited policy advice, but many also have more official roles on various kinds of ethics committees advising political decision-makers.[1]

The views put forward in this chapter have been developed through many years of friendly, but profound disagreement and discussion with John Harris, a good friend and practitioner of the virtues of mutual respect. The chapter relies on arguments I have previously discussed in Holm (2001, 2002, 2003a, b, 2004), and in Harris and Holm (2003).

[1] I was myself for six years a member of the Danish Council of Ethics, which provides advice on bioethical issues to the Danish government and parliament.

The purpose of this chapter is to discuss the issues that arise when a state or other lower public authority has to make policy decisions in areas where there is at the same time moral and scientific uncertainty.

Perhaps the most recent example of this kind of problem is the still ongoing controversy with regard to public policy in the area of reproductive cloning and the therapeutic use of stem cells (see, for instance, the thematic issues of the journals *Bioethics*, the *American Journal of Bioethics*, and the *Kennedy Institute of Ethics Journal*, all in 2002), but there are many other examples in areas like assisted reproductive technologies, abortion, euthanasia, capital punishment, funding of the health care system, and research ethics.[2] It is probably no coincidence that many of these questions touch upon moral issues where not only there are marked disagreements about moral issues, but where these disagreements are seen as fundamental by the persons involved and the corresponding views strongly held.

In these cases we often end up in a situation where each side has arguments that it sees as compelling, but which the other side rejects utterly.

In the following I will assume that the following two core features characterize the kind of societies we are discussing: (1) they are morally pluralistic, i.e. there is a variety of views concerning the moral issue at hand, and (2) they are liberal democracies, i.e. they are not dictatorships, autocracies, oligarchies, plutocracies, or populist democracies.

That they are liberal democracies does not make these societies identical at the level of political systems or ideals. Most industrialized and many industrializing countries fall within the cluster of societies picked out by these two characteristics, but each has its own specific version of a morally pluralistic, liberal democracy. This is, for instance, evident in how the generally agreed principle that religion should not directly determine public policy is implemented. Some liberal democracies have an established church (e.g. England,[3] Denmark, Norway), some have a weak separation between church and state (e.g. Sweden, Germany, Spain), and some have a strong separation between church and state (e.g. France, the United States). It is also evident at the structural level, where Montesquieu's classic separation between the legislative, the judicial, and the executive powers is implemented in quite diverse ways, and where the power balance between these three branches of government differs widely between countries.

As David Held points out, these differences concerning the meaning of the term 'liberal democracy' not only affect institutional design, they also permeate political philosophy:

In the first instance, the 'liberal' component of liberal democracy cannot be treated simply as a unity. There are distinctive liberal traditions which embody quite different conceptions

---

[2] Many of the examples in this chapter will be concerned with the stem cell debate, but I believe that the points made are generally valid.

[3] But not Scotland or Wales.

from each other of the individual agent, of autonomy, of the rights and duties of subjects, and of the proper nature and form of community. In addition, the 'celebratory' view of liberal democracy neglects to explore whether there are any tensions, or even perhaps contradictions, between the 'liberal' and 'democratic' components of liberal democracy; for example, between the liberal preoccupation with individual rights or 'frontiers of freedom' which 'nobody should be permitted to cross', and the democratic concern for the regulation of individual and collective action, that is for public accountability. Those who have written at length on this question have frequently resolved it in quite different directions.   (Held 1992: 10; notes removed)

It may be the case that political philosophy will eventually reach universal agreement on the exact form of the ideal liberal democracy, but until that happens we will be unable to base our analysis on a canonical account of the ideal society.

This multiplicity of forms of morally pluralistic, liberal democracies entails that the analysis in this chapter will have to be relatively general, and that it will therefore risk being slightly off the mark when applied to a particular jurisdiction.

Double Trouble

In morally pluralistic societies there are, by definition, many areas of moral disagreement. The scope of the current analysis is, however, only concerned with bioethical disagreements and only with those disagreements where a public policy decision has to be made. There are clearly a number of bioethical contentious issues that fall wholly within the private sphere and do not call for any public policy decisions, although it is important to remember that the extent of the private sphere is itself contentious. If the private is political, it is for instance not the case that activities wholly confined within the walls of the home necessarily fall within a protected private sphere.

The class of issues analysed here will be further restricted to encompass only those issues where there is not only moral disagreement, but also significant scientific uncertainty of relevance to the ethical analysis.

This immediately points to one potential problem for a general analysis of this type of public decision-making, since there is no general agreement on what scientific facts are of relevance to ethical analysis. Each ethical framework picks its own set of relevant facts. In the following I will, nevertheless, assume that facts about the effectiveness and usefulness of a therapy, its likely impact on major diseases, or its risks and side-effects are relevant facts of interest to most ethical analyses, as are facts about the consequences of implementing one type of policy and not another.[4]

---

[4] Is it, for instance, the case that introducing capital punishment for a given class of crimes will reduce the number of these crimes?

The chapter will initially be concerned with general issues of policy-making in liberal democracies in these circumstances, before moving on to an examination of some more specific issues where bioethical analysis and the policy-making process often clash.

LET FREEDOM REIGN

One way of solving these policy-making problems that is sometimes explicitly or implicitly invoked in bioethics writing is the idea that we should allow people to act in the ways they want to act if it does not do any harm to others. A significant part of the literature on 'reproductive freedom' or 'reproductive liberty' does, for instance, adopt this approach, as does the whole libertarian segment of moral philosophy. If we do proceed in this way, most of the policy problems engendered by ethical and scientific uncertainty can be made to go away, since we only need to estimate whether the activity we are considering is likely to cause harm, and do not have to consider its eventual benefits. The benefit estimation can be left to individual actors. This idea is often traced to Mill's dictum in *On Liberty*: 'that the sole end for which mankind are warranted, individually or collectively, in interfering with the liberty of action of any of their number, is self-protection. That the only purpose for which power can be rightly exercised over any member of a civilised community, against his will, is to prevent harm to others' (Mill 1987: 78). Philosophically this is a rather tempting idea. It is liberal, it is simple, and it seems to solve a whole range of policy-making problems in a way that happens to be in accordance with the views of many liberal bioethicists.

But it is not an idea without problems. First, it relies on us being able to define rather precisely what constitutes harms to others. When the Millian principle is used in bioethics, it is often combined with a rather narrow concept of harm, partly because this is what Mill himself does in *On Liberty*, partly because a combination with a wider or thicker concept of harm could lead to rather illiberal conclusions. But it is not self-evident that the politically (or philosophically) relevant conception of harm can be restricted in a way that does, for instance, leave out harm to the reasonable sensibilities of others, or harm to the environment, or harm to social networks and cohesiveness.

The exact demarcation of what harms should count as those kinds of 'harms to others' that can justify interference with liberty is itself a contentious issue.

Second, the call for freedom often paradoxically has to be combined with a call for state action. Many of the goals that are aimed at through an effective exercise of individual freedom can only be achieved if the legal order is arranged in such a way that the actions create the legal effects people want. Stem cell researchers want to be able to patent stem cell lines, women pursuing pregnancy through insemination with their dead husbands' sperm want the dead men named as fathers on the birth certificates, couples pursuing surrogacy arrangements want to be immediately recognized as the child's parents, etc. Whether or not legal regulations should be changed to enable people to accomplish these goals cannot be decided by a reference to their liberty interests.

A right to patent your invention is, for instance, not a natural right, but something that is granted by society in order to further the societal goals of economic prosperity and promotion of useful inventions, by creating positive incentives to invent. It is thus impossible to discuss whether stem cell lines should be patentable, without discussing whether society should promote the derivation of stem cell lines, since granting patentability would have the express aim of promoting the derivation of cell lines through the creation of larger and/or more certain economic incentives than exist without patentability.

Third, unless we adopt a libertarian approach where the state has no role in trying to promote even a thin concept of the common good, we still have to decide how the state should allocate its resources between different claims, and that question is not answered by appeal to individual liberty. What is desired is often not only the freedom to do X, but state support in the pursuit of X. Whether all taxation is theft is a large issue in itself (for an interesting new approach, see Murphy and Nagel 2002), but there is clearly a distinct subsidiary issue about state funding of contentious activities out of tax revenues. The fact that the state allows me to pursue a certain activity (e.g. bondage and domination in the privacy of my home) does not necessarily entail that it should support this activity economically in a direct way, or that it should, for instance, support education about how best to carry out the activity.

On the other hand, it is not clear either that the state should force everyone to contribute to contentious activities that the state pursues. It is now, for instance, generally recognized that there should be a right to conscientious objection to military service (for the best extant analysis, see the collected papers in Bedau 1969), as well as conscientious objection for health care professionals in the context of abortion provision (Holm 2004). Are there any good reasons for completely ruling out conscientious objection in the context of funding of these activities, apart from reasons of practicality and expediency?

A direct appeal to liberty or freedom will, for the reasons outlined above, often fail when considering the doubly contentious issues we are discussing here. Either the activity or development in question will fall within a contested area of freedoms and the liberty argument will therefore not be (politically) decisive or compelling, or what is being sought is not only the liberty to pursue the development, but 'liberty plus', liberty plus other legal change, or liberty plus public support.

DELIBERATIVE DEMOCRACY
AND LEGITIMATE POLICY-MAKING

If we cannot solve our policy-making problems by a hole-in-one approach, like a direct appeal to liberty rights as trumps, what are our options? Are we left with a choice between populist, majority rule where the winner takes all, or rule by philosophers (or perhaps theologians) as envisaged in *The Republic*, book 6? If this was our choice, we would be in trouble since both alternatives are rather unattractive. Pure majority rule often leads to highly problematic outcomes involving discrimination of minorities, and rule by philosophers is indistinguishable from other forms of, seemingly meritocratic, oligarchy. But, fortunately the dichotomy between populism and philosophocracy is a false dichotomy. Democracy has many forms and populist democracy is only one of them (Gutmann 1993).

Democracy is not only a mechanism for the aggregation of preferences, as in pure populist democracy, but also a mechanism for an examination of and societal discourse about the preferences before they are aggregated. The legitimacy of a given policy is based not only on whether it was enacted according to the current legal rules, but also on the quality of deliberation preceding the policy, on the decisive reasons for the policy, and on its congruence with basic freedoms.

Bioethicists therefore have at least to acknowledge that in liberal democracies the question of getting the right policies implemented cannot be divorced from the question of what constitutes legitimate political procedures and discourse.

As the large literature on deliberative democracy shows, specifying the conditions for political legitimacy is in itself a contentious exercise and fraught with difficulty. There are many theories of deliberative democracy, each with its own normative foundation. In the following, I will mainly draw on the Rawlsian version as proposed by Rawls in 'Political Liberalism' (Rawls 1996) and on the considerations in Gutmann and Thompson's 'Moral Conflict and Political Consensus' (Gutmann and Thompson 1990).[5] This choice is made for two reasons, first because the practical implications of this version of deliberative democracy are relatively clear, second because its theoretical framework is congruent with the mainstream analytic tradition that also encompasses much of Anglo-American bioethics. I do, however, think that very similar conclusions would be reached if we applied the other main branch of thinking on deliberative democracy developed by Jürgen Habermas (1992). There are distinct theoretical differences between Habermas and Rawls in the justification of deliberative democracy and its procedures (Habermas 1995; Rawls 1995), but very few differences at the pragmatic level of actual exercises of deliberative democracy.

---

[5] Rawls himself only argues that his approach should be applied to the setting up and modifying of the basic structures of a given society, i.e. at the constitutional level.

The basic premisses of deliberative democracy are (1) that there is an in practice irreducible plurality of reasonable comprehensive world-views in modern societies[6] because of what Rawls calls the 'Burdens of Judgment';[7] (2) that policy-making about fundamental issues should rely on public reason instead of the use of force; (3) that the aim of the use of public reason is to reach a policy that is acceptable to all as citizens because it offers them fair terms of cooperation; and (4) that 1, 2, and 3 combined justify certain restrictions on public political debate about fundamental issues, especially that it has to proceed within the confines of public reason.

Within the context of deliberative democracy it is thus important to distinguish between different kinds of debate that may all be part of the wider policy-making process. Within a comprehensive world-view, in a philosophical debate, or when thinking through the issues for oneself, the adherence to public reason is not a requirement, it is only a requirement in the public debate, between persons holding different comprehensive world-views.

What exactly are the requirements for participants in the public debate in a deliberative democracy—the features that distinguish public reason?

The main requirement is a requirement for reciprocity in public discourse. Reciprocity has two components; it entails that the principles and standards that are proposed have to be principles and standards that are viewed as reasonable for everyone to accept as fair terms of cooperation, and that there is a willingness to discuss the fair terms that others propose. As Gutmann and Thompson point out, true reciprocity can only occur if there is mutual respect, and if the participants in the debate evince two particular civic virtues: the virtue of integrity and the virtue of magnanimity[8] (Gutmann and Thompson 1990). Integrity in this context requires consistency of speech in different situations, performative consistency, and the willingness to recognize all the broader implications of the position one puts

---

[6] See the quotation at the beginning of this chapter.

[7] The burdens of judgement are those factors that lead reasonable people to hold different views on the same issues. Rawls enumerates the following six: '(a) The evidence—empirical and scientific—bearing on the case is conflicting and complex, and thus hard to assess and evaluate. (b) Even where we agree fully about the kinds of considerations that are relevant, we may disagree about their weight, and so arrive at different judgments. (c) To some extent all our concepts, and not only moral and political concepts, are vague and subject to hard cases; and this indeterminacy means that we must rely on judgment and interpretation . . . within some range . . . where reasonable persons may differ. (d) To some extent . . . the way we assess evidence and weigh moral and political values is shaped by our total experience, our whole course of life up to now; and our total experiences must always differ . . . (e) Often there are different kinds of normative considerations of different force on both sides of an issue and it is difficult to make an overall assessment. (f) Finally . . . any system of social institutions is limited in the values it can admit so that some selection must be made from the full range of moral and political values that might be realised . . . . Many hard decisions may seem to have no clear answer' (Rawls 1996: 56–7; notes removed).

[8] We will here only be discussing the civic versions of these two virtues. There are also personal virtues of integrity and magnanimity that affect our personal and intimate relations to others, but an exploration of them lie outside the scope of this chapter.

forward. Magnanimity requires the recognition of the moral status of the opposing position (i.e. treating it as a moral view and not, for instance, as mainly a politically expedient view), openness to the possibility that I might come to change my own position, and a commitment to 'search for significant points of convergence between our own understandings and those of citizens whose positions, taken in their more comprehensive form, we must reject' (Gutmann and Thompson 1990: 82).

Rawls himself summarizes the requirement of public reason in this way:

What public reason asks is that citizens be able to explain their vote to one another in terms of a reasonable balance of public political values, it being understood by everyone that of course the plurality of reasonable comprehensive doctrines held by citizens is thought by them to provide further and often transcendent backing for those values.   (Rawls 1996: 243)

When we enter the realm of public discourse concerning contentious issues, we have minimally to accept that there are other reasonable views than those we hold, and that the purpose of the public discourse is not to 'win', but to reach a solution that is mutually acceptable and respectful. In this way public discourse in a deliberative democracy differs substantially from standard philosophical discourse (see below).

Here it might be important to note that the account of reciprocity and the virtues of integrity and magnanimity is not inextricably connected to Rawls's further claim about the goal of public policy-making being an overlapping consensus. Reciprocity in public discourse is necessary even if we believe that an overlapping consensus is not realistically achievable or not the right goal at all. If we, for instance, agree with Sunstein that what we should aim for in most circumstances is an 'Incompletely Theorized Agreement' (Sunstein 1995), we would still have to discuss in a context of reciprocity to reach such an agreement.

One attempt to specify further the requirements of deliberative democracy in an important, but contested, domain of public decision-making is the framework of accountability for reasonableness in the process of policy-making on priorities in health care developed by Norman Daniels and Jim Sabin (Daniels and Sabin 1997, 2002).[9] It has four distinct components: publicity, relevance, appeals, and enforcement.

Publicity entails a call for explicitness and requires that the rationale for priority decisions be made accessible to the wider public and open for scrutiny. Relevance is a requirement to screen out irrationality in priority-setting. Priority decisions must be made only in accordance with reasons that reasonable people will agree are relevant and adequate. The appeals component is an institutional mechanism

---

[9] I owe significant parts of my account of accountability for reasonableness to a collaboration with Andreas Hasman.

that provides persons with an opportunity to dispute and challenge decisions that have gone against them, as well as providing organizations with an option to revise decisions in light of further arguments. Enforcement simply entails public or voluntary regulation of the decision process, to ensure that the three other components are maintained (Daniels and Sabin 1998).

A concrete decision process, which incorporates the components of accountability for reasonableness, will therefore have to meet requirements for both structure and content. An appropriate institutional setting must be put in place in the form of a group of reasonable people, and a procedure for appropriate deliberation amongst them established. An organizational structure that assures the dissemination of the group's reasons and decisions to the public must also be implemented. Moreover, similar but separate decision processes will have to be set up to deal with appeals and enforcement of decisions internally. These are all requirements for the structure of the process. A different set of requirements relates to the content of the process of decision-making and the specification of appropriate deliberation. Daniels and Sabin think of the relevance component as a constraint on deliberation and contend that any rationale for a decision must be reasonable. A rationale is reasonable if it appeals to reasons that are accepted by people who are disposed to finding mutually justifiable terms of cooperation, as relevant to how the varied health needs of a defined population are met under reasonable resource constraints (Daniels and Sabin 1997).

This approach has been tried in a number of health care institutions and has been shown to produce agreement around results that are seen as legitimate by the various stakeholders (Martin et al. 2003).

Is the Standard Model of Bioethics Analysis Incompatible with Deliberative Democracy?

The discussion so far raises an interesting question. Is the standard model of bioethics analysis incompatible with public discussion in a deliberative democracy?

By the standard model of bioethics analysis I mean the following process (this is clearly a simplification, but not excessively so). (1) A putative moral problem is identified; (2) it is analysed and sharpened in various ways, often to the point where it is stated that 'We can now see that the problem is essentially...'; (3) a number of solutions to this refined problem are canvassed, and counter-arguments claimed to be decisive are marshalled against all but one of them (or in some cases against all of them); (4) positive arguments in support of the remaining solution (or a new solution brought in at this stage) are presented;[10] (5) a definitive conclusion is reached.

This model is an internalized variant of what James Sterba calls the 'warmaking model of doing philosophy' and describes in the following way:

I was once asked by a well-known philosopher why I talked to libertarians. At the time, I was dumbstruck by the question, but now I believe that it reflects the dominant way that philosophy is being done these days, and maybe even the dominant way that philosophy has always been done. It sees philosophers as belonging to different groups within which there can be a significant degree of sympathetic understanding but between which there can only be hostile relations, a virtual state of war. If you believe this is the case, then there really is a question about whether you should talk to your philosophical enemies. You may perchance say something that indicates certain problems with your own philosophical view, which may in turn be used against you, and, as a result, you may lose an important philosophical battle and your reputation may decline accordingly   (Sterba 1998; 2–3)

Sterba's description is rather stark, but it is not too far off the mark.

Implicit in the standard model are a number of assumptions about the aims of philosophical analysis and the relationship between the view that is argued for, and the competing views—most importantly in the present context the assumption that most opposing views are not only wrong in some sense, but that this can also be shown decisively to be the case. The views are not only wrong; they are also irrational, or at least unreasonable. When the bioethicist enters the public debate, it is therefore with the firm conviction that most of the views being put forward by others have already been shown to be unreasonable. There is no reason to take account of them or to let them influence decision-making. Discussing them is only worthwhile as a tactical manoeuvre to get your own arguments on the table, or in order to show them to be unreasonable.

The standard model, and to an even greater extent the rhetoric of bioethics, imply that there is only one right solution to each policy-making decision, that it is possible to find this solution, and to know that it is the right decision. 'Knowing that you are right' is in general a bar to a positive engagement with the views of others,[11] but 'knowing that you are right after proper philosophical reflection' can be even more problematic.

In contrast, theorizing about deliberative democracy proceeds from the assumption that, whereas there might be a right solution, it is often impossible to find this solution or to know that it is the right solution in any absolute sense. The best we can do is to outline the area of acceptable policies, and then choose a policy within this area through a deliberative, democratic process.

---

[10] It is a feature of much bioethics writing (and of philosophical argument in general) that the negative arguments against other positions are often more convincing than the positive arguments for the author's own position.

[11] As is evidenced in many domestic rows.

If philosophers participate in the public discourse about contentious issues in the same way as they engage in philosophical discourse, they are very likely to breach many of the requirements for an engagement in public reason. But they will also have engaged in a social category mistake. Attempting to reach a legitimate public policy in a morally pluralistic liberal democracy is not a social activity of the same kind as trying to win a philosophical argument.

If all participants in a public debate adopted a war-making approach to the debate, we would eventually only have recourse to simple, non-deliberative voting for resolving our differences. Let us now move on to some more specific problems.

Hope and Hype, Doom and Gloom

A specific problem arises in those cases where our efforts of public decision-making, including public debate and deliberation, take place at such an early state of the development of a given technology that the scientific uncertainty is very large. In such cases there will typically be two scenarios painted by the proponents and the opponents of the new development, a 'Hope and Hype' scenario promising untold benefits if the technology is developed and a 'Doom and Gloom' scenario threatening all kinds of risks from the new technology. In retrospect, it often becomes evident that both of the two scenarios were wrong, and often for the very same reason—they both overestimated the new technology and its powers. In the case of human genetics it does, for instance, appear likely that Gregory Stock's *Redesigning Humans* will eventually be shown to fall within the 'Hope and Hype' category, and Francis Fukuyama's *Our Posthuman Future* in the 'Doom and Gloom' category (Stock 2002; Fukuyama 2002).

Historically it is interesting that a significant segment of the early bioethicist community in the late 1960s and early 1970s were very sceptical towards the development of new medical technologies, seeing them as potentially dangerous, either because the technologies would increase the power of the medical profession, or because they would lay our lives open to more commercial influences. This technology-sceptical stream in bioethics seems to have been somewhat marginalized in recent times, at least in Anglo-American bioethics, where it has been replaced by a marked enthusiasm for new technologies that are seen as liberating. In contrast to this development in bioethics, there is still a significant sceptical attitude towards the blessings of new technologies in environmental ethics.

Generally our ethical analysis and our policy-making are likely to go astray if we do not get the scientific facts right, a point often made in debates concerning the moral status of the embryo, but they are equally likely to go wrong if we do not get the scientific predictions right. Both too enthusiastic and too pessimistic evaluations of the science and its practical implications can seriously bias ethical argument.

John Harris has pointed out many times that it must be the ends that justify the means, but this means that if we get our prediction of the actually achievable ends wrong, we may end up allowing, or prohibiting, the use of means that should not have been allowed or prohibited.

In a society where technology is generally seen as a good, the tendency to overestimate the good effects of new technology is strong. As Khushf and Best point out, following Horkheimer and Adorno:

> Enlightened science promises the means for entering a realm of light and hope, but this means slides over into its opposite, resulting in an empty and dehumanizing rhetoric of justification. Minimally in the light of the accomplishments of science, we are forced to reassess what has been promised. One way of reading this history is to say that we should be sceptical of all utopian accounts that see the promised land emerging in this worldly terms. (Khushf and Best 2002: 37–8)

But underestimation may also occur. One example of this occurred in the ethical analysis of genetic testing. Before the development of gene-chips allowing the simultaneous detection of many gene variants, a lot of papers on the ethics of genetic testing and screening were written that explicitly relied on the empirical premiss that it was only possible to test for one or a few gene variants at the same time, and that testing and screening would therefore always be directed in the sense that one would always be looking for something specific. Worries about screening creating a genetic underclass were dismissed, because this could only happen if many genes could be screened at the same time. But we now know that the empirical premiss used in the argument was false.

Overestimation of the final impact of a given development may be a conscious rhetorical ploy, in which case it is clearly ethically problematic,[12] but it may also be an effect of a tendency to analyse new technologies in isolation from other concurrent developments. At a given point in time there will often be many different approaches to the solution of a particular problem, e.g. many different therapies being developed for the same condition. If we look at each of these in isolation we are likely to overestimate its importance,

---

[12] A subset of this issue is the ethical problems raised by far too optimistic predictions of timescale between initial scientific breakthrough and routine application. In the case of stem cells, the public was promised real benefits within five to ten years. Many years have now elapsed of the five to ten years and the promised therapies are still not anywhere close to routine clinical use. There are similarities to the initial enthusiastic presentation of gene therapy in the late 1980s and the later problems encountered, and some reason to fear that stem cell therapies will have an equally long trajectory between theoretical possibility and clinical practice.

It is clearly ethically problematic to raise false expectations in seriously ill people, and even more problematic if this is partly done from self-interest (e.g. to promote one's own research in the media).

because we bracket the consideration that one of the other concurrent developments may be developed first and corner the market, may turn out to be better overall or better for a subclass of people with the condition. Even good technologies are in a competitive race, and if we forget then we will often hugely overestimate their future positive and negative impact (an error made by many phone companies in assessing the value of third-generation cell phone licences).

All of these problems could be solved for the bioethicist and the policy-maker if it was possible to get accurate, reliable, and unbiased estimates of the likely effectiveness and long-term impact of new scientific developments. Getting such estimates is, however, exceedingly difficult. It may be the case, as in the current stem cell debate, that the best experts all have an interest to defend and that their estimates of the success of the line of research they pursue is therefore likely to be consciously or unconsciously biased. But even where this is not the case, and where it is possible to find unbiased experts, predicting long-term impact is very difficult, partly for the reasons mentioned above concerning competing technologies, partly because long-term impact will depend on and interact with the social embedding of the technology. To give an example, it was predictable that the development of really small cell phones would change our modes of communication in profound ways, and perhaps predictable that they would become fashion accessories; but no one predicted (or could have predicted?) the immense success of the cell phone, not as a phone (i.e. a device for oral communication) but as a sender of small text messages, or the rapidly growing market in ring tones.

It may even be impossible for the researchers involved in a given research programme to provide the necessary facts for a proper policy analysis, because the science is moving forward very quickly. Believing some aspect of a developing technology to be a stable feature of that technology is therefore always dangerous. One of the members of the Geron Ethicist Advisory Board describes her experiences with the information given to the Board:

The Geron board was introduced formally to the notion of the hunt for hES [human embryonic stem] cells with a careful scientific explanation of the mechanism of the research and the motivation for the science itself. . . . A second focus of concern that arose early was the use of embryos. Our understanding was that embryos were graded (1–4) with grades 1 and 2 considered useable for implantation, and grades 3 and 4 considered too physically imperfect to be used. . . . We understood at that time that no embryos would be created for the purposes of research, that embryos would be donated under the most stringent system of informed consent, and that these embryos would have been discarded in any case. . . . In the next few months the science rapidly moved forward, and hence our elaborate rationale, although certainly interesting, became archaic. Since the norm for implantation was now two instead of five, many more embryos were available but would not be used by a particular couple, giving rise to a new ethical problem of 'spare' embryos and their use and storage.[13] (Zoloth 2002: 4–5; notes removed)

Even if unbiased information can be gained, the problems are not over, because such information has to be interpreted and its significance assessed.

At approximately the same time the American National Bioethics Advisory Commission and a British government expert group reviewed the evidence concerning the need for the creation of embryos specifically for stem cell research and came to two rather different conclusions. The National Bioethics Advisory Commission concluded that

Currently, we believe that cadaveric fetal tissue and embryos remaining after infertility treatments provide an adequate supply of research resources for federal research projects involving human embryos. Therefore, embryos created specifically for research purposes are not needed at the current time in order to conduct important research in this area . . .

We conclude that at this time, because other sources are likely to provide the cells needed for the preliminary stages of research, federal funding should not be provided to derive ES [embryonic stem] cells from SCNT [somatic cell nuclear transfer]. Nevertheless, the medical utility and scientific progress of this line of research should be monitored closely. (National Bioethics Advisory Commission 1999: 71–2)

Whereas the British Chief Medical Officer's Expert Group concluded that

For some people, particularly those suffering from the diseases likely to benefit from the treatments that could be developed, the fact that research to create embryos by cell nuclear replacement is a necessary step to understanding how to reprogramme adult cells to produce compatible tissue provides sufficient ethical justification for allowing the research to proceed.   (Department of Health 2000: 40)

What was a fact for one group of experts was clearly not a fact for the other. What is at play here is a different evaluation of the available scientific evidence, but possibly also a different approach to the decision of whether a line of research should be deemed 'necessary'. Is a particular line of research only necessary if it is the only way to get the knowledge we need for stem cell therapies, or is it necessary if scientific progress will otherwise be slowed down and will be much more costly, but will eventually lead to stem cell therapies anyway even if this particular line of research is not pursued (Holm 2001)?

There is no principled way to solve the problems around scientific prediction and its interpretation. We can do better if we base our ethical and policy analysis on a range of possible developments of a technology, instead of relying on only one prediction, but we can never be sure that any of our scenarios will actually match the future. Policy decisions at the early stages of technology development should therefore almost always be seen as tentative, and not definitive.

---

[13] It would be interesting to know how this could be classified as a new problem, since it has been discussed for more than ten years; see e.g. Holm (1993).

PATH DEPENDENCE AND THE *ex ante* POSITION

Philosophical discussion of ethical issues and ethical policies sometimes takes place as if we are drawing policy on a blank slate, or deducing the right policy from first principles.

Reference to already existing regulation is only made in two situations, either to criticize it for being wrong, inconsistent, and incoherent, or conversely in consistency arguments allegedly showing that already existing policies imply certain views concerning ethics, for instance concerning the ethical status of the embryo.

But does it make sense to conceive of public policy-making as a series of unconnected acts where each can be considered on its own, without any reference to past decisions? Does where we are now, in terms of laws and policies, not at least to some extent determine where we can go and what means we should choose to get there?

There are reasons to be sceptical about the strength of consistency arguments from existing policy. In order to get the consistency argument off the ground, we almost always have to reconstruct the underlying justification for the policy, because such a justification is very rarely given explicitly, except if the decision is a judicial decision. There are usually many possible reconstructions, and committing the policy-maker to only one of these may be impossible.

Consistency arguments may, furthermore, fail completely if the policy is a result of a compromise, either because the policy-makers have openly engaged in a compromise with some other group, or because they have taken the views of some other group into account already when drafting the regulation (for instance, in order to ensure a smooth passage through the political process). If a regulation is based on a political compromise, it may well be the case that no one wants to defend or justify the position reached in the regulation, except as a legitimate result of a legitimate political process. This means that there is no argument to reconstruct, and no one saying A whom we can also commit to say B.

An example could be the abortion legislation in countries allowing abortion on demand until a certain gestational age. It is unlikely that many people would actually claim to have an argument that can justify the exact limit legislated in a specific country, but many more might be willing to accept it as a legitimate political compromise between those wanting a higher limit and those wanting a lower limit. Therefore, such laws do not necessarily imply that something radical is thought to happen to the moral status of the fetus or the moral rights of the mother when the gestational age in question is reached.

In implying further consequences of official policy we also need to take into account that there are limits to the preciseness with which one can draft regulation, and that ethically extraneous factors play a role. As Beauchamp and Childress write:

Public policy is often formulated in contexts that are marked by profound social disagreements, uncertainties, and different interpretations of history. No body of abstract moral principles and rules can determine policy in such circumstances, because it cannot contain enough specific information or provide direct and discerning guidance. The specification and implementation of moral principles and rules must take account of problems of feasibility, efficiency, cultural pluralism, political procedures, uncertainty about risk, noncompliance by patients, and the like.   (Beauchamp and Childress 2001: 8–9)

In evaluating official policy it is also very important not to forget that the ideal policy has to be both locally and globally coherent and consistent, and that maximal coherence in a body of regulations may be achieved by allowing some local inconsistencies. In many legal systems it is, for instance, accepted that a major change in legal status occurs at birth. This principle permeates many areas of law, including the laws outside those strictly dealing with reproductive matters, and it is at least arguable that global consistency is better served by upholding it in all cases, even if there are a few cases where it might seem to be locally inconsistent.

Let us look at a specific example. In the context of stem cell research, one particular consistency argument is often put forward claiming that because destructive research using embryos for certain purposes is already allowed in a given jurisdiction, consistency requires that we allow the destructive use of embryos for stem cell research (Harris 2002).

Many countries that presently allow experiments on embryos restrict these to experiments related to improving reproductive technologies and increasing our understanding of the biology of human reproduction. Many types of stem cell research fall outside this restriction and are therefore not permitted even though the jurisdictions in question allow other forms of research on embryos.

Can a restriction of embryo research to reproductive matters be justified? The decision to allow embryo research for a restricted range of research questions could possibly be reconstructed as an attempt to achieve consistency in a situation where embryo research is believed to be (somewhat) ethically problematic.[14] Most legal regulation of embryo research occurs within the broader context of regulation of assisted reproductive technologies, and it is evident that these technologies could only have been developed, and can only be improved, if embryo research is permitted. Any legislation that allows the use of assisted reproductive technologies and prohibits embryo research could therefore be charged with a form of performative inconsistency by prohibiting a necessary step in the development and improvement of a permitted technique.

---

[14] Many public policies seem to indicate that people are 'closet gradualists' with regard to the moral status of embryos and fetuses.

Would it then be inconsistent not to allow research using embryos with no connection to reproduction?

Michael Walzer has famously argued that society contains several separate 'spheres of justice' and that the application of principles of justice from one sphere to another is not necessarily warranted (Walzer 1983). Maybe there are also separate 'spheres of consistency' when we discuss the consistency of public regulations. This is not as strange an idea as it might perhaps initially seem.

Walzer's argument for different spheres of justice is that different social goods are different, and that unless we understand and take account of this difference in our analysis of justice we will go wrong. He writes:

No account of the meaning of a social good, or of the sphere within which it legitimately operates, will be uncontroversial. Nor is there any neat procedure for generating or testing different accounts. At best, the arguments will be rough, reflecting the diverse and conflict-ridden character of the social life that we seek simultaneously to understand and to regulate—but not to regulate until we understand. I shall set aside, then, all claims made on behalf of any single distributive criterion, for no such criterion can possibly match the diversity of social goods.   (Walzer 1983: 21)

In the same way as different social goods are different, the different social practices aimed at producing these social goods are different. The practices involved in reproduction and in securing the goods secured by reproduction are different from the practices involved in research. There is thus no prima facie reason to believe that arguments and conclusions valid in one of these areas can be transferred without modification to the other area.

In the area of reproductive ethics, the idea that there is a strong right to reproductive freedom or reproductive liberty has gained currency in recent years. If a given permissive legal regulation has been passed because of an appreciation of this right, then it is not immediately obvious that consistency requires the same kind of permissive regulation outside the sphere of reproduction. A right to reproductive liberty cannot, for instance, in itself support a permission to use embryos for non-reproduction-related purposes, like stem cell research!

In looking at consistency arguments in the public policy sphere we might also want to question whether 'as morally acceptable' is a transitive relation in this context. If p is as morally acceptable as q and q is as morally acceptable as r, have we therefore committed ourselves to the judgement that p is as morally acceptable as r?

Moral acceptability comes in at least two different forms, and the difference between them can be brought out by considering Tranøy's analysis of moral disagreement and consensus. If two people A and B discuss the morality of p there are, according to Tranøy, three different possible outcomes:

(1) Person A and B can agree that p is *unacceptable*, i.e. both mean *positively* that p should not be accepted.

(2) A and B can agree that *p* is *acceptable*, i.e. both mean *positively* that *p* should be accepted.

(3) A and B can agree that *p* is acceptable, but A or B might *abstain* from actively taking a stand on *p*.

(Tranøy 1998: 155)[15]

Tranøy calls the last option 'open consensus'.[16]

Let us call the kind of moral acceptability where both decision-makers positively affirm the moral acceptability of *p* 'moral acceptability' and the kind of moral acceptability where one of the decision-makers abstains from taking a stand on *p* 'moral acceptability*'. Let us assume that moral acceptability is transitive; does this entail that moral acceptability* is also transitive? Clearly not. The judgement of moral acceptability* may occur for a number of different reasons. The case *p* may for B be in a grey area between the clearly acceptable or the clearly unacceptable, or B may defer to A's judgement because the question at issue is much more important for A. Moral acceptability* is thus only transitive in those cases where B's reason for abstaining from actively taking a stand on *p* is shared by *q* and *r*, and since these reasons may be non-moral, transitivity of moral acceptability* only occurs if we can claim parity of reasoning for both the moral features and the non-moral features of *p*, *q*, and *r*.

It should be relatively obvious that the kind of moral acceptability that lies behind public regulation of controversial areas in bioethics is most often not moral acceptability but moral acceptability*. This means that purely ethical consistency arguments are often misapplied, because they assume a transitivity of moral acceptability that is often not there.

COMPROMISE, MORATORIUMS, AND ACCOMMODATION

A further reason why philosophical analysis and public policy may part company is that a number of standard political tools are not very prima facie appealing to the philosopher, since they may lead to decisions that are formally inconsistent, eclectically justified, or only legitimized procedurally through a proper democratic process. These tools include compromise, moratoriums, and various means of accommodating minority positions.

Prominent examples of successful and stable compromises are the abortion laws in many European countries that allow abortion on demand until a certain stage

---

[15] I owe the translation from Norwegian to Jan Helge Solbakk.
[16] Open consensus can also occur around the judgement that *p* is unacceptable if either A or B abstains from actively taking a stand on *p*.

in pregnancy and after that only allow abortion if certain criteria are fulfilled. The gestational age that is the legal cut-off point for abortion on demand varies between countries, as one would expect of a result of local political compromise. No one tries to defend their particular cut-off point as the uniquely right one, but the policies are remarkably stable within each society. They have given women significant reproductive freedom, they have removed the harm previously caused by illegal abortions, and they have to some degree accommodated the rather common belief that fetuses are morally significant and that this significance increases through pregnancy. This stability is clearly a political or societal and not a philosophical stability. There are strong arguments on one side to allow abortion on demand throughout pregnancy (this follows from some personhood views of moral status and from some analyses of reproductive liberty as a human right) and there are on the other side strong arguments for never allowing abortion on demand (this follows from some views giving significant moral status to all human individuals). It is, however, rather obvious that a policy implementing one of these philosophical positions would be politically highly unstable.

Instituting a moratorium can also be a very useful and legitimate political technique. If there is genuine scientific uncertainty, a well-crafted moratorium blocking certain possibly problematic uses of a technology may allow time to resolve the scientific uncertainty before a final public policy decision is made. It could even be argued that in a deliberative democracy there should always be an initial moratorium, or at least a period of cautious development, while the necessary societal deliberation about the implications of a new technology takes place. Referring the issue at hand to a national ethical council or similar body often combines two functions: it creates a moratorium-like situation while the body deliberates, and it promotes wider societal discussion.

Like all other human activities, policy-making carries opportunity costs. There are a limited number of policy decisions that can be made (e.g. because of limits on parliamentary time or on the number of issues in which the executive can simultaneously invest political capital), and this entails that it is important to get the policy right the first time and/or to have a policy that is sufficiently flexible to accommodate new technological and social developments. This is often *better* achieved if there is no rush to comprehensive regulation, but more time to assess the real implications of a given technology.

Accommodating minority positions[17] in different ways is not only politically expedient; it is also a way of showing proper mutual respect. If a society eventually decides to allow and support embryonic stem cell research, one way of accommodating those opposing this research could, for instance, be to provide generous

---

[17] In a deliberative democracy it may be the case that the policy that is implemented is not the majority position but a position that is actually only held by a minority, if for instance the policy is passed owing to moral–political agreement in the third of Tranøy's senses (see above). In that case it may be relevant to accommodate the majority position!

funding for research into adult stem cells so that there would be real competition between the two alternative sources of stem cells, or to take measures to ensure that as few embryos as possible were used in research. Both accommodations would show that the reasonable concern for embryos that was suppressed in the final public policy was nevertheless considered with respect.

CONCLUSION

Being a bioethicist myself with fairly clear and well-justified (at least in my own estimation) views on a range of contentious issues, I would have liked to be able to conclude that society ought to implement the results of good ethical analysis as public policy straight away.

However, like everyone else, I have to recognize that, despite the fact that I think I have good (and to me decisive) arguments against those who disagree with me, their disagreement is often not unreasonable, given that we are unable to agree on some of the basic premises even after all the arguments have been put on the table. They and I have to live together in the same society, and just as I would not like to have their views imposed as public policy, I should not try to impose my view, either directly or indirectly through the use of questionable rhetorical strategies in the public debate. It is only if we all adhere to the civic virtues of integrity and magnanimity that there is any chance of our finding those areas of practical convergence that allow peaceful public decision-making in a context of fundamental moral disagreement. This may require philosophers to shed some of their bad habits, but if they feel hard done by, they should think how much more difficult the task of developing these virtues will be for many politicians!

REFERENCES

American Journal of Bioethics (2002), 2/1.
BEAUCHAMP, T. L., and CHILDRESS, J. F. (2001), *Principles of Biomedical Ethics*, 5th edn. (Oxford: Oxford University Press).
BEDAU, H. A. (ed.) (1969), *Civil Disobedience* (New York: Pegasus).
Bioethics (2002), 16/6.
DANIELS, N., and SABIN, J. (1997), 'Limits to Health Care: Fair Procedures, Democratic Deliberation, and the Legitimacy Problem for Insurers', *Philosophy and Public Affairs*, 4: 303–50.
——— (1998), 'Last Chance Therapies and Managed Care: Pluralism, Fair Procedures, and Legitimacy', *Hastings Center Report*, 28/2: 27–41.
——— (2002), *Setting Limits Fairly: Can We Learn to Share Medical Resources?* (Oxford: Oxford University Press).

DEPARTMENT OF HEALTH (2000), *Stem Cell Research: Medical Progress with Responsibility: A Report from the Chief Medical Officer's Expert Group Reviewing the Potential of Developments in Stem Cell Research and Cell Nuclear Replacement to Benefit Human Health* (London: Department of Health).

FUKUYAMA, F. (2002), *Our Posthuman Future* (New York: Profile).

GUTMANN, A. (1993), 'Democracy', in R. E. Goodin and P. Pettit (eds.), *A Companion to Contemporary Political Philosophy* (Oxford: Blackwell), 411–21.

—— and THOMPSON, D. (1990), 'Moral Conflict and Political Consensus', *Ethics*, 101/1: 64–88.

HABERMAS, J. (1992), *Faktizität und Geltung* (Frankfurt am Main: Suhrkamp).

—— (1995), 'Reconciliation Through the Public Use of Reasons: Remarks on John Rawls's Political Liberalism', *Journal of Philosophy*, 92/3: 109–31.

HARRIS, J. (2002), 'The Ethical Use of Human Embryonic Stem Cells in Research and Therapy', in J. Burley and J. Harris (eds.), *A Companion to Genethics* (Oxford: Blackwell), 158–74.

—— and HOLM, S. (2003), 'Abortion', in H. La Follette (ed.), *The Oxford Handbook of Practical Ethics* (Oxford: Oxford University Press), 112–35.

HELD, D. (1992), 'Democracy: From City-States to a Cosmopolitan Order', *Political Studies*, 40: 10–39.

HOLM, S. (1993), 'The Spare Embryo—A Red Herring in the Embryo Experimentation Debate', *Health Care Analysis*, 1/1: 63–6.

—— (2001), 'European and American Ethical Debates About Stem Cells: Common Underlying Themes and Some Significant Differences', in Nordic Committee on Bioethics, *The Ethical Issues in Stem Cell Research* (Copenhagen: Nordic Council of Ministers), 35–45.

—— (2002), 'Going to the Roots of the Stem Cell Controversy', *Bioethics*, 16/6: 493–507.

—— (2003a), 'The Ethical Case Against Stem Cell Research', *Cambridge Quarterly of Health Care Ethics*, 12/4: 372–83.

—— (2003b), ' "Parity of Reasoning" Arguments in Bioethics: Some Methodological Considerations', in M. Häyry and T. Takala (eds.), *Scratching the Surface of Bioethics* (Amsterdam: Rodopi), 47–56.

—— (2004), 'Conscientious Objection and Civil Disobedience in the Context of Assisted Reproductive Technologies', *Türkiye Klinikleri Journal of Medical Ethics*, 11/4: 215–20.

Kennedy Institute of Ethics Journal (2002), 12/2.

KHUSHF, G., and BEST, R. G. (2002), 'Stem Cells and the Man on the Moon: Should We Go There From Here?', *American Journal of Bioethics*, 2/1: 37–9.

MARTIN, D., SHULMAN, K., SANTIAGO-SORRELL, P., and SINGER, P. (2003), 'Priority-Setting and Hospital Strategic Planning: A Qualitative Case-Study', *Journal of Health Services Research and Policy*, 8/4: 197–201.

MILL, J. S. (1987), *Utilitarianism, On Liberty, and Considerations on Representative Government* (London: Dent).

MURPHY, L. M., and NAGEL, T. (2002), *The Myth of Ownership: Taxes and Justice* (New York: Oxford University Press).

NATIONAL BIOETHICS ADVISORY COMMISSION (1999), *Ethical Issues in Human Stem Cell Research* (Rockville, Md.: NBAC).

RAWLS, J. (1995), 'Reply to Habermas', *Journal of Philosophy*, 92/3: 132–80.

RAWLS, J. (1996), *Political Liberalism (With a New Introduction and the 'Reply to Habermas')* (New York: Columbia University Press).

STERBA, J. P. (1998), *Justice for Here and Now* (Cambridge: Cambridge University Press).

STOCK, G. (2002), *Redesigning Humans* (New York: Profile).

SUNSTEIN, C. R. (1995), 'Incompletely Theorized Agreements', *Harvard Law Review*, 108: 1733–72.

TRANØY, K. E. (1998), *Det åpne sinn: Moral og etikk mot et nytt årtusen* (Oslo: Universitetsforlaget).

WALZER, M. (1983), *Spheres of Justice: A Defence of Pluralism and Equality* (Oxford: Blackwell).

ZOLOTH, L. (2002), 'Jordan's Banks: A View from the First Years of Human Embryonic Stem Cell Research', *American Journal of Bioethics*, 2/1: 3–11.

....

CHAPTER 7

TIERS WITHOUT TEARS: THE ETHICS OF A TWO-TIER HEALTH CARE SYSTEM

....

BENJAMIN J. KROHMAL AND

EZEKIEL J. EMANUEL

THE American health care system is a mess. The cost of the system has increased to nearly $2 trillion, over 16 per cent of the GDP (Levit et al. 2004; Smith et al. 2006). At least 45 million Americans are uninsured, while over the last few years more than 5 million jobs have lost health coverage (Holahan and Cook 2005). The demands of Medicaid are forcing the states to cut other services, especially education, forcing tuition hikes at public universities, and prompting states to consider ending Medicaid entirely (Coughlin and Zuckerman 2005; O'Dell and Goodwin 2005). The Medicare Trust Fund will be empty by 2020, and, according to the Medicare Trustees, enormous change is needed immediately to establish fiscal balance in the next seventy-five years: cutting benefits by 48 per cent or more than doubling the Medicare tax (Snow et al. 2005). While it may not be inevitable or imminent, escalating insolvency makes health care reform seem more probable. Indeed, leading conservatives including former Senate majority leader Bill Frist, Representative Bill Thomas, former chair of the House Ways and Means Committee, and Bill McGuire, chief executive of United Health Group have publicly called for comprehensive health system reform to repair inefficiency and under-coverage in the current health care system (McGuire 2004; Thomas 2004; Frist 2005).

American health care reformers face a number of ethical issues, including familiar debates over the merits of a single-payer system and publicly provided universal health insurance. No matter how these debates are resolved, a further ethical question must be addressed. Both universal coverage and a single-payer system are compatible with permitting some patients to pay more for faster, better, or more health care choices. Should the United States continue to have a two-tier health care system in which wealth grants some patients access to medical services that others with the same needs cannot obtain? Critical evaluation of both principled objections to inequalities and practical objections to anticipated social and medical consequences of a two-tier health care system are needed.

DIVERGENT VISIONS

In the United States public health coverage is currently limited. Most Americans rely upon whatever insurance they receive from their employer or can afford to purchase on their own. Many American insurance products are specifically designed with different tiers of service. For more money, people can access more services, have limited prior approvals and gate-keeping, and have greater choice of physicians and hospitals.

Israel, the Netherlands, and the United Kingdom also have two-tier systems. Each provides an extensive public tier of health care that can be supplemented with market tier coverage. Patients may pay extra for private hospital rooms or longer stays, more treatment options, and faster access by jumping queues for procedures with long waiting times, like hip replacement or cataract surgery. In Israel as much as 70 per cent of the population purchases additional coverage (Boaz Lev, personal communication, 2006).

Norway and Canada strive for a single tier of health care, though, short of draconian restrictions, completely eliminating the influence of wealth in health care may be impossible. For instance, wealth allows the affluent to obtain medical services out of country that are unavailable to their compatriots. Nevertheless, Norway and Canada each have explicitly egalitarian systems that prohibit a private market for any services covered by their universal national health care plans. However, in the 2005 decision *Chaoulli* v. *Quebec*, Canada's Supreme Court ruled some of Canada's egalitarian restrictions on health care distribution to be unconstitutional, requiring the expansion of private markets for health care. Ethical controversy in Canada pits those who support 'equal access for equal needs' against those who defend a tiered health care system that allows some medical services to be distributed by the market (Flood and Sullivan 2005).

Reformers in America must consider whether it just for a system to allow a market tier of health care services, a tier in which a set of services or amenities are available only to those who can afford them. Do Canada and Norway's prohibitions on payment for greater access to medical care provide an ethical model that the United States should follow? Does the two-tier British and Israeli model offer a more just alternative? What are the ethics of a two-tier health care system?

The remainder of this chapter reviews the main ethical arguments against a two-tier health care system, and then presents a rebuttal of those arguments (Table 1). The chapter concludes that justice not only permits but requires America to retain two tiers of health care, though significant changes are required in order to meet five criteria for an ethical two-tier system.

OBJECTIONS TO A TWO-TIER SYSTEM

Opponents of a market tier usually begin their objections by noting that health care is special. Health is 'a necessary condition for pursuing nearly all the goals around which we organize our lives' (Brock and Daniels 1994). Health care is a universally recognized need and is central to the opportunities involved in leading a normal human life (Scanlon 1975; Walzer 1983; Daniels 1995). Without good health it is difficult to achieve and enjoy valuable ends: rich family life, meaningful work, the arts, nature, athletics, hobbies, and leisure. This makes access to health care more important than access to other resources. As Descartes claimed more than 400 years ago, 'the preservation of health is undoubtedly the first good and the foundation of all the other goods in this life' (Descartes 1988: 143). While market influences on many goods may lead to inegalitarian outcomes that are nevertheless ethical, such inequality is unjust when it comes to matters as fundamentally important as health.

This conclusion is often left to stand on its own; however, it might be motivated by several considerations:

Only Need Matters

Bernard Williams argues that wealth is morally irrelevant when it comes to distributing health care (1962). Justice, notes Williams, requires treating relevantly similar cases alike, and relevance, he claims, is determined by the goal of the activity in question. In hiring a lawyer, the goal is finding qualified representation, so experience is a relevant difference but race is not. In grading students, the goal is to assess academic achievement, so demonstrated knowledge is the relevant difference

TABLE 1 Objections to a two-tier health care system and replies

Objection	Description	Response
Only need is relevant	Need should be the basis for distributing health care. Wealth is not a relevant basis for the distribution of important services	Justice requires providing a certain level of medical services to all, but the liberties of health care workers cannot be ignored. Since providers have valid claims to compensation, patients' need cannot be the only morally relevant consideration
Level of opportunity	Health must be restored for people to have a fair level of opportunity. This requires ensuring universal access to all medical services, or exhausting all public and private funds in the attempt	Health is not the only important good, and beyond a certain point further taxation and the resulting economic inefficiency limits more opportunity than it restores
Equality of opportunity	Only an equal share of opportunity is fair, and medical benefits increase opportunity. Therefore, there must be equal access to medical services	The priority of the health care system should be improving health, not equalizing it by lowering everyone to the level society can afford
Difference principle	Inequalities are only just when they are to the benefit of the worst off. A market tier of health allows inequality that does not benefit the worst off	The difference principle permits people to earn and spend unequal shares of wealth on desirable goods because it provides incentive for economic efficiency that benefits the worst off
Public good	Public funds extensively subsidize the health care system, so medical services must be equally available to all members of the public	Public health care subsidies are partial, and even full public ownership does not require that services be free or equally available
Undermining	A market tier will undermine access to health care for the disadvantaged by reducing physicians' incentive to treat the poor and by limiting the incentive of the upper class to support adequately funding public health coverage	Undermining is avoided by meeting the five criteria outlined for an ethical health care system, including public funding for universal non-means tested coverage with an adequate core benefits package

but sex is not. In treating a patient, the goal is preserving and restoring health, so medical need is the relevant criterion for distribution, but wealth, race, and sex are not. A market tier is 'straightforwardly the situation of those whose needs are the same not receiving the same treatment, though the needs are the ground of the treatment' (Williams 1962: 122). Like racial or sex discrimination, a market tier is unjust because it allows different treatment for relevantly similar patients.

Fair Opportunity

A strong entitlement to health care is most often defended by appealing to the principle of fair or equal opportunity (Daniels 1995). Rawls famously defends one version of this principle, which states that before any market produced social or economic inequalities can be just, they must be 'attached to offices and positions open to all under conditions of fair equality of opportunity' (1999: 266). Rawls argues further that society must take positive steps to ameliorate 'social contingencies and natural fortune' that arbitrarily stand in the way of opportunity (1999: 63). Ill health seems to be one component of natural fortune that arbitrarily limits opportunity. Someone who is sick will not have the same opportunity to attain advantaged offices or positions as someone who is healthy.

Fair equality of opportunity may be construed with emphasis on the *level* of opportunity or emphasis on the *equality* of opportunity. Daniels takes the former approach to health care, and Rawls has endorsed his general method (Rawls 1996: 184). Daniels holds that there is an absolute level of health—'normal species functioning'—that allows for fair opportunity when met or exceeded. Some might argue that if species' typical functioning is required for fair equality of opportunity, economic inequalities cannot be just until society does everything possible to eliminate deficits in normal species functioning; in effect to eliminate ill health. After meeting this requirement, there will either be no medical advantages over the public tier that a market tier could provide, or there will be no disposable wealth left with which to pay for them.

Alternatively, some hold that what matters for fairness is not the level of opportunity but rather that everyone have an equal share of opportunity. To the extent that health care improves health and increases opportunity, allowing a market tier of health care is unjust because it enables those who are already privileged to achieve an even more unequal share of opportunity.

The Difference Principle

Rawls argues that once fair equality of opportunity has been achieved to the extent possible, inequalities are regulated by what he calls the 'difference principle'. The difference principle states that economic and social inequalities must be 'arranged so that they are . . . to the greatest expected benefit of the least advantaged' (Rawls 1999: 1972). Unequal distributions are unjust unless the worst off are better off with the inequality than without it. Allowing the affluent to pay for greater access to a good as important as health care is unjust because it produces significant inequality without benefiting the poor. As one commentator explains Rawls's position, a market tier 'effectively severs the moral and economic bonds linking the "have nots" with the "haves". . . Whereas Rawls insists that any inequalities enjoyed by the rich should also benefit the poor' (Arras 1981: 32).

Non-mutually beneficial inequalities of this kind are made worse by undermining the self respect of the less affluent (Gutmann 1981; Dickman 1983; Daniels 1998). Social cooperation and solidarity fosters a sense of self worth, and flourishes when the advantages of the most fortunate serve also to bolster the standing of the least. On the other hand, a market tier in health services distances the fate of the ill and wealthy from the fate of the ill and poor, diminishing social solidarity. A means tested public tier of health care imposes further indignity by requiring proof of poverty before granting access to services.

A Public Good

Two further objections are raised against a market tier of health care. Some have argued that health care workers owe their products and services to all, regardless of patients' ability to pay, because of significant public subsidies of the health care system. In the United States tax revenue and deductions account for nearly half of all spending on health care (Smith et al. 2006). The American health care system is subsidized at every level—through funding research, construction of medical facilities, supplementing medical education, public health measures, and provision of medical services. Critics of a market tier object to making health care a public good in its creation and funding but a private, market good when distributed. It is claimed that 'so long as communal funds are spent, as they currently are . . . the services that these expenditures underwrite must be equally available to all citizens' (Walzer 1983: 90). And 'it is unethical [for a physician] to take publicly-provided skills and use them on behalf of only those who can pay him whatever he charges, as though his education and skills were entirely his own to do with as he likes' (Marcia Angell, personal communication, 2004). Those involved in the health care system are indebted to the public, and obligated to ensure that all medical services are equally available to all patients.

Undermining the Health Care System

Finally, many opponents of a market tier emphasize a practical argument: A market tier inevitably makes the level of health care services provided to the poor inadequate. It is an old adage in American politics that programs for the poor become poor programs because when the relatively affluent are allowed to purchase more, they have no reason to support funding an adequate public tier. At the same time as a market tier undermines funding for an adequate public tier, it produces greater demand for the best medical practitioners to treat the richest patients, 'decreasing the quality of medical care received by the majority of citizens confined to the publicly funded sector' (Gutmann 1981: 552). Rejecting a market tier is necessary to ensure the poor and others in the public tier get adequate coverage.

DEFENSE OF A TWO-TIER SYSTEM

Defenders of a market tier usually begin their arguments by noting that public funds are scarce. Though the United States is a wealthy nation and can afford to spend massive amounts on health care, the fiscal instability of Medicare and Medicaid serves as a reminder that health care is expensive, and resources are inherently finite. Even wealthy nations must make tradeoffs—overtly or otherwise—between funding for health care, economic stability, and funding for other vitally important goods that government has obligations to provide: infrastructure, food, housing assistance, the environment, security, law enforcement, and education. America can no more afford to fund every possible medically beneficial service than it can afford to fund every possible highway project, educational opportunity, or security measure. This is not to say that health care costs might not be lowered by eliminating waste or fraud, or that the current level of taxation and distribution of funds is ideal. But even a rational economy would have to make tradeoffs in which needs are weighed against needs (Daniels 1995).

Were health care available in unlimited abundance, a national health care system could provide comprehensive coverage: all medically beneficial services for everyone at any time. Unfortunately, inescapable scarcity prevents everyone from getting everything they may need or want (Eddy 1994)—which, as Rawls argues—is precisely why justice is needed to determine those goods to which people are entitled (Rawls 1999). In a nation as wealthy as the United States, there is considerable consensus that people are entitled access to a broad spectrum of health care that is both fundamentally important and compatible with providing other vital goods. But while health is clearly important, this 'does not mean that all health care is of equal importance or that every beneficial service must be provided no matter how small or unimportant the benefit and how high the cost' (Brock and Daniels 1994).

Efficiency and Incentive

Scarcity and the need for tradeoffs lead Daniels to reject interpretations of his opportunity view as requiring comprehensive health care services (Daniels 1998). In making tradeoffs between public services, absolute priority should not be given to health care. This is especially true when the same amount of resources that could restore a marginal amount of species' typical functioning could protect more opportunity for more people if spent on housing or education or some other good. After providing some level of services, society will reach a point at which further taxation and expenditure on services to promote opportunity becomes self defeating—a point at which economic inefficiency limits opportunity more than further services would restore and enhance it. A commitment to increasing opportunity requires *not* taxing every available dollar for spending on health care and other public services. This leaves medical services that are not socially guaranteed to be included in a market tier, and allows the retention of private wealth needed to pay for them.

A similar appeal to economic efficiency is at work in applying the difference principle. Rawls recognizes that allowing some inequalities is to the benefit of the disadvantaged because the prospect of greater wealth provides an incentive for greater productivity and efficiency (1999: 68). But do the disadvantaged benefit in any way if the affluent are allowed to spend their legitimately earned wealth on health care? On the face of it, there may be no direct or obvious way that the poor benefit when the rich are allowed to spend their money on most goods. This, however, is no truer of orphan drugs than of riding lawnmowers, and the difference principle permits the wealthy to spend on either for the same reason: allowing the expenditure of wealth on desirable goods is an incentive for productivity that is to the benefit of the worst off. Provided that spending money on a market tier of health care is no worse for the poor than stuffing it under a mattress, a market tier is consistent with the difference principle. The difference principle may even provide reasons to prefer that the affluent spend on market tier health care than on luxury items: additional health benefits might make the wealthy even more productive, permitting a market tier is likely to stimulate medical innovation, and the expenditure of private funds instead of tax revenue for some medical services saves the public tier money that it can devote to expanded coverage for the poor (Fried 1976; Hoel and Saether 2003).

Greater Health, Not Equal Health

A two-tier system is not compatible with a fair opportunity principle that requires equality of opportunity, but such a principle should be rejected, especially when applied to health care. In almost all cases, access to medical care is limited by fiscal scarcity, not by scarcity of material goods, like scarce vaccines or transplantable organs. When patients pay for brand name drugs or an MRI scan, they do not in any meaningful way exhaust the amount remaining; 'as much and as good' is left for others. Further, when fiscal scarcity limits access to a medical service, access to that service cannot simply be redistributed from those who can pay to those who cannot. In such cases, why should we prefer that the affluent spend on another luxury car than on an extra MRI? Should we also prohibit payment for other meaningful goods that not all can afford—like side impact airbags or Ivy League educations?

It may be reasonable to prefer that, when possible, access to scarce resources be granted to the poor. But when this is not possible, as when cost is the limiting factor for access, it is perverse to regard the receipt of good things by the affluent as an evil to be avoided. To do so runs counter to the presumptive goal of the health care system to increase the health of the population, not to make everyone equally healthy, especially when this means limiting medical benefits by prohibiting access to care. The idea that we should increase equality by making some worse off and none better—the notion that if everyone cannot have something then no one can—is the basis of the powerful 'leveling down' objection to strict egalitarianism (Parfit 2000). Increasing equality by bringing everyone down to the level that society can afford deprives the rich of liberties and benefits without regard to helping the poor. Many share the goal of increasing equality by raising the level of health care available to the disadvantaged. However, there is at least the appearance of envy and resentment in preferring that some medical services benefit nobody than that they benefit those who are willing and able to pay for them. A just health care system focuses on whether all have enough, not on preventing the rich from getting more.

Costs are Relevant

Even if medical services need not be distributed equally, however, it is still of concern that medical services be distributed on an ethically relevant basis. Patients' ability to pay is one morally relevant consideration for determining the distribution of care. The argument that the only relevant ground for distributing services is the potential recipient's need leads to the notorious conclusion that 'the only proper criterion for the distribution of barbering services is barbering need' (Nozick 1974: 234). The contention that only need is relevant fails to recognize that service providers, and not just recipients, have legitimate claims and interests. Saint-like selflessness may be a greater virtue in medicine than in barbering, but *professional* medical ethics do not demand, nor would it be just for the state to require, that physicians *never* consider compensation in accepting patients for treatment. While there is room for disagreement over what constitutes fair compensation for medical services, whether fair compensation is provided is clearly a relevant ethical concern.

No Unrestricted Access to Partial Public Goods

Health care providers should be expected to provide some measure of public service in recognition of their reliance upon public support of the health care system (Astor and Sreenivasan 2003). However, public funds have been invested in the American health care system without any agreement from or expectation that recipients of funds ensure equal access to all subsidized products and services. Further, it is not reasonable to think that participation in a system 45 per cent funded with public dollars requires health care workers to provide 100 per cent of their products and services regardless of whether patients can pay. Even if the public fully owned the health care system, Americans are reminded each time they pay the postal service for shipping that public ownership of a service provider does not require free or equal availability of the service.

Freedom of Choice

In a free society, people have the liberty to spend more of their money on enormous houses, designer clothing, travel, personal computers, and the arts. An argument claiming that private hospital rooms, shorter waiting times for cataract surgery, or Acyclovir for oral herpes are too important to be distributed by the market would, seemingly, also rule out the free exchange by market of cell phones, gourmet food, sporting goods, fancy cars, and innumerable other non-medical goods and services. At the margin, health care is simply not more important than many commodities that people should be free to buy and sell.

Among more important medical services, some require too great a sacrifice of other necessary goods to justify public funding. Education and security are fundamentally important, but this does not mean that everyone is entitled to publicly funded postdoctoral education or a personal police escort. Similarly, justice does not require socially guaranteed access to full mouth reconstruction instead of dentures, Macugen for macular degeneration, lung volume reduction surgery for emphysema, or implantable cardio defibrillators.

In distributing scarce *public* funds, justice requires consideration of the cost and value of medical services relative to other important goods. Respect for individual liberties and autonomy leads to an inherently different standard for *private* spending (Fuchs 2004). While government must avoid spending disproportionately for the value it receives in order to make prudent tradeoffs, individuals are free to spend in accordance with their own priorities. Indeed, principles of justice are devised precisely to determine what people should be socially guaranteed and what should be left to them to purchase with their own money based on their own values. Some people who are risk averse may prefer to buy coverage for every available health care service; others will prefer cooking lessons or skiing trips to a wider range of doctors or more vision coverage. So long as the objects of public and private spending are held to different standards—the state required and entrusted to make prudent policy level tradeoffs while the individual is free to pursue personal projects—there will inevitably be some medical services, including some with a substantial impact on health, that can and should be available only if patients pay for them. As a matter of individual liberty, patients should be allowed to pay for these medical services, and physicians who have worked and studied hard should be free to meet the demand for additional medical goods (Gutmann 1981; Ames 2003).

DESIGNING AN ETHICAL TIERED SYSTEM

If the current US health care system is unjust, it is not because it has a market tier, but because it fails to ensure access to adequate health care for all Americans. The proper standard for evaluating the justice of the health care system is not whether everyone has access to the exact same services, or whether the rich can buy more services, but whether everyone is guaranteed, in a sustainable manner, an adequate set of benefits—a core benefits package. In a nation with America's resources, universal coverage with a core benefits package is affordable, morally imperative, and compatible with allowing a market tier of health care (Emanuel and Fuchs 2005).

A market tier would not simply be an add-on operating in parallel to an adequate public system. There are complex interactions between the market tier and the public tier that have unfortunately been subject to little empirical analysis (Hurley 2001). Largely without the benefit of data, critics have nonetheless reasonably speculated that a market tier could undermine public coverage for the poor. On the other hand, there is good reason to think that steps can be taken that would prevent a market tier from weakening the public system, and potentially even strengthen it by increasing medical innovation and reducing the public burden of paying for the health care of the affluent (Fried 1976; Hoel and Saether 2003).

Problems arise in America's two-tier system because the public tier is viewed as a safety net for the unlucky few who slip through the cracks in what is regarded as normal market tier health coverage. Consequently, few have a stake in ensuring an adequate minimum tier, and doctors have an incentive not to treat public tier patients. The solution is for the public tier to provide a solid floor that serves as the norm for health coverage, with the market tier serving as a ladder upward for those who want and can afford more.

A sustainable and ethical tiered health care system should meet five criteria:

1. The core benefits package should cover an adequate level of health care.
2. The core benefits package should be guaranteed to all Americans, without means testing.
3. The core benefits package should be designed to attract a sizable majority of the population to use it without supplementation to the market tier.
4. Purchases of market tier services and coverage should be made with after tax dollars and should not provide exemption from tax obligations to support the core benefits package.

5. Easy adjustment of the core benefits package should be possible in response to changes in technology, data about efficacy, and demand for market tier services.

A tiered system that meets these criteria would dramatically decrease the incentive for doctors to serve only rich patients. With everyone covered by adequate health insurance, treating patients from the 'lowest' tier would no longer be a financial burden, and limiting a practice to the market tier would rarely be fiscally sound; only a small minority of physicians could be financially successful catering to the 'rich and famous'.

Political difficulties would also be avoided by making the system non-means tested, ensuring that a substantial majority of citizens have a stake in socially guaranteed service. A universal core benefits package would offer benefits to everyone, and even the minority who choose to pay for market tier services will pay less for supplemental health insurance than they would for a full health insurance plan. While means tested welfare programs face an uphill battle for popular and political support, non-means tested Medicare and Social Security enjoy broad popularity, despite the ability of recipients to upgrade with Medigap insurance and private retirement savings. Allowing a market tier would be a political strength rather than a liability (Pauly 2004).

Any concerns about the impact of tiering on social solidarity and self respect should also be allayed by a system in which the majority utilizes the public tier for their healthcare needs. Indeed, Americans prefer and regard two tiers with an adequate minimum as the most just structure for the health care system (Frohlich and Oppenheimer 1992). Eliminating means testing circumvents the need for patients to prove that they are poor in order to receive benefits, and stigma associated with the public tier would cease when the public tier is the norm.

The criteria offered are general and require elaboration. What is an adequate core benefits package? It should begin with services that, given a fair share of society's wealth, many people would pay out of pocket to cover for themselves (Eddy 1991; Nord 1996; Dworkin 2000: 307–50; Danis et al. 2002). Such a core benefits package is likely to ensure that a small proportion of Americans buy market tier services. Importantly, determining the threshold level of participation for a sustainable universal public tier will be a challenge for policy makers who have speculated but produced little data on the topic (Rashi Fein, personal communication, 2005). While encouraging widespread use of a publicly provided core benefits package should not be difficult, the requisite threshold level of participation can be sustained by providing incentives to rely upon the core package and disincentives to buy into the market tier: eliminate the current tax exemptions for purchasing more health coverage, ensure diverse choices in the core benefits package, keep co-pays low in the core benefits package, or potentially tax higher tier medical care. A single-tier system is not required to ensure adequate health care for the poor. Indeed, of the top ten rated health care systems in the United Nations' equality oriented 2000 World Health Report, all ten allow a significant market tier (World Health Organization 2000).

CONCLUSION

What sort of replacement should Americans want for their troubled health care system? Many who are rightly concerned with the ethical foundations of the American health care system look to Canada and Norway's prohibition of a market tier of health care as an ethical model for the United States to emulate. This egalitarian approach, while well intentioned, is unjust. People should not be concerned that some of their neighbors might have 'too much' access to health care, but rather that many of their neighbors might have too little. A better example is provided by Britain, the Netherlands, and Israel's two-tier systems with universal public coverage. Limited resources prevent the public from paying for access to all health care for all people at all times. Allowing a market tier of medical services above an adequate but necessarily finite universal public tier preserves freedom of choice and achieves more equitable health care by improving access for the disadvantaged, not by limiting access for the affluent. Many questions remain for American health care reformers, but on the question of tiering, justice calls for a two-tier health care system.

REFERENCES

AMES, J. T. (2003), 'Proposals for US National Health Insurance', *JAMA* 290/21: 2798.

ARRAS, J. D. (1981), 'Health Care Vouchers and the Rhetoric of Equity', *Hastings Center Reports*, 11/4: 29–39.

ASTOR, A., and SREENIVASAN, G. (2003), 'Providing Free Care to the Uninsured: How Much Should Physicians Give?', *Annals of Internal Medicine*, 139/9: W78.

BROCK, D. W., and DANIELS, N. (1994), 'Ethical Foundations of the Clinton Administration's Proposed Health Care System', *JAMA* 271/15: 1189–96.

COUGHLIN, T. A., and ZUCKERMAN, S. (2005), 'Three Years of State Fiscal Struggles: How Did Medicaid and SCHIP Fare?', *Health Affairs (Millwood)*, W5-385-98, <http://content.healthaffairs.org/cgi/reprint/hlthaff.w5.385v1>, accessed 27 June 2006.

DANIELS, N. (1995), *Just Health Care* (New York: Cambridge University Press).

——— (1998), 'Rationing Medical Care: A Philosopher's Perspective on Outcomes and Process', *Economics and Philosophy*, 14: 27–50.

DANIS, M., BIDDLE, A. K., and DORR GOOLD, S. (2002), 'Insurance Benefit Preferences of the Low-Income Uninsured', *Journal of General Internal Medicine*, 17/2: 125–33.

DESCARTES, R. (1988), *The Philosophical Writings of Descartes*, ed. J. Cottingham, R. Stoothoff, and D. Murdoch, i (Cambridge: Cambridge University Press).

DICKMAN, R. (1983), 'Operationalizing Respect for Persons: A Qualitative Aspect of the Right to Health Care', in R. Bayer, A. Caplan, and N. Daniels (eds.), *In Search of Equity: Health Needs and the Health Care System* (New York: Plenum), 161–82.

DWORKIN, R. (2000), *Sovereign Virtue: The Theory and Practice of Equality* (Cambridge, Mass.: Harvard University Press).

EDDY, D. M. (1991), 'What Care Is "Essential"? What Services Are "Basic"?', *JAMA* 265/6: 782, 786–8.

—— (1994), 'Clinical Decision Making: From Theory to Practice. Principles for Making Difficult Decisions in Difficult Times', *JAMA* 271/22: 1792–8.

EMANUEL, E. J., and FUCHS, V. R. (2005), 'Health Care Vouchers: A Proposal for Universal Coverage', *New England Journal of Medicine*, 352/12: 1255–60.

FLOOD, C. M., and SULLIVAN, T. (2005), 'Supreme Disagreement: The Highest Court Affirms an Empty Right', *Canadian Medical Association Journal*, 173/2: 142–3.

FRIED, C. (1976), 'Equality and Rights in Medical Care', *Hastings Center Reports*, 6/1: 29–34.

FRIST, W. H. (2005), 'Shattuck Lecture: Health Care in the 21st Century', *New England Journal of Medicine*, 352/3: 267–72.

FROHLICH, N., and OPPENHEIMER, J. A. (1992), *Choosing Justice: An Experimental Approach to Ethical Theory* (Berkeley: University of California Press).

FUCHS, V. R. (2004), 'More Variation in Use of Care, More Flat-of-the-Curve Medicine', *Health Affairs (Millwood)*, suppl., VAR-104–7, <http://content.healthaffairs.org/cgi/reprint/hlthaff.var.104v1>, accessed 27 June 2006.

GUTMANN, A. (1981), 'For and Against Equal Access to Health Care', *Milbank Memorial Fund Quarterly Health and Society*, 59/4: 542–60.

HOEL, M., and SAETHER, E. M. (2003), 'Public Health Care with Waiting Time: The Role of Supplementary Private Health Care', *Journal of Health Economics*, 22/4: 599–616.

HOLAHAN, J., and COOK, A. (2005), 'Changes in Economic Conditions and Health Insurance Coverage, 2000–2004', *Health Affairs (Millwood)*, W5-498-508, <http://content.healthaffairs.org/cgi/reprint/hlthaff.w5.498v1>, accessed 27 June 2006.

HURLEY, J. (2001), 'Ethics, Economics, and Public Financing of Health Care', *Journal of Medical Ethics*, 27/4: 234–9.

LEVIT, K., SMITH, C., *et al.* (2004), 'Health Spending Rebound Continues in 2002', *Health Affairs (Millwood)*, 23/1: 147–59.

McGUIRE, W. W. (2004), 'Business Opportunities in Transforming Health Care: An Interview with William W. McGuire', *Health Affairs (Millwood)*, 23/6: 114–21.

NORD, E. (1996), 'Health Status Index Models for Use in Resource Allocation Decisions: A Critical Review in the Light of Observed Preferences for Social Choice', *International Journal of Technology Assessment in Health Care*, 12/1: 31–44.

NOZICK, R. (1974), *Anarchy, State, and Utopia* (New York: Basic Books).

O'DELL, K., and GOODWIN, J. (2005), 'Work to Welfare Jarring Change', *Springfield News-Leader* (Springfield, Mo.), 28 Aug., 1.

PARFIT, D. (2000), 'Equality or Priority?', in M. Clayton and A. Williams (eds.), *The Ideal of Equality* (New York: St Martin's Press), 81–125.

PAULY, M. V. (2004), 'Conflict and Compromise Over Tradeoffs in Universal Health Insurance Plans', *Journal of Law, Medicine and Ethics*, 32/3: 465–73.

RAWLS, J. (1996), *Political Liberalism* (New York: Columbia University Press).

_____ (1999), *A Theory of Justice*, rev. edn. (Cambridge, Mass.: Belknap Press).

SCANLON, T. M. (1975), 'Preference and Urgency', *Journal of Philosophy*, 72/19: 655–69.

SMITH, C., COWAN, C., *et al.* (2006), 'National Health Spending in 2004: Recent Slowdown Led by Prescription Drug Spending', *Health Affairs (Millwood)*, 25/1: 186–96.

SNOW, J., CHAO, E., *et al.* (2005), *Status of the Social Security and Medicare Programs: A Summary of the 2005 Annual Reports, Social Security and Medicare Boards of Trustees* (Washington, DC); 2006 version available at <http://www.ssa.gov/OACT/TRSUM/tr06summary.pdf>.

THOMAS, B. (2004), *Vision for Health Care* (Washington, DC: National Center for Policy Analysis).

WALZER, M. (1983), *Spheres of Justice: A Defense of Pluralism and Equality* (New York: Basic Books).

WILLIAMS, B. (1962), 'The Idea of Equality', in W. G. R. Peter Laslett (ed.), *Philosophy, Politics and Society* (Oxford: Blackwell), 110–31.

WORLD HEALTH ORGANIZATION (2000), *The World Health Report. Health Systems: Improving Performance* (Geneva: WHO), p. v.

CHAPTER 8

....

JUSTICE AND THE ELDERLY

....

DENNIS MCKERLIE

ETHICAL concerns about the elderly are usually treated as a matter of justice. This is partly explained by the special status of the elderly in almost all economically developed societies. Public pension systems provide them with financial support, and publicly funded health care programs help to meet their health care needs. Those who are now old will have contributed to these institutions when they were younger, but it remains true that the elderly receive a degree of support from public institutions that the members of other age-groups typically do not receive. This institutional background naturally raises questions about distributive justice. Are the elderly receiving less, or more, than their fair share of health resources and economic wealth?

Moral philosophers have proposed many different theories of justice. However, it is difficult to apply their theories to the elderly. The elderly constitute a particular age-group. They are identified as people in a certain temporal stage of their lives, old age. And philosophical theories of justice are typically concerned with people's complete lives or lifetimes, not with temporal parts of lives. For example, John Rawls's influential account of justice is concerned with achieving fairness between different people's *lifetime* expectations of receiving primary goods (Rawls 1971). Thomas Nagel comments, 'Remember that the subject of an egalitarian principle is not the distribution of particular rewards to individuals at some time, but the prospective quality of their lives as a whole, from birth to death' (Nagel 1991: 69). These theories compare the complete lifetimes of different people to decide whether they have been treated fairly. Because of their broad temporal scope, these theories cannot directly answer the question of whether a person receives a fair share of income or health care during a particular temporal part of her life.

One response is just to accept that the appropriate temporal scope for a principle of justice is a complete life. I call this the 'complete lives view'. If we make this choice we cannot immediately object to treating the elderly differently from the members of other age-groups, so long as the treatment is maintained consistently over time so that everyone is treated in that way at the appropriate temporal stage of their life. For example, a policy of mandatory retirement could not be automatically criticized as unfair. If everyone at least potentially benefits from the policy when they are young, and everyone faces the same termination date of employment when they are old, the policy will not create inequalities between people's complete lives. The same would be true, for the same reasons, of a policy restricting the use of kidney dialysis to those below a certain age.

However, this does not mean that the complete lives view has nothing to say about fairness and the elderly. Certain ways of treating the elderly might be condemned as unfair because they are likely to lead to people being treated unfairly in terms of their complete lives. For example, many public pension systems—including American social security—have a degree of progressivity built into them. Poorer people contribute less to the institution than better off people, but they receive comparatively greater (although not absolutely greater) benefits in return for their contribution. A possible justification for the progressivity is that it reduces the inequality that would otherwise exist between people's complete lives. So a non-progressive pension system might be regarded as unfair.

Also, someone who holds the complete lives view can give other reasons—reasons that are not a matter of justice—for a particular form of income support or health care for those who are old. Someone who thinks that justice focuses exclusively on complete lives would probably suggest that once the requirements of justice for complete lives are satisfied we should divide resources between age-groups in whichever way would benefit people the most. For example, making a particular form of expensive health care available to the very old will be justified if this use of limited resources improves people's lives more on balance than the alternative policy of concentrating the resources on younger people. According to this view, denying that form of care to the elderly would not be an injustice, but it would be the wrong choice to make.

However, many writers believe that there are distinctive principles of justice for age-groups. For this to be the case, the principles must have a temporal scope other than complete lives. They must make claims about distribution between the temporal parts or temporal stages of lives.

The most influential view of this sort has been developed by Norman Daniels, although many other writers share the same idea and apply it to a variety of questions about fairness to the elderly (see Daniels 1988, 1996; Dworkin 2000, ch. 8; Brock 1993, chs. 11, 12). Daniels calls the theory the 'prudential lifespan account'.

The theory says that the fair social distribution between age-groups should match how a hypothetical prudentially rational individual would choose to distribute the same resources over the different temporal stages of her own life. The elderly deserve, as a matter of justice, the share of resources that prudence would award to the temporal stage of old age in considering a single lifetime.

The theory claims that the distribution established by prudence expresses genuine claims of justice concerned with temporal stages of lives. It differs from the complete lives view in holding that there can be injustice to an age-group even if the principles of justice for complete lives are fully satisfied (for example, even if people's complete lifetimes are perfectly equal). However, the theory does not completely abandon the complete lives perspective. When prudence chooses a distribution over the different temporal stages of a life, its goal is to maximize the quality of the life as a temporal whole. So the distributional constraints that apply to temporal parts of lives are derived from a consideration of a complete lifetime and a concern with maximizing the overall quality of that life. Also, Daniels supposes that the prudential lifespan account operates within the constraint of a theory of justice that is concerned with lifetimes. First we must treat people fairly in terms of their complete lives. When that goal has been realized we turn to the special kind of justice that deals with distribution between the temporal stages of different lives. So the principles of justice focused on lifetimes outweigh the principles concerned with temporal parts of lives if there is a conflict. Finally, since prudence aims at maximizing the quality of a life as a whole, it seems that the distributional conclusions this theory generates will closely resemble the conclusions drawn by the complete lives view if the complete lives view does decide to distribute resources between age-groups in the maximally beneficial way.

Those who appeal to prudence as the test of distributive fairness between age-groups characterize the prudential choice in different ways. Some (Dworkin 2000, ch. 8) allow the chooser to know her own age when the choice is made. Daniels (1988, ch. 3) suggests that the choice should be made behind a 'veil of ignorance'. The chooser should not know her age, her specific needs in terms of health care and other resources, or the goals and values that she will endorse at different stages of her life. She only has generic information about the course that human lives typically take and the health problems that people are likely to face at different ages. The restrictions are designed to rule out bias and to permit a choice made by one hypothetical individual to be used to determine the just distribution over many different actual people who will have different goals and different medical problems.

In principle the prudential lifespan account can provide specific answers to detailed questions about distribution. It is motivated by the recognition that we will not be able fully to meet all of the needs of all people of all ages. Even after we have done as much as we can to ensure that people are treated fairly when we compare their lifetimes, scarcity of resources might force us to choose between, for example, providing one kind of health care to younger people or providing a different kind of health care to people who are older. The prudential lifespan account sees this choice as involving a distinctive kind of fairness that is concerned with distribution between temporal stages in lives. It tells us that the fair or just choice is the one that prudence would see as the most beneficial to the individual concerned if a parallel choice needed to be made inside one life. The distribution that the prudential lifespan account chooses will have two features that everyone would count as merits. First, it will not create unfairness at the level of people's complete lives because the theory operates within the constraints of principles of justice for lifetimes. Second, the distribution will use the resources being distributed in the most efficient way to produce the greatest amount of benefits taking into account all of the people concerned. The distribution will have that second feature because the theory chooses the distribution between different people that would maximize lifetime well-being in the case of a single person. The distinctive and (I think) controversial claim of the prudential lifespan account as a theory of justice between age-groups is that fairness is simply *identical* to efficiency in the use of resources in the special case of justice between age-groups or justice between the temporal stages of lives. The person who would benefit most from the resources has a claim of fairness to receive them.

When we consider the specific conclusions that writers have appealed to the prudential lifespan account to justify, some seem friendly to the claims of the elderly while others strictly limit the share of resources that they would receive. Daniels suggests that the theory will stipulate that people's incomes during old age should be roughly equal to their incomes at earlier stages in their lives (Daniels 1988, ch. 7). On the other hand, in the case of health care resources, Daniels and others have argued that the prudential lifespan account would recommend (at least under certain conditions) rationing certain kinds of life-extending medical care on the basis of age (Daniels 1988, ch. 5). Some believe the prudential chooser would in general favour ensuring the availability of medical treatment during youth and middle age as opposed to old age (Dworkin 2000, ch. 8), on the grounds that treatment earlier in life would typically have a greater impact on the overall quality of a life as a temporal whole than treatment during old age. Some draw the strong conclusion that the prudential choice would prefer treatment in middle age that was not life-extending to life-extending treatment during extreme old age (Dworkin 2000, ch. 8). And some conclude that prudence would decide not to provide life-extending treatment in old age if the person were suffering from a serious form of dementia (Brock 1993, ch. 12; Dworkin 1993, ch. 8).

Yet other writers are dissatisfied with both the complete lives view and the appeal to prudence (McKerlie 2002; Temkin 1993, ch. 8). Their case against the prudential lifespan account is partly based on the suspicion that its conclusions will sometimes be intuitively objectionable. They think that the theory, if rigorously applied, will tell us to give the elderly—especially those who are very old and very ill—much less than we feel they are entitled to receive. The severity of the problems faced by such people is precisely what makes it extremely difficult and expensive to promote their well-being. Prudence will recognize this in the case of a single life, and its response will be to concentrate resources in the earlier stages of the life where they can be used more effectively and efficiently to increase well-being. Also, in budgeting resources over a single lifetime prudence will realize that resources set aside or saved for extreme old age have a low probability of actually being used, since the life in question is unlikely to last that long. If this consideration is allowed to influence the prudential choice, it is another reason for favouring the earlier stages in a life. And the critics suggest that we will reject some of the strong conclusions that advocates of the prudential lifespan account themselves draw about health care and the elderly.

The critics agree with the prudential lifespan account that there are constraints of justice applying to temporal parts of lives, as well as to complete lives. However, the prudential lifespan account derives these constraints from a prudential judgement about a lifetime made with a view to maximizing the overall quality of that complete life. The critics think that if people do indeed have moral claims based on the quality of their lives during particular temporal stages in their lives, there is no reason to expect that these claims will be revealed by such a prudential judgement.

Because it is a judgement made about one person's life, the prudential judgement aims simply at maximizing well-being. If we use it as the model for a just distribution across different lives, the view of justice that results will also aim at simply maximizing well-being across those different lives. However, the critics will contend that interpersonal justice—even the kind of interpersonal justice that is concerned with temporal stages of lives rather than lifetimes—does not aim at maximizing in the sense of producing the largest total amount of well-being taking everyone into account. It is more likely that the constraints of justice that apply to old age and the other temporal stages in our lives will be understood by applying some value that is more directly concerned with fairness in distribution—perhaps the value of having a quality of life that at least meets some minimum threshold, or the value of being given priority if one's level of welfare is very low, or the value of equality—to a temporal stage of a life rather than to a lifetime. So these writers propose a theory of justice for age-groups that takes one of these values and changes its temporal scope from a complete life to a temporal part of a life. I will call this kind of theory the 'life-stage view'.

Defenders of the life-stage view should admit that considerations of justice concerned with parts of lives need to be weighed against reasons of justice concerned with lifetimes. Often the lifetime concerns will be stronger. Nevertheless, this view still differs from the prudential lifespan account. Unlike the prudential lifespan account, the life-stage view is not compelled to hold that the lifetime considerations will always be stronger than the reasons concerned with temporal parts of lives.

If we agree with the life-stage view about the temporal scope of principles of justice for age-groups, the next step is deciding which value to incorporate in the theory. The writers who support the life-stage view tend to choose a value that is, in a broad sense, egalitarian. No doubt this partly reflects the widespread sympathy for egalitarianism in contemporary moral philosophy, but the concern that many people feel for the elderly does seem to be egalitarian in its nature. Special institutions for helping the elderly exist because we realize how badly off they would be without them, and we are anxious to spare them from living in that degree of misery.

If it does include a value like equality or priority, the life-stage view can be more generous to the elderly than either the complete lives view or the prudential lifespan account. Since it is focused on temporal parts of lives, it can tell us to help the badly off among the elderly because they are suffering *now*, during their old age. It does not limit their claim to what prudence would have provided for old age in the case of a single life, where prudence is governed by the aim of making that life viewed as a temporal whole as good as it possibly can be.

In considering that single life, the prudential choice might see happiness during youth and extreme misery during old age and then decide to assign more resources to the temporal stage of youth because that would maximize well-being over the life as a whole. When this intrapersonal judgement is transferred to the interpersonal case of comparing the current lives of a well-off younger person and a badly off older person, the judgement would recommend helping the younger person to become even better off because she is the one who can be helped the most. A view that applies equality or priority to the temporal stages of different lives would resist that conclusion. It would compare the current state of the elderly person's life and the current state of the younger person's life and think that because the older person is worse off there is a reason for making them more equal now, or a reason for giving priority to helping the older person. We might decide in the end that this consideration is outweighed by considerations of fairness dealing with lifetimes, or simply by the greater size of the benefits that the younger person would receive, but the reason would still exist.

The value of priority seems to be especially relevant to the elderly. The general notion of priority holds that benefiting a badly off person should be given a certain amount of priority over benefiting a person who is better off. Consequently, a smaller benefit for someone badly off can be more important than, or have more value than, a larger benefit for someone better off (the general notion of priority is explained in Parfit 1995). In the case of the elderly we think that the case for helping them is strongest when they are very badly off in the absolute sense, as well as being worse off than other people. We sometimes feel that we should attempt to do what we can to improve their lives, even if the resources that we devote to them could be used instead to make a greater improvement in the lives of other people. When we apply the notion of priority in the context of the life-stage view, we think that their needs should be given priority because they are worse off than other people now, considering the current state of their lives. They might not be the people who would count as the worst off if instead we compared people's complete lives.

A particular kind of priority has been regarded as a relevant consideration in the distribution of health care, apart from the debate between the three general approaches to justice between age-groups that I have described. When health resources are scarce, some people think that there is at least an apparent case for giving the health care to the person who needs it most. This person receives priority not because the quality of her life is in a general way worse than that of others, but because her medical condition is the most severe and the most urgent. There is disagreement about whether this reason can be strong enough to resist, at least sometimes, the consideration of efficiency, which tells us to distribute the medical resources to the people who will be helped the most by them so that we will produce the best outcome.

Many writers have explained the criterion of efficiency, and applied it to specific choices that arise in medical practice. Less attention has been given to criteria that might compete with efficiency, including that of medical priority. However, Frances Kamm has defended the importance of the criterion of priority (which she calls 'urgency') in an especially detailed and thoughtful way (Kamm 1993, sect. III).

This issue arises independently of concern for the elderly. Nevertheless, the elderly will frequently be among those the criterion of priority or urgency would favour. Their health care problems are frequently more serious, cause more suffering, and are more debilitating. Often they would count as the worst off in the particular respect of illness. And it will often be the case that the criterion of efficiency would support offering the health care to someone else. Because of their age, and the nature of their problems, we would not achieve the best possible medical outcome by choosing to help them.

In these choices there is a conflict between producing the best outcome and the criterion of priority. Writers about biomedical ethics seem typically to favour the criterion of efficiency. Perhaps this is due in part to the influence of a basically utilitarian moral outlook. The prudential lifespan approach also supports this answer in the end. However, an appeal to priority would at least provide a countervailing reason. There is also a case for helping the individual who needs help the most, even if this person can be helped less. If we agree with Kamm, we will see the choice as one where we must decide between competing ethical reasons that both are important and represent different kinds of moral concern.

Apart from being worse off in a general way in terms of overall well-being, and being worse off more specifically in terms of their health problems, there is another respect in which the elderly are typically worse off than other people. They stand nearer to death than others. Old age is the final temporal stage in a life, and this fact might be thought to have ethical implications.

One implication again concerns the distribution of health care resources. Institutions providing health care are compelled to choose (in distributing existing resources, and at a higher level in terms of the resources that it chooses to create) between providing life-extending treatment to the elderly and important but not life-extending health care to younger people. The latter treatment does not prevent or postpone death, but it does make a person's life better than it would otherwise have been for a certain temporal period of the life. The former treatment does prevent death, but when the treatment is provided to someone very old, death may only be briefly postponed and the quality of life during the remainder of the person's life may not be high.

Which choice should we make? To answer this question some would only consider the gain in terms of welfare that would result from each choice. In some cases, the younger person would experience a larger gain in well-being from her disease being cured than the elderly person would receive as a result of her life being extended. Then the right answer would be to treat the younger person. A theory that uses a prudential choice about a single life to answer this question would arrive at the same result.

Others would find this conclusion disturbing. They feel that it underestimates the significance of death to weigh its importance simply in terms of the amount of well-being that the person in question loses by dying. They might claim that it can be more important to delay one person's death than to improve someone else's life, even if the second option would produce a greater gain in terms of well-being. For this view to be defensible, it must be subject to certain conditions: the postponement of death would have to be for a significant period of time, and the life the person led during this period would have to be of an acceptable level of quality.

Deciding between the two views requires considering the difficult question of whether death counts as a harm or evil, and if it does, what kind of a harm it is. We need to answer the second question if we are to weigh death against other harms that people can suffer, like the harm caused by a debilitating but not life-threatening illness. There is a substantial body of philosophical literature focused on these questions (see Nagel 1979; Kamm 1993, sect. 1; McMahan 2002, sect. 2). Most writers support some version of the so-called 'deprivation view', which maintains that the badness of death, and so its gravity as a harm, is simply a matter of the good that it deprives the person of (this is true of Nagel and McMahan). However, some think that the special nature of death as a harm is not completely captured by regarding it as a loss of welfare (Kamm). If this view is correct, then the idea of priority might apply in another way to the elderly. We might think that preventing the harm of death should be given a certain amount of priority over preventing the harm involved in illness, because death belongs in a different category of harm.

Another fact about ageing raises both theoretical and practical problems in deciding what we owe to the elderly. People's goals and values change during their lives. In the case of most of us what we want and strive to achieve during our middle years will differ significantly from our most important concerns when we are old. There are some characteristic differences between the aims of middle age and the aims of old age, although we should not expect to find those differences in every life. The differences in goals and values will be more striking when extreme old age is accompanied by failing mental powers or some degree of dementia.

Changes in goals need to be taken into account when individuals make decisions that will affect their futures when their values may well be different. These changes also must be taken into account when society makes distributive choices about age-groups. This is especially so if we accept a view like the prudential lifespan account which uses a prudential decision about a lifetime as the criterion of fairness to the elderly. However, even if we endorse a different account of justice between age-groups, we might have to choose between satisfying the plans that younger people have made for their old age and helping them to achieve the goals they will actually have when they are old. This choice will be particularly difficult if we think that the goals they will aim at when they are old will be less valuable than their earlier objectives for their final years. It might seem unfair not to provide them with the kind of old age that they would relish while they lived it, but it might also seem unfair not to be guided by their own best judgement about how their lives should end.

The problem of changing goals is easier to consider in the case of a choice by an individual. What should a rational person do when a choice he makes now will significantly affect his old age, and he knows that the goals that he holds now are ones that he will reject when he is old, and that the projects he will endorse when he is old are ones that he cannot acknowledge now as having value?

One radical view is that changes in goals and values, and the other psychological changes that occur during our lives, are so fundamental that we should (although common sense does not) question whether it is really true that I am one and the same person in my youth and my old age (Posner 1995, chs. 4, 10–12). If we were to accept this suggestion, it would fundamentally change our understanding of our own lives and fairness to the elderly. Distribution across the different temporal stages of one life would then be appropriately viewed as morally equivalent to distribution between different people, and our views about justice between age-groups would have to be revised accordingly.

I will assume that this view is too extreme, except perhaps in the case of people suffering from extreme dementia when we might literally challenge the application of the notion of personal identity. A more moderate view claims that identity as such is not what matters for rationality and morality. The application of moral values and concepts of rationality depends instead on relations of psychological continuity and connectedness between the different temporal parts of a life. This continuity will vary in strength in an ordinary life, and we should take this into account in deciding what attitude it is rational for a person to take towards his old age and in making moral judgements about temporal stages in lives (such a view is defended in Parfit 1984, pt. 3, and it is applied to moral issues about the elderly in McMahan 2002, sect. 5).

However, I think myself that the variations in continuity over time in an ordinary life are not important enough to be a significant factor in understanding our moral judgements and judgements about rationality. And I believe that judgements that we do make that might seem to support this view can be explained as responses to other considerations.

Even if changes in character and values do not involve a breach of personal identity, or a serious weakening of the psychological relations that supposedly underlie identity, they do seem to be important for their own sake. How should we respond to them? Should I make provision for my pursuit of the goals I will hold when I am old, despite my current rejection of them? Or if there is something I could do now that would lock me into the kind of life in old age that I now think desirable, would it reasonable for me to make this choice despite my knowledge that my mind will change?

This issue has been discussed in a theoretical way by moral philosophers without reference to its application to ageing (see Nagel 1970, ch. 5; Parfit 1984, pt. 2; Bykvist 2003). Three responses to it have been defended. The first claims that a reasonable person should make the present decision on the strength of his present goals and values, since those are the values that he is now committed to and believes to be valid. According to the second view, a reasonable person should decide on the strength of his future goals and values, since they are the ones he will accept when the effects of his choice on his own life will eventually be realized. The third view claims that a reasonable person should make the decision by taking both sets of values into account and giving them equal weight. He should be neutral between the conflicting values.

The version of the prudential lifespan account that permits the prudential choice to be made by a young person who is aware of his present goals seems to choose the first answer. The other version of the theory appeals to a choice made by a hypothetical individual who does not know either his present or his future goals. This seems to me tantamount to requiring neutrality between present and future goals, and so amounts to a variation of the third answer.

All three answers suppose that some attitude towards the importance of time itself is distinctively rational. The first view thinks that because of the special importance of the present, it is present values that matter for a decision that will be made now. The second view thinks that in assessing a change in the future, it is future values that matter because they are the values that you will hold when the change happens. This view also gives special significance to the present, but it identifies a different present as being relevant to the decision—not the time that is the present when the decision is made, but the time that is the present when the consequences of the decision will occur. The third view holds that rationality requires us to adopt temporal neutrality, to give equal weight to all times, and it supposes that this means we should also give equal weight to the different values that we hold at different times.

I think that we should have reservations about accepting any of these answers. They all conflict with the belief that some goals and values can be objectively more important than others. If we agree with that belief, we cannot be satisfied with the claim that we should only use our present values whatever they are, or only our future values whatever they are, or that we must automatically give equal weight to both sets of values. If I am right, this would be another consideration that counts against the prudential lifespan account, which is committed to the first or the third answer.

Arguably the best answer to the problem of changing goals is reached by thinking in terms of an agent's well-being. If the agent decides on the strength of his present values then he will not approve of the change in his life when it happens, because he will then hold different values. And if he will not positively respond to the change, this will affect his well-being in the future or the quality of his life in the future. This gives him a reason to take his future goals into account now, even if they are objectively less valuable than the goals he now holds for his future. This suggestion appeals to what might be called the 'positive response condition' on well-being, an idea that has been adopted in one version or another by several recent writers on the nature of well-being (for examples, see Dworkin 2000, ch. 6; Darwall 2002, ch. 4).

The point is not just that the person will feel less contentment if his life has been designed according to standards he used to endorse but has subsequently abandoned. That is the aspect of well-being that depends on hedonic goods. Some believe that the positive response condition can also matter in a different, and perhaps more important, way. They think that endorsing an activity that you perform enhances the value of the activity so that it makes a greater contribution to the quality of your life. A significant artistic achievement might increase the well-being of its creator even if she herself does not value what she has produced or her own actions in producing it. But it will do more to enhance the quality of her life if she herself appreciates what she has done. On this view, there are two factors to consider in deciding how much the activity will contribute to her well-being: the objective value of the activity, and whether she will endorse the activity when she performs it.

The condition applies to choices that we must make about our future selves. A creative writer might correctly think that the most valuable goal she could pursue in old age would be to preserve her legacy as a writer. When she can no longer produce new fiction she can at least lecture on university campuses, prepare new editions of her works, and mentor young writers. Still, suppose she knows that when she is old she will instead think—wrongly—that relaxing with television, games, and socializing is more important. If her interest is in making her old age go as well as possible, she has a reason for planning her old age to fit the values that she will hold when she is old. The objective value of golfing might be less than the objective value of helping young writers, but if she will positively respond to the former activity, but not the latter, playing golf might contribute more to her well-being.

It may seem that the explanation in terms of well-being is identical to what I originally called the third solution to the problem of changing goals. The goals that matter are the goals the person holds at the time of the event or change in his life that we are evaluating. But the two views are not the same. The well-being view does not claim that because of the special importance of the present we are rationally required to evaluate the change in terms of the goals that the person holds when the change occurs. It explains the relevance of those goals in terms of the positive response condition on well-being, not in terms of the rationality of a particular attitude towards time itself. And the well-being explanation is compatible with the thought that if the person's present goals are less valuable than his past goals, it might be better for his present life to match his past goals, despite the positive response condition.

It has been suggested that younger people tend to disvalue or disparage the characteristic goals of old age. If so, the view that I have explained gives them a reason to change their attitude. However, it is an advantage of the view that it can lead to respect for the goals of the elderly even if we are willing to admit (as I believe many elderly people themselves would) that these projects are not as objectively important for the value of a life as the characteristic goals of middle age.

There is another way—a sadder way—in which changes of goals are relevant to the ethical treatment of the elderly. The very old are sometimes afflicted by severe mental disabilities. The problems can take many different forms and arise in very different degrees of seriousness. The most tragic cases involve dementia, more specifically Alzheimer's disease in its moderate and extreme forms. The frequency with which this disease attacks the elderly, and the increasing number of people who will live long enough so that it will pose a serious threat to them, mean that coping with the illness is now and will continue to be a major issue of public health.

The illness affects characters and minds in complex ways. Impairment of short-term memory, or rather the loss of the capacity to convert short-term memories into long-term memories, is the most familiar symptom, but radical changes in personality and deep cognitive impairments of other kinds are also experienced in more severe cases.

One aspect of the problem is whether we should believe that the most problematic cases involve a change in a person's goals or values at all. Some believe that in the worst cases the sufferer has become incapable of having goals, of having interests that take the form of valued projects rather than unreflective or automatic desires. And some believe that the afflicted person can no longer be regarded as an autonomous agent with the ability to control her life, and so cannot be regarded as possessing a moral claim to be left free to make her own choices about her own life.

If this picture is correct, it obviously has profound consequences for how those who suffer from these diseases should be treated. It might lead us to give broad decision-making powers over their lives to relatives or medical personnel. If the patients had settled goals before their illness and had then expressed their wishes about questions that might arise later in their lives, it might lead us to give authority to their past decisions, even if there is some apparent evidence in their current behaviour that they are now of a different mind. And some would argue that if they lack autonomy and the capacity to hold values, this limits the value that would be gained (meaning value for those suffering from the disease themselves, not value for others) by a prolongation of their lives in a state of dementia. Here some conclude that we should not save their lives if they acquire a life-threatening but curable disease, especially if there is an advance directive from their earlier self requesting this lack of treatment. They would stand by this conclusion if the person seems placid and contented in their present state, and is not experiencing any pain or emotional distress.

Sorting out these issues requires both settling difficult factual questions about precisely what capacities the people in question have and do not have, and answering broader ethical questions about the nature of autonomy and the source of its value, and about what if anything is special about endorsing something as a value as opposed to merely having a desire. This makes worthwhile and sensitive work on the problem very difficult indeed, but a number of writers have made valuable—though conflicting—contributions.

Ronald Dworkin defends the strong thesis that a person afflicted with moderate or extreme Alzheimer's disease lacks an autonomous will (Dworkin 1993, ch. 8). If before the onset of the disease she wished that her life would end without a final stage of dementia, that choice must be regarded as remaining in place as her standing will and it should determine what medical treatment she receives. Dworkin grants that the person can enjoy the circumstances of her limited life with the disease, and that if she experiences contentment, this counts as a good for her. Dworkin characterizes this as satisfying her experiential interests. However, he believes that the disease has rendered her incapable of holding values and applying them to her own life. She cannot form evaluative beliefs about her life as a whole—beliefs like her former view that her life would be better without the final state of dementia. So Dworkin considers her incapable of having what he calls 'critical' interests. Or rather he believes that her past evaluative beliefs, including her view about how her life should end, are still in force and constitute her present critical interests. Since Dworkin thinks that critical interests are more important than experiential interests, he thinks that allowing her life to end is in her best overall interest. According to Dworkin, the two considerations of implementing the patient's will and doing what is best for her both support the conclusion that we should not provide her with life-extending medical treatment.

Dworkin's critics contest his view of the capacities of such a patient (Jaworska 1999; Shiffrin 2004). They think that in the Alzheimer's sufferer who is undeniably contented, we can discern something that deserves to be called a desire to go on living, even if she is no longer capable of thinking about her life as a temporal whole or capable of articulating her desire to others (at least they believe this about many sufferers from moderate Alzheimer's disease and perhaps some patients with extreme forms of Alzheimer's—they might concede that Dworkin's view does fit the most extreme cases). And some also believe that when this desire is present it should be respected as representing her will. So they think that her will has changed, has taken a new direction, as a result of the disease. Respect for her autonomy should motivate us to implement what is in fact her current will, not what her will used to be.

They also think she is capable of more than being pleased by her current experiential states. Her present interests are partly determined by values that she does hold now. In other words she possesses critical interests as well as experiential interests, and the critical interests that now belong to her might differ significantly from those she held before the disease. If she finds value in the conditions of her new life, these critical interests will support the continuation of her life. In effect the Alzheimer's patient has undergone a change in her critical interests or values. Those who see the patient in this light will be tempted to think that what is in her best interest is determined by her new critical interests as well as her experiential interests, but not by the critical interests that she held in the past. So they would think that providing her with the medical treatment that will prolong her life is really what is best for her.

It is not easy to decide between the two views. Most of us will be disturbed at setting aside the careful provisions that the person made, when her mind was clear, for just this eventuality. But we will also be disturbed by not offering life-extending treatment to a person who is now contented with her life and wants it to continue, even if she had previously wished not to live a life of that sort.

Perhaps the issue about autonomy can be answered, assuming that we agree that the patient should be credited with an autonomous will that has as one of its objects the continuation of her life. She now wishes to live, and it seems to me that her wish should be honoured. Since her new will takes the direction it does partly because of the damage the disease has done to her, we might think that her new will is less reasonable—objectively less reasonable—than her previous will. Still, the value of autonomy counts in favour of respecting a person's wishes—meaning by this the person's current wishes—even if they are less reasonable than her past objectives and even if respecting them would be against her best interest. As a value, autonomy seems to operate in this 'present tense' way. Perhaps we would not respect a person's current wishes if their will was grossly irrational, or disastrously opposed to their best interests. But this does not seem to be true of the Alzheimer's patient. Given her condition, it is not grossly irrational of her to want the life she enjoys to continue, even if we think that it is against her interest for reasons that she can no longer understand. If we accept these ideas, we will feel obligated to provide the life-extending medical treatment on grounds of respecting autonomy, regardless of how we may answer other questions about her condition and interests.

However, we might not find as ready an answer when we turn to the question of what would be in the patient's best interest. Our judgement about the patient's good might differ from our judgement about her autonomy, because autonomy and considerations about a person's good are different moral reasons that might work in different ways. In considering the Alzheimer's patient's best interests, the crucial thing is the status of the critical interest represented by the patient's past conviction that her life would be better if it ended without the postscript of a period of dementia. Does this conviction still apply to her life after she has been changed by the disease in precisely the way that she feared?

On the one hand, it is clear that she no longer explicitly adheres to the conviction. We can suppose that she could not even begin to understand this belief if it were expressed to her. And I would agree with Dworkin's critics that she may now have other interests, no doubt of a much simpler sort, that nevertheless count as critical interests because they involve a kind of valuing—for example, her desire for the company of individuals who love her, even if she might be uncertain of their identities or their role in her past life. Some would conclude that her critical interests have simply changed. The critical interest that Dworkin appeals to has been replaced, and it should not be applied to an assessment of her life with the disease. It is not relevant to a judgement of the value or quality of that life, or in deciding how much well-being she can enjoy. If we think of the change in the patient in this way we will suppose that her life will be better if it continues, so long as she is contented and the limited but important interests that she still possesses are satisfied.

This is how we react to a self-conscious change of values during an ordinary life. We appeal to the person's new values, not to the supplanted values, to determine what is in the person's best interest from now on. We do this even if we think that the new values are less reasonable than the old ones, or that the person changed his mind for bad reasons.

However, this comparison should lead us to challenge the view. The patient did not change her mind, her mind was changed by the disease. She did not reconsider the question of the shape she wanted her life to have and then decide (perhaps for inadequate reasons) that the years of dementia would not after all make her life worse. Rather, the disease took away from her any capacity to even think in those terms. The cause of the change in her—Alzheimer's disease—is a disease or impairment, a condition that does not merely initiate changes in a non-rational way but destroys valuable abilities and damages its victim. In fact the person did not change her mind at all. In virtue of that, it is not clear that the old critical interest fails to apply to her current life. Arguably it remains one of her critical interests, although she is now unable to understand or express it.

The point is easier to see in an example that does not involve deciding whether to save a life. We can suppose that the Alzheimer's sufferer had lived as a devout Roman Catholic until the disease destroyed her ability even to think in those terms. Perhaps in her final years she took pleasure in the cheerful non-denominational religious services in the nursing home. Her appreciation of them might amount in its own way to a critical interest, but I think we would feel that when her life ends she should be buried according to the rites of the Roman Catholic Church, not with a simple service in the nursing home. In this example, her previous critical interest has not been supplanted by the new one, and it continues to matter in determining what would be in her best interest.

If we agree, then this interest must be taken into account in deciding what would be best for her. It is true that it must compete against the 'new' critical interests and experiential interests that might support enabling her life to continue. But it should be remembered that her own view, before the disease took hold, was that this critical interest was more important than whatever good she might be able to enjoy in the state of dementia. Her new critical interests do not include a revised view about the question of respective importance. So we might be led back towards Dworkin's conclusion that a peaceful death is what is really in her best interest, although we are not basing the conclusion on Dworkin's reasons.

However, this tentative conclusion should not lead us to withhold the treatment if we also believe that the patient's will is that her life should continue. As I have suggested, thinking about autonomy is different from thinking about what is in her best interest. I believe that her new will does supplant and replace her old will, even if her will changed because of the cognitive damage the disease did to her. By contrast we should conclude that her original critical interest was not simply replaced by her new critical interests, when we consider why her interests changed. The old critical interest still applies to her, with at least some degree of force, in her altered condition.

Consequently those who find it unconscionable to withhold treatment in such a case should appeal to autonomy. This means being convinced of two things: that the Alzheimer's patient does currently possess a will capable of some degree of autonomy, and that her will is directed at the continuation of her life. Some might grant the first but question the second. They might argue that because of her cognitive impairment she cannot be said to have as an object of her will something as complex as the prolongation of her life, even if it is true that she is living happily in her current state. According to this view we cannot be accused of frustrating her will if we withhold the medical treatment. If we agree then, as I understand the applicable reasons, we might after all be forced to the conclusion that the treatment should not be provided, assuming that we have decided that it would be against her best interest.

I have discussed a series of issues that I believe involve a special kind of justice holding between the young and the old. Even if we agree that there is a distinctive problem of justice concerned with age-groups, we should also acknowledge that it differs in a fundamental way from justice between different races or different genders. At any given time, the age-groups of the young and the elderly will contain different people, but those who are now old were once young, and those who are young now will eventually be old. So the young should not understand a view about the claims of the elderly as simply a proposal about how they should treat someone *else*. In time that view will determine their own claims. The issues I have discussed—issues about distributing health care and other resources fairly and issues about deciding which goals and values to respect when they differ in significant ways at different times in a person's life—are ones that we will experience from both sides.

The difficult question for moral philosophy to answer is whether there is a way of giving the proper weight to this fact without retreating to the complete lives view and concluding that justice is only concerned with complete lifetimes. The prudential lifespan account responds to this fact in a distinctive way. When a young person views an elderly person, he sees someone who used to be young and someone who is now in the stage of life that he himself will eventually occupy. It is as though he is seeing himself in old age. According to the prudential lifespan account, this makes it fair for him to decide what if anything he now owes to that elderly person by thinking about a single life containing both youth and old age and asking how prudential rationality would divide resources between those two temporal stages. The single life can stand in for both his own complete lifetime and the elderly person's complete lifetime. The result of the theory will be the distribution of resources that would maximize the well-being of the single life considered as a temporal whole, and I have tried to describe the apparent advantages and the apparent disadvantages of this solution to justice between the young and the old.

However, that might not be the only way of responding to the fact that we all have lives that over time will contain the different temporal stages. When the young person sees that the elderly person is experiencing misery now, he may think that there is a reason to help, even if the resources that he contributes would create a larger amount of well-being were he to use them himself. This reason—if we are willing to suppose that it might exist—would naturally be expressed by a value like equality or priority applied to temporal stages in lives.

Critics will object that we will only see this reason—or think that we see it—if we mistakenly regard this choice as a simple choice between the welfare of two different people in exactly the same way that a choice between two members of different races would be a choice between the welfare of two different people. I am not persuaded by their claim. I think the choice is concerned with interpersonal justice, even if it is not exactly the same as a choice between the members of different races. When the young person views the elderly person, he sees someone else living in a distinctive temporal stage of a human life.

Moreover, I also believe that if we see the reason for helping when we compare the current life of the young person and the current life of the elderly person, it might lead us to change our mind about the prudential choice made about a single life. A concern like that of priority might apply inside lives as well as across lives. If I recognize that my own old age will contain the same kind of misery that the elderly person feels now, I might decide that it would be better to alleviate some of my future suffering even if some other choice would maximize the total amount of well-being in my lifetime.

Applying the value of priority to my own life does not require thinking of my elderly self as being virtually a different person. I am not suggesting that we should appeal to a view about personal identity or a view about the extent of the psychological unity of a human life over time in order to justify this way of using priority. The basic thought is that a benefit is more important when it is received by someone who is badly off, as it is in the case when we apply priority to a choice between benefits for different people. However, if this proposal is reasonable, it reverses the order of explanation of the prudential lifespan account. Instead of learning what fairness requires between the temporal stages of different lives by considering a prudential assessment of the diachronic temporal stages in one life, we might begin by considering how resources should be divided between the simultaneous temporal stages of different lives and discover something about the best way to allocate resources inside our own lives.

References

Brock, D. B. (1993), *Life and Death: Philosophical Essays in Biomedical Ethics* (Cambridge: Cambridge University Press).

Bykvist, K. (2003), 'The Moral Relevance of Past Preferences', in H. Dyke (ed.), *Time and Ethics: Essays at the Intersection* (Deventer: Kluwer Academic Publishers), 115–36.

Daniels, N. (1988), *Am I My Parents' Keeper?* (New York: Oxford University Press).

—— (1996), 'The Prudential Lifespan Account of Justice Across Generations', in Daniels, *Justice and Justification* (Cambridge: Cambridge University Press), 257–83.

Darwall, S. (2002), *Welfare and Rational Care* (Princeton: Princeton University Press).

Dworkin, R. (1993), *Life's Dominion* (New York: Knopf).

—— (2000), *Sovereign Virtue* (Cambridge, Mass.: Harvard University Press).

Jaworska, A. (1999), 'Respecting the Margins of Agency: Alzheimer's Patients and the Capacity to Value', *Philosophy and Public Affairs*, 28/2: 105–38.

Kamm, F. M. (1993), *Morality, Mortality*, i (New York: Oxford University Press).

McKerlie, D. (2002), 'Justice Between the Young and the Old', *Philosophy and Public Affairs*, 30/2: 152–77.

McMahan, J. (2002), *The Ethics of Killing* (New York: Oxford University Press).

Nagel, T. (1970), *The Possibility of Altruism* (Oxford: Clarendon Press).

NAGEL, T. (1979), 'Death', in Nagel, *Mortal Questions* (Cambridge: Cambridge University Press), 1–10.

—— (1991), *Equality and Partiality* (New York: Oxford University Press).

PARFIT, D. (1984), *Reasons and Persons* (Oxford: Clarendon Press).

—— (1995), 'Equality or Priority?', Lindley Lecture (Lawrence: University of Kansas Press).

POSNER, R. A. (1995), *Aging and Old Age* (Chicago: University of Chicago Press).

RAWLS, J. (1971), *A Theory of Justice* (Cambridge, Mass.: Harvard University Press).

SHIFFRIN, S. (2004), 'Autonomy, Beneficence and the Permanently Demented', in J. Burley (ed.), *Dworkin and His Critics* (Oxford: Blackwell), 195–217.

TEMKIN, L. S. (1993), *Inequality* (New York: Oxford University Press).

PART III

BODIES AND
BODILY PARTS

CHAPTER 9

ORGAN TRANSPLANTATION

RONALD MUNSON

In 1954 the first successful kidney transplant was performed by Joseph Murray at the Harvard Medical School's Peter Bent Brigham Hospital (Merrill *et al*. 1956). At that moment, we entered a new age.

We had acquired, after decades of work by a small number of researchers, the power to snatch someone out of the grasp of death by replacing a vital organ. Since 1954 researchers have consolidated and extended that power. Improvements in surgical techniques, crossmatching tissues, experience in medical management, and, above all, the advent of Cyclosporin and other powerful immunosuppressive drugs have elevated transplantation to the category of standard therapy.

Kidney transplants offered a preferable alternative to dialysis by the late 1970s, and the list of organs that can be transplanted with significant success has now expanded to include the heart, liver, lungs, intestines, and pancreas. Corneas, bone, bone marrow, blood, cells, blood vessels, heart valves, and skin are also transplanted, but because they are not functional wholes, they are not considered organs. Discussions of organ transplants are thus typically restricted to what are known as *solid*, or *vital*, organs.

A SUCCESS—WITHIN LIMITS

Each year about 50,000 Americans have their lives extended by receiving new organs. (Statistics are from United Network for Organ Sharing 2004 unless otherwise cited;

transplant and waiting-list numbers are estimates from 2003 data.) This is a number equal to the combined enrollments, graduate and undergraduate, of Columbia, Harvard, and Princeton universities. The number is particularly striking because three decades ago virtually all those now saved by transplants would have died. No matter how healthy the rest of a person's body, without a functioning kidney, liver, or heart, death is the outcome.

Yet transplants are not perfect fixes. Completely successful transplants would give people replacement organs without turning them into patients who must be treated with powerful immunosuppressive drugs for the rest of their lives. The drugs have disagreeable side effects, make recipients prone to infections, and increase their risk of cancer and other diseases. Chronic rejection remains a constant threat, and an organ that has functioned well for five or six years may, suddenly and unaccountably, be attacked by the recipient's immune system and damaged so severely it has to be removed.

A perfect transplant would restore a patient to health, be a one-time, long-term fix, and as free of negative consequences for the recipient as changing batteries is for a flashlight. Stem-cell technology may make this possible by engineering organs to be genetically identical with the ones they replace (Munson 2002, ch. 10). Yet while we wait for this marvelous future, transplants, though far from perfect, save lives right now.

A SHORTAGE

Every year nearly 10,000 people on the United States' United Network for Organ Sharing (UNOS) national waiting list die without getting the organ they need to survive. They depart quietly, with little public notice. Yet the total of their deaths is roughly equivalent to *three times* the number of people who died in the 11 September 2001 terrorist attack on the World Trade Center.

Almost 100,000 people are on the waiting list at any given time. Some are not as sick as others and, with medical help, are able to wait for months or even years. Those who are lucky may get a needed organ within weeks or a few days. But waiting is not always rewarded, and not everyone who needs an organ, no matter how desperately, receives one.

The waiting list is growing at a rapid rate. A new name was added every eighteen minutes in 1998, every sixteen minutes in 1999, every fourteen minutes in 2001, and by 2005 it may be every ten minutes. Given our aging population, the list will grow longer at an increasing rate, and even now more names are put on the list than are removed from it.

The need for organs is constant, pressing, and escalating. It may already be greater than can be met, even assuming complete efficiency in recovering organs from those recently dead (Evans 1989: 15). No more than 15,000 brain-dead potential donors are available annually, and even if the current average of 3.6 organs were recovered from each, this would amount to only 54,000 organs—less than half the number needed now. What makes the situation more desperate is that nothing like this number is actually recovered; hardly more than 50 per cent of those asked to donate the organs of a deceased family member agree to do so.

Every organ transplanted may translate into a life extended. Thus, the failure of the present system of altruistic donations to secure enough organs to meet even current needs has produced recommendations for making the system more efficient. It has also led to more radical proposals to recover organs by 'presuming' consent and to supplement voluntarism with some sort of market scheme to reward donors or donor families. Then, too, animal organs, organs grown from stem cells, or artificial devices might ultimately eliminate or severely reduce the need for donor organs (Munson 2002, chs. 9–11). Such prospects are at best long-term, however.

The ethical and social issues raised by transplants are so interrelated that the thread of any problem eventually leads to the whole tangled ball. I will, however, limit discussion to topics involving living donors in the United States. This restriction is not dictated solely by space constraints. Rather, the rise in the number of living donors gives a particular urgency to questions about informed consent, donor protection, and recipient needs. How we resolve conflicts of interest, address issues of consent, and define the scope of autonomy will shape the policies and practices that determine whether donors are protected and whether lives are lost or saved.

LIVING-DONOR TRANSPLANTS

The most effective measure to reduce the shortage of the organs in greatest demand, kidneys and livers, is to increase the number of living donors (Spital 1989, 2001). Although several attempts were made during the 1940s and 1950s to transplant a kidney taken from a patient's mother or father, all efforts failed until 1954 when Joseph Murray took a kidney from Ronald Merrick and transplanted it into his identical-twin brother Richard (Munson 2002: 125–9). A series of sixty successful twin transplants followed (Tilney 1986), but it was not until the advent of effective immunosuppressive drugs and crossmatching tissues that using kidneys from unrelated donors became feasible.

Kidneys are no longer the only vital organ that—at least in part—can be donated by a living person. People can donate a liver lobe, lung lobe, or pancreas segment.

I will additionally restrict this chapter by focusing on issues associated with the living donors of kidneys and livers. Not only do these organs jointly constitute 80 per cent of all transplants; the ethical issues concerning donors are basically the same for other organs.

Sixty per cent of all transplants are of kidneys. More than 14,000 of the 23,000 organs transplanted in 2001 (the latest year with complete figures) were kidneys. With 50,000 people waiting for a kidney transplant, the kidney is the organ with the highest demand and shortest supply.

Liver transplants number about 5,000 a year, some 20 per cent of all transplants. Nearly 20,000 people are on the waiting list for a liver, making it the organ with the second highest demand and the second lowest supply. Only about 10 per cent of liver transplants use lobes contributed by living donors, but this number will likely increase as the surgical techniques involved become standardized and spread to more transplant centers. Pressure to increase living-donor liver transplants comes from the fact that there is no effective way to replace the liver's function (unlike that of the kidney and the heart) for even a few days or weeks.

The number of living donors increased by a factor of 2.5 during the period 1992–2000. Living donors constitute 52 per cent of all kidney donors, but they contribute only 40 per cent (6,000) of transplanted kidneys, because they can donate only one kidney. Most strikingly, the number of unrelated donors has reached 1,600, ten times the 1966 figure. The importance of living donors can be appreciated by the fact that if only one of every 3,000 people became a kidney donor, the kidney shortage would be solved.

Easing the organ shortage is not the only reason for valuing living donors. Transplant surgery can be planned; organs are disconnected from their blood supply for a shorter time and thus remain in good condition; recipients may spend little or no time on the waiting list or undergoing dialysis, so their health does not deteriorate; organs from a living donor will be healthy and undamaged; and good immunological compatibility between donor and recipient can often be arranged. Also, when cancerous liver nodules prompt a transplant, the patient needs a new liver before the cancer metastasizes. A living donor can save the patient from a long wait for a deceased-donor liver and thus perhaps from developing metastatic disease.

Kidney recipients benefit significantly from a living-donor organ. The one-year survival with a deceased-donor kidney is 94 per cent, but with a living-donor kidney, survival rises to 98 per cent. Five-year survival increases from 80 to 90 per cent.

Liver recipients do not gain as much. Those getting a deceased-donor liver do slightly better (86 v. 85 per cent) during the first year. Yet by the fifth year the situation is reversed, with living-donor recipients significantly surviving longer (86 v. 73 per cent). These figures may change as living-donor transplants become routine and more frequently performed.

BENEFITS TO RECIPIENTS, RISKS TO DONORS

Living donors reduce the organ shortage and directly benefit transplant recipients, but what are the consequences for the donor? Donors risk death, as well as temporary and permanent injuries. They undergo abdominal surgery, and, in addition to the accompanying pain, they risk infection, blood clots, and a damaging or fatal reaction to the anesthesia. Removing a donor kidney via laparoscopy, as is now becoming more common, may reduce pain and shorten recovery, but risks remain.

A UNOS survey of transplant centers and a twenty-plus-year follow-up study of living kidney donors show that the risk of dying from a kidney donation is 0.03 per cent (Najarian *et al.* 1992). (This is about 3 out of 10,000 donors or one donor death every four years.) Also, 56 kidney donors (as of 2004) have later required a kidney transplant themselves. Life-threatening or permanent complications occur in about a quarter of one per cent (0.23 per cent) of donors. No long-term difference between the longevity of donors and non-donors has been determined (Najarian *et al.* 1992; Park *et al.* 1996). Donors must also be prepared to alter their behavior (e.g. giving up contact sports) to reduce the chance of damaging their remaining kidney.

Living-donor liver transplants are relatively recent. The first was performed in 1987, when surgeons at Brazil's São Paulo Medical College transplanted the left lobe of a mother's liver into her 4-year-old child (Crouch and Elliot 1999: 276). The procedure was restricted to children for the next few years, then several centers began transplanting the right lobe of an adult donor into an adult recipient. About 1,000 living-donor liver transplants are now performed every year.

Because the number of cases is comparatively small and the procedure relatively recent, risks to liver donors are not yet well understood (Miller *et al.* 2001). The donor has 25–60 per cent of the liver removed (the left lobe for children and the larger right lobe for adults). The liver begins to grow back, but during the first several weeks the donor may develop liver failure so severe as to require a transplant. The gall bladder is removed when the lobe is removed, and bile leaks occur in 2–5 per cent of donors and may require additional surgery. Problems, major or minor, occur in 15–30 per cent of all donors. The mortality rate is estimated to be 0.2 per cent or 2 deaths per 1,000 donors. So far only two people are known to have died as a result of being liver-lobe donors.

The following case called the public's attention to the risks of becoming a donor and raised the question of what policies transplant centers ought to adopt with respect to living liver donors.

Case 1. Mike Hurewitz, a 57-year-old Albany, New York, journalist, died at Mount Sinai Hospital in New York City on 13 January 2002 following an operation to remove a lobe of his liver. Hurewitz was in good health when he volunteered to donate part of his liver to his younger brother Alan. Alan made a good recovery from the surgery and continues to do well.

Vickie Hurewitz, Mike's widow, sued the hospital and six physicians, alleging negligence and malpractice. She also claimed that her husband had not been properly informed about the risks of becoming a liver donor. She recommended that transplant centers declare a national moratorium on the procedure until its value and safety could be established.

Neither federal nor state laws specify who is eligible to become a living donor, how informed consent should be obtained from a donor, nor how a donor's interests should be protected. These are all matters determined by policies at transplant centers. Legislation, state or federal, will likely replace local rules soon, and this makes framing ethically justifiable procedures particularly pressing. We need to be sure that any new regulatory laws are grounded on sound moral reasoning.

SHOULD LIVING DONORS BE ALLOWED?

Thomas Starzl, who pioneered both kidney and liver transplants, argues against the use of living donors on the grounds that, in his experience, the weakest or least valued member of a family is targeted as the donor. Others in the family then manipulate the person into volunteering. Starzl's view can be generalized into the claim that the risk that the decisions of candidate donors will not be voluntary is too great to permit the practice of using living donors.

Surveys of donors provide no evidence that they believe their decisions were manipulated or coerced. The studies show that donors are motivated by a desire to help, take satisfaction in their role in benefiting another person, and experience an increase in self-esteem. They are pleased with their decision and would make the same one again. (See Riether and Mahler 1995: 338; Rhodes 1994: 78; Spital 1996: 376.)

Yet surveys necessarily reflect how donors feel after the fact. Surveys cannot prove that donor decisions were not compromised. After all, an unconsenting person shoved off the platform at a bungee jump may later report a good experience. Also, some donors may have been so subtly manipulated that they were never aware of the factors influencing their decisions.

Like Starzl, we tend to think of family members or the recipient doing the controlling. Siblings Sue and Tom look to their younger sister Beth to volunteer a lobe of her liver for their mother. Beth is unmarried, has no children, and works only part-time. She is not regarded by her siblings as worth as much as they are, because they are married, employed, and have young children. Beth, in her siblings' and maybe her mother's view, seems to owe it to the family to become a donor. Many similar scenarios are possible (Dwyer and Vig 1995), and, as Fox and Swazey (1978) point out in their classic study, where living donors and families are concerned, the potential always exists for moral blackmail.

Less appreciated is that physicians, nurses, or others at transplant centers may unintentionally evoke guilt and so maneuver candidates into becoming donors. Candidates may be 'actively encouraged' (Spital 1996: 374) to become donors. This may involve something as simple as a nurse pointing out that 'If you donated a liver lobe, your mom could beat her cancer.' Or the encouragement may be a conversation with the patient's physician, who urges the necessity for quick action to save a loved one.

Autonomy as the Basis

Living-donor transplants can be morally legitimate, if the donor's autonomy can be guaranteed. We act autonomously when our actions are the result of our own decisions, when they are self-determined. Autonomy is thus infringed when our behavior is coerced or manipulated.

Our society is committed to recognizing the determining power of the individual in making self-regarding decisions. We thus let people decide how to live their lives, including deciding which risks to take. Some people, knowing the facts about becoming a donor, may be willing to undergo suffering and risk their lives to help a sister, mother, friend, or even a complete stranger. Others, for a variety of reasons or no reason at all, may decide otherwise.

Autonomy, if it is to be exercised, must be protected, and that is the purpose of informed consent. Informed consent is a way to minimize the chance that, when it comes to decision making, people will be deceived, exploited, tricked, misled, duped, manipulated, or pressured so that their autonomy is violated. If a significant violation of autonomy occurs, the resulting decision is not, in a real sense, the individual's. Informed consent is thus a means of making sure that the agent of an action is also its true author.

For informed consent to be legitimate (valid, genuine, etc.), we require that adults be competent to make decisions—that their powers to understand not be compromised by drugs, mental confusion, disabilities, injury, or depression. We then demand that these competent people be provided with information relevant to the decision at hand and that the information be understandable and sufficient to allow them to weigh the character and consequences of the actions open to them. We require, finally, that people be protected from coercive forces, deception, situational pressures, or other factors that infringe on their autonomy and thus take away some of their decision-making power. To emphasize the importance of this requirement, we often speak redundantly of consent that is '*free* and informed'.

Requiring informed consent is a way of making sure that people understand what they might be getting into if they become a living donor, a participant in a clinical trial, or merely a patient considering surgery. The function of informed consent is not to protect people from the consequences of their actions. Rather, it is to make sure that they can know (so far as anyone does) the nature and results (the potential risks and benefits) of each course of action open to them before they make their decision.

The generalized Starzl objection that people always risk being manipulated into becoming donors does not entail that using living donors is inherently wrong. Rather, it is a condemnation of any process of securing consent from a candidate that fails to guarantee the protection of the candidate's autonomy. To be morally legitimate, any transplant program that permits living donors must meet the practical challenge of securing informed consent in a way that protects donor candidates from family and situational pressures and permits them to refuse consent (or withdraw it later) without suffering adverse personal consequences. (See 'Summary: Rules Regulating Living Donors' below for measures to protect autonomy.)

INHERENT COERCION

Some bioethicists suggest that where the life of a patient is a stake, someone strongly emotionally attached to the patient is not free to decide to become a donor. The attachment plus the patient's grave condition (it is suggested) make the situation inherently coercive for the potential donor. Caplan, in commenting on liver-lobe transplants when a parent is confronting the potential death of a child, asks, 'Does anyone really think parents can say "No" when the option is certain death for their own son or daughter?' Annas echoes this opinion: 'The parents basically can't say no' (both quoted in Crouch and Elliott 1999: 276). If 'The parents can't say no' is construed to mean something like 'The parents dare not say no, because they will be berated as bad parents', the argument has merit. Our society expects parents to make sacrifices for their children, and this includes enduring suffering and, if required, running the risk of injury and death. We do not admire a father who refuses to be a liver-lobe donor and so fails to give his child the chance to live. Yet we also acknowledge that it would be wrong for us to violate his autonomy by forcing him to become a donor.

Given our commitment to respecting autonomy, the most we can do is present the father with the option of becoming a donor and spell out its benefits and risks. Indeed, given the role of informed consent in preserving autonomy, we must make it possible for the father to refuse to be a donor without suffering rebuke. Even if we feel disapproval, we must avoid pressuring the parent into making a positive decision. (Whether the parent may later regret his decision is not our concern.) Expressing autonomy is not necessarily doing what others think is right, but exercising control over one's actions.

Crouch and Elliott (1999: 277) suggest, alternatively, that the 'can't say no' of Caplan and Annas may be construed as invoking a certain notion of moral agency according to which agents are completely free only when they have no ties to others and so every decision considers only the agent's interests. The authors rightly reject this notion, pointing out that the only people who fit such a description are sociopaths. Moral and emotional commitments, they write, 'are not constraints on freedom, but are rather part of ordinary human life' (Crouch and Elliott 1999: 278). I take this to mean that acting for the sake of someone we love does not make us less free. Deciding to act out of love is not a constraint on autonomy but an expression of it, and the Caplan–Annas claim rests on an error.

'Can't say no', in a third interpretation, may be taken to mean 'For anyone emotionally attached to the patient, no option other than becoming a donor is worth considering.' Under this construal, when a transplant offers the best chance of saving the patient's life, the volunteer donor is not interested in other possibilities. He knows at once what he wants to do and is ready to make an immediate decision. 'Can't say no' means, in effect, 'Doesn't want to say no', and if this is what Caplan and Annas are claiming, I find it unobjectionable. (The volunteer must be informed of risks and options and given a chance to consider them, of course, for otherwise his consent is not informed.)

It is a mistake to believe, though, as Caplan and Annas may be asserting, that when a decision must be made in a stressful situation in which we care very much about the outcome, the decision is necessarily compromised. This confuses the external pressure that illegitimately influences a decision (family expectations, for example) with the pressure inherent in a situation that requires making a decision. Calling both 'coercive' obscures the crucial difference. Being forced to decide is not the same as being forced to decide a certain way.

Buying a house is stressful for most people, and while we use laws to shield customers from being coerced into buying the house they are considering, we have no way to shield them from the need to make the decision to buy that house, another house, or no house at all. Similarly, while we can use the consent process to protect parents or others from being pressured into becoming donors, we cannot protect them from the need to make the decision in an inherently stressful situation. They are coerced (by the situation) into having to make a decision, but the decision whether to become a donor is not necessarily (and should not be) coerced.

HEROIC DONORS

Because autonomy is the justifying foundation for using living donors, discussions of the practice usually focus on ways of making sure that candidates are free to decide if they want to take the risks. (See e.g. Gutmann and Land 1999: 516.) But what are we to say when volunteers insist on becoming donors against medical advice? Is it acceptable for a physician to reject a candidate who demands to become a donor because the risks would be greater than usual for donors? The case below illustrates how the question arises.

> *Case 2*: Donald Astrid's wife died from a pulmonary embolism in childbirth, and his newborn daughter was diagnosed with biliary atresia. Surgery to bypass the child's bile ducts by attaching a loop of intestine to her liver failed, and without an immediate liver transplant, she would die.
>
> Astrid is assessed as a donor at Bayshore Transplant Center and found medically unacceptable. He has a heart arrhythmia, diagnosed and treated with drugs for three years, that puts him at a higher than usual risk of suffering a stroke or dying during the surgery. Astrid insists on becoming a donor, despite the outcome of the assessment and against the recommendation of his physician.

Spital refers to people like Astrid as 'heroic volunteers' and argues that if a physician had to accept a volunteer 'against his best judgment', this would mean the volunteer 'has an absolute right to donate', because the volunteer's wishes 'would be determinative'. The physician would have to do the transplant, 'even though he considers donation to be dangerous and ill-advised' (Spital 2001: 193).

Spital's talk about an 'absolute right' is difficult to interpret in the absence of a definition. What Spital appears to mean is: If A has an absolute right to do D, we must permit A to do D whatever the circumstances or consequences. But it is unreasonable to believe that a heroic volunteer is asserting anything so strong. A volunteer who insists on donating against the 'best judgment' of his physician is merely rejecting the advice of his physician. He is not claiming that no consideration will alter his decision and that he must be allowed to do D just because that is what he wants to do. He would, presumably, drop his demand if he learned that his blood type is incompatible with his child's so that if his child received a lobe of his liver, the child would die. It is, furthermore, doubtful that anyone holds that we have any absolute rights in the sense Spital seems to mean.

Spital's argument seems beside the point, in any case. The real issue arises when we ask who is entitled to make the final decision about whether a volunteer can become a donor. Spital sees the autonomy of the heroic volunteer as conflicting with the autonomy of the physician who must carry out the volunteer's wishes. Thus, 'the physician must agree with the volunteer that the potential benefits of the procedure are worth the risks, as is true for any medical procedure' (Spital 2001: 193).

Potential benefits have to be worth the risks, Spital says. But whose benefits and whose risks is Spital talking about? The potential *medical* benefits of being a donor are never worth the risks. Indeed, the donor suffers medical harms. By contrast, the potential medical benefits of being the recipient of a healthy organ are *always* worth the risks, because without it the recipient will either die (in cases like Astrid's daughter) or experience additional suffering. The benefit the donor achieves has to be something other than medical.

The physician, on Spital's view, must then have to balance the risk and non-medical benefit of the donor against the benefit of the recipient. But this means that the physician is put in the position of deciding whether she is willing for the volunteer to take the risks. The result is that, in making it her decision, she is denying the volunteer the opportunity to decide how much risk he is willing to take for the benefit he seeks. Rather than the physician's exercising her autonomy, as Spital suggests, she is exercising paternalistic power over the volunteer.

It would be wrong for a physician to agree to kill even a willing volunteer for the sake of obtaining an organ for a recipient, even if the transplanted organ would save the recipient's life. (Removing vital organs and thereby causing death would violate the dead-donor rule, which is the moral and social cornerstone of the practice of organ transplantation. While it is possible to challenge the rule on the ground that perhaps six lives might be saved by sacrificing one willing subject, it is not clear that rejecting the rule and permitting this would allow more lives to be saved. Indeed, the entire enterprise might collapse. I assume here, without argument, the legitimacy and utility of the rule.) Short of this extreme, however, the donation decision ought to be the volunteer's. The physician should, of course, advise the volunteer of the risks to his health and life. It would even be appropriate for the physician to warn the heroic volunteer against becoming a donor on the grounds that he will be taking a greater than usual risk.

Ultimately, though, the physician must let the volunteer decide whether he wants to put his life on the line. The physician may, as is the case with all medical treatment, exercise her autonomy by refusing to accept the heroic volunteer as a patient, but it is not clear, given her role as a physician, how she could justify her refusal.

Spital offers what can be taken as an attempt to address this issue. 'Physicians are responsible for the welfare of their patients, and should act in their best interests . . .', he writes. But the problem with this view, as with the initial one, is that because transplant surgery *always* causes harm to the donor, it can never be in the best medical interest of anyone to become a donor. This can be the case only if 'best medical interest' is understood to include a commitment to the welfare of the recipient. While this was the position taken by Justice Counihan (see below) in the first of the twin-transplant cases, this construal of 'medical' seems arbitrary and no more than a dodge to permit causing medical harm.

'Best interest', as understood by the heroic volunteer, may include a commitment to the welfare of the recipient, despite the fact that the volunteer's medical best interest will not be served. Thus, Astrid's concept of his best interest will include doing whatever he can to save the life of his daughter. He will not find it acceptable, then, for a physician to refuse to let him become a donor because the physician does not consider it in his best interest. Why should the physician's concept of the volunteer's best interest always trump the volunteer's concept? Why should the volunteer's decision about the risk he is willing to take be supplanted by the physician's decision? Spital offers no answer to these questions.

Spital accepts the notion that a heroic volunteer rejected as a donor by one physician may legitimately find another who will accept him. This concession is enough to permit, in principle, heroic donors to take whatever risks they consider appropriate to further their concept of their best interest. But 'in principle' does not necessarily translate into 'in fact'. What if a heroic volunteer cannot find any physician willing to accept him as a donor?

We are then back in the position that Spital characterized as a conflict between the autonomy of the would-be donor and the autonomy of the physician. The donor cannot act to promote his understanding of his best interest (e.g. saving the life of his child) without the participation of the physician, while the physician believes she should not act, because it would not serve what she considers the best interest of the patient.

Once again, I hold that the patient's concept of his best interest should trump the physician's. The physician has a duty to inform the volunteer that he would be taking a greater than usual risk, but the decision about whether to take it should ultimately be the donor's, not the physician's. This would be no more than a case of acting against medical advice, something long acknowledged to fall within the scope of patient autonomy. While the physician may regret the patient's decision, refusing to abide by it would amount to a violation of the patient's autonomy for paternalistic reasons.

I also hold that, where living donors are concerned, an appropriate understanding of what it means for the physician to be committed to promoting the interest of the volunteer–patient makes clear that there is no conflict between the autonomy of the volunteer–patient and the physician. Ordinarily, the physician's commitment to promoting the best interest of the patient is understood as limited to the diagnosis and management of disease in the medical context. But the practice of using living donors requires extending the notion of 'best interest' beyond that context. The volunteer's best interest must include his non-medical wants and values. Thus, the physician's commitment to promote the volunteer–patient's best interest is a commitment to promote the broadened notion, the one that includes the volunteer–patient's decisions about what is important and what risks he is willing to run to secure ends he values.

A physician *qua* physician must act for the sake of the patient's best interest, and, given the practice of using living donors, this means accepting the broadened notion of best interest as determined by the volunteer–patient. The physician, therefore, has an obligation to accept a heroic volunteer as a donor, even though the volunteer acts against medical advice. Because the physician *qua* physician is acting in the best interest of the volunteer, the physician's autonomy is not in conflict with the volunteer's. It would be in conflict only if 'best interest' is understood by the physician as limited to the medical best interest.

Even if this argument is correct, finding a physician willing to operate on a willing heroic volunteer may remain a practical problem. This is not, however, a circumstance unique to transplant ethics. During the early years of the AIDS epidemic, some physicians refused to treat HIV-positive patients. While physicians lack moral grounds for refusing to accept heroic volunteers, given the circumstances in which transplants take place, the volunteers may not be permitted realize their intention to become donors.

STRANGERS AS DONORS

The initial basis for accepting living donors was a broadly construed concept of 'medical interest' (the sort of construal Spital needs to make his argument work). The purpose of medical treatment is to benefit the patient, but when surgeons remove an organ from a living donor, only the recipient appears to benefit. How then can physicians justify causing harm to a healthy person for the sake of someone else?

Surgeons at Boston's Brigham Hospital grappled with this question in 1957 at the dawn of kidney transplantation. Leonard Marsden, a 17-year-old, eagerly consented to donate a kidney to his identical twin, Leon. The surgeons then hesitated, questioning whether by subjecting Leonard to surgery they would be providing him with any benefit. Hoping to clear the way, the twins' parents petitioned the Massachusetts Supreme Judicial Court to rule on the question. Justice E. A. Counihan, after hearing testimony about the brothers, decided that if the transplant were not done and Leon died, Leonard would suffer an emotional disturbance that would adversely affect his health and well-being (Curran 1959: 893). The surgery would thus confer a 'medical benefit' on both brothers. Consequently, the surgeons would not be harming Leonard just to benefit Leon.

The judge's insight was that benefit should not be understood too narrowly, even in the medical context. That the benefit for Leonard should be viewed as 'medical' was never persuasive. Without much discussion, as the frequency of kidney transplants increased, centers began to construe Counihan's 'medical benefit' as equivalent to the donor's having an 'emotional relation' to the recipient. Thus, donors were limited by most centers to parents, spouses, siblings, or other blood relatives. In the 1980s and 1990s, however, as transplants became safer and deceased-donor organs scarcer, centers expanded the notion of 'emotional relation' and started accepting friends of recipients as donors.

While some centers still adhere to such a policy, others have decided to accept also 'altruistic strangers' or 'Good Samaritan donors' (see Case 3 below). The transplant community, even when dealing with family donors, has always stressed altruism as a reason for becoming a donor, and some recent writers have claimed altruism as the sole basis for organ donation. This has occasioned a debate about how the altruism of family and friends ('intimates') compares with that of strangers. At stake is thought to be how much risk each group ought to be permitted to take.

Ross and co-authors (Ross et al. 2002: 426) argue that intimates cannot be purely altruistic, because, given their sense of duties and obligations, they are both other-regarding and self-serving. Thus, intimates should be permitted to run higher risks than strangers, because intimates both act out of duty and do not identify their interest as being completely different from that of a recipient. Daar (2002) shows, however, that this conclusion depends on accepting the authors' definition of an altruistic act as 'one motivated primarily or solely by respect and concern for the preferences and needs of others, freely chosen rather than done out of a duty or obligation' (Ross et al. 2002: 426). Daar argues persuasively that, even if we accept the definition, 'altruism does not negate every element of self-interest' and even strangers may have their own sense of intimacy and duty (Daar 2002: 424). Each potential donor, Daar holds, should be treated as an individual person and his or her acceptability based on such considerations as the level of risk, not on intimacy or degree of altruism.

While Daar's rejection of the Ross position is warranted, the debate itself rests on a misconception. Altruism may be a motive for organ donation and serve as an explanation for why people become donors, but it is not the moral basis for allowing living donors. Altruism is a value, but it is neither a duty nor an ethical principle, and it is a mistake to look to it to justify donation policies. Rather, it is our commitment to the autonomy of the individual, protected by the process of informed consent, that makes the use of living donors morally legitimate.

Volunteers are given the opportunity to become informed and protected from pressures. They are given the chance to deliberate, with the opportunity to change their minds later, and then allowed to decide whether they wish to become donors. Perhaps some, maybe even the vast majority, will be moved by the wish to benefit others. But a misanthrope who wants to become a donor is as acceptable as an philanthropic superstar, so long as the process of informed consent is followed.

While we may be curious about people's motives (and may want to appeal to them to increase the number of donors), it is not motives that determine whether the selection of volunteers is legitimate. When the conditions of informed consent are satisfied, living donors, whether strangers or intimates, can reasonably be viewed as promoting their own interest. They are exercising their autonomy in deciding what is important to them and what they are willing to risk to secure it. They are deciding how they want to shape their lives.

The assertion that altruism, rather than autonomy, is the basis for organ donation is a way of blocking what some see as an unacceptable consequence of allowing unrelated donors. The major objection to using such donors is that the practice may encourage the commercialization of transplantation (Kaplan and Polise 2000: 520). A mother is not likely to sell a kidney to her son, but a stranger might sell hers to the same person. Commercialization, which entails self-interest, is inherently incompatible with altruism. Thus, if altruism were required to legitimize donation, the very possibility of commercialization would be ruled out.

Yet even if compelling reasons could be given against commercializing organ procurement, merely asserting that altruism must always be the basis for donation is not persuasive. We need an argument to show that there is something about selling organs that is morally different from selling cars or blood plasma.

PAYING LIVING DONORS

The idea of paying donors or selling organs has been denounced by the transplant community, politicians, and religious leaders since the early 1980s (Munson 2002: 98–110), coincidental with the time that transplants were becoming successful. The United States National Organ Transplantation Act of 1984 makes buying and selling organs, whether from living or deceased donors, illegal, as do the laws of Great Britain, all European countries, China, India, Russia, Mexico, and South Africa. The World Health Organization condemns paying for organs under any circumstance (World Health Organization 1991), and, although trade in transplant organs takes place in parts of Asia, the Middle East, and South America, it is illicit (Cameron and Hoffenberg 1999: 727).

The world ban on organ sales has been defended over the decades by a number of ethicists, lawyers, and transplant professionals who have generated a laundry list of objections to paying donors. (I shall limit discussion to living donors of kidneys; selling organs from deceased donors raises different issues.) Prominent and recurrent objections include: a paid donor loses the psychological benefits that reward an altruistic donor; paid donation reduces altruism in society; the quality of donated kidneys will decline; the donor may suffer harm and become a burden to society; paying donors may reduce the number of donations from deceased donors; organ selling puts the human body in the same moral category as slavery; organ selling involves putting a price on the priceless; paying for organs exploits the poor;

organ selling treats the human body as a commodity and thus violates our respect for persons. (See Phadke and Anandh 2002; Radcliffe-Richards *et al.* 1998; Russo and Brown 2003, for a review of objections.)

Most of these complaints are about institutionalizing the buying and selling of transplant organs—that is, making organs goods in the market economy. Such objections are, for the most, consequentialist, and while the numerous issues raised are important, they go beyond the scope of this chapter. The question logically prior to the market and consequentialist issues is whether there is something about paying kidney donors that makes it inherently wrong.

I claim there is not. If the autonomy of the individual is the basis for recognizing that, when the conditions of informed consent are met, donating a kidney to someone is a morally legitimate act, it must also be morally legitimate for the individual to be paid for donating the kidney. Either act follows as a result of a decision made freely by the person. In the first case, the individual decides to be altruistic, in the second case, she decides she wants money.

Individuals may be said to own (or, at a minimum, have legitimate control over) their bodies in substantially the same sense in which they own their diamonds. Thus, in the way that individuals are free either to sell or give away one of their diamonds, they are free either to sell or give away parts of their bodies. Altruism might move someone to donate a diamond to a charity or to donate a kidney to a stranger; or he might decide to sell both. (I consider someone's selling his own organ and being paid to be an organ donor as equivalent.)

While differences between diamonds and body parts are numerous, I suggest that none is morally relevant with respect to the matter of getting paid to become an organ donor. Once we have agreed that autonomy is the ground for legitimizing an individual's decision to donate a kidney, we must also acknowledge it as legitimizing his decision to sell a kidney.

But what if someone wants to sell both his kidneys? Or his heart, liver, or lungs? While we may agree that, as their owner, he may dispose of his organs in any way that he sees fit, this does not mean that we are free to remove them or to buy them. We are constrained by the fact that by taking both his kidneys or his vital organs, we would be killing him. We would (to put the point another way) be violating the dead-donor rule, which requires us to establish that a donor is dead before any organ needed to sustain his life is removed. It is prima facie wrong to kill someone, even if he wants us to, and even if we could use his organs to save several lives.

The most common defense of the claim that selling a kidney is morally wrong in itself is based on the Kantian view that it does not show respect for one's humanity. Selling a kidney expresses disrespect for oneself and, as a consequence, disrespect for what it means to be human (Morelli 1999: 320). Gill and Sade (2002: 26) reject this complaint, justifiably, on the ground that it is not persuasive to consider one's humanity as dependent on one of one's kidneys. One's humanity may be viewed, more reasonably, as dependent on one's rationality and one's capacity to follow self-given laws (autonomy) dependent on it. Selling a kidney thus has no destructive effects on one's humanity. Hence, it cannot express disrespect for all humanity.

A second and similar Kantian-type objection is that it is wrong to sell kidneys because human beings are not property, and, as Cohen says, to sell them 'and those bits and pieces integral to them is to violate that which is essential to them' (Cohen 2002: 28). While Cohen is right that to sell human beings violates their inherent worth, she wrongly assumes that the 'bits and pieces' of their bodies are likewise of inherent worth. If 'integral' means 'essential' or 'indispensable', a kidney fails to meet the description. Unlike selling oneself into slavery, selling one's kidney will have no consequences on one's capacity for self-governance. Indeed, Cohen's argument appears to be a case of the fallacy of division.

Gill and Sade (2002: 25) point out that even if the Kantian argument that selling one's kidney violates the categorical imperative, because it involves treating oneself as a means only, were correct, it would not follow that paying a donor should be against the law. We do not base our laws on the Kantian duty to respect humanity by respecting oneself. The laws we make aim, rather, at protecting the (non-Kantian) autonomy of individuals. We protect their freedom to make personal decisions about self-regarding acts, and, if the decision they make is to follow their understanding of a rational moral law (Kantian autonomy), they are free to do that as well. No one need sell a kidney.

The transplant community is now in the process of rethinking its long-time condemnation of paying donors (Joralemon 2001; Cameron and Hoffenberg 1999: 724–5). The initial impetus for disapproval, in my opinion, was the fear of alienating the public by associating transplants with money and the unseemly business of trading in body parts. The community was afraid that a loss of public approval, due to bad associations, would result in a decline in the number of people donating their organs at death. Without donated organs, the entire transplant enterprise would then collapse. To sustain the system, the community has always stressed altruism and downplayed the commercial aspects of transplantation. That hospitals, surgeons, coordinators, laboratories, transport services, and organ procurement organizations make money from transplants is not a shameful truth, yet it is rarely mentioned in public. Inspiring stories of transplant miracles are the preferred sort of publicity.

Yet now that the organ shortage is desperate and the public is more familiar with transplants (and perhaps more tolerant of commerce), some are saying that we need to reconsider the issue of paying donors. Extolling altruism has not produced nearly enough donors, so thousands of people are dying who might be saved. (The situation is especially critical in countries that cannot afford to buy and maintain the dialysis equipment required to sustain the lives of thousands in kidney failure.) Many do not find the arguments against paying donors compelling and believe that we could devise mechanisms to protect consent and prevent the exploitation of the poor and disadvantaged. Because so many lives are at stake, the resolution of this issue is of more than academic concern.

Protecting the Donor: Promises Unkept

Protecting a living donor must be understood as involving more than securing informed consent and guaranteeing the volunteer's autonomy at the time of decision making. The following case points to a problem that needs solving.

> *Case 3*: Arielle Dove was so moved by the selfless acts displayed in the aftermath of the 9/11 terrorist attacks that she decided to donate a kidney to a stranger (Meckler: 2003). She located a living-donor web site and arranged for one of hers to be removed and transplanted into someone she had never met.
>
> After the surgery her life took a turn for the worse. More than a year later she still had episodes of vomiting and felt dizzy and listless. She was also very angry. The man who received her kidney assured her he would pay for her expenses not covered by his insurance. But he didn't keep his promise. 'I volunteered to put my life on the line, and I guess I've given up my good health for this, and nobody seems to care,' she said. 'It's really hard not to cry.'

Living donors may develop long-term medical problems, may not be able to work for weeks or months, may require a liver or kidney transplant themselves, may run up medical bills not covered by their insurance or a recipient's. Who is going to pay for the donor's post-transplant expenses? Will it be the recipient? The transplant center? Or will the donor herself have to find some way? These are among the questions that need to be settled before a potential donor becomes an actual one. Yet often the questions are neither asked nor answered.

No one, as matters stand, is committed to looking out for the longer-term interest of the donor. Some donors complain that once they have had a kidney or liver lobe removed and are out of the hospital, transplant centers no longer take any interest in their welfare. Promises that the donors thought were made are not kept, and their future health problems are not recognized as possibly related to the surgery or the loss of an organ. To make sure that the practice of using living donors functions in a morally legitimate way requires that we introduce into general practice three measures to protect the welfare of donors and future donors.

1. *Living-donor advocate: medical.* Some transplant centers provide donors with a medical advocate, and this should be required of all centers that accept living donors. (This is also a recommendation of United States Department of Health and Human Services Advisory Committee on Organ Transplantation 2002: 3.) A medical advocate should be a physician with expertise in transplantation who is not

involved in the care of a potential recipient. An advocate should assist a candidate donor in understanding the process, risks, and benefits of becoming a donor and help the candidate frame appropriate questions and gather information relevant to making a decision. The advocate should, in general, take the measures needed to guarantee that consent is free and informed.

If a volunteer becomes a donor, the advocate should then be responsible for making sure that the medical interest of the donor is served. This means not only seeing to it that the donor–patient receives appropriate hospital care, but making sure that she receives whatever follow-up care she needs. The advocate should serve as the donor's medical advisor and champion, though not as her physician.

2. *Living-donor advocate: legal.* The Dove case illustrates, taking Dove at her word, what can happen to a donor when commitments made to her are only an informal understanding. A properly written consent document spells out the potential risks and benefits to the donor, alternatives to donation, and the opportunity to withdraw consent, but its usefulness is limited.

It serves the dual purposes of informing the volunteer and offering partial proof that a donor's choice was appropriately informed and risks were voluntarily undertaken. This (among other things) helps protect centers and physicians from lawsuits and professional censure, but the document, other than informing, provides little help to the donor. The center or the recipient's insurer may agree to provide the donor with medical care that is immediately associated with the surgery, but if the donor loses income due to the hospitalization, will the money be reimbursed? And if the donor develops medical problems six months or a year later, will she be provided with free care? If, as Dove alleges happened to her, the recipient agrees to pay for costs not covered by insurance, then fails or refuses to do so, what remedy does the donor have?

What the donor requires to protect her interest is a legally enforceable agreement—a contract—with the transplant center and with the recipient. The donor needs a legal advocate, as well as a medical one. The advocate should be an attorney whose fees are paid by the center, the recipient, or the recipient's insurer, but whose client is the donor.

The legal advocate, with the medical advocate, should consult with the potential donor as part of the consent process. The advocates should go over the consent document with the candidate, and the legal advocate should be available to offer advice before the volunteer makes the consent decision. (A potential donor may refuse legal advice or act against it.)

Either as part of the consent document or in an additional document, commitments made to the donor with respect to such matters as financial compensation for time lost while hospitalized, the assumption of responsibility for health-care costs of the donor for donation-related problems, how a dispute about whether a complaint is donation-related should be resolved, and the limits of assumed responsibility should be addressed.

The legal advisor should consult with the donor after the donation is completed and the donor hospitalized. If either advocate questions whether the kind or quality of care promised is being delivered, then the attorney should advise the donor about the availability of appropriate legal remedies.

Physicians and centers, fearing unwarranted litigation, are not likely to welcome legal advocates into the donation process. Yet donors put themselves at risk, and they deserve to be assured that guarantees made to them have the status of a legally enforceable contract.

The addition of a legal advocate will add to the cost of a transplant. Quite apart from protecting the interests of donors, however, the knowledge that a legal advocate will be assigned to each donor may make becoming a living donor an acceptable option for many more people. This opens the possibility of saving more lives than can be saved at present.

3. *Living-donor registry*. Data about living donors are mostly from kidney donors. Even here, the data are for the most part confined to statistics about operative mortality and survival (Park *et al.* 1996). Liver-lobe donation is sufficiently untried that even the mortality rate associated with it is uncertain. Data for lung-lobe and pancreas-segment donors are similarly sparse.

The long-term effects of becoming a living donor of any organ or organ-part have been little studied (Najarian *et al.* 1992). Thus, the information needed by donor candidates is not as good as it should be. Perhaps better information would do little to change the decisions parents make to donate to their children, but it might have a significant impact on others, particularly on those who want to deliberate before making a decision about donating an organ to a stranger. Because the liver regenerates, data showing that harmful results are rare over the long term would likely increase the number of living liver donors.

Also, if donors develop serious medical problems years later that are shown to be donation-related, we need to decide how to compensate the donors and establish who has responsibility for doing so. Further, if some problems are serious and occur often, we need to decide whether our commitment to individual autonomy requires transplant centers to accept donors who are likely to develop diseases that will compel us to spend considerable public resources for treatment.

Such considerations show that because we allow living donors, establishing a national living-donor registry is a compelling need. (For a similar recommendation, see United States Department of Health and Human Services Advisory Committee on Organ Transplantation 2002: 3.) The registry would keep track of donors and collect and preserve medical information about them over the years. The registry could take the form of a database operated and financed either by a federal agency or by an organization like UNOS, which works under a federal contract. Computers and the Internet make it possible for hospitals, transplant centers, and physicians to supply the information needed at relatively little cost. That the time has come to establish such a registry is a belief widely shared in the transplant community (Ochs 2002).

DONORS OF LAST RESORT

A basic rule of donor selection is that children and others incapable of consenting ought to be donors of last resort. Those able to consent are (by definition) capable of looking out for their welfare, but those incapable of doing so are open to exploitation. Hence, we have a duty to protect them.

When primarily living donors were employed in the 1950s–1970s, whether it was legitimate to use a child as a donor was often a life-or-death issue. The situation has eased but not disappeared. Kidneys remain in short supply, and children benefit from being removed from dialysis as soon as possible. Thus, families continue to be pressured by circumstances to make wrenching decisions about risking the health and safety of one child to benefit another. The scope of the problem may also be increasing. While now only adults are accepted as liver-lobe donors, when the transplants become better established, children and other 'incompetents' may become regarded as potential donors for siblings or other family members.

Circumstances in which a child might be the only available liver-lobe donor for a sibling are easy to imagine. The surviving parent, for example, might not have a blood type compatible with that of the child in need. Or the parent might be too ill to become a donor. More distant relatives, if any, might fail to qualify as donors or might refuse. The child's sacrifice could be all that stands between her sibling and death.

Important Interest at Stake

The fundamental requirement to be met in justifying a child's becoming an organ donor, I suggest, is that the child must have something important at stake in the use made of the organ. (I will refer to children here, yet most considerations apply also to incompetent adults.) Becoming a donor must be in the child's best interest, and this may require that the child suffer surgical injury and run some risk of death. The child's best interest can be understood as the child's having a significant stake in the welfare of the organ's intended recipient. (As mentioned above, Leonard Marsden, with respect to his brother's welfare, had at stake something affecting his own 'health and physical well-being'.)

No matter how slight the risk, a child (or other incompetent person) cannot be required to donate an organ to help a stranger, even if the organ would save the stranger's life. The child has no direct stake in the stranger's welfare, and thus the donation would not serve the best interest of the child. By contrast, an intimate who is not a relative may be of crucial importance to the child's welfare, as Anne Sullivan was to Helen Keller.

Reasonable Risk

It is appropriate to subject a child to some risk to protect her best interest. Thus, in cases where the life of a person important in the child's life is at stake, it is reasonable to put the child at risk for the benefit she may gain. We put children at risk for expected benefits in other medical contexts, even when their lives are not endangered—surgery to correct club foot, cleft palate, or amblyopia, for example.

What we know of risks at present indicates that it is sometimes justifiable to make children into kidney donors, but not liver-lobe or lung-lobe or pancreas-segment donors. We do not yet know enough about the effects and risks of such donations to subject children to them, even when a child has an important stake in the life of a recipient. The American Medical Association's Council on Ethical and Judicial Affairs puts the point tersely: 'Children should not be used for transplants that are considered experimental or non-standard' (American Medical Association 1996–7: 35).

Where the chances of death or suffering serious harm are considerable or unknown, we lack justification to put a child at risk, even to save the life of a person important to the child. We are free to decide to risk our own lives for anyone, because we are able to understand our alternatives and the consequences of our actions. Children cannot. Hence, when we decide for them, we must take the most conservative stance compatible with their interest.

Deciding About Donors of Last Resort

An asymmetry exists between those competent to consent and those who are not. Children are not competent to decide to become donors, but they are also not competent to decide *not* to become donors. (I will not address here issues of assent connected with older children.) A decision belonging to competent people belongs to someone else in the case of incompetent people.

This asymmetry offers the potential for exploitation. Suppose Sue Crane needs a kidney transplant. High blood pressure eliminates her husband, Sam, as a donor, but their healthy 22-year-old son Bob, now in law school, has the same blood type and is a good antigen match. The Cranes's retarded 16-year-old son, Tom, is also a good match, however.

Bob is willing to be the donor, but he is the pride of the Crane family, and his parents do not want to interrupt his education and subject him to the risks of surgery. Tom is a constant source of difficulty. 'Now he has a chance to do something to help the family,' Sam says. Sam and Sue then instruct Bob to refuse to volunteer when he is interviewed at the transplant center. Sam is medically unacceptable, Bob refuses, and no one else steps forward. Thus, Tom becomes the donor of last resort.

The duty to protect incompetent people from exploitation rests with whoever has the responsibility to decide what is in their best interest. The courts already decide for institutionalized and demonstrably incompetent adults. With respect to children, parents are the obvious candidates to make the decision, but two considerations rule them out. First, parents like the Cranes can conspire to sacrifice the weakest member of the family to protect a favored one. The person who needs the most protection thus becomes, ironically, the one who is the most vulnerable.

The situation is not improved if, as Ross (1993) recommends, the family as a whole is given the power to decide. While this could, as she says, promote intimate relations and allow the family to draw upon its own values, religious beliefs, and sense of itself, it leaves children with no protection from family pressures. Indeed, Ross's process of family decision making describes exactly the situation Starzl (1985) considered so inherently manipulative as to lead him to recommend against the use of even adults as living donors.

A second difficulty is that parents can be forced into a Sophie's-choice situation requiring them to help one child (or family member) only at the expense of another. This faces them with a conflict of interest, so that whatever decision they make will be suspect (even to themselves) and open to charges of unfairness and favoritism.

Decisions about accepting competent adult candidates as donors are now made by committees at transplant centers, and this same approach might be taken with children. Williams (1995: 499) advocates the use of ad hoc groups to make decisions about children as potential bone marrow donors and describes how, at a Honolulu hospital, a staff committee interviews children in an informal way and determines if they understand 'their role in the transplant procedure' and if their willingness to be a donor is 'free from duress and based on adequate information'. Depending on the judgment of the committee, a child is accepted or rejected as a donor. The committee process, Williams observes, is inexpensive, efficient, and offers a way to consider the best interest of a child.

Despite these virtues, a committee approach has drawbacks so serious as to make it unacceptable. First, committees work effectively only when children are old enough to grasp what is being asked of them and assent to it. This leaves open the question of how we should deal with younger children.

Committees are also limited in their powers to obtain data relevant to the decision they must make. If a family member withholds information or lies to the committee (claiming he has a close relationship with a child, for example), the committee can impose no sanctions and must make its decision on the basis of whatever data it can gather or surmise.

More is at stake, furthermore, for an organ donor than for a bone marrow donor. Harvesting bone marrow involves discomfort and the risk of infection, but no significant danger is associated with it. Being a kidney donor requires extensive surgery, greater risk of infection, and a chance of dying or long-term effects. Because more is at stake for organ donors, more protection for vulnerable potential donors is required.

Decision of the Court

Williams's observation that court proceedings can be time consuming and costly is correct, but protecting people from serious exploitation is sufficiently important to warrant additional time and money. The courts, more than any other institution, are in the best position to guarantee that stringent criteria for a child's becoming a donor are satisfied and that the best interest of the child is served.

Courts of law, unlike committees, however constituted, operate within a tradition of protecting the rights of individuals by invoking a variety of procedural and substantive safeguards. Should a 6-year-old girl contribute a kidney to her teenage sister? A court can conduct discovery proceedings and gather relevant medical and personal information, using its subpoena powers if necessary, and thus put itself in the position of answering the question.

Experts can be called to offer opinions, and family members required to testify under oath. Rules of evidence, relevance, and proof can be brought to bear on the basic question. Most important, a court can appoint an attorney (a guardian *ad litem*) to represent the child to make sure everything recognized as relevant to her interest is brought forward for the court to consider.

Because courts have powers committees lack, committees are never able to delve so thoroughly into issues affecting the welfare of candidate donors. At the end of hearings, when the evidence and arguments for and against a child's becoming a donor have been presented, a court's deliberations offer the best chance of getting an independent and objective decision. A committee might have arrived at the same decision, but where protecting the vulnerable is concerned, process and safeguards matter.

The presiding judge of a Massachusetts court made this point forcefully in the 1977 *Saikewicz* decision:

We take a dim view of any attempt to shift the ultimate decision-making responsibility away from the duly established court ... to any committee, panel, or group, ad hoc or permanent.... questions of life and death seem to us to require the process of detached but passionate investigation and decision that would form the ideals under which the judicial branch of government was created. Achieving this ideal is our responsibility ... (*Superintendent of Belchertown State School, et al. v. Saikewicz*, 417)

I have argued, to recapitulate, that a child (or other incompetent person) may become an organ donor when: it is in the child's best interest; risk to the child is reasonable; the child is the donor of last resort; a court of law, rather than parents or any sort of committee, is making the decision.

Summary: Rules Regulating Living Donors

Perhaps the most useful way to summarize the above discussions is to state rules or guidelines. Yet because several important questions were not addressed and guidelines must always be interpreted, the following rules are not offered as either exhaustive or definitive.

1. A potential donor must be competent to make decisions. This includes being able to understand the nature and likelihood of the risks involved in becoming a donor.

2. A potential donor must be provided with information adequate for making the donation decision. The need to provide information about the nature and likelihood of risks and benefits is clear. Less obvious is the need to supply the candidate with information about the alternatives available to the potential recipient (e.g. dialysis, continued medical support, waiting for a deceased-donor organ, or waiting for another living donor).

3. Potential donors should not be solicited. A center may inform the patient and others that those who want to consider becoming donors should contact a designated person who is uninvolved with the patient. Russo and Brown endorse this rule (Russo and Brown 2003: 27), and Biller-Andorno and Schauenburg suggest that a volunteer should identify herself 'without any action on the part of the physician' (2001: 163).

4. A potential donor must be protected from pressures to volunteer. A willingness to become a donor ought to be considered a necessary condition for being a 'suitable' candidate. The assessment team should determine in a private interview if the candidate is willing. The candidate needs to be told that, no matter what he may have said to others nor what others may expect him to do, if he decides he is not willing to be a donor, this will remain confidential. If the candidate says he is unwilling, the assessment team will then declare him an 'unsuitable' candidate, with no details made public. This will protect the candidate from the anger, recriminations, or blame that might have been directed at him for publicly refusing to help the patient needing the transplant.

A candidate must also be permitted to change his mind about becoming a donor until the last moment before surgery. This may result in great inconvenience and disappointment and even put the intended recipient at greater risk than if no apparent donor had become available, but it would be a serious violation of an individual's autonomy to remove one of his organs after he has withdrawn his consent.

5. Assessment of the suitability of a potential donor should not be done by physicians or others involved in the care of the potential recipient. This will eliminate the conflict of interest inherent in a relationship in which those caring for a patient needing a transplant also select a donor.

The assessment should be done by a team (e.g. hepatologist or nephrologist, psychiatrist or psychologist, social worker, etc.) able to determine whether the candidate is medically and psychologically suitable to become a donor. The assessment should also consider a potential donor's social and economic situation so that the candidate can be provided with information about the impact that becoming a donor might have on his or her life.

6. Potential donors should be provided with medical and legal advocates. Both advocates should advise a candidate before she makes a decision. If she decides to becomes a donor, the legal advocate should represent her interests in making contractual arrangements with the center and with the intended recipient. The medical and legal advocates should monitor her welfare after the transplant.

7. A registry should be established to gather longitudinal data about the health of living donors. The database in the United States could be operated by UNOS under a contract with the federal government. The information could be medically important to donors, and it would be relevant in informing potential donors about potential risks.

8. Donors incompetent to consent may become donors if it is in their best interest, the risk to them is reasonable, no other donors are available, and the decision permitting them to become donors is made by a court of law.

Conclusion

Organ transplants save thousands of lives every year, yet thousands more die because of the shortage of organs. While increasing the number of organs from deceased donors would be of considerable value, the best hope for saving the lives of tens of thousands of people who would otherwise die is to increase the number of living donors.

The autonomy of the individual legitimizes an individual's decision to become a living organ donor. This does not relieve transplant centers of the responsibility for seeing to it that donors are genuine volunteers and have the information they need to assess their risks and options. Measures are needed to protect the autonomy of the individual in deciding whether to become a donor, but additional measures are needed to protect the welfare of living donors. These include appointing donor advocates and maintaining a registry of living donors.

The prospect of saving so many thousands of lives requires us to take seriously the moral and the practical issues centering around the use of living donors. Yet we do not have time to discuss those issues indefinitely. The sooner some matters are settled, such as the moral legitimacy of paying donors, the more lives will be saved. The issues are urgent, for literally life and death are at stake.

REFERENCES

AMERICAN MEDICAL ASSOCIATION, COUNCIL ON ETHICAL AND JUDICIAL AFFAIRS (1996–7), 'The Use of Minors as Organ and Tissue Donors', in *Code of Medical Ethics: Current Opinions with Annotations* (Chicago: American Medical Association), 34–6.

BILLER-ANDORNO, N., and SCHAUENBURG, H. (2001), 'It's Only Love? Some Pitfalls in Emotionally Related Organ Donation', *Journal of Medical Ethics*, 27: 162–4.

_____ (2001), 'Who Shall Be Allowed to Give? Living Organ Donors and the Concept of Autonomy', *Theoretical Medicine*, 22: 351–68.

CAMERON, J., and HOFFENBERG, R. (1999), 'The Ethics of Organ Transplantation Reconsidered: Paid Organ Donation and the Use of Executed Prisoners as Donors', *Kidney International*, 55: 724–32.

COHEN, C. (2002), 'Public Policy and the Sale of Human Organs', *Kennedy Institute of Ethics Journal*, 12: 47–64.

CROUCH, R., and ELLIOTT, C. (1999), 'Moral Agency and the Family: The Case of Living Related Organ Transplantation', *Cambridge Quarterly of Healthcare Ethics*, 8: 275–87.

CURRAN, W. (1959), 'A Problem of Consent: Kidney Transplantation in Minors', *New York University Law Review*, 34: 891–8.

DAAR, A. (2002), 'Strangers, Intimates, and Altruism in Organ Donation', *Transplantation*, 74: 424–6.

DWYER, J., and VIG, E. (1995), 'Rethinking Transplantation Between Siblings', *Hastings Center Report*, 25: 7–12.

EVANS, M. (1989), 'Organ Donations Should Not Be Restricted to Relatives', *Journal of Medical Ethics*, 15: 15–20.

FOX, R., and SWAZEY, J. (1978), *The Courage to Fail: A Social View of Organ Transplants and Dialysis* (Chicago: University of Chicago Press).

GILL, M., and SADE, R. (2002), 'Paying for Kidneys: The Case Against Prohibition', *Kennedy Institute of Ethics Journal*, 12: 17–45.

GUTMANN, T., and LAND, W. (1999), 'Ethics Regarding Living-Donor Organ Transplantation', *Langenbeck's Archives of Surgery*, 384: 515–22.

JORALEMON, D. (2001), 'Shifting Ethics: Debating the Incentive Question in Organ Transplantation', *Journal of Medical Ethics*, 27: 30–5.

KAPLAN, B., and POLISE, K. (2000), 'In Defense of Altruistic Kidney Donation by Strangers', *Pediatric Nephrology*, 14: 518–22.

LINDSAY, D. (2002), 'An Organ, Stem Cells, and Blood Are Precious Gifts of Life', *Online Washingtonian Community Service*, <http://www.washingtonian.com/schools/savealife_give>.

MECKLER, L. (2003), 'The Dark Side of Organ Donation', *Associated Press*, <www.cbsnews.com/stories/2003/08/12/health>.

MERRILL, J., MURRAY, J. E., HARRISON, J. H., GUILD, W. R.. (1956), 'Successful Homotransplantation of the Human Kidney Between Identical Twins', *JAMA* 160: 277–82.

MILLER, C., *et al.* (2001), 'One Hundred Nine Living Donor Liver Transplants in Adults and Children: A Single-Center Experience', *Annals of Surgery*, 234: 301–10.

MORELLI, M. (1999), 'Commerce in Organs: A Kantian Critique', *Journal of Social Philosophy*, 30: 315–24.

MUNSON, R. (2002), *Raising the Dead: Organ Transplants, Ethics and Society* (Oxford: Oxford University Press).

NAJARIAN, J., CHAVERS, B. M., McHUGH, L. E., and MATAS, A. J. (1992), 'Twenty Years or More of Follow-Up of Living Kidney Donors', *The Lancet*, 340: 807–10.

OCHS, R. (2002), 'Live-Donor Procedures Carry Risks', *Newsday.com*, <http://www.news day.com/health/ny-hsmed1928302117aug1>.

PARK, K., *et al.* (1996), 'A 16-Year Experience with 1275 Primary Living Donor Transplants: Univariate and Multivariate Analysis and Risk Factors Affecting Graft Survival', *Transplantation Proceedings*, 28: 1378–9.

PHADKE, K., and ANANDH, U. (2002), 'Ethics of Paid Organ Donation', *Pediatric Nephrology*, 17: 309–11.

RADCLIFFE-RICHARDS, J., *et al.* (1998), 'The Case for Allowing Kidney Sales', *The Lancet*, 352: 1950–2.

RHODES, R. (1994), 'A Review of Ethical Issues in Transplantation', *Mount Sinai Journal of Medicine*, 61: 77–82.

RIETHER, A., and MAHLER, E. (1995), 'Organ Donation: Psychiatric, Social, and Ethical Considerations', *Psychosomatics*, 36: 336–43.

ROSS, L. (1993), 'Moral Grounding for the Participation of Children as Organ Donors', *Journal of Law, Medicine, and Ethics*, 21: 251–7.

____ GLANNON, W., JOSEPHSON, M. A., and THISTLETHWAITE, J. R., Jr. (2002), 'Should All Living Donors Be Treated Equally?', *Transplantation*, 74: 418–22.

RUSSO, M., and BROWN, R. (2003), 'Ethical Issues in Living Donor Liver Transplantation', *Current Gastroenterology Reports*, 5: 26–30.

SPITAL, A. (1989), 'Unconventional Living Kidney Donors: Attitudes and Use Among Transplant Centers', *Transplantation*, 48: 243–8.

____ (1996), 'Do U.S. Transplant Centers Encourage Emotionally Related Kidney Donation?', *Transplantation*, 61: 374–7.

____ (2001), 'Ethical Issues in Living Organ Donation: Donor Autonomy and Beyond', *American Journal of Kidney Diseases*, 38: 189–95.

____ and SPITAL, M. (1990), 'The Ethics of Liver Transplantation from a Living Donor', *New England Journal of Medicine*, 322: 549–50.

STARZL, T. (1985), 'Will Live Organ Donations No Longer Be Justified?', *Hastings Center Report*, 15: 5.

Superintendent of Belchertown State School, et al. v. *Saikewicz*, 370 NE 2d 417(MA), 1977.

TILNEY, N. (1986), 'Renal Transplantation Between Identical Twins: A Review', *World Journal of Surgery*, 10: 381–8.

UNITED NETWORK FOR ORGAN SHARING (2004), <http://www.unos.org>.

UNITED STATES DEPARTMENT OF HEALTH AND HUMAN SERVICES ADVISORY COMMITTEE ON ORGAN TRANSPLANTATION (2002), 'Organ Donation: Recommendations to the Secretary', <http://www.organdonor.gov/acotrecs>.

WILLIAMS, R. (1995), 'Consent for Children as Organ Donors', *Hawaii Medical Journal*, 54: 498–500.

WILLIAMS, S. (1986), 'Long-Term Renal Function in Kidney Donors: A Comparison of Donors and Their Siblings', *Annals of Internal Medicine*, 106: 1–8.

WORLD HEALTH ORGANIZATION (1991), 'Guiding Principles on Human Organ Transplantation', *The Lancet*, 337: 1470–1.

CHAPTER 10

BIOBANKING

LOUISE IRVING AND JOHN HARRIS

INTRODUCTION

THE possession, storage, and display of human tissue has until recently been a relatively non-contentious issue. Henry Wellcome, founder of one of the largest pharmaceutical companies in the world and an inveterate collector of all things unusual, had in his display, shrunken heads, a tuft of hair from King George III, two fine tattoos complete with arm skin, and a piece of the philosopher Jeremy Bentham (Gosden *et al.* 2003). Peter the Great's collection of monstrosities and malformations in organisms keep the visitors flocking to the Kunstkammer in St Petersburg.

It is not just public collections that hold such an assortment of human body parts. There is currently a thriving market for shrunken heads, the most prized specimens being made by the Shuar people of Ecuador, so prized because of their method of carefully crushing the skulls before extracting bone fragments through the neck.

Museums everywhere hold the bodies of the long dead. In ancient Egypt the belief that the journey to the afterlife could only be made if the body was preserved required ancient embalmers to remove the internal organs and store them in jars. The pharaohs presumably consented to this, although their poor attendants, accompanying the dead and themselves condemned to a lingering death, may not have consented so willingly. Indeed, the boy pharaoh Tutankhamun is currently having his remaining DNA studied by scientists, and while he may have consented to the original burial and mummification, it is unlikely that he envisaged the eventual use to which his remains have been put. (See Holm 2001 for an excellent discussion of how we might think about an ethical framework for applying new genetic testing techniques to ancient tissue samples.)

From these ancient archives, medical anthropologists can tell us that much of the same afflictions that blight lives today were around in the past. In a similar vein, relics of the Christian saints and martyrs are to be found in cathedrals and churches across Europe; likewise it is claimed that the blood of Christ can be found on fragments of the true Cross. We are very familiar with the astonishing range of human tissue, bodies, bones, and bits that form much of our cultural, religious, and anthropological heritage, and are usually undisturbed by such collections.

Collections with the moral purpose of attempting to elucidate the nature of health and illness can be dated to the time of the Italian anatomists in the fourteenth century, when human tissue started to be systematically collected, stored, and studied. This long history of the research of human biological materials is the basis of much of our knowledge and understanding of disease causation and progression. 'The human tissue archive' is a name that has been given to the sum total of collections of human tissue worldwide, and these have been, with some justification, called 'a research resource that is rich, unique, irreplaceable, and virtually indestructible' (Korn 1998: 41). The practice originated in Renaissance Italy, when physicians first began systematically to perform autopsies, as a method of completing their case records. Pathology, as it is undertaken now, is generally agreed to have originated in mid-nineteenth-century Germany, where Professor Rudolph Virchnow began the systematic study of diseased tissue through the use of light microscopy. The availability of tissue archives has meant that when a connection is made between a disease and its possible causation, the requisite samples are at hand to test the theory. If such speculative research required the collecting of relevant tissue samples *de novo*, then many of the breakthroughs in understanding disease causation and prevention could not have occurred.

It is possible that this system, responsible for so much enlightenment in the history of medicine, may be under threat from two corners (Harris 2002). First, in an increasingly individualized society, proprietorial sensibilities are raised, encouraged by various scandals involving unauthorized organ and tissue retention. Secondly, with the rise of genetic medicine and the personally identifying nature of genetic information, citizens are likely to be more cautious regarding granting permission for the storage and undefined use of their tissue samples. We believe that any diminishing of tissue archiving or any threat to its continuation would be a retrograde and severely damaging trend.

In this chapter we will look at some of the chance discoveries and elegant ideas that were borne out through the availability of archived tissue samples. We then discuss some of the planned changes to the method and purpose of tissue storage and collection. The changes are in the form of new types of tissue bank, or biobank as they are conceived. These banks are part of a trend to move towards a preventative approach to public health rather than the current costly interventionist model. This approach is not without its problems and it is these that threaten the unfettered continuation of the tissue archive. The sophistication of new research tools can uncover information about individuals that may have a detrimental effect on their well-being in various ways. We analyse these possibilities in the context of how health care might develop. Much of the disquiet centres on the fact that the information held has a genetic component. This leads us to consider the nature of genetic information. We discuss some social and cultural trends that have contributed to the idea of genetic 'essentialism' and 'exceptionalism'. The former is the idea that persons are reducible to, or held captive by, their genetic components. Genetic exceptionalism is a corollary of this and insists that medical information with a genetic component is different in kind from other medical information and therefore requires different treatment. This ideology, if accepted, brings with it an assortment of individualistic concepts such as property rights in human biological materials and litigation avoidance strategies that will manifest themselves as consent hurdles. This is a clear threat to the centuries-old practice of the altruistic donation of human tissue for the advancement of the common good. We close with a brief discussion of an appropriate approach to biobanking and our moral obligation to participate in research.

The Legacy of Tissue Archives

In the United States the National Bioethics Advisory Commission was moved to consider the rights and welfare of human research subjects and the management and use of genetic information. These deliberations also occurred in the United Kingdom, where the issues were considered by both the Human Genetics Commission and the Nuffield Council on Bioethics. The catalysts for such deliberations are new technologies for the study of human biological materials. The sophistication of the new research tools can uncover information about individuals, which may impact upon their privacy in various ways. The need to increase knowledge about human disease in order to develop better diagnostic and prevention tools needs to be balanced with appropriate protection from unwarranted harms for those who participate in medical research by donating their tissue. To give an indication of the scale of the human tissue archive, the archive in the United States alone is thought to run to more than 282 million samples in laboratories, tissue repositories, and health care institutions.

Tissue samples can be collected specifically for research purposes, as part of diagnostic procedures such as biopsies, appendectomies, or blood samples. The storage may be appropriate for secondary analysis, quality control, or research purpose. The astonishing worth of such enormous tissue archives is beautifully mapped out by David Korn in his commissioned paper for the NBAC (Korn 1998).

This work is impressive in its scope and detail and we draw on it liberally in this first section.

Atherosclerotic cardiovascular disease has long been the leading cause of death in the United States. In fact figures supplied by the World Health Organization state that cardiovascular disease kills an estimated 17 million people a year worldwide through its effect on the functioning of the heart and blood vessels. Before the mid-twentieth century it was generally believed to be a condition that accompanied middle through old age. In 1963, during the Korean War, military pathologists documenting chest wounds from artillery noticed something interesting. Approximately three out of every four young male American soldiers showed signs of atherosclerotic changes in their coronary arteries. Comparative studies on Korean prisoners of war and Japanese civilians showed a different pattern. The careful documenting and conclusions reached through tissue analysis led to a breakthrough in the understanding of the relationship between atherosclerotic lesions and cholesterol, diet, smoking, and blood pressure. Instead of being a late-onset disease, in Western subjects it develops at a significantly early age and progresses in both severity and extent. As a result of these chance findings and the use of stored human tissue samples, changes in both surgical and medical therapies and in individuals' approach to their health, primarily through stopping smoking, and dietary modification, brought about a revolution in preventative medicine and public health.

The collection and storage of biological samples has proved invaluable for the tracking and identifying of virus breakouts. In the American south-west during the early 1990s young people started dying from a pneumonia-like illness. Analysis of tissue from the archives of the Centers for Disease Control and Prevention, which contain global samples of viruses, serum samples, and proteins, enabled initial tests of serological screening. Testing turned up the possibility of a Hantavirus. Then autopsy tissue samples were tested with relevant Hantavirus monoclonal antibodies and genetic probes to identify the presence of Hantavirus and its source.

The above example relied on the combination of the tissue archives with the observations of 'a suspicious clinician, an astute epidemiologist [and] observant Navajo elders' (Korn 1998: 40). The suspicions of individuals are a common theme in Korn's report. The existence of comprehensive and available tissue archives speeded up the recognition of the carcinogenic influence of certain chemicals used in pesticides. For example, recognition that a vinyl chloride monomer (MVC) was a carcinogen causing liver tumours started with the concern of the factory physician employed where polyvinyl chloride was manufactured. The physician's suspicions were validated through the availability of pathologic archival materials collected from collections of the tumour type. Similarly, the tissue archives of underground uranium workers led to an understanding of the maximum allowable environmental radiation exposures for workers and to the encouragement of methods of cancer prevention.

Understanding of the aetiology and pathogenesis of brain and muscle diseases is critically dependent on archives of pathological samples from the central nervous system and skeletal muscle samples. Rodent models were long used for research into multiple sclerosis (MS). The use of these models led to some misleading conclusions. Only recently have studies of acute and chronic lesions in human brain samples been able to illuminate the sequence of events in the causation and progression of MS. A more sophisticated understanding of muscular dystrophy has occurred through advanced techniques and the study of human tissue. The histopathological features can now be separated into different gene mutations.

There are, then, countless examples of how tissue archives have benefited mankind. The availability of archived and accessible human tissue samples permits the rapid evaluation of disease. As Korn writes:

To try to initiate prospective studies de novo for each new promising candidate marker for each of the many varieties of human neoplasia would not only be extraordinarily costly in dollars and human effort, but would require study periods of many years, or even decades before definitive endpoints could be reached. In contrast, being able to apply such new technologies to archival materials, where clinical course, therapeutic response and outcome are already known, represents an incredible collapse of time and money, to say nothing of the human suffering required to evaluate the technologies, launch the necessary corroborative community trials, and possibly bring entirely new screening strategies into general application.   (Korn 1998: 11–12)

This fact is not particularly well appreciated or understood, and it may be that this under-awareness of the benefits attached to tissue banking may threaten its future.

TISSUE ARCHIVING NOW: BIOBANKING

There are now changes affecting traditional tissue archiving. It has long been known, by patient groups at least, that medicines do not have set standards of efficacy for all patients. Currently, drugs for Alzheimer's disease work in fewer than one in three patients, whereas those for cancer are only effective in a quarter of patients. Only half the sufferers of migraine, osteoporosis, and arthritis can hope to be helped by prescription medication. The answer to this problem is thought to lie in pharmacogenetics, which is the application of human genetics to drug development. That not all people respond in the same manner to prescription drugs is due to individual genetic differences—different susceptibilities to the effect of the drug. It is speculated that those who do benefit from drugs could be identified by a genetic test which could then be used to eliminate those people who would not respond; they, in turn, might be able to benefit from other medication.

The inefficiency of many drugs and the ever-increasing cost of maintaining the health of populations mean that a more progressive and innovative approach to public health is desirable. This would ideally be towards a model of prevention. It has become apparent that a smart thing to do would be to collate genetic and lifestyle information on a large scale in an attempt to discern how genetic susceptibility combines with environmental influences to impact health and longevity. National biobanks have been set up in countries with typically small gene pools such as Estonia, Iceland, and Tonga. This idea is not limited to small gene pools. The United Kingdom, with its multicultural population, has the benefit of a National Health Service and therefore the possibility of tracking the health records of individuals, and is undertaking a similar venture. To call it 'biobanking' is no misnomer; the plan is truly to build a bank, a resource, rather than to undertake certain particular studies. The new biobanking seeks to hold the anonymized human tissue and lifestyle information of individual volunteers as a resource for multiple users and researchers. These new-style tissue banks, which have raised awareness about the importance of tissue archives, have also raised fears about the storage and use of such data. We shall briefly map out the expected potential of ventures such as national population biobanks; detail the possible downside or fears of such a project; and then consider how the balance of potential goods might be weighed against the concerns we have highlighted.

New-Style Biobanks

It is thought that the elusive nature of the interaction between nature and nurture might be elucidated by comprehensive analysis of individuals' lifestyle habits, environmental influences, and a sample of some type of biological material—blood or tissue yielding the complete genome. Most, and perhaps all, conditions detrimental to well-being and our susceptibility to infectious diseases have some genetic component. Cancer, diabetes, asthma, and degenerative neurological diseases are prime candidates for investigation. Finding the genetic factors involved is naturally complicated by the myriad environmental influences. Biobanking projects are large-scale and long-term in order to be able to see correlations between lifestyle, susceptibility, and disease. The method is to collect information from volunteers on environmental and lifestyle factors and then link these to medical records and biological samples. Considerations will be of risk factors, diagnoses, what illnesses are suffered, any disabilities, which treatments were used, and which outcomes achieved. The samples will be stored in a central database so they can be analysed by scientists undertaking ethically approved research projects.

There are some fears about what types of research might be undertaken. Projects of such scale and novelty cannot anticipate the identities of all the research users or estimate their purposes. Traditionally, tissue samples removed for research and archiving have been done under sparing consent language. Indeed, guidelines in the United Kingdom developed by the Nuffield Council on Bioethics proposed that, providing there were no adverse consequences for the patient, consent to remove tissue for therapeutic reasons implied consent to any subsequent ethical use of the tissue (Nuffield Council on Bioethics 1995). Nevertheless, concerns have been raised that research may be undertaken to try to find genetic causes for behavioural characteristics such as violence or antisocial behaviour. There is validity in these concerns. Past claims for genes linked to schizophrenia, manic depression, homosexuality, and alcoholism have all eventually been withdrawn, but without the press attention that accompanied their 'discovery'. It may be that all characteristics or illnesses have a genetic component, but the tendency to link, in the mind of the public at least, a single gene and an affliction or characteristic contributes to the idea of 'genetic essentialism'. The notion supporting essentialism is that human beings are reducible to, or held captive by, their genetic components. It is partly the lingering nature of this discredited notion that threatens tissue archiving, and we discuss genetic essentialism in more detail later in the chapter.

WHAT IS GENETIC INFORMATION?

In order to understand how genetic information might be thought to threaten individual privacy, it may be helpful to know how genetic information works at the basic level. There are different types of genetic information and different ways of obtaining it. The genotype itself is simply the genetic constitution of an organism. A gene is actually a section of sequence of the chemical DNA that goes into making a particular protein. In other words, a gene is the protein coding sequence. Proteins are the class of chemicals that largely determine the structure and function of the self. At fertilization, egg and sperm, which hold a single set of twenty-three chromosomes each, join to form the double set of forty-six chromosomes which are then replicated as each new cell is formed. Chromosomes are largely made up of DNA but only a small percentage of this DNA forms our genes. The rest is termed non-coding, or 'junk', DNA. The function of this junk DNA is unknown at this time. The genotype gives details, from the basic DNA or protein, of the precise variations inherited from both parents. The phenotype is how these variations are expressed, for example, height, eye colour, blood pressure. It is this pattern of inheritance of different phenotypes that also supplies the information about the families of individuals. Obtaining genetic information can be achieved by analysing either the DNA or proteins or blood.

Genetic information is sensitive in a number of ways. Not only can it reveal information about the individual concerned, it can also reveal information about their family. It may be able to say what that person's susceptibility to disease is—and there is lively and robust debate in the bioethics literature about whether one has a right *not* to know information about one's future health (Takala 1999, 2001; Harris and Keywood 2001; Bennett 2001). Personal genetic information is thought to differ from other types of information in several respects. Most important is considered to be its uniquely identifying nature, which can confirm, deny, or reveal family relationships. Also, genetic information can be taken from the smallest amount of biological material. This capacity means that genetic material can be secured without the consent of the person. It is this potential of genetic testing to provide information about the individual that is of interest to others—family, insurers, or employers.

The question that needs to be considered is: Does the fact that genetic information can affect others and that it can potentially be used to the detriment of the person mean that it is different in kind from regular medical information? What needs to be determined is whether the difference involved requires a change to the way human tissue is thought of and managed. To discover what might be different about genetic information as opposed to regular tissue we can look at some of the issues it has raised.

TRENDS INVOLVING GENETICS

It is not merely the nature of genetics that poses a threat to tissue storage and collection. There have been other social and cultural changes that influence how individuals perceive both their own biological materials and even their obligations to others in the form of a shared interest in scientific advance. We live in a climate where ownership is the fundamental framework for protecting interests. That this is stretched to human biological materials is probably somewhat natural. This is quite obviously seen in the idea and practice of patenting genes. The complexities of the necessary protection required by biotech and pharmaceutical companies who invest heavily in research and development are often subsumed to the notion that the importance of human tissue or the development of cell lines lie in their inherent value. The perceived importance of genetics and biology and the difference inherent therein are given a further boost by legislation supporting such perceived importance. For example, at the time of writing, the UK government has just announced a legislative change that will deny anonymity to sperm and egg donors. This is based on the primacy of the rights of individuals to know their genetic heritage. The ruling seeks to parallel the right of adopted children to this knowledge, despite the fact that children born naturally have no 'right' to know their genetic heritage.

Should people have knowledge of their genetic origins? We know that there are significant non-paternity rates in the United Kingdom and other countries. Non-paternity refers to births where the children of the family are not in fact genetically related to the person they believe to be their father and who usually believes he is their genetic father. Non-paternity rates are quoted with wildly differing values (from less than 1 per cent to more than 30 per cent). A modest, and probably reliable, figure is 2 per cent. However, even at a modest rate of 2 per cent, non-paternity rates in the United Kingdom account for over 12,000 births registered annually to men who are not in fact the genetic father. Thus, if there is such a thing as a 'need for children to know their genetic background and true identity', then on the grounds of numbers alone we should start with normal families. This might imply an obligation for paternity testing in all families.

Also, in a climate that stresses the importance of determination over one's biological materials, the issue of broad consent to tissue collection and archiving is problematic. For example, it may be that many people would be happy to give their tissue samples for most research activities, but not for any research into human intelligence. But if nature and nurture cannot be separated, if they are inextricably combined and our knowledge of their relationship is in its infancy, then it may be that perfectly respectable, ethical, and innovative research into the complex nature of intelligence is legitimate. It is not possible or desirable, with all our prejudices and ill-informed suppositions, to attempt to exclude or determine in advance which research can proceed.

In his report on the contribution of the human archive, David Korn relates the example of Kaposi's sarcoma (KS), a strange spindle cell and vascular tumour now associated with the HIV virus. Previously endemic in parts of Africa, it had not been associated with any specific predisposition, including predisposing infectious diseases. However, KS was identified as an early defining feature among HIV patients. Researchers at Columbia University, led by Dr Yuan Chang, used analysis of archival tissue from HIV patients to discover a unique human herpes virus, HHV8, in KS cells. The discovery of this association led to many further studies on the molecular and cellular mechanisms by which HHV8 drives the precursor cells of the KS lesions into neoplastic proliferation. For Korn this research 'demonstrates the remarkable utility of large human tissue archives, well characterized pathologically and clinically, in supporting novel kinds or research, not predictable at the time the tissue samples were originally collected, but of significant public benefit' (Korn 1998: 38).

These cultural and social changes emphasizing individual rights and the notion that genetic information is different in kind have fuelled the debate about privacy and discrimination. It is supposed by some that the interests of individuals regarding their tissue samples would be better served by some form of property rights over their tissue (Erin 1994; also, for a discussion of the arguments surrounding this issue, see Gold 1988). Property rights are an attractive framework in that they encompass several rights. They include the right of use, transfer, possession, management, and usually the right to receive any capital value and income generated by such property. Such a framework would permit individuals to sell their genetic material, and if the material was found to be of particular value then it could be sold to the highest bidder. This individualistic approach could see the replacement of altruistic donation by a system whereby researchers bid for access to tissues. This would severely impact academic researchers and increase the research and development costs of the private sector.

The availability of genetic information has potentially serious adverse emotional, social, and financial consequences. It may threaten the ability of those, already unlucky in the genetic lottery, to access decent insurance coverage or employment contracts. It is these threats that support the growing lobby of those who seek to make genetic information a different class of medical information. This trend is known as 'genetic exceptionalism', and we shall discuss the merits, implications, and validity of such a concept in the next section.

GENETIC EXCEPTIONALISM

Genetic exceptionalism is the idea that genetic information is so importantly different that it deserves classification as exceptional. In her informative paper on the subject Lainie Friedman Ross (2001) tracks the history and content of the debate surrounding genetic exceptionalism from its origins in the early 1990s. It arose out of the early stages of mapping the human genome, when tests for dispositions were in development despite there being no possible interventions. The term 'exceptionalism' in relation to medical matters came into being as a result of HIV. New practices, such as pre- and post-HIV-test counselling, the development of new consent forms, and strict requirements of confidentiality, were brought into being. The rationale was that testing would prevent the spread of the disease and those at risk might be reluctant to be tested if complete confidentiality was not assured. Confidentiality was thought to be the only way to avoid the stigmatization associated with the illness. Many of the same issues, fear of discrimination and stigmatization, apply to genetics, hence genetic exceptionalism.

Ross maps out the proposed justifications for genetic exceptionalism and considers their merits. The rationale of commentators who insist that genetic information is *sui generis* and thus deserving a separate and stringent legislative framework is that

- genetic information is immutable;
- it can be detrimental to the individual;
- it poses implications for familial relationships.

Taking these in turn, we will elaborate on the above and, in agreement with Ross, ultimately reject these justifications for genetic exceptionalism.

The immutability of genetic information is actually a rather dated concept. It was supposed that genetic testing only had to be done once in order for one's genetic status to be known for ever. But, as is often the case, the more that becomes known about genetics, the more we realize that this is less likely to be the case. The prophetic potential of genetic information is not cast in stone. Mutations occur, and little is known about the variations within gene combinations. Ross (2001: 141) explains that this means that 'what geneticists share with their patients about their genetic make-up cannot be considered immutable'. Even if all the alleles are known, this would still leave the question of why the gene translates into illness. There are very few single gene disorders and myriad environmental influences. Genetic testing is not the accurate forecaster that reductionist models of genetic medicine or imprecise science journalism have implied.

So how might the exceptionalists fare with the discrimination argument, which, at least according to measures taken to assess public sensibilities, has the most force? Most concerns centre on the possibility of an individual's genetic information being somehow accessible by virtue of the fact that the information is stored. We will leave aside the obvious point that one does not imply the other and the relative ease with which this can be made unlikely by appropriate access regulations, the anonymization and encryption of data, and strict penalties for abuse. It is inconceivable that employers or the insurance industry could have access without consent to an individual's medical information. Different rules may well apply in law enforcement, but that's a debate for another time. It may be that employers wish to test employees for susceptibility, particularly if they will be exposed to known carcinogens. As nice as it would be if no one had to be exposed to carcinogens, it may be a prudent and preventative measure for both employees and companies alike. As for insurance companies, it may be that, in the paradigm shift from interventionist medicine to preventative medicine, different models of insurance need to be introduced. Again, possible alternatives to standard models of insurance coverage are being debated in the bioethics literature (Burley 1999; also see Knoppers 1999). After all, why should it be acceptable for those who have a good indication of their likely future health condition to be able to use that as an unfair advantage against their insurers? This aside, the main reason that the threat of discrimination, victimization, and stigmatization cannot be considered justification for genetic information to be treated differently is that these sorry conditions exist wherever there is difference. Age, gender, ethnicity, religion, social class are all characteristics by which people can be discriminated against. With the proper safeguards in place, genetic information should be considerably less likely to be used as a tool for discrimination than obvious characteristics such as gender.

Finally, the implications for families and kin. The justification for exceptionalism here is that genetic knowledge is likely to reveal familial relationships and risk implications. Well, that is true, and perhaps one of the reasons that it is difficult for us to accept the responsibility for the kin and risk elements of genetic information, and thus to treat it differently, is that the sacred cow of individual autonomy results in a tendency to think one's own interests are always paramount when it comes to medical matters. But medicine is not just about individual interests, as our first section on the value of tissue archiving testifies. Public health policy, particularly in countries where the state foots the bill, needs to have strategies not solely based on individual need. Ross (2001) points out that transplantation and public health issues such as vaccinating populations are testament to health care beyond individual patients. Instead of legislative frameworks that take individuals and their desires as a prime good, Ross (2001: 141) acknowledges that there is a need for 'an ethic that can accommodate patients as members of families and communities'. That aside, the argument against exceptionalism is that implications for families are not limited to genetic information. Sexually transmitted diseases and infectious diseases require the disclosure of what may be very uncomfortable information to family members and spouses. How to assess risk within families, and issues of how and whom to tell, need to be approached through the appropriate genetic counselling mechanisms and the application of judgement and compassion. Issues of paternity have been problematic probably as long as families have existed.

FURTHER THREATS TO TISSUE ARCHIVES

It is not just the genetic factor that has changed our conception of human tissue. Those seeking a property framework have had their case strengthened by two very damaging scandals in the United Kingdom. In both cases, public inquiries were held into allegations that the organs and tissues of children were taken and stored without proper consent. Lawsuits abound. Ironically, although the scandals caused a dip in tissue donations, this was compensated by increased public awareness of the importance and need for tissue sample contributions (Dickson 2002). But such stories serve to confirm a link between human tissue and possession, and thus ownership. Furthermore, the emotive nature of the scandal serves to elevate the importance of tissue, in itself. For example, many families exhumed the bodies of their children, sometimes more than once, to bury the retrieved body and tissue parts. This had a direct impact on the availability of tissue and a perhaps more damaging secondary effect. The problem lies in the now over-cautious approach taken by medical intermediaries. The prominence of the principle of valid informed consent is taken as such a primary good that intermediaries such as pathologists and ethical review boards insist that 'Removal of a piece of tissue during surgery requires that informed consent be obtained from the patient, that an independent research ethics committee approve the supply of tissue to researchers and companies, and that patient confidentiality be maintained' (Dickson 2002: 543). It has resulted in risk-averse procedures within hospitals and other traditional centres of tissue collecting, and the vitiating of liability means that the consent hurdles are much greater.

We commented earlier that the UK's Nuffield Council on Bioethics, in its report on the ethical and legal issues surrounding human tissue, argued that, providing there were no adverse consequences for the patient, consent to remove a tissue for therapeutic reasons implied consent to any subsequent ethical use of the tissue. The rise of individual autonomy as the prime moral good in bioethics, combined with decreasing expectations of social responsibility and the organ retention scandals, mean that this presumption is no longer the case (Furness 2003). The position autonomy demands now is that the patient should have control over the use to which their excised tissue or blood is put. But it has been pointed out that patients who have given informed consent to their tissue being used for research or teaching should not have these wishes overridden by research ethics committees (Furness 2003).

There is confusion caused by the tension between patient as arbiter of their tissue samples and the need for good access and availability of tissue samples. Much of the tension is between researchers and the research ethics committees that are required to approve their proposals. There are guidelines and mechanisms in place to permit research where consent is difficult to obtain—for example, in cases where the patients are unable to be contacted (Medical Research Council 2001). But the primacy of patient autonomy perceived by many research ethics committees has resulted in the ignoring of such mechanisms and guidelines. This confusion extends to the researchers themselves, with many imposing restrictions on their own work by 'an unnecessary commitment to exclude samples from patients who had died or were lost to follow up' (Furness 2003: 39).

That research in the United Kingdom has been damaged in the wake of organ retention scandals is not in doubt. It created a substantial reduction in the numbers of post mortems undertaken with the consent of relatives. The effect of this is an increasing difficulty in obtaining tissue samples (Underwood 2001). The decrease has been unnecessary as many of the parents of children who died have spoken of their willingness to donate organs for use in research if only they had been asked.

THE NATURE OF GENETIC INFORMATION

These ideological positions undercut the social purpose and requirement of human tissue archiving. The very nature of genetic information is a denial of our individuality and separateness. In fact, it is about how very similar we are and in itself displays the connections and responsibilities we hold to others. All threats to privacy and non-discrimination can be secured against by the appropriate legislation. In fact when polls have been taken determining the public reaction to the holding, by anyone, of genetic information, there are very strong Rawlsian 'veil of ignorance' responses made. These intuitions of what would be just—i.e. no discrimination on top of being unlucky in the genetic lottery—are fairly unanimous. They should be used to make the foundation of appropriate legislative conditions under which altruism can flourish without penalty. It should also be borne in mind that demands for individual property rights come from persons who, like all of us, have been advantaged by past medical discoveries. Why they should think it appropriate that such benefits should not be extended to future generations is indicative of the mean-spirited nature of much individualistic thought.

There should be no genetic exceptionalism—it is medical information like any other—and can be accommodated by appropriate moral principles and concepts. The very same familial consequences cause alarm should also remind us of our deep connection and therefore our responsibilities to each other. Personal genetic information, rather than being something detrimental or alarming, is actually beneficial for all of us. The sharing of genetic information within families can help people avoid serious illness. To be informed of one's susceptibility to a genetic disorder may permit a therapeutic intervention or allow the individual to make lifestyle changes in order to lessen the possibility of contracting a disease or disorder. But, the main importance of research in genetics is the resulting therapeutic advances gained from such research. As this benefits all individuals, we perceive there to be a corresponding responsibility by individuals to continue with altruistic participation.

When this question was raised most recently in the United Kingdom, it fell to the Human Genetics Commission to consider the implications of genetic information. Their consultation document 'Inside Information' canvassed public attitudes to personal genetic information and how it should be treated (Human Genetics Commission 2002). They concluded that there was strong public support for research into human genetics and the benefits it is expected to bring. It was widely held that public, rather than private, ownership of genetic knowledge is preferable, and the majority of people believe in the central role of consent for the obtaining and storing of genetic information. There was considerable opposition to the use of genetic information by insurance companies or employers. The Commission concluded that the public do not wish to see people disadvantaged by their genetic characteristics.

We believe that genetic knowledge and the nature of genetic information creates a moral relationship between people. Concepts and moral principles have been proposed to give guidance to all parties in regard to genetics. The Human Genetics Commission has proposed the concepts of genetic solidarity and altruism that promote the common good. It states that

We all share the same basic human genome, although there are individual variations which distinguish us from other people. Most of our genetic characteristics will be present in others. This sharing of our genetic constitution not only gives rise to opportunities to help others but also highlights our common interest in the fruits of medically-based genetic research.   (Human Genetics Commission 2002: 2.11)

As virtually all medical facts have a genetic component, genetic information should have the same robust protections that exist for all medical information.

Finally, it may be that the fears surrounding the new type of biobanking is actually less of a threat to individual privacy. The goal of large-scale tissue banks is to predict the risk of disease in populations and subgroups rather than individuals.

How to Proceed

The need to continue tissue archiving is paramount. Korn writes that advances in therapeutics, diagnostics, and understanding do not obviate the need for the continuation of tissue archiving and research. The most striking example of the need for this is to be seen in respect to the central nervous system and neuromuscular disorders. This is for several reasons. There are still no tissue culture or animal models accurate enough to supply parallels to the human brain. Also the most effective way of trying to determine the aetiology and pathogenesis of the brain is still based on the 'meticulous investigation of human tissue samples in correlation with equally meticulous clinical evaluation of patients over relatively long periods of time' (Korn 1998: 17). As with the chance discoveries we noted at the start of this chapter, the application of new technologies or invention to the study of neurological and central nervous system disorders is completely dependent on the existing tissue archives to make the necessary experiments.

Good concepts and moral principles are available to us to take us into a new era of preventative medicine. Furthermore, personal genetic information may or may not be significant for the individuals involved, therefore a 'one size fits all approach', such as property rights in tissue, is inappropriate. There is no reason for genetic information, in itself, to be treated as being particularly sensitive. Historically and culturally, it is understood that medical information is confidential. Medical information with a genetic component is not different. In both cases the information has the potential to disclose a patient's vulnerability.

Appropriate principles can be used to enlighten the frameworks for biobanking and the utilization of genetic information. Principles of respect for persons affirm the 'equal value, dignity and moral rights of each individual. Each individual is entitled to lead a life in which genetic characteristics will not be the basis of unjust discrimination or unfair or inhuman treatment' (Human Genetics Commission 2002: 2.20). This reflects the instincts and intuitions received from polls of public opinion.

The principles identified as appropriate for guiding legislative and other frameworks are still concerned with safeguarding individuals—as they should be. Other secondary principles advocated by the Human Genetics Commission include the principle of privacy, the principle of consent, the principle of confidentiality, and the principle of non-discrimination. Instead of a persistent debate about the individual versus society, the nature of genetics and medical progress require individuals to be seen, and to see themselves, as members of a society with shared interests in the improvement of health.

CONCLUSION

When we consider the history of tissue archiving and appreciate the great gains it has brought individuals and society, we should appreciate that removing tissue samples for research and archive was done so under sparing consent language. We cannot foresee what research ideas will spring from the elegant ideas, inspiration, lateral thinking, or observations of medical researchers. Tissue archiving must remain a 'rich, unique, irreplaceable, and virtually indestructible' resource (Korn 1998: 41). Our fears of threats to the privacy and fair treatment of individuals must be tempered by our experience of the great good of medical research, which seeks to improve the lives of mankind as a whole. Medical information that is genetic in nature is neither necessarily nor fundamentally different, in itself. Vigilance and appropriate legislation can safeguard individuals. The thorny problems that arise from the obligations engendered by familial connections are an addition to the bioethical canon of problems to be dealt with through robust debate.

THE OBLIGATION TO UNDERTAKE RESEARCH

Finally, it must be emphasized that we, all humankind and all societies, have the strongest of obligations to pursue promising therapeutic research and that to fail to pursue research that might save these and many other lives would be both tragic and truly immoral. Two separate but complementary lines of argument lead to this conclusion. First, it follows from one of the most powerful obligations that we have, the obligation not to harm others. Where our actions will probably prevent serious harm, then if we reasonably can (given the balance of risk and burden to ourselves and benefit to others), we clearly should act because to fail to do so is to accept responsibility for the harm that will then occur (Harris 1980). This is the strong side of a somewhat weaker but still powerful duty of beneficence, our basic moral obligation to help other people. Most, if not all, diseases create unmet needs in those who are affected, and because medical research is often a necessary component of relieving those needs, furthering medical research becomes a moral obligation.

We all benefit from living in a society, and indeed in a world, in which serious scientific research is carried out and which utilizes the benefits of past research. It is both of benefit to patients and research subjects and in their interests to be in a society that pursues and actively accepts the benefits of research and where research and its fruits are given a high priority. We all also benefit from the knowledge that research is ongoing into diseases or conditions from which we do not currently suffer but to which we may succumb. It makes us feel more secure and gives us hope for the future, for ourselves and our descendants, and others for whom we care. If this is right, then we all have a strong general interest that there be research, and in all well-founded research. The human tissue archive in the past, and biobanking in the future, together constitute one of the most powerful research tools available to humankind. To turn our backs on the research that might save so many lives is literally to acquiesce to participation in the sacrifice of those lives.

References

Bennett, R. (2001), 'Antenatal Genetic Testing and the Right to Remain in Ignorance', *Theoretical Medicine and Bioethics*, 22/5: 461–71.

Burley, J. (1999), 'Bad Genetic Luck and Health Insurance', in J. Burley (ed.), *The Genetic Revolution and Human Rights* (Oxford: Oxford University Press), 54–60.

Dickson, D. (2002), 'Human Tissue Samples More Difficult to Obtain for Academics', *Nature Medicine*, 8/6: 543.

Erin, C. (1994), 'Who Owns Mo? Using Historical Entitlement Theory to Decide the Ownership of Human Derived Cell Lines', in A. O. Dyson and J. Harris (eds.), *Ethics and Biotechnology* (London: Routledge), 157–78.

Furness, P. N. (2003), 'Use and Abuse of Consent', *Bulletin of the Royal College of Pathologists*, 123 (July 2003), 38–9.

Gold, R. E. (1988), *Body Parts: Property Rights and the Ownership of Human Biological Materials* (Washington: Georgetown University Press).

Gosden, C., Olsen, D., *et al.* (2003), *Medicine Man: The Forgotten Museum of Henry Wellcome* (London: British Museum Press).

Harris, J. (1980), *Violence and Responsibility* (London: Routledge & Kegan Paul).

—— (2002), 'Law and Regulation of Retained Organs: The Ethical Issues', *Legal Studies*, 22/4: 527–49.

—— and Keywood, K. (2001), 'Ignorance, Information and Autonomy', *Theoretical Medicine and Bioethics*, 22/5 (Sept.), 415–36.

Holm, S. (2001), 'The Privacy of Tutankhamen: Utilizing the Genetic Information in Stored Tissue Samples', *Theoretical Medicine*, 22: 437–49.

Human Genetics Commission (2002), 'Inside Information: Balancing Interests in the Use of Personal Genetic Data', <http://www.hgc.gov.uk/UploadDocs/DocPub/Document/insideinformation_summary.pdf>.

Knoppers, B. M. (1999), 'Who Should Have Access to Genetic Information', in J. Burley (ed.), *The Genetic Revolution and Human Rights* (Oxford: Oxford University Press), 39–53.

Korn, D. (1998),'Contribution of the Human Tissue Archive to the Advancement of Medical Knowledge and the Public Health', in National Bioethics Advisory Commission (ed.), *Research Involving Human Biological Materials: Ethical Issues and Policy Guidance*, ii: *Commissioned Papers* (Rockville, Md.: NBAC).

MEDICAL RESEARCH COUNCIL (2001), *Human Tissue and Biological Samples for Use in Research: Operational and Ethical Guidelines*, <http://www.mrc.ac.uk/pdf-tissue_guide _fin.pdf>, accessed 19 June 2006.

NUFFIELD COUNCIL ON BIOETHICS (1995), 'Human Tissue: Ethical and Legal Issues', <http://www.nuffieldbioethics.org>, accessed 19 June 2006.

ROSS, L. FRIEDMAN (2001), 'Genetic Exceptionalism vs. Paradigm Shift: Lessons from HIV', *Journal of Law, Medicine and Ethics*, 29: 141.

TAKALA, T. (1999), 'The Right to Genetic Ignorance Confirmed', *Bioethics*, 13: 288–93.

____ (2001), 'Genetic Ignorance and Reasonable Paternalism', *Theoretical Medicine and Bioethics*, 22/5: 485–91.

UNDERWOOD, J. (2001), Vice-President of the Royal College of Pathologists in interview with the BBC, 31 Jan. 2001, <http://news.bbc.co.uk/1/low/talking_point/forum/1144293. stm>, accessed 19 June 2006.

CHAPTER 11

·············

FOR DIGNITY OR MONEY: FEMINISTS ON THE COMMODIFICATION OF WOMEN'S REPRODUCTIVE LABOUR

·············

CAROLYN MCLEOD

RACHEL is a beautiful woman who is faced with a difficult choice. She is in love with a handsome man; yet if she chooses to be with him, she may be happy but she won't be rich. She could choose to be without him, however, and take a million dollars instead, in which case she would be rich but alone. What to do? If you think women only face this sort of question on the hit American reality television

I am grateful to Amanda Porter for her research assistance and to Bonnie Steinbock, Andrew Botterell, and Françoise Baylis for their comments on drafts of the chapter. I would also like to thank the Stem Cell Network, a member of the Networks of Centres of Excellence program, for support in the way of funding, and the Lupina Foundation for giving me a fellowship at the Munk Centre for International Studies (University of Toronto), which gave me much-needed time to write the chapter. In many ways, this chapter is a companion piece to a paper I co-wrote with Françoise Baylis (McLeod and Baylis 2006). One section of this chapter, namely 'On Commodification and Alienability', is a version of what appears in that other paper.

show *For Love or Money* (which is the inspiration for the title of this chapter), think again. The premise of the show is more real than it may first appear. If, unlike most undergraduate students in North America, you have never seen the show and think the above question might be an idle academic one, think again also. Love—for men, for children, or for themselves—has often been something women could choose only if they were willing to sacrifice their financial independence. Good women put their partners' careers first and do not pursue demanding careers if they have small children at home. Good women, dignified women, also do not sell their sexual or reproductive services (e.g. by becoming prostitutes or contract pregnant women), even if doing so could get them out of poverty or serious debt. For women, being 'for money' has often meant being against love or dignity.

The dilemma of dignity or money presents itself to women in new ways in the current age of technological reproduction. In some legal jurisdictions,[1] women can now sell forms of reproductive labour that in the past were non-existent: they can undergo oocyte retrieval for the purpose of selling oocytes, or they can engage in commercial, gestational contract pregnancy. Oocyte vendors respond to a demand for oocytes used in treating some forms of female infertility, or for research, particularly human embryo research done on embryos that are created for the research itself (which would include some embryonic stem cell research). As oocyte vendors, women commit themselves to performing the laborious task of oocyte retrieval, and consent to use this reproductive labour not for their direct reproductive benefit, but for the reproductive benefit of others, as women do with contract pregnancy.[2] While women who sell such labour may get healthy sums of money in return, they also may sacrifice their dignity as women. Traditionally at least, dignified women did not treat their reproductive potential as a source of cash.

At issue here is the moral permissibility of commodifying women's reproductive labour, particularly given the double bind, or binds, that such commodification poses for women. Should women be able to treat their own reproductive labour as a commodity, that is, as something that can be traded for a price? Should others encourage them to do so, despite the difficulty many women would find in choosing whether to sell such labour? Assuming that ethical restrictions exist on what things can properly be commodified, it is an open question whether women's reproductive labour is among these things. This question is both open and difficult, for a number of reasons. For example, while the financial independence that the selling of such labour could offer women is in some sense empowering, the work

---

[1] These include many states in the United States, but exclude, for example, all areas of Canada, Britain, France, and Australia.

[2] Following Donna Dickenson (2001: 211), I assume that when women sell or donate oocytes or embryos, they are engaged in a form of *labour*, since the oocyte retrieval process involves mental or physical exertion as well as physical pain on the woman's part (see below for a description of this process). Labour is simply the 'exertion of the faculties of the body or mind, especially when painful or compulsory' (*Oxford English Dictionary* online).

itself seems to be degrading. Feminists need to sort through such difficulties, and do it soon, because of the growing market in, and the growing pressure on women to provide, reproductive service through oocyte vending and commercial contract pregnancy.

Some feminists have tried to provide answers to this problem; but unfortunately, their answers tend to conflict. Whether the subject is oocyte vending or commercial contract pregnancy, some feminists argue that being able to sell reproductive labour is empowering for women in general (i.e. not just financially); to deny women this right would be to treat them in a manner that is inconsistent with their status as autonomous persons. By contrast, other feminists claim that allowing women to sell reproductive labour is degrading, and hence ultimately disempowering, for women. The debate is reminiscent of feminist debates about pornography and prostitution. Are oocyte vending and commercial contract pregnancy *reproductively* liberating for women, just as pornography and prostitution are sexually liberating for women, according to some feminists (Vance 1984)? Or is the liberation really just disguised subordination? For ease of exposition, and borrowing some terminology from *For Love or Money*, I will say that those who claim the former are *for money* or in favour of commodification, which may or may not be compatible with being *for dignity* (i.e. women's dignity) or against women's subordination.

My main purpose in this chapter is to lay out the 'for money' and 'for dignity' arguments that *feminist* ethicists have given about the reproductive labour women perform in providing oocytes or in getting pregnant for others.[3] Feminist arguments about the morality of these two practices overlap significantly because, from a feminist perspective, the morally relevant facts about them are quite similar. Still, there are dissimilarities, stemming from the obvious fact that one practice involves giving up oocytes while the other involves giving up a baby after a pregnancy (Steinbock 2004: 255). Some arguments by feminists reflect this core difference, in that they apply specifically to one practice but not to the other. I shall highlight when the relevance of a particular argument differs for these different reproductive practices.

The structure of the chapter is as follows. I begin with a discussion of the meaning of 'commodification' and of a related term, 'alienability', followed by a description of the commodification of women's labour in providing oocytes and in undergoing contract pregnancies. I then elaborate on why having to choose dignity or money with respect to such labour is a double bind for women. In the next part of the chapter, which is the bulk of it, I explain how feminists have dealt with this dilemma of dignity or money. The chapter ends with a summary of the state of the feminist literature on this topic, along with recommendations for future feminist inquiry.

---

[3] My exposition covers only the feminist literature, and thus excludes such non-feminist arguments as religious arguments against 'sinful' uses of one's reproductive capacity (see Steinbock 2004: 256).

On Commodification and Alienability

To begin: when exactly is women's reproductive labour *commodified*? And is commodifying it a bad thing, given the nature of commodification? In other words, is commodification *inherently* bad? It turns out that commodification can be, morally speaking, malign or benign. Whether one commodifies something malignly depends in part on whether that thing is normatively alienable to persons (or to other beings with moral worth). Something is alienable to us if it is separable from us; and something is normatively (or benignly) alienable to us if it is separable without causing us harm or degradation. When we treat something that we possess as a commodity, we treat it as an 'item of trade' (*OED*), that is, as something that we can trade away and therefore separate from ourselves, to some degree at least. But we cannot separate everything from ourselves and remain intact as persons; therefore, we cannot commodify everything benignly. Understanding commodification and alienability, and how they connect up with one another, is crucial for navigating smoothly through the ethical debate on commodifying women's reproductive labour.

Commodification

First consider commodification: when we commodify something, we 'take that which is not already a commodity and make it into, or treat it as though it were, a commodity. Simple enough, but what the heck is a commodity?' (McLeod and Baylis 2006: 3). Marx (1867/1954: 43) wrote that 'A commodity is, in the first place, an object outside us, a thing that by its properties satisfies human wants of some sort or another.' The satisfaction of human wants is the use value of the commodity for Marx. As he notes, however, something can have use value without its being a commodity. For example, I might (poorly) design a coat and only wear it myself, to satisfy my desire for warmth, rather than sell it or trade it. In that case, the coat is not a commodity. 'To become a commodity a product must be transferred to another, whom it will serve as a use-value, by means of an exchange' (Marx 1867/1954: 48). In other words, a commodity is fundamentally an item of trade. As such, it has exchange value as well as use value.

In his description of commodities, Marx (1867/1954: 43–87) speaks of commodities as though they were essentially objects, which is not obviously the case. Arguably, a service can be a commodity, and a service is not an object. With some services, the true commodity may just be the product of the service (e.g. a clean house in the case of cleaning as a service); but with other services, such as reproductive services, there may be no product in the end (i.e. no baby or no oocyte), yet the person who performs the service may be compensated nonetheless, which suggests that the service itself is a commodity. For example, some women who enter into contract pregnancies are remunerated to some degree for their reproductive service even if the pregnancy ends in a miscarriage or a stillbirth.

Thus, a commodity is an object or service that one trades for something of equal value, typically money. To *commodify* something, then, is typically to turn it into, or treat it as though it were, an object or service that one trades for a price. As Margaret Radin (1996) emphasizes, this process can be complete or incomplete; one can commodify something only to a degree.

Commodification can also be morally benign or malign (not unlike objectification; see Nussbaum 1995). Relevant factors in determining moral permissibility with commodification include the following: (1) 'whether the thing commodified has intrinsic value that is incompatible with its being' treated as a commodity, where an example might be a religious artifact; (2) 'whether moral constraints exist on the alienability of the thing from persons,' as they do in the case of life-sustaining organs; (3) 'whether the consequences of making the thing alienable and of commodifying it are' unfavourable, which may be true for non-life-sustaining organs, such as second kidneys (McLeod and Baylis 2006: 3). (2) and (3) both concern (normative) alienability, which is the focus of the feminist literature on the permissibility of commodifying women's reproductive labour.[4] Should the labour be commodified, given that women will have to alienate it from themselves, along with the products of their labour?

Alienability

Alienability is related to commodification in that it shapes whether the latter is benign, as illustrated above. A legitimate commodity *is* an object or service that is normatively alienable to persons, meaning they could transfer or forfeit it without doing damage to their selves (Radin 1996: 17; Bartky 1990: 34). For example, people can transfer their savings into mutual funds without harming or degrading themselves. Yet they cannot exchange for money the protection afforded by their basic human rights without causing such harm.

Alienating something from the self that is not normatively alienable to it brings on a state of alienation. Here, the self is so fragmented from what is constitutive of it that it cannot be itself, cannot be psychologically integrated, or cannot be truly human. Marx thought that alienation occurs when workers are forced to engage in productive activity that is neither free nor creative. Doing the opposite of such activity—that is, doing truly stimulating and imaginative work—was definitive of humanity for Marx (1844/1964).

---

[4] (1) applies to whether the products of this labour (i.e. oocytes, embryos, fetuses, and babies) have such intrinsic value that they should not be commodified, which relates directly to the commodification of *them*, as opposed to the labour that goes into creating them. This chapter deals only with issues that directly concern the latter.

In the Western philosophical tradition, our humanity resides primarily in our autonomous agency, and in what sustains that agency, although what does sustain it is a subject of considerable controversy. Feminists tend to disagree with mainstream moral theorists on this point about sustainability; they tend to define autonomous agents as more relational (i.e. sociopolitically constituted), more embodied, and more emotional than non-feminists do (Mackenzie and Stoljar 2000). What might count, therefore, as benign commodification based on what is normatively alienable to persons may differ for feminists compared with non-feminists. As we shall see, some feminists base their moral analyses of the commodification of women's reproductive labour on feminist accounts of autonomous agency, and, more specifically, on whether women can maintain their autonomy, or personhood, while separating themselves from the emotional and embodied aspects of their labour.

THE REALITY OF 'DIGNITY OR MONEY' WITH RESPECT TO WOMEN'S REPRODUCTIVE LABOUR

Before turning to feminist arguments in favour of dignity or money, we should be clear on what the facts are concerning real practices of commodifying reproductive labour. What are the morally relevant facts, particularly from a feminist perspective? When women engage in oocyte vending or commercial contract pregnancy, what do they trade away, for what, why, under what conditions, and with what consequences to themselves?

First of all, *what* do *women trade away*? The most obvious answer perhaps, assuming that their labour fulfills its purpose, is, in the case of oocyte vending, their own oocytes, and in the case of contract pregnancy, a baby that is their own in the sense that they gestated the baby (and would also be genetically related to it if their contract pregnancy were traditional or genetic, as opposed to gestational). But women also give away a lot of their own sweat and, possibly, tears when they perform reproductive labour for others. Even to get chosen in the first place to do such labour, women have to fill out forms that can be longer 'than college applications' (J. Cohen 2002); and they often have to undergo a series of medical tests, including psychological tests to rule out mental health problems (McShane 1996: 32; Serafini *et al.* 1996: 38, 39). The serious work begins, however, only if they succeed in getting chosen: they must have oocytes retrieved in the case of oocyte vending, or get pregnant, carry the pregnancy to term, and deliver a baby in the case of contract pregnancy. The process of oocyte retrieval involves uncomfortable daily hormone injections, frequent blood tests and ultrasound examinations, and the often painful procedure of retrieving the eggs, which proceeds by laparoscopy or vaginal ultrasound normally while the woman is under partial sedation (see Fielding *et al.* 1998: 274; New York State Task Force 2002). Gestational contract pregnancy includes weeks of hormone injections, as well as uncomfortable tests to assess potential blockage in Fallopian tubes, and the sometimes painful procedure of embryo transfer.

What do women get in exchange for this labour? Aside from possibly feeling good about themselves for helping others, they can receive large sums of money. With oocyte vending, the going rate is anywhere from \$1,500 to \$5,000 in the United States, if the women are paid only for their 'time, effort, and discomfort' (New York State Task Force 2002). Yet sometimes the women are paid also for their oocytes, that is, if they provide them to couples who want a 'designer baby': often one who is intelligent, musical, and good-looking. Some of these couples are willing to pay thousands of dollars for oocytes (e.g. \$50,000), at least according to advertisements in Ivy League college newspapers (Steinbock 2004: 259). Such payments resemble those given for gestational contract pregnancy, for which payments tend to run between \$18,000 and \$25,000 (again in the United States).[5]

Why do women perform the labour? Do they just really need the money? In general, women who vend their services of oocyte retrieval and pregnancy are not desperate for the money, although they could certainly use it. Oocyte vendors and contract pregnant women tend to be less well off financially than the couples who pay them. Sometimes, they are in university and face the prospect of large student debts. But often they are working class women, with little to no postsecondary education, who have children of their own to support (Fielding *et al.* 1998: 276; Ragone 1994: 54–5). Many reproductive labourers say that financial reward is an important consideration, but not their primary motive for performing the relevant service (Ragone 1994: 57; 1999: 78). More often than not, they *want* to do what they are doing because it helps people or because, in the case of contract pregnancy in particular, it makes them feel special (perhaps because they get to be pregnant, and being pregnant is special) (Anderson 1993: 180).[6]

Under what conditions are women performing this labour? Usually, with oocyte vending and contract pregnancy, a power differential exists between relevant parties, which does not favour the woman as reproductive labourer. The differential can be based on gender, class, or race. For example, traditional or genetic contract pregnancies often occur against a background of gender- and class-based inequalities,

---

[5] Source: David Smotrich, reproductive endocrinologist and medical director of La Jolla IVF in San Diego, California; personal communication, 2 Oct. 2004. These amounts are what contract pregnant women get paid only if they produce a baby in the end.

[6] Other possible reasons include, with oocyte vending, wanting 'to know if [one's] eggs are "good"' (Steinbock 2004: 258), and, with contract pregnancy, seeking to resolve guilt feelings about a past abortion (Anderson 1993: 180), presumably by carrying a fetus to term this time, rather than ending its life.

since the contracts exist between the sperm provider, a man who is usually well off, and the contract pregnant woman, who is usually not so well off. With gestational contract pregnancy, racial inequality can occur, and in a way that benefits the paying couple, because of racial differences between them and the woman who bears a child for them (see Ragone 2000: 65–6). Such inequalities *may* not at all compromise the moral legitimacy of these contracts; but they could do so because of how vulnerable they can make the reproductive labourer.

The conditions under which women exchange their reproductive labour for money can also involve manipulation or deception. Reproductive labourers are manipulated when information about the nature of the relevant medical procedures is withheld from them, and when the 'downstream commodification' (Holland 2001) of their labour is withheld. Recent studies show that withholding information about procedures (and consequently undermining informed choice) is common in oocyte 'donation' programs in the United States (Gurmankin 2001; New York State Task Force 1998). For instance, in preliminary attempts to gather information from many of these programs, prospective vendors will receive either no information about risks or inaccurate information (Gurmankin 2001). Often, they will not be told about the potential risk of ovarian cancer from the hormone injections, and about the risks of infertility or of ovarian hyperstimulation syndrome, which in severe cases is life-threatening (Fielding *et al.* 1998: 274; Serafini *et al.* 1996: 37). The motivation to manipulate or coerce women to sell their reproductive labour can be quite strong because of a shortage of 'desirable' labourers or simply because reproductive labour is big business for the intermediaries involved, that is, for those who run the programs.[7] Enterprises in oocyte 'donation' are highly lucrative if the labour is commodified downstream from payment to the actual labourers (Mahoney 2000). Oocytes may be sold in this way to researchers or to infertile couples for significant profit, often without the woman who originally sold the oocytes knowing about that profit (Holland 2001: 266).

What are the consequences for women as reproductive labourers? In particular, what are the emotional consequences? Reportedly, they can include regret or shame for agreeing just to perform the labour or for agreeing to specific acts outlined in the contract (e.g. genetic abortion). For example, a woman might regret her consent to be an oocyte vendor after she discovers how painful the process of retrieval can be.[8] A woman who serves as a contract pregnant woman might wish that she had never consented to abort her pregnancy if the fetus has a genetic abnormality, to reduce her pregnancy selectively if it is a multiple one, or just to give 'her' child away.[9] Of course, not all women who sell or donate their reproductive labour experience

---

[7] See J. Cohen (2002) and Ragone (2000: 61) on the difficulties that couples can have with finding the labourer they want.

[8] A student of mine had that experience.

[9] Consents to both genetic abortions and selective reductions are common in pregnancy contracts. Selective termination is an issue with gestational contract pregnancy, because multiple pregnancies are

regrets; presumably the ones who say they would do it again feel little to no remorse about doing it the first time.[10]

Women who respond to the market for reproductive labour can also experience rejection that threatens to undermine their dignity, or others' dignity. While programs can reject a prospective labourer for reasons that are not morally troubling—for example, the woman's health is truly poor—they can also reject a woman for reasons that *are* troubling—for example, she is not pretty enough, smart enough, or talented enough. Such standards may be appropriate for beauty contests or college admissions, but they are arguably inappropriate as standards for determining whose gametes to use when creating a new human being. The reason is that, in this context, the standards imply that some lives (including that of the gamete provider herself) were not, or are not, worth creating.

The abovementioned facts suggest that in consenting to oocyte vending or commercial contract pregnancy, women might alienate from themselves more than just the physical act of reproductive labour. They might also lose some autonomy owing to manipulation, some integrity owing to regret, and some dignity owing to rejection. Since such qualities are normally deemed inalienable to persons, their loss is morally regrettable to say the least.

THE DOUBLE BIND OF CHOOSING DIGNITY OR MONEY

Given the negative impact that the market in reproductive labour can have on women, one might wonder why feminists are so divided about it. Why not just ban the market? What would we be sacrificing if we did that? It has to be something important, unless in disagreeing with one another so strongly, feminists are way off track. On the contrary, I think they are right on track in struggling so much with this issue, which is quite complex. Let me explain, drawing on Radin.

In having to decide whether to endorse the commodification of women's reproductive capacities, feminists are in a serious double bind. In other words, as feminists, they are damned if they allow the commodification of women's reproductive labour and damned if they don't. If they do the former, they risk allowing women to be exploited, especially if substantial downstream commodification occurs. Exploitation is an issue for all potential reproductive labourers, but particularly for poor or economically deprived women, who may find the payment

common in such arrangements, since multiple embryos are transferred to the uterus of the contract mother during the IVF process (Ragone 2000).

[10] In one study of oocyte donors, 60 per cent of them said they would donate again (Fielding *et al.* 1998: 279).

for oocyte retrieval or contract pregnancy irresistible. A further problem with commodification is that it would 'seem to treat [women's reproductive capacities] as ... fungible market commodities', which 'in this culture ... [could] diminish the personhood of women' (Radin 1991: 349). In other words, women could be objectified as breeders when their reproductive labour is commodified. Women may themselves go to market, as cows do.

But banning commodification would not obviously serve women's interests either. For one thing, being able to sell their reproductive labour gives women market power, which *is* power within capitalism. Yet women have 'historically been denied [this power]', and currently have a lot less of it than men, which suggests that barring women from it in the realm of reproduction could really harm women (Radin 1991: 349). In particular, it could harm poor women who might better their situation a lot by responding to the market for oocytes or for contract pregnancies. Sometimes, guidelines for the latter require 'that the candidates not be poor women who need the money' (Radin 2001: 309). Besides being paternalistic—perhaps 'in the worst way'[11] since the paternalism involves wealthy people telling poor people what they cannot sell—such measures force poor women to 'remain in bad circumstances' (Alpers and Lo 1995: 42). They prohibit 'desperate exchanges' (Walzer 1983) because exchanges founded on the desperation of one party are wrong; but they do nothing to ease the desperation.

Moreover, if banning commodification meant encouraging more altruism (i.e. altruistic donation or contract pregnancy), then women would not necessarily benefit. Women have traditionally been the 'care-takers of the world' (Mahoney 2000: 188), which has probably brought them more toil and suffering than joy. Relying on women's acculturated desire to help others as a way to ensure that oocytes and babies are available to infertile people would simply perpetuate sexism.

Thus, various things that are bad from a feminist perspective could happen if we banned commodification, and if we did not. While a ban would do nothing to alleviate, and might even encourage, the disempowerment of many women, the absence of a ban leaves women open to exploitation and to breeder status.

This dilemma of dignity or money exists largely because of women's oppression. If women as a social group were not so oppressed that they were taught to be self-sacrificing nurturers, were excluded from powerful positions in the market economy, or were regularly forced into poverty upon divorce and becoming single mothers, the issue of commodification would not be so troubling for feminists. Oppression has this effect of creating double binds (Frye 1983); it keeps people down by ensuring that they repeatedly face choice situations in which the only available options are grim oncs.

One might argue that rather than choose one side of the bind of dignity or money, we could simply work toward eliminating the oppression of women—that

---

[11] Alta Charo put it to me this way in conversation.

is, toward removing the conditions that create the bind. Do we not just promote women's oppression anyway if we accept the awful choice situations that it puts women in? Still, do we really have the choice *not* to respond to these situations? If, instead, we simply worked toward 'ideal justice'—that is, no oppression but rather real reproductive and economic freedom for women—we might miss the chance to create 'nonideal justice', or a situation that is at least more just than our current one. Radin calls this broad dilemma of ideal versus nonideal justice '*the* double bind' (1996, ch. 9; my emphasis). Feminist activists come up against it all of the time, in having to balance 'their aspirations for a right world' with their ability to right some wrongs 'in the here and now' (Shultz 1990: 337).

Feminists who do embrace one side of the bind of whether to commodify women's reproductive labour are sensitive to varying degrees to the strength of this bind and to the need to fight against the oppression that causes it. Let me outline their arguments, starting with those that are for money.

For Money

Past feminist arguments for money focused on contract pregnancy (e.g. Shultz 1990; Shalev 1989), while present arguments deal mostly with oocyte vending (e.g. Mahoney 2000; O'Donnell 2000). Further, most of the arguments—past and present—apply equally well to both practices. Some of them are merely arguments for money, while others are arguments for both dignity *and* money—assuming that being for money is compatible with being in favour of women's dignity. (Who would admit to being against it?) I deal with the latter sort of arguments in the next section, and focus on the former here.

Arguments that are (merely) for money say that commodifying women's reproductive labour is preferable to the alternatives. And the alternatives include: (1) a system of donation that relies upon *altruism*; (2) *being paternalistic* toward women and telling them that they cannot perform reproductive labour for others at all; and (3) having a *black market* crop up in response to a ban on commodification. Arguments for money exist that address each of these possibilities.

Altruism

Feminists for money claim that a commercialized system is preferable to an altruistic one, because the latter would prey upon the socialization of women as 'care-takers of the world' (Mahoney 2000: 188, 192; Shultz 1990: 380). Most programs for oocyte vending and contract motherhood prey upon this socialization process now. They weed out women who apply because of the money rather than the opportunity to help others in need. For women who do become 'donors' or contract pregnant women, the programs tend to characterize the compensation they receive as 'reimbursement' rather than purchase (Mahoney 2000: 188), presumably to avoid the bad press the programs would get by admitting that they buy and sell women's reproductive labour. According to feminists for money, the programs *should* be buying and selling the labour, and be open about that fact, because otherwise they exploit women (especially if they profit themselves from downstream commodification), and they promote sexist stereotypes about women. On the second point, Julia Mahoney writes that, 'the implication that young *women should* desire to undergo a series of highly uncomfortable procedures that pose both short-term and long-term risks to their physical well-being for which they [may not or] will not collect the market clearing price threatens to reinforce stereotypes of females as generous rather than self-interested' (2000: 188; my emphasis on 'women').

The fact that we are asking *women* to be generous in this area is significant, given our history of relying on women to respond to others' needs, especially surrounding childbearing and -rearing; and given that we do not have similar expectations of men (for whose sperm we pay).

Paternalism

Some feminists would agree that we should not expect women to do reproductive work for free, especially when we pay men for much less arduous 'work' (as if masturbating in a cup was work!); but better yet, they would argue that we should not expect women to do the work at all. On their view, we should discourage women from becoming reproductive labourers because of how unlikely it is that women will choose to do so autonomously. Barriers to women's autonomy in this area lie in sexist norms about women, the nature of the relevant work (particularly with contract pregnancy), and poverty. For example, norms about women's worth residing in their reproductive potential, which could make a woman want to be pregnant even if she cannot keep the child she bears or even believe that the child is *hers* during the pregnancy (a common attitude amongst women in gestational contract pregnancies; Ragone 2000: 69), can profoundly shape a decision to undergo a contract pregnancy. Moreover, as some argue, entering into a contract to relinquish a child at birth before it has even been conceived is not something women can do freely, for they cannot predict how they will feel about a pregnancy once it occurs.

In response to these objections about autonomy, feminists for money say two things: first, such arguments give too little credit to women as autonomous agents, and, second, they reinforce stereotypes that women lack autonomy. In other words, the objections support a form of paternalism that is profoundly disrespectful of women. Women are not dupes in the face of pronatalism, according to these feminists; women can rationally weigh the risks and benefits of contract pregnancy and of oocyte vending, and critique their own reasons for wanting to do either. Similarly, with contract pregnancies, women can anticipate and factor into their decision-making possible shifts in their perceptions of their pregnancies, especially if they have been pregnant before, which is true of most contract pregnant women (Ragone 1994: 54). The opposite idea—that women cannot enter into pregnancy contracts because they might have a change of heart—encourages a view of women as 'unstable, as unable to make decisions and stick to them, and as necessarily vulnerable to their hormones and emotions' (Shultz 1990: 384). The worry that they will change their minds *in favour* of keeping a baby that they gestate in a contract pregnancy also reinforces the view that 'some kind of instinctive maternal bonding to the fetus' occurs in pregnancy, which would be true only if women were maternal by nature (Shalev 1989: 121). But since most feminists reject reproductive essentialism for women, they should also reject paternalistic stances toward contract pregnancy in general. Or so say feminists for money.

Black Market

In the view of these feminists, banning commodification would only lead to a black market in women's reproductive labour anyway, which could not be good for women. With a black market, there may be little incentive, if any, to ensure that women's participation is autonomous. There may instead be a strong incentive to coerce women into participating because of the ability either to reap large profits if one is an intermediary, or to get the oocyte vendor or contract pregnant woman of one's dreams if one is a buyer. Moreover, a black market would almost inevitably heighten inequalities in power between women, including class- and race-based inequalities. While it is true that what the market will bear would determine payment, surely classism and racism would shape what the market will bear. Lower-income women of colour would be paid less than middle-income white women either because the latter's genes or wombs are deemed more desirable (because of classism and racism) or because the former may be desperate and take whatever money they can get.[12] The net result of a ban on commodification, according to these feminists, is a situation that would be much worse than what we get with commodification.

Feminists for money generally favour a *regulated* market in oocytes and contract pregnancies, compared to a black market or a system of donation. (Hence, what

---

[12] With respect to oocytes specifically, Ann Alpers and Bernard Lo refer to a two-tiered market that may already exist: 'one high-priced market for the eggs of white middle-class women to be sold to infertile couples seeking IVF treatment and another for the eggs of lower-income women of color whose ova are valued for research purposes only' (1995: 42). In the latter case, the ova may be used to create embryos that will ultimately be destroyed, adding, perhaps, further insult to the injury of getting a relatively low price for one's oocytes.

they actually endorse is *incomplete* commodification. One does not commodify anything completely if one regulates the market for it. With regulation, non-market values are at play determining what the regulations are, which in turn limit property rights in the commodified item or service.) Feminists for money also tend to believe that regulation could solve many of the problems that people often see with commodification. For example, governments or medical associations could impose a cap on payments for reproductive labour so that no group of women gets considerably more than any other group and no woman finds the payments irresistible. The American Society of Reproductive Medicine already recommends a cap of $5,000 (an amount that may be too high) on compensation for oocyte 'donation' (ASRM 2000). In addition to policies that concern payment, we could have ones about informed choice that ensure oocyte vendors and contract pregnant women are always free, informed, and competent. The process of informed choice for either practice could always occur in the presence of a feminist counsellor even, who would be attuned to how pronatalist norms *can* (but do not necessarily or even frequently!) undermine autonomy for women in reproductive choice situations. With policies like these in place, women who are reproductive labourers would not be disempowered breeders. They would not be the handmaids of Margaret Atwood's *Handmaid's Tale* (1985).

We have seen that a regulated market in women's reproductive labour is preferable to various alternatives, according to feminists for money. We will now see that they defend such a market as well because it is a good or a just option, rather than simply the best amongst a host of possibly bad or mediocre options.

For Dignity and Money

Feminists for money assert that receiving payment for reproductive labour is dignifying for women for three main reasons.[13] (1) Within capitalism, being paid to do things for other people is a sign of *respect*. (2) Getting paid to do reproductive labour for others can also enhance women's *autonomy* by fulfilling autonomous desires they may have to sell that labour. (3) Such payment *disrupts patriarchal ideals* of motherhood or womanhood. Let me deal with each of these points in turn.

Respect

Financial compensation and respect are intimately connected, whether the person who receives the compensation desires it or not (Shultz 1990: 336; Mahoney

---

[13] These feminists are therefore for dignity *and* money; but since they are the same feminists as those who we were just discussing, for simplicity's sake, I will continue to refer to them as 'feminists for money.'

2000: 205). While according to one strand of thought, monetary exchanges are *less* valuable than gift exchanges, 'In fact, there is a strongly competing truism suggesting that that which we reward with money is that which we value. In particular, the inability of women to gain monetary recognition for the things they uniquely or preeminently do is one of the core causal factors in the exploitation of women' (Shultz 1990: 336).

Paying for things suggests that we value them; but more to the point, paying *people* for what they do for us can show that we acknowledge them not as mere instruments for our use, but as people. Not paying others, especially when we reap substantial profits from their work (as some programs or clinics do that facilitate oocyte 'donations' or contract pregnancies) is exploitative. Marjorie Shultz implies that women are already exploited in many of the things they do for others. On her view, we should avoid adding reproductive labour to the list.

Autonomy

We should also respect the autonomy of women who freely agree to relinquish their oocytes for a price or to bear a child for someone else, according to feminists for money. We should do so because women's dignity demands it, not only because the alternative of being paternalistic is bad. Permitting the commodification of reproductive labour acknowledges that women can do what they want with their lives and with their bodies. Some theorists frame the moral issue of commodification as an issue of respect specifically for women's *bodily* autonomy. Richard Arneson writes that 'legal toleration of surrogacy presupposes that the woman's body is hers and hers alone unless she consents to some particular use of it' (1992: 162). In other words, if reproductive labour is commodified so that the women who perform it get to trade it for money, women's bodies must be their own. Donna Dickenson (2001) and Kath O'Donnell (2000) make the same sort of claim but in the reverse: women's bodies *will* be their own if we grant them some sort of property right in their bodies. Such a right would give reproductive labourers some control over who profits from their labour and some ability to protect themselves from exploitation. Whichever way they put the point, a strong connection exists for these feminists between commodifying reproductive labour and viewing women as the rulers of their own bodies specifically, and of their own fates more generally.

Disrupting Patriarchal Ideals

Finally, we honour women's dignity by paying them for reproductive labour performed for others, in the view of feminists for money, because payment, especially for contract pregnancy, helps to dismantle patriarchal ideals of motherhood and womanhood that are undignifying for women. According to these ideals, women undergo the 'emotionally volatile condition' of pregnancy (Shalev 1989: 121) for its own sake or in order to feel fulfilled as women. While pregnant, they develop 'sacred bonds' (Chesler 1988) with their unborn children that make it impossible for them to be separated from their children upon birth and for many years to come. Thus, with gestation comes motherhood, whether the pregnant woman intended to be a mother or not. In stark contrast to this picture, we have the practice of commercial contract pregnancy, in which women rationally choose to enter into and then honour a contract to bear a child for someone else in exchange for money, and not for mere feminine fulfillment. The contract pregnant woman acts rationally and need not bond so emotionally with her unborn child that she could not imagine life without it. (Gestation, therefore, does not entail motherhood.) Moreover, the mother of the child in the end (i.e. if the child is to have a mother, as opposed to one or two fathers) will not be the person who gave birth to it, but rather someone who paid someone else to give birth to it. Clearly then, with contract pregnancy, especially of the commercial variety, motherhood and womanhood cannot be what they are under patriarchy. For example, the 'standard of motherhood' must be 'intent-based' as opposed to gestational (Anderson 1993: 183), which is as it should be according to Shultz and Carmel Shalev. A parent of a child should be someone who *intended* to raise that child, or to bring him or her into existence. Shultz and Shalev object to the gestational standard because it does not allow women the dignity to choose their own life path. It binds women to children in circumstances in which women did not intend to be mothers, which is true of women in contract pregnancies and in unwanted pregnancies.

Thus, feminists for money suggest that women not only maintain the level of dignity they currently have, but in fact gain some dignity when their reproductive labour is commodified. If commercial reproduction were normalized, less of a connection would exist in people's minds between women's reproductive activity and motherhood. The end result would be tangible freedom for women to pursue goals other than becoming a mother. While this outcome would benefit all women, the actual compensation for reproductive labourers would support them specifically. It would show respect for these women as subjects rather than objects to be used by others, and as autonomous beings, assuming that they autonomously choose to sell their labour.

For Dignity

Underlying feminist arguments for money is the belief that we should deal with women's reproductive labour as we do other forms of labour for which a market exists (e.g. university teaching, rough carpentry). As with other labour markets, the reproductive one should be regulated to prevent discrimination as well as forced or coerced labour. People who respond to that market by offering their reproductive services to others should be paid what the market will bear and what the relevant regulations will allow, according to feminists for money. To put a label on their view, these feminists defend a 'symmetry thesis' with respect to women's reproductive labour: our treatment of it should be symmetrical with our treatment of other forms of labour.[14] Feminists for dignity (alone) defend instead an *asymmetry* thesis. They contend that women's reproductive labour is special, in that, unlike other forms of labour, no one should sell it, nor consent to perform it for others for free perhaps. The labour is special either because of *inherent* features of it, which is the view of some feminists for dignity, or because of *contingent* features that exist when the labour is performed in environments that oppress women, which is Satz's (1992) view.

The Labour Is Inherently Special

So some arguments for dignity (alone), or against the commodification of women's reproductive labour, say that because of inherent features of such labour, the commodification of it is always malign. Let me consider two such arguments. One defends what I will call the 'identity thesis': that because a woman's reproductive activity is so intimately tied to her identity, it can never be an item of trade. The other argument, which is relevant only to contract pregnancy, concerns a thesis that I discussed earlier: that a woman's autonomous perspective on her pregnancy may evolve in such a way that she could no longer perceive the child within her as one that belongs to someone else; and the possibility that such a shift in perspective will occur suggests that she should not treat pregnancy as labour like any other form of labour. Let me call this thesis the 'autonomy thesis'.

The Identity Thesis

According to the identity thesis, reproductive activity is tied to the identity of women either as women or as persons. Feminists have used versions of this thesis to object first to contract pregnancy and then to oocyte vending and embryo donation. For example, Carole Pateman is described as asserting, in opposition to contract pregnancy, that 'a woman's self is intimately connected to her body in its reproductive function' (Arneson 1992: 161; Pateman 1988). A woman's identity as a woman is so tied to her reproductive activity, according to Pateman, that when she sells it, she 'sell[s] herself in a very real sense' (1988: 207; Satz 1992: 114). More recently, some feminists have stated, mostly in response to the growing market in oocytes and embryos, that women's identity *as persons* is tied

---

[14] This terminology is from Debra Satz (1992). She explores in her paper whether the opposite thesis, the asymmetry one, is true. She also discusses how feminists are split on the issue of symmetry or asymmetry.

to their reproductive activity or to their reproductive bodily tissues, including oocytes and embryos. For example, Radin suggests that reproductive activity is not a 'severable fungible object', but an essential attribute of persons (1996: 127). Suzanne Holland maintains that gametes and embryos have such 'an intimate connection to [our] personhood' (2001: 265) that they are inalienable from us and are therefore non-commodifiable (see also C. Cohen 1999). Notice that if reproductive tissues or activity are inalienable to us, not only should they not be sold, they also should not be donated to others. The identity thesis rejects both donation and vending.

Unfortunately, feminist claims about identity and women's reproductive activity or tissues tend to lack sufficient argument. Sometimes feminists take the claims to be sufficiently obvious that they are stated without argument, as they are in Pateman and Radin. At other times, the arguments that feminists provide are deeply flawed. For example, Holland defends her version of the identity thesis by saying that gametes and embryos have a special connection to us as persons because they are parts of our bodies, which themselves are 'intimately connected to . . . who we are' (2001: 273). Just as we should not be treated as mere commodities, our gametes and embryos should not either. The flaws in this argument are serious. They include not distinguishing body parts that are somehow essential to persons from those that are not (surely 'spit and fingernail parings' do not count; C. Cohen 1999: 291), and failing to defend the view that gametes and embryos in particular are essential to persons.

Feminist claims about why our reproductive activities or parts are inalienable to us tend to be not only unsound, but also pronatalist. If a woman's identity is intimately connected to her reproductive potential, then she can never escape her fertility. On the contrary, she should embrace it and discover part of who she is by actualizing her reproductive potential (McLeod and Baylis 2006). But such a conclusion supports the status quo, according to which women and men (but women in particular) are not free to lead a life in which reproduction does not occur, or is a non-issue. Satz made this sort of objection against Pateman's work in the early 1990s. Since then, feminists such as Holland and Radin have simply reproduced Pateman's mistake.

The Autonomy Thesis

A further attempt to establish that women's reproductive labour, particularly in pregnancy, is inherently different from other forms of labour concerns the need to restrict the autonomy of contract pregnant women to ensure that they maintain a certain relationship to their 'product' (the child): that is, a non-parental relationship. Women in contract pregnancies will have to manipulate themselves, or be manipulated by others, into having, or continuing to have, a perspective on their labour that fits with their contractual obligations; otherwise, a couple will lose their child. Either contracts for other forms of labour (at least for morally legitimate forms) do not require for their fulfillment the same degree of control over the labourer's perspective on what he is doing, or what's at stake with their fulfillment is not important enough to warrant profound manipulation. It follows that the asymmetry thesis is true. Elizabeth Anderson makes this sort of argument in 'Is Women's Labor a Commodity?' (1993). She explains that a woman in a contract pregnancy must agree at the outset not to view her pregnancy relationship as a parental one, which the woman may well do. But,

Regardless of her initial state of mind, she is not free, once she enters the contract, to develop an autonomous perspective on her relationship with her child. She is contractually bound to manipulate her emotions to agree with the interests of the adoptive parents. Few things reach deeper into the self than a parent's evolving relationship with her own child. Laying claim to the course of this relationship in virtue of a cash payment constitutes a severe violation of the mother's personhood and a denial of her autonomy. (Anderson 1993: 178)

As noted above, according to feminists for money, this line of argument itself denies women's autonomy by suggesting that their minds waver too much in pregnancy for them to enter into pregnancy contracts, or by implying that 'sacred bonds' inevitably develop during pregnancy.

But there are responses that feminists for dignity could give to these objections. First, changing one's mind about a decision at some point during a nine-month period does not indicate a lack of autonomy, since people who are autonomous will in fact reevaluate and often revise their decisions. Thus, a true autonomy thesis *would* respect a change of heart by a woman in a contract pregnancy. Second, it could do so while acknowledging that not all women bond with their fetuses. ('Some women abort them,' as Satz reminds us; 1992: 117.) Feminists could construct the autonomy thesis so that it says only that a woman *may* bond with her fetus, not because of some gender-wide instinct, but because she has cared for this being for months at a time. And whether a woman will bond with her fetus is not something of which she can be certain ahead of time, since women's perspectives on their pregnancies do tend to evolve as their pregnancies progress, and the evolution need not occur in the same direction as previous pregnancies (see Mackenzie 1992). Further, when bonding does occur, it *can* reach so deeply into the self that forcing the woman to relinquish the child would be cruel.

This autonomy thesis is weaker than Anderson's, however (which assumes that the pregnancy relationship *will* reach deeply into the woman's self); and it is not clear whether or not this weaker thesis supports the asymmetry thesis. Unless most pregnancy contracts required for their fulfillment that the labourer's perspective on her labour be seriously manipulated (which would be the case only if sacred bonds were inevitable), such manipulation would not need to be common practice. And therefore perhaps the labour, in this respect, would not have to be treated differently from other (legitimate) forms of labour. But even though manipulation may not need to be common, one might argue that it would have to occur in some cases and it would not be known ahead of time which cases (i.e. if the weaker autonomy thesis were true), which itself could make pregnancy contracts unique and morally problematic. In other words, perhaps the weaker thesis *does* support the asymmetry thesis.

The Labour Is Contingently Special

Satz maintains that both the autonomy thesis and the identity thesis are totally indefensible. Nevertheless, she contends that an asymmetry exists between women's reproductive labour and other forms of labour. For Satz the asymmetry is contingent upon the reproductive labour being performed in an environment that is sexist, racist, and classist.

Satz's main criticism of pregnancy contracts is that they strengthen gender inequality. They feed on an environment in which women earn significantly less than men, live in poverty more often than men, are more confined to the home because of an unequal distribution of child care and other domestic work, and, in general, have less opportunity to better their lives (1992: 124). Gender inequality extends as well to reproduction, where men have historically had more control than women over when, and how, women reproduce. Contract pregnancy reproduces this pattern by having women relinquish significant control to others (sometimes specifically to men) over their own bodies in pregnancy (Satz 1992: 124, 125). The practice is troubling for this reason, and because it reinforces a pronatalist connection between women and reproduction, and a further connection between women and the home, since women in contract pregnancies tend to stay at home. Satz claims that while some women may prefer to be at home and to make money by selling their reproductive labour, 'we need to pay attention to the limited range of economic opportunities available to these women and to the ways in which these opportunities have shaped their preferences' (1992: 127).

For Satz, contract pregnancy involves increased subordination rather than autonomy for women, in addition, because it shores up rather than dismantles the core foundation of parenthood under patriarchy, which is genetic rather than gestational. With a genetic standard for parenthood, men are at least equal parents to women, although, traditionally, their 'seed' meant more than a woman's in defining whose child a particular child was. Women were simply 'the incubators of men's seeds' (Satz 1992: 128). On the genetic model, gestation does little to shape whom a child will become, although it may do a lot to determine how a woman will feel toward that child. Women are mostly just the 'maternal environment' during pregnancy; and if their genes were no part of the fertilization process, then they are no parent at all. In settling disputes about pregnancy contracts, the courts in the United States have supported this picture; they will grant parental rights to a woman who bore a child as a result of a genetic (or traditional) contract pregnancy, but not as a result of a gestational contract pregnancy (Satz 1992: 127).

Satz concludes that the loss of dignity for women is profound, but not inevitable with contract pregnancy. Many of us recall images of women as incubators or breeders when we contemplate this practice, and for good reason, according to Satz. Contract pregnancy reinforces sexist stereotypes that prescribe undignified social roles for women. But if these stereotypes did not exist—that is, if our society were non-sexist—the practice would be more benign, morally speaking, in Satz's view. It may not be completely benign, only because it could still flourish as a result of inequalities that are class- or race-based, rather than gender-based (Satz 1992: 128, 129).[15]

Moving Forward

In broad summary, most feminists who are for dignity alone—that is, against commodification—are at the opposite pole of feminists who are for money, or in favour of commodification. Whereas the latter say, 'Pay the women, not only because it is the best option given the circumstances (of poverty for women etc.), but because it is the most dignified option for women', the former assert that it is simply undignified for women to sell their reproductive labour: they sacrifice too much of their identity or their autonomy in doing so. With her work on contract pregnancy, Satz is somewhere in between these two poles, for she claims that selling reproductive labour could be dignified, or at least not undignified, in an egalitarian society. Satz's work is important because it cautions against the reproductive essentialism that is embedded in some feminist claims about women's reproductive labour being inherently special. In discussing how contract pregnancy promotes gender inequality, Satz also exposes the naivety of some feminists for money in thinking that this practice could actually liberate women.

Still, it is not clear that Satz responds adequately to the double bind of dignity or money that I outlined earlier. She says that we should discourage pregnancy contracts by making them legally unenforceable, for example (1992: 129), which is the logical conclusion to her argument. But, on its own, this solution does little to address the 'limited range of economic opportunities available to [women for whom the contracts are attractive]' (Satz 1992: 127), a range that Satz herself identifies. Are we justified in restricting this range, so that it excludes reproductive labour, while doing nothing to expand it? If not, could our plans be for long-term expansion alone, or would we have to introduce some short-term relief in exchange for eliminating the opportunity of selling one's reproductive potential? Further, how serious is the risk of a black market arising in which female reproductive

---

[15] A refusal to grant parental rights to a woman who underwent a gestational contract pregnancy because she lacked a genetic tie to the child (children in fact, since there were twins) has occurred in Canada as well; see *J.R.*v. *L.H.*, [2002] OJ 3998 (QL).

labourers have even less dignity than they do now? Feminists need to address these practical matters, or, in other words, confront head on the main oppressive aspect of commodification: that it creates a double bind for women.

Moving forward with the feminist debate on commodification will also require that feminists learn from what other feminists, or non-feminists, have written on topics similar to their own. Even amongst feminists writing on women's reproductive labour, there has been little cross-pollination of ideas. The newer debate on oocyte vending does not respond well to progress in the older debate on contract pregnancy. For example, just as reproduction should not be seen as inherent to women's identities, perhaps neither should oocytes or embryos. But if that is true, the question remains whether oocyte vending is morally problematic; and if it is problematic, is the problem contingent on the practice occurring in certain sociopolitical environments, or is it inherent to the practice itself?

Feminists writing on oocyte vending or commercial contract pregnancy could also draw valuable insights from feminists who have theorized not about these practices, but about others that raise similar moral issues for feminists. For example, feminists have done detailed work on what it means to say that women are autonomous in choosing cosmetic surgery (Morgan 1991) or medical interventions in pregnancy (Sherwin 1998; McLeod 2002). They have discussed how myths of beauty or of pronatalism can shape women's preferences for these interventions such that the preferences are not fully autonomous, but may be *rational* nonetheless given how much easier it is to get by in a sexist world if one conforms to its expectations. Such subtle distinctions—for example, between autonomy and rationality (or a form of rationality)—are important for any nuanced discussion of the autonomy of women who engage in gendered pursuits such as selling their reproductive labour.

Thus, while feminist debate on commodifying women's reproductive labour is surely intricate, there is room for even more depth and sophistication. In particular, the debate could progress more toward concrete solutions that genuinely promote women's autonomy if the situation of potential reproductive labourers was analogized with that of potential consumers of cosmetic surgery, for example, or potential sex trade workers. The promise of such a turn in the literature is a greater appreciation of how choosing between dignity and money with respect to women's reproductive labour is a classic double bind.

REFERENCES

ALPERS, A., and LO, B. (1995), 'Commodification and Commercialization in Human Embryo Research', *Stanford Law and Policy Review*, 6/2: 39–46.

ANDERSON, E. S. (1993), 'Is Women's Labor a Commodity?', in Anderson, *Value in Ethics and Economics* (Cambridge, Mass.: Harvard University Press), 168–89; first pub. in *Philosophy and Public Affairs*, 19/1 (1990), 71–92.

ARNESON, R. J. (1992), 'Commodification and Commercial Surrogacy', *Philosophy and Public Affairs*, 21/2: 132–64.

ASRM (AMERICAN SOCIETY OF REPRODUCTIVE MEDICINE), ETHICS COMMITTEE (2000), 'Financial Incentives in Recruitment of Oocyte Donors', *Fertility and Sterility*, 74/2: 216–20.

ATWOOD, M. (1985), *The Handmaid's Tale* (Toronto: McClelland & Stewart).

BARTKY, S. L. (1990), 'Narcissism, Femininity, and Alienation', in Bartky, *Femininity and Domination: Studies in the Phenomenology of Oppression* (New York: Routledge), 33–44.

CHESLER, P. (1988), *Sacred Bond: The Legacy of Baby M.* (New York: Times Books).

COHEN, C. (ed.) (1996), *New Ways of Making Babies: The Case of Egg Donation* (Bloomington: Indiana University Press).

—— (1999), 'Selling Bits and Pieces of Humans to Make Babies: *The Gift of the Magi* Revisited', *Journal of Medicine and Philosophy*, 24/3: 288–306.

COHEN, J. (2002), 'Grade A: The Market for a Yale Woman's Eggs', *Atlantic Monthly*, 290/5: 74–6.

DICKENSON, D. (2001), 'Property and Women's Alienation from Their Own Reproductive Labour', *Bioethics*, 15/3: 205–17.

FIELDING, D., HANDLEY, S., DUQUENO, L., WEAVER, S., and LUI, S. (1998), 'Motivation, Attitudes and Experience of Donation: A Follow-Up of Women Donating Eggs in Assisted Conception Treatment', *Journal of Community and Applied Social Psychology*, 8: 273–87.

FRYE, M. (1983), *The Politics of Reality: Essays in Feminist Theory* (Freedom, Calif.: Crossing Press).

GURMANKIN, A. D. (2001), 'Risk Information Provided to Prospective Oocyte Donors in a Preliminary Phone Call', *American Journal of Bioethics*, 1/4: 3–13.

HOLLAND, S. (2001), 'Contested Commodities at Both Ends of Life: Buying and Selling Gametes, Embryos, and Body Tissues', *Kennedy Institute of Ethics Journal*, 11/3: 263–84.

KITTAY, E. F. (1999), *Love's Labor: Essays on Women, Equality, and Dependency* (New York: Routledge).

MACKENZIE, C. (1992), 'Abortion and Embodiment', *Australian Journal of Philosophy*, 70/2: 136–55.

—— and STOLJAR, N. (eds.) (2000), *Relational Autonomy: Feminist Perspectives on Autonomy, Agency, and the Social Self* (New York: Oxford University Press).

MCLEOD, C. (2002), *Self-Trust and Reproductive Autonomy* (Cambridge, Mass.: MIT Press).

—— and BAYLIS, F. (2006), 'Feminists on the Inalienability of Human Embryos', in R. Kukla (ed.), *Hypatia*, suppl. vol. 21: *Maternal Bodies*, 1–14.

MCSHANE, P. M. (1996), 'Oocyte Donation Service at IVF America–Boston, Waltham, Massachusetts', in Cohen (1996: 29–34).

MAHONEY, J. D. (2000), 'The Market for Human Tissue', *Virginia Law Review*, 86/2: 163–223.

MARX, K. (1844/1964), *The Economic and Philosophic Manuscripts of 1844*, ed. D. J. Struik, trans. M. Milligan (New York: International Publishers).

—— (1867/1954), *Capital*, ed. F. Engels, trans. S. Moore and E. Aveling (Moscow: Progress Press).

MEYERS, D. T. (1989), *Self, Society, and Personal Choice* (New York: Columbia University Press).

MORGAN, K. P. (1991), 'Women and the Knife: Cosmetic Surgery and the Colonization of Women's Bodies', *Hypatia* (Fall), 25–53.

New York State Task Force on Life and the Law (1998), 'Assisted Reproductive Technologies: Analysis and Recommendations for Public Policy', Executive Summary, <http://www.health.state.ny.us/nysdoh/taskfce/execsum.htm>.

—— (2002), *Thinking of Becoming an Egg Donor? A Guidebook*, <http://www.health.state.ny.us/nysdoh/infertility/pdf/1127.pdf>.

Nussbaum, M. (1995), 'Objectification', *Philosophy and Public Affairs*, 24/4: 249–91.

O'Donnell, K. (2000), 'Legal Conceptions: Regulating Gametes and Gamete Donation', *Health Care Analysis*, 8: 137–54.

Pateman, C. (1988), *The Sexual Contract* (Stanford, Calif.: Stanford University Press).

Radin, M. (1991), 'Reflections on Objectification', *Southern California Law Review*, 65: 341–54.

—— (1996), *Contested Commodities: The Trouble with Trade in Sex, Children, Body Parts, and Other Things* (Cambridge, Mass.: Harvard University Press).

—— (2001), 'Response: Persistent Perplexities', *Kennedy Institute of Ethics Journal*, 11/3: 305–15.

Ragone, H. (1994), *Surrogate Motherhood: Conception in the Heart* (Boulder, Col.: Westview Press).

—— (1999), 'The Gift of Life: Surrogate Motherhood, Gamete Donation, and Constructions of Altruism', in L. L. Layne (ed.), *Transformative Motherhood: On Giving and Getting in a Consumer Culture* (New York: New York University Press), 65–88.

—— (2000), 'Of Likeness and Difference: How Race Is Being Transfigured by Gestational Surrogacy', in H. Ragone and F. Winddance Twine (eds.), *Ideologies and Technologies of Motherhood: Race, Class, Sexuality, Nationalism* (New York: Routledge), 56–75.

Roberts, D. (1997), *Killing the Black Body: Race, Reproduction, and the Meaning of Liberty* (New York: Pantheon Books).

Satz, D. (1992), 'Markets in Women's Reproductive Labor', *Philosophy and Public Affairs*, 21/2: 107–31.

Serafini, P. D., Nelson, J. R., Smith, S. B., Richardson, A., and Batzofin, J. (1996), 'Oocyte Donation Program at Huntington Reproductive Center: Quality Control Issues, Pasadena, California', in Cohen (1996: 35–48).

Shalev, C. (1989), *Birth Power: The Case for Surrogacy* (New Haven: Yale University Press).

Sherwin, S. (1998), 'A Relational Approach to Autonomy in Health Care', in Feminist Health Care Ethics Research Network, *The Politics of Women's Health: Exploring Agency and Autonomy* (Philadelphia: Temple University Press), 19–47.

Shultz, M. M. (1990), 'Reproductive Technology and Intent-Based Parenthood: An Opportunity for Gender Neutrality', *Wisconsin Law Review*, 297: 287–398.

Steinbock, B. (2004), 'Payment to Egg Donors', *Mount Sinai Journal of Medicine*, 71/4: 255–65.

Vance, C. S. (ed.) (1984), *Pleasure and Danger: Exploring Female Sexuality* (Boston: Routledge & Kegan Paul).

Walzer, M. (1983), *Spheres of Justice: A Defense of Pluralism and Equality* (New York: Basic Books).

PART IV

THE END
OF LIFE

CHAPTER 12

THE DEFINITION OF DEATH

STUART J. YOUNGNER

INTRODUCTION

UNTIL the invention of the stethoscope and the acquisition of knowledge about human anatomy in the early nineteenth century, physicians were unable to diagnose death with precision. The ability to do so provided them with great credibility from a public that had, until then, been concerned about premature burial.

Significant uncertainty and debate about the definition and determination of death did not resurface until the latter half of the twentieth century, again owing to the state of medical science. But this time, physicians knew too much, rather than too little, about the pathophysiology of the dying process. In the modern intensive care unit (ICU), they have been increasingly able to break down the dying process, teasing apart each of its component parts and supporting some functions while providing technological replacement for others. In the intensive care unit, death approaches as much on the electronic screens of heart, brain, and blood pressure monitors as it does in the failing bodies of patients.

These developments have had two important consequences. First, the cascade of events that previously led to death is no longer inevitable. Before, if one vital function ceased, the others quickly followed, removing the necessity of choosing one as more 'vital' than the other. Today, the mechanical ventilator, the cardiac pacemaker, drugs that maintain blood pressure, and many other interventions keep the body 'going' after loss of innate functions that formerly would have meant the cessation of them all. The second consequence is the incredible control such monitoring and support gives physicians, patients, and families over the timing of death. Once thought to be in the hands of God or fate, the time of death is now most often a matter of deliberate human decision. This understanding and control, while never able to defeat death, gives human beings the illusion of control over death and an uneasy sense of responsibility, however it arrives.

Two factors, medical science's growing control over the timing of death and the increasingly desperate need for organs, have led to a reopening of the debate about the definition of death and have forced consideration of aspects of the determination of death that had never been addressed before. Without the pressing need for organs, the definition of death would have remained on the back shelf, the conversation of a few interested philosophers or theologians.

In the discussion that follows, we will examine some new questions raised by medical technology and the frantic search for new, morally acceptable sources of human organs over the past thirty years. This examination will lead us to conclude that death itself is a social construct and that, in a pluralistic society such as ours, a conclusive definition of death or determination of the moment of death is out of the reach of both medical science and philosophy.

PHILOSOPHICAL DEFINITIONS OF DEATH

Philosophers have argued convincingly that the definition of death, while grounded in human biology, is, ultimately, a philosophical question. To define death, one must answer the question 'What function(s) is (are) so essential that its (their) irreversible loss signifies (signify) the death of the human being?' Once a correct *definition* of death is chosen, an operational *criterion* can be selected for determining that the definition has been fulfilled. At an even more operational level, specific clinical tests can be done to assure that the criterion has been fulfilled.

Specific criteria and tests are valid only because they fulfill a philosophically defensible definition. So, for example, if one argued that consciousness and cognition were the unique functions that differentiated a living person from a corpse, the corresponding criterion would be loss of functioning of the higher brain. Specific tests to demonstrate that this criterion had been fulfilled might include non-responsiveness of the patient, a flat EEG, and a brain scan showing destruction of those parts of the brain responsible for consciousness and cognition. If this definition, loss of consciousness and cognition, is wrong, then the corresponding criteria and tests are 'wrong' as well. Conversely, no criterion can stand alone. It must be supported by a philosophically sound concept answering why it measures the difference between a living human being and a corpse. For example, a claim that irreversible loss of all liver function was the correct criterion for measuring death would be absurd. Persons with no liver function may be dying, but they breathe, their hearts pump blood, and they can still talk, read, and suffer.

In addition to loss of consciousness and cognition, there are two other philosophical notions of what it means to be dead. The first is *loss of vital fluid flow*—the circulation of blood and oxygen through the body. The corresponding criterion is irreversible cessation of cardiopulmonary function that might be tested by listening for breath sounds, feeling for a pulse, or performing an electrocardiogram. The vital fluid flow definition dominated from the early 1800s until the early 1970s. The other definition is *loss of functioning of the organism as a whole*. The corresponding criterion is irreversible loss of all brain function, including that of the brain stem. Tests to see that that criterion has been fulfilled might include examination of brain stem reflexes, EEG, or scans to see if all blood flow to the brain has ceased.

Each of the three definitions has its adherents in the United States and the rest of the world, although the whole brain formulations have been enshrined in law in the United States and many European countries through recognition of so-called 'brain death'. Before going on to discuss brain death in greater detail, an observation is in order.

The Implications of Stretching Out the Physiologic Events Surrounding Death

Until the advent of the mechanical ventilator and the modern intensive care unit, when one vital function ceased, the others stopped quickly and, to the unsophisticated eye, simultaneously as well. It all happened at once. For example, if someone had a sudden heart attack and cardiac arrest, the person stopped breathing and lost consciousness (owing to lack of oxygenated blood to the brain). Similarly, if breathing ceased, loss of consciousness quickly followed, and the heart, also deprived of oxygen, stopped beating within minutes. If someone sustained a massive head injury (stroke, gunshot wound), he or she immediately stopped breathing because spontaneous respiration is controlled by a center in the brain stem. The heart, deprived of oxygen, stopped within minutes. Thus, we never had to choose between vital fluid flow, function of the organism as a whole, or consciousness and cognition as the key function that distinguished life from death.

With medical intervention, these events no longer take place simultaneously. If a person has a heart attack, we can resuscitate them, put them on a mechanical ventilator, and shock or pump on the chest to restore circulation to the brain. Respiratory arrest can be treated with mechanical intervention. Most relevant here, following an acute and catastrophic brain injury, we can now mechanically ventilate a patient, preserving heart but not brain function.

This latter category, patients who have lost all brain function, including that of the brain stem, but are maintained with life support, is called brain death. Brain-dead patients' hearts continue to beat spontaneously, they breathe with the aid of a ventilator, and, in many other ways appear to be alive. Their kidneys produce urine, their pancreases produce insulin, their livers metabolize waste products in the blood, etc. In the early stages of pregnancy, such 'dead' patients can gestate fetuses for months until they are capable of living *ex utero*. Although initially considered very unstable, better technology, persistence, and demands of family members have kept some brain-dead patients 'alive' for up to ten years.

As we shall see, the 'discovery' of so-called brain death was a direct consequence of the invention and employment of the mechanical ventilator in patients who had sustained catastrophic head injuries. Maintaining such patients provided both a problem and an opportunity. The problem was that when ventilators were first deployed in the late 1960s, we had no legal, professional, or cultural experience with turning them off. To many, it seemed that to do so would mean killing the patient. Coincidentally, the severely brain-damaged patients, now maintained on ventilators, were a potential source of organs for transplantation.

BRAIN DEATH IN THE UNITED STATES

In 1968 an ad hoc committee at the Harvard Medical School proposed 'a new criterion for death': total and irreversible loss of functioning of the whole brain (Ad Hoc Committee 1968). This proposal came as a result of a new class of patients inhabiting intensive care units—patients with massive brain injuries who were being sustained by mechanical ventilators and aggressive ICU staff. Interestingly, the Harvard Committee proposed only a *criterion* of death with no corresponding *definition*. In other words, they did not ask or answer the question 'What is the critical characteristic of brain-dead patients that makes them dead?' Instead, they made it explicitly clear that they were trying to solve two practical problems: (1) to relieve the 'burden' imposed by severely brain-damaged patients; and (2) to quell the 'the controversy in obtaining organs for transplantation'. Let us examine these practical problems in order.

Relieving the Burden

Mechanical ventilators had just come into use in the 1960s. In many instances, they were able to stabilize patients not otherwise able to breathe, allowing critical medical treatment, removal from the ventilator, and discharge home from the hospital. In other cases, however, patients could not be 'weaned' from the ventilator. Examples included people at the end-stages of terminal illnesses such as metastatic cancer or heart failure, or, more to the point here, patients with massive head injuries whose lungs and hearts were working fine.

It may be hard to imagine now, fifty years later, when 'terminal' discontinuation of mechanical ventilation is an everyday event in modern ICUs, but in the 1960s our society had no legal, clinical, or cultural experience with turning off ventilators. There were no court cases, no laws, no professional guidelines, and no hospital policies. The Harvard Committee clearly believed that reclassifying some of these patients as 'dead' would avoid charges of homicide when they were allowed to die by 'pulling the plug'.

Quelling the Controversy

By the late 1960s organ transplantation was becoming a reality. One of the obstacles was (and remains) a shortage of potential donors. Patients who died of cardio-respiratory arrest were not adequate organ sources. After the heart and lungs stop, oxygenated blood no longer flows to the body's organs and tissues. However, the cells in those tissues and organs continue to metabolize in the cooling, but still warm, body, but without the benefits of oxygen, nutrients, and a way to get rid of waste products. Thus, warm ischemic (without blood) damage occurs and, as a result, by the time they are removed, organs are no longer fit for transplantation. Until the invention of brain death, organs came primarily from live donors, and, at first (because of immunologic incompatibility), only from identical twins.

As noted earlier, patients with massive brain destruction, maintain their heart-beats on ventilators, and have healthy and functioning hearts, kidneys, livers, lungs, and pancreases. It was precisely these characteristics that made them an attractive new source of organs. But, if they were not dead, removing vital organs would surely kill them, violating an unwritten but powerful rule that governs organ transplant to this day—the *dead donor rule*. The dead donor rule states that patients may not be killed by or for removal of their organs for transplantation. Violating this rule would have provoked the controversy the Harvard Committee proposed to 'quell'.

Amazingly, their radical new proposal was embraced by the legal and medical communities in the United States, all major religious groups, and, seemingly, the public—with very little controversy or even discussion. Within two decades, brain death became a legal standard of death throughout the United States and allowed a tremendous expansion in organ transplantation. Why this was so is an interesting question. In Japan, as we shall discuss in detail later, the opposite is true. Japan has only recently adopted a highly controversial and, largely, ineffective law linking brain death and transplantation.

It is likely that a number of factors combined to ease acceptance in the United States. First is the practical or utilitarian bent of American society, with its great enthusiasm for the 'advances of medical science'. Second, there was no natural political constituency to oppose it. As Courtney Campbell (1999: 199) has written:

It can be questioned why such religious opposition did not emerge . . . The time frame is very important. One cannot speak of a politically mobilized and socially active fundamentalist movement until after the *Roe v. Wade* decision legalizing abortion in 1973, some 5 years after the report of the Harvard committee. Nor was euthanasia a realistic end-of-life option for patients until very recently.

Campbell notes that the current cultural climate is quite different. Currently, religious conservatives criticize today's social ethos as an embrace of the 'culture of death' and apply a much more vigorous and carefully developed analysis to the issues of abortion and euthanasia than they ever did to brain death.

Lastly, although brain death is, as we shall see, tremendously flawed from a philosophical and clinical perspective, it has practical characteristics that make it acceptable to different people for different reasons. First, unlike its cousin condition, persistent vegetative state (PVS), with which it is often confused, brain death is a relatively quick and easy diagnosis to make. Patients can reliably be pronounced brain-dead within hours of initial diagnosis. Moreover, once the diagnosis is made, the prognosis is entirely clear. Brain-dead patients will never wake up and they will never breathe on their own. In fact, they are notoriously unstable and, even maintained on ventilators, will often suffer cardiac arrest and cardiovascular collapse within hours or days of diagnosis. So, the diagnosis of irreversibility is certain and, even if one believed in a cardiopulmonary criterion of death, cardiac arrest would predictably come very soon on the heels of a brain death diagnosis. For the vast majority of people, the quality of life for brain-dead patients, ICU dependent and forever unconscious, is unacceptable. Finally, although the Harvard Committee attempted no definition of death with which to justify its criterion, the brain death criterion can actually satisfy two competing definitions, making it acceptable to a wider number of persons.

The first definition to justify the whole brain criterion was proposed by Bernat and his colleagues in 1981—*thirteen years after* the whole brain criterion was first proposed by the Harvard Ad Hoc Committee, surely the case of a criterion in search of a definition (Bernat *et al.* 1981). Bernat said that the quality absent in brain-dead patients that made them dead was 'permanent cessation of functioning of the organism as a whole', that is, 'the spontaneous and innate activities carried out by all or most subsystems' and 'the body's capacity to organize and regulate itself'. Examples given included neuroendocrine control, temperature regulation, and the ability to maintain blood pressure and fluid and electrolyte balance—all functions of the brain stem. Thus, Bernat saw the critical brain function as the ability to integrate the body's non-cognitive vegetative functions, thereby maintaining homeostasis. Although justifying a 'whole brain' criterion, Bernat gave no significance to another important brain function, consciousness and cognition. Bernat's definition was quickly endorsed by a President's Commission whose report facilitated the widespread acceptance of brain death (President's Commission for the Study of Ethical Problems in Medicine and Biomedical and Behavioral Research 1981).

In a simplified way, the brain has two major functions: the integrative functions of the brain stem so important to Bernat and the President's Commission, and the capacity for consciousness and cognition. The integrative capacity resides primarily in the brain stem, the smaller, more primitive part of the brain buried beneath the much larger cerebral hemispheres where cognitive capacity largely resides. These are sometimes referred to as the lower brain (brain stem) and higher brain (cerebral hemispheres). Many persons think that permanent loss of consciousness and cognition is the critical one that makes brain-dead patients dead. However, when patients become brain-dead, they lose both consciousness and cognition and integrative capacity. Thus, a brain-dead patient satisfies both camps and does not force a choice between higher and lower brain functions as necessary and sufficient for death.

There has been little intellectual support in the philosophical and bioethics literature for Bernat's position. In fact, in the twenty-five years since Bernat's whole brain formulations were introduced, philosophic thought and clinical experience have largely refuted them. However, because of its wide appeal for a variety of practical reasons, rejection of brain death has been confined primarily to academic circles; in the United States there have been no significant challenges to brain death as public policy.

Philosophical and Clinical Challenges to the Whole Brain Formulations

Philosophers have savaged the formulations of Bernat and his colleagues on several counts. First, while they agree that the ability of the brain stem to integrate the body's subsystems is necessary to maintain life and that without it the person would die very quickly, dying is not the same as death. Moreover, integrative function hardly defines what it means to be a living human being. Consciousness and cognition alone, they argue, are the necessary and sufficient conditions (Bartlett and Youngner 1988; Gervais 1986).

Consider the following thought experiment. A patient has severe damage to the brain stem but not cerebral hemispheres and, therefore, has lost *only* the innate integrative brain functions so dear to Bernat. However, these brain stem functions are being carried out by the mechanical ventilator and a highly trained ICU staff. For example, the nurses monitor blood pressure; when it drops, the patient is given drugs to raise it. However, unlike a 'brain-dead' patient who has lost *all* brain function, this patient remains conscious and can respond to our questions. She has lost all the spontaneous and innate functions Bernat identifies as essential, yet she is aware and can communicate. So, while the patient does not meet Bernat's criterion of death, since she still retains some brain function, she does meet his definition—the loss of integrating capacity. His formulations are inconsistent and illogical. He should either include consciousness and cognition as essential functions for his definition or drop the cerebral hemispheres from his criterion.

Another problem with Bernat's definition is that he insists the essential functions must be 'innate and spontaneous'. But, why? During bypass surgery, the functions of circulation of blood and oxygen (vital fluid flow) are not spontaneous and innate, but rather done quite effectively by a so-called heart–lung machine. In the case of the brain-dead patient, the function of integration is not innate and spontaneous either. It is taken over by the machines and health professionals in the ICU. But, the critical *function* continues. Why does the critical function have to be innate and spontaneous in the brain-dead patient, but not so for the patient undergoing cardiac bypass?

Clinical experience has identified a third problem with the brain death formulations. Some functions, identified as critical by Bernat, remain in the brains of many patients declared brain-dead. Physicians simply do not test for them. For example, routine tests for brain death do not include tests for an important neuroendocrine function—production of antidiuretic hormone. Presence of this hormone is integrative in the true sense that Bernat suggested. In fact, he specifically mentioned neuroendocrine function in his 1981 paper. There seems an easy way to reconcile this inconsistency. In addition to the current tests for brain death (that included testing for the reaction of pupils to light and a gag reflex) we could also test for adequate vasopressin levels in the blood. If they remained, the patient could not be declared dead. But this policy would add to the cost of care, and, more importantly, would exclude some patients who are currently organ donors.

Bernat takes another way out. In response to criticism, he modified his definition to include only 'critical' functions and insisted that production of antidiuretic hormone is not one of them because 'patients without such secretion can survive for long periods without treatment' (Bernat 1998). But what about other functions that we currently do test for such as the gag reflex and the reaction of pupils to light? Surely, patients can survive even longer without these functions. Bernat's defense gives no logical way to order brain functions as more or less critical. Moreover, all state laws require loss of *all* brain functions, and the word 'all' has without doubt been instrumental in public acceptance of brain death. Accepting Bernat's position would require either changing all the state laws or maintaining the fiction that they were being followed.

Problems with Alternative Definitions

The loss of consciousness and cognition has its adherents, but also its problems. Mayo and Wikler argue that the definition of death should include only those characteristics that are common to all living things (Mayo and Wikler 1979).

Another problem with the higher brain definition is that while it could explain why patients who had lost all brain function were dead, its application would logically require declaring PVS patients dead. If brain-dead patients retain many signs usually associated with life, PVS patients retain even more. PVS patients, as mentioned earlier, have sustained severe damage to their cerebral hemispheres and are permanently unconscious but have fully functioning brain stems. Thus, they breathe without assistance. They even have periods each day when they open their eyes. The only technology they require is a feeding tube. Thus, to many observers, calling them dead is counterintuitive, regardless of how logical the argument that they are dead.

Public Confusion and Disagreement About the Definition and Criterion of Death

Bernat and his colleagues made an empirical claim (without any empirical evidence) that 'what the layman actually means by death' is loss of integrating function. However, empirical studies do not support their claim. When asked if a brain-dead patient was dead, 95 per cent of 195 physicians and nurses likely to be involved in organ procurement for transplantation said yes (Youngner *et al.* 1989). However, when asked why the patient was dead, 36 per cent gave loss of consciousness and cognition as the explanation while only 26 per cent chose loss of integrating capacity. Interestingly, 32 per cent gave answers such as 'the quality of the patient's life is unacceptable' or 'they will die soon no matter what you do'—indications that they believed the patient was as good as dead, rather than dead. Moreover, fully 38 per cent of respondents believed that a patient in PVS was dead.

A more recent study of the general public had similar results. A survey of 1,351 randomly selected residents of the state of Ohio found that only 40.4 per cent personally believed that a brain-dead patient is dead, while 43.3 per cent thought they were 'good as dead' and 16.3 per cent thought they were alive (Siminoff *et al.* 2004). Similarly, to the health professionals in the earlier study, about 34 per cent of Ohio residents personally believed that a patient in PVS is dead.

The findings of the two studies hardly support Bernat's contention that loss of integration is 'what is commonly meant by death'. To the contrary, the studies demonstrate the persistence of a variety of personal beliefs about the definition of death, including the traditional loss of vital fluid flow. In addition, both studies found a considerable level of ignorance about factual matters related to death. Among health professionals, for example, only 35 per cent were able to identify correctly the legal and medical criteria for determining death. Among the general public, only one third knew that brain death was legal death in Ohio, 28 per cent mistakenly thought that brain-dead patients can hear, and nearly 60 per cent incorrectly thought that organs were retrieved from brain-dead patients after, not before, the ventilator is turned off.

This data suggests that, while brain death currently seems to be working as public policy, the public hardly has a monolithic view about what it means to be dead. Moreover, considerable confusion remains about the legal and clinical status of brain-dead patients.

Irreversibility: New Issues and New Debates

As discussed earlier, brain-dead patients provided transplanters with a valuable new source of organs. However, the increased supply of organs and the growing success of organ transplantation spawned an even greater demand. Today, there are over 80,000 people waiting for organs. As a result, the transplant community revisited the idea of taking organs from patients who died of cardio-respiratory arrest by devising a strategy for removing organs before they had suffered warm ischemic damage. The strategy, formerly called non-heart-beating donation, is now called donation after cardiac death (DCD) and works as follows (Arnold *et al.* 1995). Often, patients with devastating head injuries still retain enough brain function to preclude a diagnosis of brain death. Yet, the prognosis for recovery is nil and families want to discontinue ventilatory support. Sometimes they are disappointed that they cannot donate organs. DCD works as follows. Instead of discontinuing ventilatory support in the ICU, patients are taken to the operating room, where they are draped, their skin is disinfected, and they are otherwise prepared for surgery. The patients, already unconscious from their injuries, are carefully monitored with electrocardiogram machines and blood pressure censors. When all is ready, the ventilator is turned off. Deprived of oxygen, the heart soon stops. Depending on the protocol, death is declared between two and ten minutes later by cardiopulmonary criteria. At this point the surgeons quickly open the patient and remove the desired organs—most often kidneys but sometimes liver. Once removed, the organs are quickly cooled on ice.

The DCD protocols produce viable organs because they are structured to take the organs out as quickly as possible after the declaration of death in order to keep warm ischemic time to a minimum. However, there are no clinical guidelines upon which to make such a declaration. No law, textbook, or medical school lecture has indicated how long after cessation of breathing and heartbeat death occurs. It never used to matter because either death was declared after lengthy resuscitation efforts had failed, or at the end of a long dying process in patients for whom comfort measures only were being provided. In the latter cases, when there were no resuscitative efforts after cardiopulmonary arrest, there was a significant time interval when the patient was visited by the family and cleaned and prepared for transfer to the hospital morgue by the nursing staff. During this interval, if the heart began beating again for a few seconds, no one knew and there were no bad consequences.

With DCD, however, patients are closely monitored. It would not do for surgeons and nurses to see cardiac activity after they had begun to remove organs. There is some evidence, although incomplete, that the heart will not autoresuscitate (start beating on its own) after two minutes of stopping. More troublesome is the fact that many patients qualifying for organ removal under DCD protocols could have their hearts restarted if given external electric shocks. Of course, without ventilation, the hearts would soon stop again, but the fact remains that, however briefly it beats, a beating heart is not consistent with a pronouncement of death for patients who have not been pronounced brain-dead. This situation has forced physicians and bioethicists to revisit the meaning of 'irreversible'.

Although irreversibility is part of every clinical and legal determination of death, it has never been defined. In order to examine this issue comprehensively, let us consider the following case.

> Mr Smith is walking down the street and has a massive heart attack resulting in cardiopulmonary arrest and loss of consciousness at time T_1. Four minutes later, at T_2, he is discovered lying on the sidewalk, is not breathing, and has no pulse. Cardiopulmonary resuscitation is begun and a 911 call is placed. The EMS squad arrives and continues the resuscitation efforts as they transport the patient to the emergency room, where it is continued for a total of forty-five minutes following T_2 when the patient was found on the street. After forty-five minutes of resuscitation, there is no resumption of spontaneous heartbeat so the emergency room physicians stop and declare the patient dead at T_4. Since there is no good data on how long resuscitative efforts must continue before declaring them a failure, it is likely that the situation became hopeless sometime earlier, between T_2 and T_4. Let us call this time T_3.

When did Mr Smith die? At T_1 when he lost cardiopulmonary function? Four minutes later, at T_2, when it is determined that he has lost cardiopulmonary function? At T_4, when physicians decided to give up resuscitative efforts, or did he die at T_3, when his arrest really became irreversible? Again, the answer cannot be found in either the law or medical texts (Lynn and Cranford 1999). And, aside from the bizarre kinds of cases used to teach law students, nothing much has ever hinged on this decision. However, in DCD cases a great deal is at stake because there is a premium on getting organs out as quickly as possible without killing patients by violating the dead donor rule. Because DCD patients are being closely monitored, T_1 and T_2 are the same. The critical question is about T_3, the moment when irreversibility is determined.

Supporters of the DCD protocols argue that even though the cessation of cardiac beat could be reversed with electric shocks at two or five minutes, the fact that a morally acceptable decision not to do it has been made means that the cessation is irreversible. Is this position defensible? Most philosophers who have tried to tackle this question say no. In fact, David Cole has argued that irreversibility is not part of the ordinary concept of death and should be dropped from the definition and criteria (Cole 1993). 'Irreversibility', argues Cole, is hopelessly ambiguous. It belongs to a class of modal terms that have always resisted analysis in logic and philosophy of language. More specifically, 'irreversible' invites such questions as: By whom? When? And under what circumstances? While it is unlikely that law and medical guidelines will abandon their insistence on irreversibility, Cole outlines three different construals of the term.

The first and strongest construal of 'irreversible' is that 'a lost function cannot be restored by anyone under any circumstances at any time now or in the future'. For example, if a person's entire body is frozen upon death with the hope that sometime in the future they could be thawed and restored to life, the loss of function would not be irreversibly lost. Others reject this strongest construal of 'irreversible', arguing that 'Magical, or futuristic scenarios are the sort of concepts to be contrasted with rather than being illustrative of ordinary ones' (Bartlett 1995: 272). The philosopher David Lamb agrees with Bartlett. 'In the real world,' he says, 'logical possibility without the check of plausibility is a worthless guide to action' (Lamb 1992: 32).

The second construal of 'irreversibility' is that loss of function cannot be reversed by those present. This construal would preclude taking organs in DCD protocols after two to five minutes because electric shock could restore heartbeat.

The third construal, the weakest, is that a function is irreversibly lost if a morally defensible decision has been made not to try to reverse the loss. Tom Tomlinson has defended this construal, writing that patients in DCD protocols are dead after two minutes because 'irreversible . . . is best understood not as an ontological or epistemic term, but as an ethical one' (Tomlinson 1993: 157). This position has been effectively attacked by others. Bartlett argues that Tomlinson's analysis justifies active euthanasia to obtain organs but does not support a determination of death.

Youngner, Arnold, and DeVita argue that basing a declaration of death on a moral analysis rather than on ontological arguments or biological phenomena leads to several problems (Youngner *et al.* 1999). First, while removing a ventilator with family consent has been increasingly accepted as ethical in the United States, other countries do not turn off ventilators as a matter of social policy. Using Tomlinson's standard, a patient who is considered dead in the United States would be alive in Spain or Italy. Second, moral judgments about the acceptability of stopping life-sustaining treatment often depend on secondary issues such as adequacy of informed consent that are themselves subjective and prone to controversy. Disagreement about non-medical details of a particular case could force discussion further and further from commonsense notions about what it means to be dead. Consider the following case in the context of brain death.

> A 70-year-old patient with end-stage metastatic cancer is rushed to the hospital, comatose. She meets all other clinical criteria for brain death but is found to have high levels of barbiturates (a central nervous system depressant) in her blood. A note is found that says the patient took an intentional overdose and wants to be allowed to die.

According to current medical standards, such a patient could not be declared dead. If she were supported while barbiturates cleared from her system, she could wake up with no damage whatsoever to her brain. Yet, according to Tomlinson, such a patient could be declared dead while the drug is still in her system *if we thought her suicide attempt was morally justified*. But our society is hopelessly divided about the issue of whether or not suicide, or assisted suicide, in such circumstances is morally acceptable. Tying the decision about whether someone is dead to public opinion or individual attitudes about the acceptability of various practices would hardly make for sound public policy.

On the other hand, defenders of the DCD protocols note that when patients are not to be resuscitated, and their hearts stop beating, it is common practice to declare them dead right away. They also question whether if someone suffered cardiac arrest on a camping trip with no medical technology available, we would be obligated to wait five, ten, or more minutes to declare them dead simply because we would have had to wait longer in an ICU?

Is There a Solution?

We have seen that there are at least three competing definitions of death that are accepted by health professionals and the general public. We have seen that philosophers and bioethicists continue to defend plausible, but competing, definitions of death. We have also seen that the medical criteria and tests for declaring brain death are applied inconsistently with each other. Moreover, the term 'irreversible', the reassuring adjective wedded to all definitions and criteria of death, is itself hopelessly vague and context-dependent.

Is there a way to resolve these conflicts and contradictions? Will one philosophical view of what exactly constitutes death emerge that is so persuasive that competing views will fall by the wayside? Will medical science become so sophisticated that it can locate the moment of death when philosophy cannot? The answer to each of these questions is no. Proof of the correct definition will not arrive as proof that the world was round instead of flat. New medical technology and the knowledge it brings will only confound society's understandable wish to have a definitive moment of death.

However, death is a social construct. Medical science can better illustrate (or complicate) the biological context in which it takes place. Philosophy can present more or less cogent arguments to choose one loss of function as conceptually more important than another. But culture and context will always be the final arbiter. Brain death may have been 'grandfathered' into American culture, but a look at other modern societies illustrates that belief in and acceptance of brain death are not inevitable.

Defining Death in Other Cultures

If one were to assume that the course of public acceptance of brain death in other highly industrialized liberal democracies would parallel that in the United States, the assumption would prove incorrect. For example, the Danish parliament passed a law recognizing brain death only in 1990, after long public debate and education encouraged by the Danish government (Rix 1999). Surveys showed, however, that, despite the education, the public still had trouble distinguishing between brain death and PVS. Moreover, open discussion about the ambiguities surrounding brain death may well have contributed to an actual decline in organ donation.

Until the National Transplant Act in 1997, brain death in Germany was recognized de facto in clinical practice. However, the 1990s saw a tremendous debate about brain death and its inevitable connection to organ transplantation. Opposition came from several sources, but as Schöne-Seifert (1999: 267) has observed, 'a core objection is the claim that brain death supports a reductionistic view of human beings'. This core objection was part of a more general 'anti-bioethics' sentiment that accused bioethics of an unacceptable utilitarian ethic that, argued the critics, resonated uncomfortably with Germany's Nazi past.

Of all the industrialized countries, the debate has been deepest and most bitter in Japan. In her book *Twice Dead*, the anthropologist Margaret Lock (2002) traces the roots of organ transplantation in the United States and Japan. Unlike the United States, problems in Japan emerged from the beginning, when, in 1968, a transplant surgeon, Wada Jiro, performed the world's thirteenth heart transplant in Sapporo. Wada both pronounced the donor (an 18-year-old boy who had drowned) dead and performed the transplant surgery. The Japanese news media, involved from the beginning, questioned both whether the surgery was needed by the recipient and if the donor was really dead when his organs were removed. Wada was charged with intentional homicide and professional negligence. It came to light that Wada had tampered with the recipient's discarded heart to make it look more damaged than it really was. It was also widely noted that Wada had obtained much of his training in the United States.

A second heart transplant was not performed in Japan until 1999. In the interim, an incredible public debate ensued. Lock describes it as an unprecedented effort to reach consensus about an issue that had caused 'national angst'. More than 100 books for the general public were written on the topic. Brain death was the subject of numerous television news specials. The effort to debate and educate included children. Lock (2002: 143) writes:

Manga (comics) have an enormous popularity in Japan; their influence on the young is arguably as great as that of television . . . The best-selling Black Jack series . . . read by millions of Japanese, has vividly depicted the living death of brain-dead and PVS patients and the moral dilemmas they pose, and the children's page in major newspapers put out cartoon pages educating young readers about brain death.

Such a social practice is unimaginable in the United States. Lock paints a complicated picture of the roots of opposition to brain death in Japan, including: deep ambivalence about the 'West'; the lingering presence of animism in Japanese culture; the absence of Christian charity as practiced in the West; mistrust of medicine; and that death is seen as more of a process in Japan, with the family more fully in control. As proof of its deep ambivalence, Japan did not legally recognize brain death until 1997, and then only grudgingly. Brain death must not only be rigorously established (in contrast to the United States, where the diagnosis is less and less rigorously conducted), but if the patient or family does not accept brain death, the medical diagnosis is not enough to take organs or even to declare death. Both donor and family must have signed donor cards. It is not surprising that the new law has yielded only a handful of donors in the seven years since its inception.

Lock argues that while brain death is seemingly accepted in North America and Europe, 'historical and multi-sited ethnographic research make plain the ambiguities and doubts that have surrounded living cadavers during nearly half of century of existence' (Lock 2002: 42).

The Japanese have an unnerving word for taking organs from brain-dead patients, *autaguari*, which means harvesting green rice. While no such word use exists in the United States, the stubborn persistence of the term 'brain death' may be a less jarring version of the same phenomenon.

For two decades transplant surgeons and organ procurement personnel have been arguing that the adjective 'brain-dead' should be dropped in favor of the simpler 'dead'. After all, the argument goes, if you call patients brain-dead instead of dead, it implies that they are different categories. Perhaps the implication is intentional, if not always conscious, and the persistence of the term 'brain death' represents a deep-seated sense among lay persons and health professionals that they are *not* the same. Our use of language often betrays other instances of the 'ambiguities and doubts' to which Lock refers. For example, it is commonplace for news reporters, families, and health professionals to talk about 'brain-dead' patients being 'kept alive' by machines.

Perhaps, as the neurologist Alan Shewmon has written, we have simply not developed the proper language with which to understand death in the modern ICU. 'Instead of proceeding via logical deduction from some preconceived,

abstract "concept of death"', Shewmon (2004: 279) proposes 'a phenomenological approach: to step back from linguistically constrained notions... and simply
look afresh at the spectrum of realities surrounding what people call and have
called "death"—as though we had never heard of the term "death" and have no
compulsion to label any particular phenomenon "death"'.

Shewmon argues that in the pretechnological era, when the events surrounding
death occurred simultaneously, the single word 'death' sufficed. It no longer does,
and our use and insistence on discovering the one correct meaning of death may
grow from a

delusion that our concepts of life and death are simply generalized from everyday experience
and labeled by linguistic convention with the words 'life' and 'death' when in actuality
those very concepts have been shaped by our language, and more importantly *constrained*
by it... no wonder that the death-debate is so full of logical inconsistencies and failures to
communicate, because people use the same word to express different concepts, not quite
realizing (precisely *because of* the single word) that the concepts *are* different.   (Shewmon
2004: 279)

Shewmon points out that in the west Greenlandic language there are at least
forty-nine different words referring to snow and ice—snow on the ground, snow
falling in air, air thick with snow, feathery clumps of falling snow, newly fallen
snow—that are perceived and conceived by natives of western Greenland as significantly different things. These distinctions are important for a way of life and
survival and

should be reflected in linguistic distinctions; for those of us for whom snow is but a wintry
nuisance or source of fun, the words 'snow', 'slush' and 'ice' probably suffice. Now imagine
that pioneers from the tropics migrated to the arctic and suddenly had to learn how to
survive there. Their very language, which allows them to see only 'snow' and 'ice' all around,
would be detrimental to survival.   (Shewmon 2004: 280)

We are today, says Shewmon, in a similar predicament regarding death.

We have migrated through human history into the modern ICU, bringing with us the
linguistic baggage of a relatively simple concept of death for which the one word has always
sufficed. Now we find ourselves in a situation for which medically real and ethically critical
distinctions lack words in the common vocabulary. The best we can do is to speak in
awkward paraphrases, such as 'the point in time beyond which cardiac autoresuscitation
is impossible'. To ask which of these technological mumbo-jumbos is *really* death may
perhaps be as linguistically and epistemologically inappropriate as asking an Eskimo which
of *sullarniq, aput, qantiit, nittaalaq*... is really 'snow'.   (Shewmon 2004: 280)

CONCLUSIONS

It is clear that the pressing need for more organs will continue to test the limits of
the dead donor rule. Public policy in this regard has several choices. The first is

a dramatic redefinition of death to include patients in PVS as a way to 'quell' the controversy that taking organs from them would cause. This is not likely. Vehement objections from religious fundamentalists and disability rights activists such as the group Not Dead Yet would make any major gerrymandering of the line between life and death impossible. Even the late Pope John Paul II declared there should be no judgments about the quality of life of PVS patients and that removing a feeding tube from patients in PVS is immoral and constitutes 'true euthanasia by omission'. The implications of the Pope's pronouncement for end-of-life care in PVS are uncertain, but is unlikely that the Catholic Church will embrace taking organs from PVS patients anytime soon.

A second choice for social policy is to have a public discussion about whether the dead donor rule can be violated under circumstances in which: (1) the donors or their surrogates have authorized removal; and (2) no tangible harm (e.g. pain and suffering) can come to the donor as a result of organ removal. This course would be likely to galvanize the same religious and political forces mentioned above who are wedded to the notion of clear dichotomies—between life and death, killing and letting die, and good and evil. Furthermore, public acknowledgement that patients were being killed by organ removal would likely alienate other groups who already have great mistrust of the health care system.

In fact, public discussion about either choice, redefining death yet again or abandoning the dead donor rule, is likely to erode what has appeared to be a workable social consensus, however flawed, about brain death. Most probably, the ongoing shortage of organs will force a gradual erosion of the line between life and death so that ambiguous states are increasingly and quietly included in the dead category or that little fuss occurs when severely compromised but living patients are killed by organ retrieval. The general acceptance of DCD protocols is an example of how this has happened already. If our society really insisted on maintaining a bright line between life and death and between killing and allowing to die, it would reject a two- to five-minute waiting period after heartbeat ceases because there is no proof or agreement about irreversibility at that point. There seems to be a passive acceptance that not much is lost either way.

Perhaps, as Shewmon has suggested, we will begin adopting new words or phrases to describe such states and contexts. Perhaps these new words will allow us to avoid the traditional battles about who is 'alive' and who is 'dead' and whom we are 'killing' and whom we are 'allowing to die'. The new words might improve on current phrases such as 'good as dead', 'euthanasia by omission', 'morally irreversible', and 'critical function', which, to some degree, reflect human feeling and practice, but, in the end, fail to capture the complexities of life and death as they are experienced in the modern intensive care unit.

References

AD HOC COMMITTEE OF THE HARVARD MEDICAL SCHOOL (1968), 'A Definition of Irreversible Coma', *JAMA* 205: 337–40.

ARNOLD, R. M., YOUNGNER, S. J., SCHAPIRO, R., and SPICER, C. M. (eds.) (1995), *Procuring Organs for Transplant: The Debate Over Non-Heart-Beating Cadaver Protocols* (Baltimore: JHUP).

BARTLETT, E. T. (1995), 'Differences Between Death and Dying', *Journal of Medical Ethics*, 21: 270–6.

_____ and YOUNGNER, S. J. (1988), 'Human Death and the Destruction of the Human Cortex', in R. M. Zaner (ed.), *Beyond Whole Brain Criteria* (Dordrecht: Kluwer Academic Publishers), 199–216.

BERNAT, J. L. (1998), 'A Defense of the Whole-Brain Concept of Death', *Hastings Center Report*, 28/2: 14–23.

_____ CULVER, C. M., and GERT, B. (1981), 'On the Definition and Criterion of Death', *Annals of Internal Medicine*, 94: 389–94.

CAMPBELL, C. S. (1999), 'Fundamentals of Life and Death: Christian Fundamentalism and Medical Science', in S. Youngner, R. Arnold, and R. Schapiro (eds.), *The Definition of Death: Contemporary Controversies* (Baltimore: JHUP), 194–209.

COLE, D. J. (1993), 'Statutory Definitions of Death and the Management of Terminally Ill Patients Who May Become Organ Donors After Death', *Kennedy Institute of Ethics Journal*, 3: 145–55.

GERVAIS, K. G. (1986), *Redefining Death* (New Haven: Yale University Press).

LAMB, D. (1992), 'Reversibility and Death: A Reply to David J. Cole', *Journal of Medical Ethics*, 18: 31–3.

LOCK, M. (2002), *Twice Dead: Organ Transplants and the Reinvention of Death* (Berkeley: University of California Press).

LYNN, J., and CRANFORD, R. (1999), 'The Persisting Perplexities in the Determination of Death', in S. Youngner, R. Arnold, and R. Schapiro (eds.), *The Definition of Death: Contemporary Controversies* (Baltimore: JHUP), 101–14.

MAYO, D., and WIKLER, D. (1979), 'Euthanasia and the Transition from Life to Death', in W. L. Robinson and M. S. Pritchard (eds.), *Medical Responsibility: Paternalism, Informed Consent, and Euthanasia* (Clifton, NJ: Humana Press), 195–211.

PRESIDENT'S COMMISSION FOR THE STUDY OF ETHICAL PROBLEMS IN MEDICINE AND BIOMEDICAL AND BEHAVIORAL RESEARCH (1981) *Defining Death* (Washington, DC: US Government Printing Office).

RIX, B. A. (1999), 'Brain Death, Ethics, and Politics in Denmark', in S. Youngner, R. Arnold, and R. Schapiro (eds.), *The Definition of Death: Contemporary Controversies* (Baltimore: JHUP), 227–38.

SCHÖNE-SEIFERT, B. (1999), 'Defining Death in Germany: Brain Death and Its Discontents', in S. Youngner, R. Arnold, and R. Schapiro (eds.), *The Definition of Death: Contemporary Controversies* (Baltimore: JHUP), 257–71.

SHEWMON, A. (2004), 'The Dead Donor Rule: Lessons from Linguistics', *Kennedy Institute of Ethics Journal*, 14: 277–300.

SIMINOFF, L., BURANT, C., and YOUNGNER, S. J. (2004), 'Death and Organ Procurement: Public Beliefs and Attitudes', *Social Science in Medicine*, 59: 2325–34.

TOMLINSON, R. (1993), 'The Irreversibility of Death: Reply to Cole', *Kennedy Institute of Ethics Journal*, 3: 157–65.

YOUNGNER, S. J., LANDEFELD, C. S., COULTON, C. J., *et al.* (1989), 'Brain Death and Organ Retrieval: A Cross-Sectional Survey of Knowledge and Concepts Among Health Professionals', *JAMA* 261: 2205–10.

—— ARNOLD, R. M., and DEVITA, M. A. (1999), 'When Is Dead?', *Hastings Center Report*, 29: 14–21.

CHAPTER 13

THE AGING SOCIETY AND THE EXPANSION OF SENILITY: BIOTECHNOLOGICAL AND TREATMENT GOALS

STEPHEN G. POST

OF the many topics worthy of discussion regarding older adults and bioethics, two seem to provide an especially pointed opportunity for reflection on our aging society. First, is aging itself something that biomedical researchers should focus on as a deficit to be overcome through eventual anti-aging treatments? While aging may not fall neatly into the disease category, it is clearly the primary susceptibility factor for the innumerable diseases of older adults, and therefore its potential deceleration consistent with the compression of morbidity might constitute a salutary biomedical goal. The aging society is no panacea to those who suffer from a host of chronic illnesses and feel overwhelmed by the burden of years. Perhaps we must now take scientific steps that may allow an escape from widespread frailty and senility, or such costly demographics will drive us toward inordinate filial, economic, and social responsibilities. Such thoughts raise broad questions about endeavors to modify human nature along 'posthumanist' lines. Second, we must concentrate on the most challenging problematic of our current aging society, assuming that anti-aging technologies will only become available in future decades. One immense problem is the harsh reality of irreversible progressive dementia, which will serve here as an example of the rise of chronic illness, for which age itself is the primary risk factor. While this second focus overlooks the many older adults who age well and are functional until their final days, these examples of 'successful aging' pose no unique issues worthy of special bioethical consideration. And so this chapter is framed around the more unfortunate realities of an aging society, and the related question of whether we ought to strive to ameliorate these realities by developing anti-aging interventions.

DECELERATED AGING AND THE AMELIORATION OF AGE-RELATED DISEASE

The possibility for significant deceleration of human aging can be ethically assessed in a variety of frameworks. The outcome of this assessment is a direct result of the ethical theory and assumptions that disparate camps bring to the debate. Two theories that currently shape a rather acrimonious discussion are natural law and equalitarianism, each of which presents a deeply critical perspective on the goal of prolongevity. Yet despite valid natural law cautions that human goods are violated by anti-aging goals, and meaningful equalitarian concerns that anti-aging treatments would create immense class disparities, there is one extremely powerful ethical argument that may outweigh such criticisms: i.e. the principle of beneficence, which supports the deceleration of aging so long as this significantly diminishes the onset of the many chronic diseases for which aging is the primary risk factor. This assumes that the deceleration of aging will achieve this purpose, rather than the harmful protraction of decrepitude.

Ethical theories do have consequences. A resurgence of natural law ethics, which asserts the goodness of human nature and aging as we know it, has of late given rise to a significant set of criticisms of the goal of prolongevity, in particular through the work of Leon R. Kass and the President's Council on Bioethics, for which he serves as chair. The equalitarians, on the other hand, do not engage in the moralization of human nature as we know it, but nevertheless cannot support the goal of prolongevity until the vast inequalities that currently plague the world—including access to basic healthcare—are corrected. These are both important frameworks for critique of decelerated aging, should this ever become possible.

At first glance, however, it is difficult to see why the deceleration of human aging presents a major ethical concern. There are four reasons for this.

1. Aging may not be a 'disease' by most definitions, but it is the major risk factor for innumerable diseases of old age, and is therefore so closely associated with disease that it is not completely implausible to think of it as such.

2. While the concept of 'aging as disease' might be thought to reinforce existing stereotypes of older adults, and so contribute to 'ageism', there is no logical connection between 'anti-aging' research and prejudice. The goal of prolongevity through deceleration of aging has the more obvious inclusive aspect of making old age more enjoyable and acceptable by mitigating the frailties and infirmities that make the increase of years unwelcome.

3. The goal of decelerated aging and prolongevity does not obviously violate the ethical principle of nonmaleficence. Unlike abortion, infanticide, suicide, and euthanasia, the goal of prolongevity does not violate respect for, or sanctity of, life. It is difficult to see how the addition of healthy years to old age could be anything but 'pro-life'. While moral criticism of therapeutic stem cell cloning is based on the unavoidable destruction of embryos in the process of procuring stem cell lines, there is no such destruction associated with prolongevity.

4. The goal of longer and healthier lives is hardly new and we have been acculturated to it. Life expectancy has risen dramatically over the past two centuries and has been embraced as progress. Public health, sanitation, reduction of infant mortality, antibiotics, and many other factors have contributed to our current level of prolongevity, which some might have deemed an 'unnatural' goal a century or more ago. In other words, the genie is in many respects already out of the bottle. This progress in life expectancy might be hampered by sedentary lifestyles, fast foods, obesity, and related diabetes, all of which are viewed as public health problems to be overcome.

And yet deeply thoughtful bioethicists are concerned with the implications of anti-aging research and related prolongevity. Kass prepared a discussion paper for members of the Council on Bioethics prior to their meeting on 16–17 January 2003. Entitled 'Beyond Therapy: Biotechnology and the Pursuit of Human Development', it established the Council's future agenda (Kass 2003).

Biogerontologists, one of whom is with the National Institute on Aging, can embrace the ideas of 'The Serious Search for an Anti-Aging Pill' that would mimic the effects of caloric restriction as an approach to the eradication of disease (Lane *et al.* 2002). Aging is the prominent risk factor for so many diseases, and the best way to prevent such debilitation is to alleviate aging. The removal of this risk is not obviously contrary to human dignity. In fact, we would all agree that removing the major risk factor for diseases such as Alzheimer's or osteoporosis would do quite a bit for the preservation of human dignity, for the control of health care costs, and for the alleviation of sometimes overwhelming adult filial duties. Still, Kass's natural law ethics are to be taken seriously, a topic to which attention now turns.

Natural Law Criticisms

Natural law places moral value on human nature as we know it, and represents a necessary reaction to post-humanism. One reason why natural law, a form of anti-posthumanism, has an immediate appeal is because many of the major defenders of posthumanism are rather cavalier (see e.g. www.betterhumans.com; www.transhumanism.org; www.foresight.org). Websites reflect the enthusiasm of the young convert to some new image of the human future that is liberated from biological constraints but lacking in wisdom. More reverence for human nature and aging itself as the product of millions of years of evolutionary selection would be the necessary corrective, and this is just what natural law theorists offer.

The posthumanist embraces decelerated and even arrested aging, but only as a small part of a larger vision to re-engineer human nature, and thereby to create biologically and technologically superior human beings (Hayles 1999). Posthumans are the much more advanced models that we humans today will design for tomorrow, not unlike new models of automobiles. Genetics, nanotechnology, cybernetics, and computer technologies are all part of the posthuman vision, including the downloading of synaptic connections in the brain to form a computerized human mind freed of mortal flesh, and thereby immortalized. Posthumanists do not take biology to be destiny, and see human nature as an obstacle to be overcome (Hook 2004). They see the next great step in evolution as our own re-creation by human ingenuity.

The posthumanist may be irreverent of human nature, but within the boundaries of the technology of the day, humans have been reinventing themselves anyway for millennia. And what is natural and what is unnatural, when the human condition has already been so deeply impacted by technological innovation? Where do we draw lines? As Freeman Dyson writes, 'the artificial improvement of human beings will come, one way or another, whether we like it or not', as scientific understanding increases, for after all, such improvement has always been viewed as a 'liberation from past constraints' (1997: 12). After all, the idea of human flight was once deemed heretical hubris in the light of eternity and nature. So it is that Gregory Stock writes a book entitled *Redesigning Humans: Our Inevitable Genetic Future*, in which he introduces the idea of 'superbiology' as we take full control of our own biology in turning toward perfectibility (2002).

Thus did George Bernard Shaw, in his remarkable *Back to Methuselah* (1921), take up the variations in lifespans between species such as parrots and dogs, or turtles and wasps, and ask that science rise to the redemptive occasion by vastly increasing human longevity. Indeed, Francis Bacon, a founder of the scientific method four centuries ago, in his essay *The New Atlantis* (1996), set in motion a biological mandate for boldness that included both the making of new species, or 'chimeras', organ replacement, and the 'Water of Paradise' that would allow the possibility to 'indeed live very long'. Three centuries before Francis Bacon the English theologian Roger Bacon argued that in the future the 900-year-long lives of the antediluvian patriarchs would be restored alchemically. Like many Western religious thinkers, both Bacons saw death as the unnatural result of Adamic fall into sin. These Western dreams of embodied near-immortality could only emerge against a theological background that more or less endorses them.

The modern goals of anti-aging research and technology are historically emergent from a pre-modern religious drama of hope and salvation. Longings for immortality within a religious context are understandable in light of existential anxiety over finitude and mortality, and the goal of prolongevity may be—at least historically—shaped by such passions. Renaissance science transferred the task of achieving immortality from heaven to earth in the spirit of millennial hopes. The economy of salvation presented by Dante was replaced by the here and now. There is a vibrant millennialist optimism in the responsible biogerontologists, for they have proclaimed aging itself to be surmountable to degrees through human ingenuity.

At the end of *The New Atlantis*, Bacon lists more specifically among the goals of science 'the retardation of age', which is taken with great seriousness by today's biogerontologists who create scientific breakthroughs with fruit flies, roundworms, rodents, and monkeys, but with an eye toward the alleviation of senility in an already aging society plagued by chronic age-related diseases.

But the natural law theorists attempt to stem such rash tides. One of the wiser minds of the last century, Hans Jonas (d. 1993), an intellectual inspiration for today's natural law anti-posthumanists, first articulated deep questions about the prolongevity agenda. How desirable would this power to slow or arrest aging be for the individual and for the species? Do we want to tamper with the delicate biological balance of death and procreation, and preempt the place of youth? Would the species gain or lose? Jonas, by merely raising these questions, meant to cast significant doubt on the anti-aging enterprise. His later essays raising many of these same questions were published posthumously (1996).

Many of these questions are echoed in the writings of Kass, who for the most part accepts biotechnological progress within a therapeutic mode; his issue is with efforts to enhance and improve upon the givens of human nature.

There is arguably a tone of solipsism in grasping at extended life rather than accepting old age and celebrating youth in the lives of our offspring. Responsibility to future generations precludes a clinging to our own youthfulness. There is wisdom in simply accepting the fact that we evolved for reproductive success rather than for long-lived lives. Without such wisdom will we lose sight of our deepest creative motives? Possibly. And so it is written, 'teach us to number our days that we may get a heart of wisdom' (Psalm 90).

The possibility of fundamentally modifying the rate of human aging and thereby altering the perennial process of generational transition could prove destructive of all the human propensities to nurture and elevate the young. Perhaps the improvement of the human condition lies not in modifying the human vessel, but in developing the treasures within, such as compassion, justice, and dignity.

In summary, the natural law traditions represented by anti-posthumanists exhort us to live more or less according to nature, and warn that our efforts to depart from what we are will result in new evils that are more perilous than old ones. To use an analogy, we are like the sailor who climbs as high on the mast as one can in order to rise high above the waters of nature, but only to see the boat capsize under our weight tipping the mast into the waves below. How can we presume that the brave new world will be a better world? Should not the burden of proof be on the proponents of radical change? Who are we today to impose our arbitrary images of human enhancement on future generations?

Thus are anti-posthumanist thinkers critical of biogerontology to the extent that it seeks to slow the aging process. Our focus, argue the anti-posthumanists, should be on the acceptance of aging rather than on its scientific modification. The intergenerational thrust of evolution, by which we are inclined toward parental and social investment in the hope, energy, and vitality of youth, provides the basis for a natural law ethic that requires us all to relinquish youthfulness.

I agree with the anti-posthumanists that a decision for or against decelerated aging based on superficial thinking and a commitment to individual freedom is a formula for the easy destruction of what is good in being human. They are right to place an emphasis on Aristotelian 'final causes' and human goods. Unless we are radical relativists, it can and must be asked whether any scientific aspiration contributes to the human condition or detracts from it. There is truth in the claim of anti-posthumanists that a contemporary bioethics that does not ask such questions is inadequate. And yet the natural law criticism of the goal of prolongevity does not leave me quite convinced. In the context of posthumanism, the religion of technology, and scientific hubris, efforts to slow or arrest human aging appear morally ambiguous at best. And yet one aspect of human nature has always been freedom over itself. Freedom causes us to break the harmonies of nature and establish new harmonies, especially when confronted with severe risks that require a creative solution.

A Solution to the Chronic Illnesses Associated with Aging?

If we bracket out this ancient debate between the natural law and its detractors, there is another context that is more immediate. The stark reality of our already aging societies is that, factoring out infant mortality, people can expect to live into their eighties. Many will experience chronic illness for which old age is the dominant risk factor, ranging from Alzheimer's and Parkinson's to osteoporosis and vascular disease. Our demographic transition to greatly increased life expectancy through means that do not involve the deceleration of aging has resulted in a scenario that is clearly not idyllic, and the solution may rest with advances in the basic science of aging that would achieve even greater prolongevity but without the perils of massive debilitation. In other words, to resolve the problems of senility and dementia, brought on chiefly by enhanced life expectancy absent anti-aging interventions, we must now develop those interventions or suffer the immense negative consequences.

Among those consequences are future generations of young people extremely burdened with the direct and indirect support of tens of millions of citizens who require demanding, complex, constant, and expensive care.

When one considers the goal of decelerated aging in this context, it begins to appear more rational, salutary, and necessary. No longer the bizarre dream of superficial technology zealots, decelerated aging appears to be a more reasonable aspiration. Indeed, the biogerontologists hard at work in serious research are much less the children of posthumanism than they are of a will to benefit a common humanity regrettably caught between the old world of relatively short and 'natural' life expectancy and the future world of the nonfrail and nonsenile.

So, the individual confronted with the possibility of decelerating his or her aging process may not ask the question of the dignity of human nature as we know it, or of whether we humans are wise enough to control our future development, or of equalitarian justice. Instead, he or she may reflect on loved ones who have struggled with a syndrome that strips away memory and self-identity, such as dementia, and quickly declare that his or her true dignity lies in decelerated aging consistent with the retention of cognitive temporal glue between past, present, and future.

It may well be that the only real progress we will see in ridding the world of such debilitating diseases as Alzheimer's is through slowing the process of aging because old age is by far the most significant risk factor. Currently there is no reason for strong optimism about scientific breakthroughs to cure this disease, or to stabilize symptoms in the long term, although there are some compounds in use to ameliorate some symptoms for a limited period. Thus, basic scientific advances in the area of aging itself could, if successful, significantly reduce the incidence of diseases associated with old age that are too complex to be solved on their own terms. It is, then, unfair to responsible anti-aging researchers to suggest that they are engaged in an effort that will only radically protract the lives of the most deeply forgetful. Maybe greatly enhanced prolongevity is not all bad if a number of conditions can be met regarding preserved memory and other dimensions of health and rigor. It might also be that, given the realities of the old age boom, anti-aging research will prove curative where all else has failed.

Will anti-aging researchers provide the solution? Two respected researchers from the University of London conclude in *Nature* that ultimately we will find the human lifespan to be quite plastic, and scientific progress in this area 'may allow us to reduce the impact of ageing-related diseases as the limits on the human lifespan recede' (Partridge and Gems 2002: 921).

While I share natural law concerns over the unleashed powers of biotechnology to influence what increasingly appears to be a somewhat malleable human nature, and while I too cringe at immature millennialist enthusiasm over the remaking of the species, I nevertheless can appreciate the goal of eradicating our modern epidemic of chronic illness, which grows more extensive and costly with every elevation in average life expectancy.

Indeed, it is because of the potential positive health consequences of anti-aging treatments that they will probably not be easily restrained in the name of natural law or equalitarianism. It may well be that, in the process of decelerating aging with the intent of ameliorating chronic diseases, the human lifespan will be extended. We do not have much choice but to move forward. The goal of prolongevity is rooted in the reality of the 80-year-old who has struggled with hip replacements, a diagnosis of dementia, retinopathy, and related depression. Perhaps Kass is correct that under conditions of prolongevity many of us would lose interest and engagement in life, seriousness and aspiration, and virtue and moral excellence centered on a generative relationship with the young. Yet more surely, a potential solution to the widespread problem of the death of the mind before the death of the body may rest with the anti-aging technologies of the future, and we must at least seriously grapple with this important and very real problem.

A number of scientists convened in 1999, under the auspices of the National Institute on Aging, for a conference entitled Caloric Restriction's Effects on Aging: Opportunities for Research on Human Implications, where they charted a bold new therapeutic research agenda focused on slowing or 'retarding' the aging process, which implies the extension of the lifespan (Masoro 2001). The driving motivations expressed, however, were focused on slowing aging in order to prevent the many diseases for which old age puts people at risk. This scholarly meeting sparked no significant public debate, although few things could be more deserving of critical reflection on human aspirations than this. A principal topic was the research to develop a treatment to prolong life and youthful vigor through imitating the remarkable effects of caloric restriction, which for more than sixty years has been documented for its dramatic ability to slow aging in nonhuman mammals and significantly extend their lifespans.

More research on the basic science of aging will hopefully give rise to the ability to decelerate this natural process. People will be attracted to this technology because they know how burdensome are the diseases to which old age makes us all susceptible. Should they wish to select this medical option, as a way of insuring a better quality of life for themselves and for those loved ones who would otherwise have to provide long-term care, few would condemn them unless the problem of prolonged senescence arises. We simply cannot predict the future, but over the last century we have seen a dramatic rise in life expectancy, and it is hard to imagine that the addition of more healthy years would be widely deemed contrary to human dignity.

But there is reason to urge extreme caution. The technology to slow the aging process may be coming nearer to reality, yet the goal of prolongevity has not been carefully considered (Juengst *et al.* 2003). In a time when biotechnology is allowing for the reconstruction of both nature and human nature, all thoughtful citizens must ponder the implications of potentially dramatic change. Of the many possible biotechnological goals on the horizon, which ones are likely to enhance the human condition, and which ones are likely to diminish human dignity? We think of the provocative developments in therapeutic cloning, in fertility and reproduction, in organ procurement and transplantation, in genetic testing and therapy, or in the treatment of a myriad of illnesses, and our collective breath is taken away by the pace of change. But we are also rightly haunted by the reality that, while biotechnological powers grow, human nature has in no obvious way progressed with regard to unselfish behavior, humility, peace, and equality. Thus, we raise the question of the very nature of goodness, and whether some biotechnological developments divert us from growth in virtue, or even tempt us to create a new class of an ageless elite that inevitably begins to look down upon the ordinary older adult as a misfit.

Should we move forward in the twenty-first century as bold new 'co-creators' of our somewhat malleable human nature, or should we accept a more humble approach that endorses a caring and just stewardship over human nature more or less as it is, seeking therapies rather than transformations? At least in the area of decelerated aging, where therapy and enhancement merge, we will probably move forward. Progress takes creativity, and in the meanwhile, we must deal as humanely as possible with the major moral, social, economic, familial, and medical challenges of an aging society—the death of the mind before the death of the body.

DEATH AND DEMENTIA

The syndrome of dementia is an irreversible decline in cognitive abilities that causes significant dysfunction. Like most syndromes, dementia can be caused by a number of diseases. In the nineteenth century, for example, a main cause of dementia was syphilis. Currently, as a result of dramatic increases in average human life expectancy, dementia is caused primarily by a number of neurological diseases associated with old age. Dementia is distinguished from 'pseudo-dementia' because the latter is reversible; for example, depression, extreme stress, and infection can cause dementia but with treatment a return to a former cognitive state is likely. Dementia is also distinguished from 'normal age-related memory loss', which effects most people by about age 70 in the form of some slowing of cognitive skills and a deterioration in various aspects of memory.

Although dementia can have many causes, the primary cause of dementia in our aging societies is Alzheimer's disease (AD). Approximately 60 per cent of dementia in the American elderly and worldwide in industrialized nations is secondary to AD (US General Accounting Office 1998). This discussion will focus on so-called 'Alzheimer's dementia' in order to illustrate ethical issues that pertain to all progressive dementias. Epidemiologists differ in their estimates of late-life AD prevalence, but most studies agree roughly on the following: about 1–2 per cent of older adults at age 60 have probable AD, and this percentage doubles every five years so that 3 per cent are affected at age 65, 6 per cent at age 70, 12 per cent at age 75, and 24 per cent by age 80. While some argue that those who live into their nineties without being effected by AD will usually never be affected by it, this is still speculative. According to a Swiss study, 10 per cent of nondemented persons between the ages of 85 and 88 become demented each year (Aevarsson 1996). There are very few people in their late forties and early fifties who are diagnosed with AD. Without delaying or preventive interventions, the number of people with AD, in the United States alone, will increase to 12 to 14 million by 2050. These numbers represent a new problem of major proportions and immense financial consequences for medicine, families, and society.

Various stage theories of disease progression have been developed. However, in clinical practice, professionals speak roughly of three stages. In *mild stage dementia*, the newly diagnosed patient has significant cognitive losses resulting in disorientation and dysfunction, and often displays affective flatness and possibly depression. In *moderate stage dementia*, the patient forgets that he or she forgets, thereby gaining relief from insight into losses. Some patients will at this point adjust well emotionally to a life lived largely in the pure present, although some long-term memories are still in place. The recognition of loved ones is usually still possible. However, as many as a third of patients in the moderate stage will struggle with emotional and behavior problems, including agitation, combativeness, paranoia, hallucinations, wandering, and depression. The *advanced stage of dementia* includes a loss of all or nearly all ability to communicate by speech, inability to recognize loved ones in most cases, loss of ambulation without assistance, incontinence of bowel and/or bladder, and some weight loss due to swallowing difficulties. The advanced stage is generally considered terminal, with death occurring on average within two years. AD, however, is heterogeneous in its manifestations, and defies simplistic staging.

A Fundamental Moral Question: Do People with Dementia 'Count'?

Despite the seriousness of dementia and the responsibilities it creates for care-givers, it is ethically important that the person with dementia not be judged by 'hypercognitive' values (Post 2000). The self is not cognition alone, but is rather a complex entity with emotional and relational aspects that should be deemed mor-ally significant and worthy of affirmation (Sabat 2001). A bias against the deeply forgetful is especially pronounced in 'personhood' theories of moral status in which persons are defined by the presence of a set of cognitive abilities (Kitwood 1997). After discussion of the disparities in bioethical thinking about what constitutes a person, Stanley Rudman concludes, 'It is clear that the emphasis on rationality easily leads to diminished concern for certain human beings such as infants . . . and the senile, groups of people who have, under the influence of both Christian and humanistic considerations, been given special considerations' (1997: 47). Often, the personhood theorists couple their exclusionary rationalistic views with utilitarian ethical theories that are deeply incoherent with regard to life and death. As Rudman summarizes the concern, rationality is too severe a ground for moral standing, 'allowing if not requiring the deaths of many individuals who may, in fact, continue to enjoy simple pleasures despite their lack of rationality' (1997: 57). Of course, in the real world of families, love, and care, personhood theories have no practical significance.

The philosophical tendency to diminish the moral status or considerability of people with dementia is also related to a radical differentiation between the formerly intact, or 'then', self and the currently demented, or 'now', self. The reality is that until the very advanced and even terminal stage of AD, the person with dementia will usually have sporadically articulated memories of deeply meaningful events and relationships ensconced in long-term memory. It is wrong to bifurcate the self into 'then' and 'now', as if continuities are not at least occasionally striking (Kitwood 1997; Sabat 2001). This is why it is essential that professional caregivers be aware of the person's life story, making up for losses by providing cues toward continuity in self-identity. Even in the advanced stage of dementia, as in the case presented at the outset of this chapter, one finds varying degrees of emotional and relational expression, remnants of personality, and even meaningful nonverbal communication as in the reaching out for a hug.

The fitting moral response to people with dementia, according to classical Western ethical thought and related conceptions of common human decency, is to enlarge our sense of human worth to counter an exclusionary emphasis on rationality, efficient use of time and energy, ability to control distracting impulses, thrift, economic success, self-reliance, self-control, 'language advantage', and the like. As Alasdair MacIntyre argues, we have made too much of the significance of language, for instance, obscuring the moral significance of species who lack linguistic abilities, or human beings who have lost such abilities (MacIntyre 1999). It is possible to distinguish two fundamental views of persons with dementia. Those in the tradition of Stoic and Enlightenment rationalism have achieved much for universal human moral standing by emphasizing the spark of reason (*logos*) in us all; yet when this rationality dissipates, so does moral status. Those who take an alternative position see the Stoic heritage as an arrogant view in the sense that it makes the worth of a human being entirely dependent on rationality, and then gives too much power to the reasonable. This alternative view is generally associated with most Jewish and Christian thought, as well as that of other religious traditions in which the individual retains equal value regardless of cognitive decline. As the Protestant ethicist Reinhold Niebuhr wrote, 'In Stoicism life beyond the narrow bonds of class, community, and race is affirmed because all life reveals a unifying divine principle. Since the principle is reason, the logic of Stoicism tends to include only the intelligent in the divine community. An aristocratic condescension, therefore, corrupts Stoic universalism' (1956: 53).

Diagnostic Truthtelling

Diagnostic truthtelling in the context of dementia should be handled as it is in other medical contexts: be as truthful as information permits while attending to the patient's need for social, emotional, spiritual, and practical support. Compassionate diagnostic disclosure is a moral act of respect for persons, an opportunity for human resilience and community, and a necessary practical step toward future planning.

In serving on more than 120 ethics panels organized by Alzheimer's Association chapters across the United States and Canada in the late 1990s, comprised of leading physicians and other health professionals caring for those with dementia, as well as of family caregivers and affected patients, I did not find a single individual among an estimated 880 who thought that compassionate honesty was not the best policy. There were disagreements about optimal emotional and relational supports, precise wording and approach, and whether to inform the patient together with the family or independently.

There are some poor excuses for deceit and nondisclosure:

Anxiety. The idea of denying the truth to protect a patient from anxiety underestimates the remarkable human capacity to deal creatively and resiliently with the implications of serious diagnoses, and denies the power of a caring family or community to provide emotional healing. Many patients, when provided with a diagnosis, are actually relieved of the anxiety that stems from uncertainty. The ways in which people cope with a diagnosis need to be empirically examined, but if we were to argue that anxiety-related behaviors justify nondisclosure or deceit, then in the final analysis no patient would be told of any serious diagnosis, with disastrous results. Clinically significant depression, however, indicates a more cautious and gradual approach than might otherwise be the case. Secondly, a diagnosis and its emotional challenges to the patient mobilize family and community to provide the care and acceptance without which only further isolation is possible.

Culture. The physician may encounter some patients from cultures in which the model of nondisclosure to the patient is still in place, and families still operate in a highly 'protective' manner. However, it is well documented that individuals often want diagnostic information despite cultural pressures to the contrary. A physician should never presume to withhold information unless the patient specifically requests this. Professional commitment is to patients, not cultures. Moreover, cultures can have moral blind spots that are only gradually modified through interacting with other traditions, including the tradition of diagnostic truthtelling on the basis of human dignity.

Lack of objectivity. The syndrome of dementia is comprised of a cluster of symptoms. The core feature of dementia is decline in cognitive abilities that causes significant dysfunction. Such cognitive dysfunction is reasonably objective. Like most syndromes, dementia can be caused by a number of diseases. All possible conditions—e.g. pseudo-dementia, dementia, and Alzheimer's disease (AD)—can and should be supportively discussed with patients, and, when possible, treated with consent. Not to present reasonably clear diagnostic information is to disenfranchise the person who is experiencing an illness—and usually is well aware of some losses—and to create a climate of distrust that will ultimately serve no good purpose.

Diagnostic truthtelling is the necessary beginning point for an ethics of 'precedent autonomy' for those who wish to implement control over their futures through advance directives such as durable power of attorney for health care, which allows a trusted loved one to make any and all treatment decisions once the agent becomes incompetent. This can effectively be coupled with a living will or some other specific indication of the agent's material wishes with regard to end-of-life care. Unless the person knows the probable diagnosis in a timely way while still competent to file such legal instruments, the risk of burdensome medical technologies is increased. Even in the absence of such legal forms, however, many technologically advanced countries will allow next of kin to decide against efforts to extend life in severe dysfunction. This is important because many patients suffer incapacitating cognitive decline long before having a diagnostic work up; those who are diagnosed early enough to exercise their autonomy can become quickly incapacitated.

In the United States the Alzheimer's Disease Association does not support mandatory reporting of a probable diagnosis of AD to the Department of Motor Vehicles. There are a number of reasons for this caution, one of which is patient confidentiality. Reporting requirements might discourage some persons from coming into the clinic for diagnosis at a time early in the course of disease when drug treatments are most clearly indicated. Eventually all people with AD must stop driving when they are a serious risk to self or others. Family members must know that if a loved one drives too long and injures others, they may even be held financially liable and insurers may not be obliged to cover this liability. Ideally, a privilege is never limited without offering the person ways to fill in the gaps and diminish any sense of loss. An 'all or nothing' approach can and should be avoided. Compromise and adjustments can be successfully implemented by those who are informed and caring, especially when the person with AD has insight into diminishing mental abilities and loss of competence. The affected person should retain a sense of freedom and self-control if possible (Alzheimer's Disease Association 2001).

Truthtelling, which is clearly the accepted norm in modern medical care, has been encouraged by the emergence of new treatments such as cholinesterase inhibitors, and by an appreciation for the rights and needs of patients as they and their families plan for the future, financially and otherwise. The Association's statement (2001) includes the important argument that disclosing the diagnosis early in the disease process allows the person to 'be involved in communicating and planning for end-of-life decisions'. Diagnostic truthtelling is the necessary beginning point for responsible stewardship over one's future through advance directives such as durable power of attorney for health care, which allows a trusted loved one to make any and all treatment decisions once the agent becomes incompetent. This can effectively be coupled with a living will or some other specific indication of the agent's material wishes with regard to end-of-life care. Unless the person knows the probable diagnosis in a timely way while still competent to file such legal instruments, the risk of burdensome medical technologies is increased.

With early treatments available, with options for research participation, with the availability of support groups where these exist, with many patients already having a significant knowledge base through informational technologies, with the need to be protected against the aggressive use of burdensome medical technologies as the disease progresses, and with the importance of financial, family, and career planning, it is simply impossible to defend the old paternalistic model of the physician–patient relationship. It is the job of the physician and the health care team, including pastoral care as requested, to disclose a diagnosis of dementia and, when possible, the disease cause underlying it, in a sensitive and supportive way. In individual cases, this may require different approaches, timing, and venues, but there is no alternative consistent with human dignity, resilience, and care. Where the patient can no longer retain information in a sustained and meaningful manner, diagnostic truthtelling is impossible and uncalled for. For those whose ability to retain information is unclear or fast fading, one trusts in the physician to improvise as the case merits.

Quality of Life

Emotional, relational, aesthetic, and symbolic well-being are possible to varying degrees in people with progressive dementia (Kitwood 1997). Quality of life can be much enhanced by working with these aspects of the person.

Kitwood provides indicators of well-being in people with severe dementia: the assertion of will or desire, usually in the form of dissent despite various coaxings; the ability to express a range of emotions; initiation of social contact (for instance, a person with dementia has a small toy dog that he treasures and places it before another person with dementia to attract attention); affectional warmth (for instance, a woman wanders back and forth in the facility without much socializing, but when people say hello to her she gives them a kiss on the cheek and continues her wandering). In enhancing quality of life it is crucial to accept the reality of the person with dementia rather than try to impose one's own reality. In the mild stage of AD there is much to be said for trying to orient a person to reality; at some point in moderate AD, however, it becomes oppressive to impose reality upon them. The aesthetic well-being available to people with AD is obvious to anyone who has watched art or music therapy sessions. In some cases, a person with advanced AD may still draw the same valued symbol, as though through art a sense of self is retained (Firlik 1991). The abstract expressionist de Kooning painted his way through much of his fourteen-year struggle with AD until his death in 1996. Good caregivers know how to work with remaining capacities in the person with dementia, rather than against them.

In general, quality of life is a self-fulfilling prophesy. If those around the person with dementia see the glass as half empty and make no efforts to relate to the person in ways that enhance his or her experience, then quality of life is minimal. Steven R. Sabat, who has produced the definitive observer study of the experience of dementia, underscores the extent to which the dignity and value of the person with dementia can be maintained through affirmation and an existential perspective (Sabat 2001).

A Relatively 'Good' Dying

AD is on the leading edge of the debate over physician-assisted suicide and euthanasia. The policies that emerge from this debate will have monumental significance for people with dementia, and for social attitudes toward the task of providing care when preemptive death is cheaper and easier. The Association affirms the right to dignity and life for every Alzheimer patient, and cannot condone suicide (Alzheimer's Disease Association 2001).

The Association asserts that the refusal or withdrawal of any and all medical treatment is a moral and legal right for all competent Americans of age, and this right can be asserted by a family surrogate acting on the basis of either 'substituted judgement' (what would the patient when competent have wanted) or 'best interests' (what seems the most humane and least burdensome option in the present).

The Association concludes that AD *in its advanced stage should be defined as a terminal disease*, as roughly delineated by such features as the inability to recognize loved ones, to communicate by speech, to ambulate, or to maintain bowel and/or bladder control. When AD progresses to this stage, weight loss and swallowing difficulties will inevitably emerge. Death can be expected for most patients within a year or two, or even sooner, regardless of medical efforts. One useful consequence of viewing the advanced stage of AD as terminal is that family members will better appreciate the importance of palliative (pain medication) care as an alternative to medical treatments intended to extend the dying process. All efforts at life extension in this advanced stage create burdens and avoidable suffering for patients, who could otherwise live out the remainder of their lives in greater comfort and peace. Cardiopulmonary resuscitation, dialysis, tube-feeding, and all other invasive technologies should be avoided. The use of antibiotics usually does not prolong survival, and comfort can be maintained without antibiotic use in patients experiencing infections. Physicians and other health care professionals should recommend this less burdensome and therefore more appropriate approach to family members, and to persons with dementia who are competent, ideally soon after initial diagnosis. Early discussions of a peaceful dying should occur between persons with dementia and their families, guided by information from health care professionals on the relative benefits of a palliative care approach (Alzheimer's Disease Association 2001).

Avoiding hospitalization will also decrease the number of persons with advanced AD who receive tube-feeding, since many long-term care facilities send residents to hospitals for tube placement, after which they return to the facility. It should be remembered that the practice of long-term tube-feeding in persons with advanced dementia began only in the mid-1980s after the development of a new technique called 'percutaneous endoscopic gastrostomy' (PEG). Before then, such persons were cared for through assisted oral feeding. In comparison with assisted oral feeding, however, long-term tube-feeding has no advantages, and a number of disadvantages (Alzheimer's Disease Association 2001).

Gastrostomy tube-feeding became common in the context of advanced dementia and in elderly patients more generally after 1981, secondary to the development of the PEG procedure. The PEG procedure was developed by Dr Michael Gauderer and his colleagues at Rainbow Babies and Children's Hospital in Cleveland (1979–80) for use in young children with swallowing difficulties. The procedure required only local anesthesia, thus eliminating the significant surgical risk associated with general anesthesia and infection (Gauderer and Ponsky 1981). Gauderer wrote, two decades later, that while PEG use has benefited countless patients, 'in part because of its simplicity and low complication rate, this minimally invasive procedure also lends itself to over-utilization' (Gauderer 1999). Expressing moral concerns about the proliferation of the procedure, Gauderer indicates that as the third decade of

PEG use begins to unfold, 'much of our effort in the future needs to be directed toward ethical aspects' (1999: 882). PEG is being used more frequently even in those patients for whom these procedures were deemed too risky in the past.

For over a decade, researchers have underscored the burdens and risks of PEG tube-feeding in persons with advanced dementia. The mounting literature was well summarized by Finucane *et al.*, who found no published evidence that tube-feeding prevents aspiration pneumonia, prolongs survival, reduces risks of pressure sores or infections, improves function, or provides palliation in this population (Finucane *et al.* 1999; Gillick 2000; Post 2001).

Families often perceive tube-feeding as preventing pneumonia or skin break-down, and many assume that it extends survival. These perceptions are erroneous. The main benefit of PEG is that it makes life easier for the informal family caregiver who, for reason of competing duties or perhaps physical limitation, cannot find the time or energy to engage in assisted oral feeding. Yet PEG use is not really 'easy', because it has its technological complexities, and the recipient will usually have diarrhea. In some cases, physical restraints are used to keep a person from pulling on the several inches of tube that extend out of the abdomen. One wonders if assisted oral feeding is not easier after all. Regardless, purported technical ease and efficiency do not mean that these technologies should be applied. Should persons with advanced progressive dementia ever be provided with PEG? In general, assisted oral feeding and hospice are the better alternative to tube-feeding, although in practice there will be some cases in which the limited capacities of an informal family caregiver do justify tube-feeding as the ethically imperative alternative to starvation when the ability to swallow has begun to diminish. Ideally home health aides would make assisted oral feeding possible even in these cases, but this is not a priority in the current health care system. Institutions, however, should uniformly provide assisted oral feeding as the desired alternative to tube-feeding, a measure that would profoundly obviate the overuse of this technology.

There will be many family caregivers who have no interest in PEG use and who feel that they are being loyal to their loved one's prior wishes. A physician should expect this response. A study included in-person interviews of eighty-four cognitively normal men and women aged 65 years and older from a variety of urban and suburban settings (including private homes, assisted-living apartments, transitional care facilities, and nursing homes). Three-fourths of the subjects would not want cardiopulmonary resuscitation, use of a respirator, or parenteral or enteral tube nutrition with the milder forms of dementia; 95 per cent or more would not want any of these procedures with severe dementia (Gjerdingen *et al.* 1999). These subjects were adequately informed of the burdens and benefits of such interventions.

Physicians and other health care professionals should recommend this less burdensome and therefore more appropriate approach to family members, and to persons with dementia who are competent, ideally soon after initial diagnosis. Early discussions of a peaceful dying should occur between persons with dementia and their families, guided by information from health care professionals on the relative benefits of a palliative care approach (Volicer and Hurley 1998).

As we move forward to overcome the problematic of a partial mental death that precedes physical death, a degree of moral complexity arises that is quite distinct from death due to conditions that leave the autobiographical self intact.

A CONCLUDING CALL FOR PROGRESS

While I have argued that we should care for the deeply forgetful by enhancing the quality of their lives, I have also suggested that openness to efforts to decelerate aging—the key risk factor associated with so many debilitating morbidities—should move forward to the extent that such deceleration is found to significantly reduce, rather than protract, said morbidities. Even for the anti-posthumanists, the direct goal of anti-aging research and interventions should be the amelioration of those morbidities, including AD, while a secondary unintended effect is the further expansion of life expectancy, and even of maximum lifespan.

Aging itself may not be easily categorized as a disease, although it is most certainly a process of natural deterioration. In a time when average life expectancy was low, people who survived birth and childhood could expect to live into their sixties, although always some individuals lived well beyond that. Now, as most people live into their late seventies and beyond, the implications of aging as a susceptibility factor for innumerable diseases and chronic conditions become more vivid. Our aging society becomes a complex of widespread deterioration, dysfunction, and dependence.

Unless we create anti-aging interventions that also reduce morbidity and dysfunction to a considerable extent, we will continue on in the halfway house that we have created, in which many lives are burdened with the illnesses of old age, at great cost to their adult children and to society. Beneficence requires that we take the final bold step of freeing ourselves from decrepitude, should this become possible, for reasons of individual well-being and intergenerational covenant. For the adult children who sacrifice so much for a parent with dementia, and for a society that must care for the senile, the move toward a more long-lived society through unlocking the basic cellular mechanisms of aging and decelerating it consistent with the compression of morbidity must be welcomed.

REFERENCES

AEVARSSON, O., and SKOOG, I. (1996), 'A Population-Based Study on the Incidence of Dementia Disorders Between 85 and 88 Years of Age', *Journal of the American Geriatrics Society*, 44: 1455–60.

ALZHEIMER'S DISEASE ASSOCIATION (2001), *Ethical Issues in Alzheimer's Disease* (Chicago: Alzheimer Disease Association).

BACON, F. (1996), *The New Atlantis*, in *Francis Bacon: A Critical Edition of the Major Works*, ed. B. Vickers (Oxford: Oxford University Press), 457–89.

DYSON, F. J. (1997), *Imagined Worlds* (Cambridge, Mass.: Harvard University Press).

FINUCANE, T. E., CHRISTMAS, C., and TRAVIS, K. (1999), 'Tube Feeding in Patients with Advanced Dementia: A Review of the Evidence', *JAMA* 282: 1365–70.

FIRLIK, A. D. (1991), 'Margo's Logo', *JAMA* 265: 201.

GAUDERER, M. (1999), 'Twenty Years of Percutaneous Endoscopic Gastrostomy: Origin and Evolution of a Concept and Its Expanded Applications', *Gastrointestinal Endoscopy*, 50: 879–82.

—— and PONSKY, J. L. (1981), 'A Simplified Technique for Constructing a Tube Feeding Gastrostomy', *Surgery in Gynecology and Obstetrics*, 152: 83–5.

GILLICK, M. R. (2000), 'Rethinking the Role of Tube Feeding in Patients with Advanced Dementia', *New England Journal of Medicine*, 342/3: 206–10.

GJERDINGEN, D. K., NEFF, J. A., WANG, M., and CHALONER, K. (1999), 'Older Persons' Opinions About Life-Sustaining Procedures in the Face of Dementia', *Archives of Family Medicine*, 8: 421–5.

HAYLES, N. K. (1999), *How We Become Posthuman: Virtual Bodies in Cybernetics, Literature and Informatics* (Chicago: University of Chicago Press).

HOOK, C. C. (2004), 'Transhumanism and Posthumanism', in S. G. Post (ed.), *The Encyclopedia of Bioethics*, 3rd edn., 5 vols. (New York: Macmillan Reference).

JONAS, H. (1985), *The Imperative of Responsibility: In Search of an Ethics for the Technological Age* (Chicago: University of Chicago Press).

—— (1996), *Mortality and Morality: A Search for the Good After Auschwitz* (Evanston, Ill.: Northwestern University Press).

JUENGST, E. T., BINSTOCK, R. H., MEHLMAN, M., and POST, S. G. (2003), 'The Social Implications of Genuine Anti-Aging Interventions: The Need for Public Dialogue', *Science*, 299: 1323.

KASS, L. R. (2003), 'Beyond Therapy: Biotechnology and the Pursuit of Human Development', <http://www.bioethics.gov/material/kasspaper.html 2003>, accessed 12 Mar. 2003.

KITWOOD, T. (1997), *Dementia Reconsidered: The Person Comes First* (Buckingham: Open University Press).

LANE, M. A., INGRAM, D. K., and ROTH, G. S. (2002), 'The Serious Search for an Anti-Aging Pill', *Scientific American*, 287: 36–41.

MACINTYRE, A. (1999), *Dependent Rational Animals: Why Human Beings Need the Virtues* (Chicago: Open Court).

MASORO, E. J. (2001), *Caloric Restriction's Effects on Aging: Opportunities for Research on Human Implications*, *Journal of Gerontology*, ser. a, 56a, special issue 1.

NIEBUHR, R. (1956), *An Interpretation of Christian Ethics* (New York: Meridian).

PARTRIDGE, L., and GEMS, D. (2002), 'A Lethal Side-Effect', *Nature*, 418: 921.

POST, S. G. (2000), *The Moral Challenge of Alzheimer Disease: Ethical Issues from Diagnosis to Dying*, 2nd edn. (Baltimore: Johns Hopkins University Press).

—— (2001), 'Tube-Feeding and Advanced Progressive Dementia', *Hastings Center Report*, 31/1: 36–42.

_____ et al. (1997), 'The Clinical Introduction of Genetic Testing for Alzheimer Disease: An Ethical Perspective', *JAMA* 277/10: 832–6.

RUDMAN, S. (1997), *Concepts of Persons and Christian Ethics* (Cambridge: Cambridge University Press).

SABAT, S. R. (2001), *The Experience of Alzheimer's Disease: Life Through a Tangled Veil* (Oxford: Blackwell).

SINGER, P. (1993), *Practical Ethics* (Cambridge: Cambridge University Press).

STOCK, G. (2002), *Redesigning Humans: Our Inevitable Genetic Future* (Boston: Houghton Mifflin).

US GENERAL ACCOUNTING OFFICE (1998), *Alzheimer's Disease: Estimates of Prevalence in the U.S.*, HEHS-98–16 (Washington, DC: GAO, 28 Jan.).

VOLICER, L., and HURLEY, A. (eds.) (1998), *Hospice Care for Patients with Advanced Progressive Dementia* (New York: Springer).

CHAPTER 14

....

DEATH IS A PUNCH IN THE JAW: LIFE-EXTENSION AND ITS DISCONTENTS

....

FELICIA NIMUE ACKERMAN

> My hospice room is rose and blue.
> The blue is like the sky.
> They think that if you're happy here,
> You'll be content to die.
> They proffer comfort, warmth, and peace,
> All shining like the sun.
> They strive to meet your every need.
> They meet all needs but one.
> So now I have another scheme,

I thank James Dreier, Sara Ann Ketchum, Christine Overall, and Bonnie Steinbock for extremely helpful discussions; James Dreier, David Estlund, and Bonnie Steinbock for extremely useful advice about background reading; Antonio Ramirez for extremely adept research assistance; and Zelda Sondack Ackerman, soon to embark on her second century, for extremely sharp-eyed proofreading.

My object all sublime.
I've gotten on a transplant list,
And so I bide my time.

(Ackerman 2005*b*)[1]

GRADUATE students in my department run a weblog that has solicited suggestions for 'the worst philosophical position ever' (Ichikawa 2004). When I suggested the position that 'illness and mortality are good things [and] it is bad to do research on extending the human life span',[2] Jonathan Ichikawa wrote, 'Do philosophers really hold [that view]? I find that so absurd that I have a hard time imagining anyone seriously thinking otherwise.' I replied by citing the most powerful bioethicist in America, Leon Kass, then head of the President's Council on Bioethics, whom the *New York Times Book Review* described as 'among the most respected authorities in the field' (Nuland 2002: 49).[3] Kass has said that 'the finitude of human life is a blessing for every human individual, whether he knows it or not' (Kass 2002: 264). He also opposes attempts to extend the maximum human lifespan, i.e. 'the outer limit of human longevity' (Overall 2003: 7), which 'has remained more or less fixed at about 120' (Overall 2003: 10). This chapter will argue that Ichikawa's common-sense intuition is basically right. The achievement of greatly extended human life and even (or especially) immortality would be like the discovery of electricity. It would bring many problems and dislocations and would even do some people more harm than good, but overall it would be an enormous boon to humanity.

Like other secular philosophers who write on this topic, I will assume there is no afterlife and hence that death is 'the unequivocal and permanent end of our existence' (Nagel 1979: 1). Except where indicated, I use 'immortality' to mean earthly immortality rather than immortality in a religious sense. This assumption accords with what I believe, but my reason for making it here is to delimit the scope of this chapter. It is hardly surprising that, after seeing 'a part of the adventures of the [Holy Grail]', Sir Galahad 'fell in his prayer long time to Our Lord, that at what time he asked, that he should pass out of this world', because of the 'great

---

I dedicate this chapter to my mother, Zelda Sondack Ackerman (b. 1912), in anticipation of a time when nonagenarians will have most of their lives ahead of them.

The chapter title comes from the following letter of mine in the Arts and Leisure Section of the *New York Times* (Ackerman 2002). 'William Hurt, a star of the film "Tuck Everlasting", is quoted as saying, "Most people think of life as the story of life and death. Death is a bookend. If you take that bookend away, what have you got?" This is typical of attempts to sugar-coat death. Here's an alternative metaphor: Death is a punch in the jaw. Take away the punch and what have you got? An [unpunched] jaw.'

[1] Also see 'Flourish Your Heart in This World' (Ackerman 1998*b*) and n. 10 below. (This poem first appeared in *Ragged Edge Online* and is reprinted by permission.)

[2] I actually wrote 'so' rather than 'and', but that was a poor formulation.

[3] Many assessments of Kass are more critical, however. For example, see Mooney (2001) and McGee (2003). Even Nuland's largely admiring review expresses reservations, acknowledging that 'most [readers] will . . . recognize the need for [more] flexibility' (Nuland 2002: 49) than Kass offers.

joy [he anticipated at seeing] the Blessed Trinity every day, and the Majesty of Our Lord' in the afterlife (Malory 1969: 367, 368). Admittedly, belief in an afterlife does not always bring willingness to leave earthly life. Believers may be unwilling to leave their familiar lives and loved ones, or they may fear ending up in hell. But when believers and unbelievers talk about death, they are talking about two entirely different things.[4] Richard Momeyer points out that views that do 'not regard death as final, as the complete cessation of consciousness and personhood' should be 'regarded as but sophisticated forms of death denial' (Momeyer 1988: 8). Amusingly illustrating this point is the career of Elisabeth Kübler-Ross, who began by combating the 'denial of death' and finished by denying that death ends one's conscious existence.[5]

Why is death bad? What Nagel calls the 'natural' answer is that 'death is an evil [not] because of its positive features, but only because of what it deprives us of' (Nagel 1979: 1), i.e. 'all possibility of satisfying experience' (Momeyer 1988: 50). Why, then, would anyone object to greatly extended human life? Such objections fall into two categories.[6] Objections in the first category hold that greatly extended life would harm the person living it. Objections in the second category hold that greatly extended human life would bring some other sort of harm; for example, harm to society or to the human species.

I will consider these types of objection in turn. My discussion will deal both with greatly extended finite life and with immortality and will use the term 'greatly extended life' to cover both. Except where indicated, I will proceed from some assumptions adapted from Christine Overall (2003: 96, 128 ff.). First, people would know the life expectancy in their society or would know (or at least have good reason to believe) that they were immortal. Second, everyone would have the opportunity to choose greatly extended life. Third, greatly extended life would not be mandatory; people would be able to opt out at any point.

WOULD GREATLY EXTENDED LIFE BENEFIT OR HARM THE PERSON LIVING IT?

If there is one position on which secular bioethicists approach unanimity, it is that life is worth extending only if the quality is satisfactory. As David Gems puts it, 'Most of us would agree that it makes little sense to postpone death once our quality of life has diminished beyond a certain point' (2003a: 34). This seemingly unproblematic statement covers up some crucial questions. What is that point? Who decides? The conventional wisdom that we should avoid 'endlessly prolonging

---

[4] See Overall (2003: 178–9).   [5] See Momeyer (1988: 9) and Rosen (2004).
[6] See Singer (1991); Overall (2003, ch. 1); President's Council on Bioethics (2003a, ch. 4).

the morbid phase of our lives' (Gems 2003a: 34) should be assessed in light of the fact that many seriously ill people find the 'morbid phase' of their lives well worth prolonging. 'Study after study has concluded that many healthy people often say they would never want to die in an intensive care unit, but may change their minds when they are very sick' (Kolata 1997). One study found that 'The majority of [a group of 244 patients with various serious illnesses] wanted to receive a life-sustaining treatment if it would prolong life for any length of time' (Danis et al. 1996: 1813). Another study, emphasizing the disparity of values between the healthy and the ill, found that 'Patients with cancer are much more likely to opt for radical treatment [a grueling course of chemotherapy] with minimal chance of [cure or if it offers as little as three months of life-prolongation] than people who do not have cancer, including medical and nursing professionals' and also including healthy controls matched with patients for 'age and sex, as well as for occupation and hence educational and social class' (Slevin et al. 1990: 1458, 1460), i.e. a control group selected to represent the attitudes of the patients before they had cancer. And a study of patients with end-stage kidney disease concluded that 'chronically ill people cherish their lives, despite the appearance [to outsiders] of inadequate quality' (Gutman 1988: 899).

Here it is crucial to recognize that expertise lies with the patients. They have first-hand knowledge of what it is like to be seriously ill. So their desire to extend the 'morbid phase' of their lives seems prima facie rational. This point will resurface in my discussion of resource allocation. For the present, note that even Overall—who perceptively warns against assuming that 'life with chronic health problems or disabilities is not worth living', and stresses that decisions about 'the minimum conditions of quality of life that make existence worth sustaining' should be made by competent patients, 'not their families and not their health-care providers'—says, 'If the available medical, social, and material resources are so limited that one's extra stretch of time is lived in misery, then that is a problem, and *no prolongevist advocates the extension of human life if it can be lived only in poverty, pain, and ill health*' (2003: 188, 191, 192, 41; italics added).[7] She is mistaken. I advocate this (for people who desire it). Of course, I believe that wealth, comfort, and good health are better than poverty, pain, and ill health. But the blanket presumption that the latter states bring 'misery' that is worse than death is disrespectful to those who, having experienced them, disagree. (Perhaps they disagree because they have found that these states, far from entailing living in misery, do not preclude such pleasures as love, friendship, television, music, reading, and thinking.) Thus, the popular phrase 'compression of morbidity', i.e. 'reduction of . . . the end of life morbidity characteristic of old age'

[7] Elsewhere in her book she offers the more moderate formulation 'Prolongevists . . . advocate the extension of life only if it will not involve the severe illness, unrelieved pain, or disablement *that undermine an individual's capacity to pursue his or her life's projects*' (Overall 2003: 65–6; italics added). This formulation is more respectful of individual differences in values. Also see Overall (2003: 96).

(Battin 1987: 328), glosses over the difference between curing a sick person and denying him treatment that would extend his 'morbid' life.[8] And Overall's claim that 'medical treatments that . . . extend an end-state of suffering, extreme dementia, *or* relentless deterioration must be recognized as pointless or even, at worst, as harmful' (2003: 190; italics added) conflicts with her above-quoted views about patient self-determination, given that some competent people choose 'relentless deterioration' over death.

This consideration is particularly important in view of some ideas behind the conventional wisdom about when life is worth prolonging. Thus, M. Pabst Battin identifies 'increasing debility, dependence . . . loss of communication and affection . . . isolation' as part of an 'unfortunately realistic picture of old age' constituting 'human degradation' that can lead to a sick old person's 'increasingly poor self-image' and desire to die (1980: 274). By contrast, other philosophers, such as Susan Wendell, question independence as an ideal, pointing out that no one is completely independent and that ' "independence" . . . is defined according to a society's expectations about what people "normally" do for themselves and how they do it' (Wendell 1996: 145). Overall says, 'There are varying patterns of dependence throughout the life span' and 'to the extent that [old people] are dependent, their dependence should not be interpreted as evidence that increased longevity is bad' (2003: 188). Such views are more logical as well as more humane than the view that 'dependence' is characteristic of only some people's lives or is inherently degrading.

Three more points are worth noting here. First, the 'increasingly poor self-image' of the old, ill, and disabled, like the poor self-image some blacks may have in a racist society, arises 'from the low value . . . society places on people of a certain sort, rather than from anything inherent in the person's condition' (Ackerman 1998a: 151–2). Second, present-day society over a quarter-century after Battin's article appeared, offers the old, ill, and disabled a new opportunity to bypass ageism and ableism and to overcome isolation 'in a better world, where there is neither young nor old, healthy nor crippled . . . On the Internet' (Ackerman 2005c: 43)[9] or in online relationships with people who have chosen to identify themselves online as old, ill, and/or disabled. Third, I am not claiming that all sick people want to extend their lives even if they cannot be cured, just that many bioethicists have shortchanged those who do.

Overgeneralization is hardly rare in discussions of whether greatly extended life would benefit the person living it. For example, Kass, whose opposition to attempts to extend the maximum human lifespan rests partly on his *ad hominem* 'For most of us . . . the desire to prolong the lifespan (even modestly) must be seen as expressing a desire never to grow old and die',[10] suggests the following 'virtues of mortality':

---

[8] See the discussion in Battin (1987: 328–36).

[9] This reference is to a short story about a crippled old woman who does just that.

[10] See also President's Council on Bioethics (2003a: 162, 186). For a dissenting view, see Blackburn and Rowley (2004: 0420). (Of course, I also reject Kass's view that there is something wrong with a

interest and engagement, seriousness and aspiration, beauty and love, and virtue and moral excellence (Kass 2002: 263, 266–9).[11] I will discuss these in turn.

As to the first, Kass offers mainly not arguments but rhetorical questions designed to suggest that interest and engagement would decline as life proceeded endlessly. The most plausible answers, however, are far from what he supposes. Thus, his question 'Would the Don Juans of our world feel better for having seduced 1,250 women rather than 1,000?' (Kass 2002: 266) receives this apt reply from Gems: 'on his deathbed, the extra 250 women might not seem that important to Don Juan. But if he was at only number 1,000 and was offered an extra 250, one can only imagine his joy' (2003a: 35). Kass's view that greatly extended life would bring diminishing interest and engagement pays scant attention to individual differences. The same problem is evident in his famous anti-cloning slogan 'Shallow are the souls that have forgotten how to shudder' (Kass 2002: 150)—a slogan that 'invites this reply: Narrow are the souls that cannot comprehend that different souls shudder at different things. I shudder at the thought of being denied lifesaving technology because it violates Kass's particular conception of dignity' (Ackerman 2005a).[12]

Kass's scant respect for individual differences is ironic in view of his criticism of bioethics as 'Universalist in conception [and thus caring] little for the variety of human types' (2002: 65).[13] His discussion ignores the large philosophical literature on whether greatly extended life would lead to boredom. Such literature is often very sensitive to differences among various types of people and various types of pleasures. Thus, Overall says, 'The perceived value of endless life could well be closely related to the general type of person one is and the sort of life one chooses to live' (2003: 179). Gems says, 'Some people seem especially able to enjoy endless repetition of the same experience' (2003a: 35).[14] Moreover, there are some experiences whose repetition few people find boring. As Momeyer points out, 'so long as appetite remains strong, food and sexual union remain satisfying' (1988: 19).

desire never to grow old and die.) Note also Robin Marantz Henig's castigation of patients who seek to combine the comforts of hospice care with the opportunity for life-prolonging medical treatment. She claims they are 'indulg[ing] the fantasy that dying is somehow optional' (Henig 2005: 28). But she gives no evidence that they are indulging such an (at-present) irrational fantasy, rather than pursuing the rational goal of living longer without sacrificing comfort care. In fact, it seems a matter of basic human decency not to force patients into the cruel choice between comfort care and life-prolonging care (see Ackerman 1990: 315). But none of the twelve published letters commenting on Henig's article criticizes her on this score and some even praise her for 'compassion' (Libert 2005) and 'great sensitivity' (Rogatz 2005). This is a chilling illustration of how public opinion seems to be out of sympathy with terminally ill people who seek to prolong their lives rather than accept death.

[11] The President's Council on Bioethics suggests that these 'virtues of mortality' might be endangered not only by immortality 'but even [by] more modest prolongations of the maximum lifespan, especially in good health, that would permit us to live as if there were always tomorrow' (President's Council on Bioethics 2003a: 297).

[12] See also the discussion in Naam (2005).

[13] Even Daniel Callahan, who calls Kass 'one of the most stimulating people I have ever known', has criticized Kass's 'distorted, out-of-date picture of the present field of bioethics'; see Callahan (2002).

[14] Also see Overall (2003: 147 ff.).

But sensual satisfactions are far from all that can keep immortals from boredom. People can also be continually learning new things, at least in so far as their mental capacities are up to the task (which hardly seems an implausible supposition in a world scientifically advanced enough to achieve immortality).[15] Gems distinguishes among relatively static life plans, 'such that the desired future is essentially a continuation of things as they are' (and which may lead to boredom in those unable to enjoy repetition), fixed goal life plans, where 'the value of life extension will depend on whether the plan is realizable' (Gems 2003a: 38), and open-ended life plans (such as that of a medical researcher who wants to help as many people as possible), where the value of greatly extended life is high. Overall suggests that the pursuit of various excellences 'could . . . occupy us during earthly immortality. Is it so far-fetched to suppose that a deep understanding of this infinite universe would take an eternity?' (2003: 151). James Lindemann Nelson distinguishes between Margaret Walker's notion of a career self, who sees his life 'as a unified field in which particular enterprises, values, and relationships are (in principle) coordinated in the form of a "rational life plan" . . . or a "quest" . . . or a "project"' and a 'seriatim self', deriving from Hilde Lindemann Nelson's concept of 'living life seriatim', where life is seen 'less as an overall unified project and more as a set of fits and starts' (Nelson 1999: 121, 122). Overall points out that either type of self can appreciate greatly extended life. The career self may 'value continued survival, for the career self sees human existence as an open-ended set of challenges' and thus may 'continue to seek opportunities for activity, striving, self-development, and the achievement of goals' (Overall 2003: 186). 'The seriatim self might choose . . . to enjoy a life lived without further conquests' (Overall 2003: 181). Overall discusses the possibility of personal transformation while retaining one's core identity, as happens in our society to people who undergo religious or other conversions (Overall 2003: 158–61). Clearly, the issue is far more complex than Kass's discussion recognizes, especially since, as Overall points out, the career self and the seriatim self are not mutually exclusive (Overall 2003: 235–6 nn. 15, 16) and, as Gems points out, life plans can change (Gems 2003a: 38).

But Overall also expresses reservations about immortality. She suggests that perhaps, given the limits of people's abilities, eventually, 'Although the repetition of old familiar activities would still be possible for the immortal . . . every activity he undertook would eventually be "used up" . . . and he would feel ready to die', a problem that would 'apply most clearly to the life of the career self' (2003: 166, 176). However, when she contemplates the reply that 'the physical capacities of the immortal [could be] increased gradually and indefinitely' so as to permit 'the acquisition of greater and greater abilities and talents' (2003: 171), she makes some problematic objections. For one thing, she finds this scenario difficult to imagine.

---

[15] See the speculative discussions in Puccetti (1978), Gems (2003a: 36–7), Overall (2003: 167–73), Kurzweil (2005: 64–5), and Naam (2005, ch. 9).

A world of immortals, though, would be scientifically advanced way beyond our present level. Why couldn't we imagine such continued human development?[16]

Overall further objects that in such a scenario we would have godlike abilities and hence not be living a 'recognizably human life' (2003: 173). And Kass holds that 'to argue that human life would be better without death is . . . to argue that human life would be better being something other than human' (2002: 265). This makes me wonder what people in the time of Sir Thomas Malory (the fifteenth century) would have said about beings who went to the moon, received new hearts, talked with others thousands of miles away, and held it to be self-evident that all men are created equal. Progress means change.[17] Why shouldn't scientific progress cause people to have characteristics previously deemed beyond human possibility? Why should we be 'defining humans in terms of our limitations rather than by our ability to supersede our limitations' (Kurzweil 2005: 67)? Consider also Nagel's apt observation 'A man's sense of his own experience . . . does not embody [an] idea of a natural limit. His existence defines for him an essentially open-ended possible future' (1979: 9–10).

Two further points are important here. First, since I am assuming that immortality would be optional and reversible, people who found their greatly extended lives unsatisfactory would be as free to commit suicide as are people in our world. Although some who long for death might have scruples against suicide just as some do in our world, there could be an equivalent of 'passive euthanasia', where immortality would be maintained by a substance that people could simply choose to stop taking.[18] Second, even in cases where Kass is right that eternal life brings diminishing returns, the real question is not whether this extra life is as fulfilling as the early part, but whether it is better than nothing. If boredom is taken to be a reason against immortality, see how high the bar for acceptable quality of life has been raised. 'Bored to death' is a figure of speech. How many people deem boredom a fate literally worse than death?[19] Overall considers the possibility that the boredom could be so extreme as to make 'the experience of immortality . . . analogous to the experience of severe insomnia, in which, having been awake for seemingly endless hours without respite, one feels tired of being awake and exhausted by being oneself and wants only the nothingness of unconsciousness that is afforded, temporarily, by deep sleep' (2003: 145). This certainly does not correspond to my own experience of severe insomnia, which has led me to long for sleep not as a temporary escape from consciousness but as a means to an improved state of consciousness upon awakening. Moreover, the unpleasant state of intense physical exhaustion, which frequently accompanies severe insomnia, seems less characteristic of boredom.

Kass's other 'virtues of mortality' are equally problematic. He asks, 'Could life be serious or meaningful without the limit of mortality?' and cites the Greek gods as living 'shallow and rather frivolous lives' (Kass 2002: 266). But he himself admits

---

[16] See the references in n. 15.   [17] See Bostrom (2003, 2005) and Naam (2005).
[18] For a case of this sort, see Williams (1975).   [19] Also see Steele (1976).

that learning does not require finitude as a spur. In addition, his suggestion that 'real friendship [may] depend in part on the shared perceptions of a common fate' (Kass 2002: 267) not only is unsubstantiated but overlooks the fact that immortality would count as a common fate just as much as death does. Finally, should religious believers conclude that God lives a shallow and frivolous life or that the religious vision of life in heaven is neither serious nor meaningful? As Roland Puccetti says, 'That death is *spiritually* desirable is incomprehensible ... since in many of the great living religions, at least, it is the (other-worldly) conquest of death that gives them much of their attraction and *rationale*' (1978: 173).[20] Although Kass says his discussion of the 'virtues of mortality' is intended to apply 'entirely in the realm of natural reason and apart from any question about a life after death' (2002: 265) and also that he is 'at best an agnostic on heaven' (President's Council on Bioethics 2003*b*: 33), it is worth asking whether his concerns would preclude worshiping an immortal God or valuing an eternal afterlife in heaven.

Equally dubious is Kass's pronouncement that beauty and love require mortality. His suggestion that 'natural beauty ... depends on its *im*permanence' (Kass 2002: 267) overlooks the fact that, relative to our lives, stars are permanent, which does not impede our appreciation of their beauty. Kass's suggestion that perhaps 'only a mortal being, aware of his mortality and the transience and vulnerability of all natural things, is moved to make beautiful artifacts' (2002: 267) is particularly odd from a religious believer,[21] as it fails to allow for God's being moved to make beautiful things. A similar objection applies to Kass's rhetorical question 'How deeply could one deathless "human" being love another?' (Kass 2002: 267). Should believers in heaven believe God cannot love angels deeply or that people cannot deeply love a God with whom they expect to be eternally in the afterlife?[22] One could just as well argue that knowledge of impermanence undermines beauty and love, making them ultimately meaningless.[23]

Kass's final 'virtue of mortality' is that mortality is necessary for virtue and moral excellence. He maintains that 'for ... nobility, vulnerability and mortality are the necessary conditions. The immortals cannot be noble' (Kass 2002: 268). This errs in equating immortality with invulnerability.[24] As Overall points out, immortality does not entail that death is impossible, just that it is not inevitable (Overall 2003: 131). Immortality also does not mean one cannot lose things he values or make

---

[20]   Also see Ackerman (1999: 85); Overall (2003: 125). Philip Larkin (1999) puts the matter more tartly when he describes religion as 'That vast moth-eaten musical brocade | Created to pretend we never die.'

[21]   Kass is an observant Jew. Interestingly, he grants that, unlike him, 'Jewish commentators on ... medical ethics nearly always come down strongly in favor of medical progress and on the side of life—more life, longer life, new life' (Kass 2002: 258).

[22]   See Overall (2003: 160).

[23]   I am not endorsing this sort of argument, which Nagel (1971) criticizes effectively. My point is that this argument is no weaker than Kass's.

[24]   See Overall (2003: 131–2).

sacrifices to aid another person, even another immortal one. Religious believers may further wonder whether they are supposed to conclude that an immortal God lacks virtue and moral excellence.

In addition to telling us what we ought to want, Kass tells us what we actually do want: 'man longs not so much for deathlessness as for wholeness, wisdom, goodness and godliness—longings that cannot be satisfied fully in our embodied earthly life' (2002: 270). Having always longed for deathlessness, I offer myself as one counterexample. Different people want different things. The safest conclusion is that greatly extended life is likely to benefit many. Recall again that in the scenario under consideration, those who find greatly extended life unsatisfactory can opt out at any time. Of course, people who opt out of greatly extended life would still find their world changed by it. Like those in our society who opt out of cyberspace, such people may feel unhappy and displaced. But their loss seems small when measured against the gains for those who choose greatly extended life.

WOULD GREATLY EXTENDED HUMAN LIFE BRING SOME OTHER SORT OF HARM?

I begin with the simplest problem: Some people benefit from the prompt demise of some particular others. Anyone who longs for the death of an enemy or rival, like any 'adult child' who values his anticipated inheritance more than he values his parents, will hardly regard everyone's greatly extended life as a blessing. But not all desires for other people's death are similarly unworthy. Concerned about the 'chilling . . . prospect of power concentrated relentlessly into the hands of a few undying individuals—and particularly into the hands of tyrants' (Gems 2003a: 38), Gems argues that a greatly extended lifespan is 'a very serious threat to humanity in the long term' (2003a: 34). A parallel objection, however, could have been made to any life-saving medical advance, including chemotherapy and antibiotics. Surely, a tyrant who dies of an infection at 30 will do less harm than one who lives vigorously into his seventies. But it seems cruel to object to medical advances for fear that such advances might prolong the active lives of some dreadful people. Moreover, a short lifespan is hardly an effective deterrent to tyranny, for one tyrant can replace another and often does. Particularly inappropriate for his argument is Gems's admonition 'Remember the words of O'Brien to Winston Smith in Orwell's *1984*: "If you want a picture of the future, imagine a boot stamping on a human face—forever" ' (2003a: 34). No increased longevity was envisioned in *1984*. Tyranny arose from a totalitarian system[25]—and is most effectively prevented by a democratic one.

[25] These objections come from my (2003) letter commenting on Gems's article. See Gems's reply (Gems 2003b). Note that Gems's article acknowledges that 'perhaps with effective legislation to prevent such accumulations of power . . . such threats may be disarmed' (Gems 2003a: 34).

Another potential problem involves overpopulation. Here it is important to distinguish greatly extended but finite longevity from immortality. I will consider the former case first. Peter Singer suggests that if an anti-aging drug doubled the human lifespan in a world unable to support an increased population, an increase could be avoided 'by persuading people to have fewer children, and that one of the means of achieving this is by persuading them to start their families later—say, only when they reach about 50, rather than when they reach about 25, as they do now' (Singer 1991: 138). He adds that, in the scenario he is envisioning, the drug will make this biologically possible. Note that although population increase can be avoided if people have fewer children, it can also be avoided if people have the same number of children but have them later in life, thereby preventing increased longevity from increasing overlap between generations. This point is especially important if instead of considering Singer's hypothetical doubled human lifespan, we consider a finite lifespan that is multiplied tenfold or more. People who live to be 800 can, without risking overpopulation, have as many children as we do—provided that their reproductive period occurs no farther from the end of their lives than our reproductive period occurs from the end of our lives.

Would this harm society or the human species? Obviously, much depends on what these long-lived people would be like. Singer, asking 'how . . . to quantify the benefits of the freshness of youth as against the benefits of the wisdom of accumulated experience', reasonably replies that 'we do not know' (1991: 138). I also doubt we know that the 'freshness of youth' and 'wisdom of accumulated experience' are actualities rather than simplistic cultural stereotypes on a par with women's altruism or blacks' sense of rhythm.

One of Singer's main concerns is that in his scenario fewer people would come to exist over the course of, say, a century. He rejects the intuitively plausible objection that we should take no account of the interests of 'those who *might* have existed, if we had not opted for the anti-aging drug' (Singer 1991: 144). His reason for this rejection involves imagining our adopting the following strategy in response to the moral imperative of not condemning future generations to a life unsustainable by our planet's remaining resources. Suppose we all decide to avert ecological disaster for future generations by ensuring there will be no future generations; i.e. suppose we all decide to refrain from reproducing and to enjoy a fling as the last generation on earth. Singer comments, 'Those who refuse to take into account the interests of merely possible people seem committed to saying that this would be right' (1991: 144). This seems mistaken. Holding that the end of human life and human civilization would be catastrophic does not entail locating the catastrophe in the violation of the interests of merely possible people. Consider the following three scenarios: (1) the 'last generation' scenario Singer envisions; (2) a scenario where members of that generation reproduce at the average rate of one replacement per person; (3) Scenario 2 with the following changes: first, in the generation under consideration, the average replacement rate is two people per person; second, the world's resources are adequate to sustain this population increase. It seems incontrovertible that the difference in desirability between Scenarios 1 and 2 is much greater than that between Scenarios 2 and 3. But anyone accepting this intuition must find the source of this discrepancy in something other than the interests of merely possible people.[26]

At this point it may be tempting to suggest that a society scientifically advanced enough to achieve greatly increased longevity might find a way to sustain a greatly increased population. Perhaps this could occur, as Overall suggests in her discussion of immortality, through migration 'to other planets, perhaps planets in other solar systems' (Overall 2003: 140).[27] For the sake of argument, however, I have been accepting Singer's background assumption that available resources would be inadequate to support a population with increased longevity that continued our present pattern of reproduction. This problem intensifies once we consider immortality rather than greatly extended but finite longevity, at least if we assume that problematically many people will opt for immortality. Overall discusses various ways of dealing with this problem. One is to confine the opportunity for immortality 'to a select few' (Overall 2003: 139). Her objections here—the moral problem of unfairness and the practical problem of resentment—might be obviated if the 'few' were selected by lottery.[28]

Another approach is John Harris's suggestion that we might 'offer people life-prolonging therapies only on condition that they did not reproduce, except perhaps posthumously, or that they agreed if they did reproduce to forfeit their right to subsequent therapies' (Harris 2000: 59). Overall objects that 'it is hard to see that making pregnancy a capital offense could be justifiable' (Overall 2003: 137). But this approach, which allows each person to choose what he or she values most, seems preferable to more coercive alternatives, such as either outlawing pregnancy altogether or setting 'some definite upper limit on the duration of one's right to live' (Woods 1978: 128). Suppose everyone, given the choice, opted for immortality over reproduction. Overall maintains that if reproduction were to cease, 'the culture as a whole . . . would suffer a staggering loss of relationships and interactions with babies and children and the invigoration and renewal provided by the presence of young people' (2003: 137). Although elsewhere expressing skepticism of clichéd claims about the 'freshness of youth' (Overall 2003: 44), here she seems to take it for granted that those who are no longer young would be inadequate to provide 'invigoration and renewal'. Harris, who identifies 'fresh ideas' with 'new human

[26] For further discussion of the moral status of merely possible people, see Woods (1978: 128) and Overall (2003: 137–9).

[27] See also Sawyer (2005: 88–9).

[28] Then, again, they might not be. In discussion, Sara Ann Ketchum has pointed out that many people consider the 'natural lottery' unfair in its distribution of beauty, talents, etc. and might resent the outcome of a socially engineered lottery as well. But I doubt that many who find immortality desirable would prefer no chance at immortality to a lottery for it. (For a more optimistic view of the population problem, see Kurzweil 2005: 65–6.)

individuals' (Harris 2000: 59), rather than with youth, escapes this objection. Once again, however, we should keep in mind that a society capable of achieving human immortality will be scientifically advanced beyond ours in other ways as well. Perhaps, as already suggested, these ways will enable the same people to keep generating new ideas from their vast experience. This is not to deny that cessation of reproduction would be a significant loss. People who choose immortality over reproduction, however, are indicating that they find loss of their own lives even more significant.[29]

To better appreciate this, imagine a society of non-reproducing immortals who know no other sort of existence but are suddenly told they must die in order to make way for new people. Would their outrage be surprising? Or unjustified?[30] Although John Stuart Mill's 'Everything which is usual appears natural' (Mill 1970: 4) is an obvious exaggeration, we often feel outraged at the prospect of losing the good things we have taken for granted. Overall recognizes that 'it is probably too much to expect that immortals would freely choose to abandon their immortality', that it is unclear 'why the right to reproduce [should] trump the right to go on living', and that 'it is hard to see that . . . limiting the amount of time that people are permitted to live, is justified' (Overall 2003: 139, 138). Why should the onus of keeping the population down fall on the old? As John Woods says, 'None of us . . . need feel obliged to pay with our lives for the consequences of an out-of control population' (1978: 130).[31] Furthermore, Gems points out that 'advances in

[29] There is an intriguing parallel here to the claim that the loss of Jews to assimilation and intermarriage amounts to a 'silent Holocaust', as if the decline of Judaism through lack of interest could in any way be equated with the decline of Judaism through the murder of Jews. See the discussion in Buchwald (n.d.). In this case, as in the case of the end of human reproduction, the distinction between an end that comes about through individual choice and an end that comes about despite it will seem crucial only to those who give individual choice high priority.

[30] Upon reading a draft of this chapter, Bonnie Steinbock mentioned her 'son's comment (age 2½): "I don't want to die; I want the new people to die"'.

[31] Note the relevance of this point to the common view that even though compulsory retirement is now illegal for professors in America, elderly professors should retire in order to free up space for 'new blood'. Remaining unanswered is the question of why the onus should fall on the elderly. Why not instead have it fall on professors who are too experienced to count as 'new blood' but are still young enough to train for other careers without running great danger of age discrimination, or on married professors who could afford to live on the income of their spouses while taking extended sabbaticals to devote their energies to child-rearing? It is noteworthy that those urging retirement on elderly faculty overlook the contribution elderly professors make to the goal, much trumpeted in America, of 'diversity'. Of course, there is no perfect correlation between attitudes and age, just as there is no perfect correlation between attitudes and dimensions on which American colleges and universities prize diversity, such as race or gender. But, as a bioethicist, I have attended conferences where no one (except me) favored high-tech life-extending care for the old and ill—and no one appeared to be much (if at all) over 70. (Full disclosure: At the time of this writing, I am only (?) 58.) What would we say about a conference of white men who assured one another of the wrongness of affirmative action? Note also that, as Ketchum has pointed out in discussion, different generations may provide diversity of perspective through having lived through different historical events, such as the Cold War. Note further that Kübler-Ross justifies compulsory retirement on the grounds that it benefits the young

medicine along with improved nutrition and hygiene have greatly reduced infant mortality during the last century. This has led to dramatic increases in population, but no one has called reducing infant mortality undesirable' (Gems 2003a: 34).[32]

Kass also emphasizes the tension between immortality and reproduction. He says that 'in all higher animals, reproduction *as such* implies both the acceptance of the death of self and participation in its transcendence' (Kass 2002: 271).[33] But it is far from obvious that having children automatically makes people more willing to die. Overall reasonably suggests just the opposite, saying that her children are among 'the best possible reasons for me to want to live a very long life' (2003, p. xi). Kass's claim that 'to covet a prolonged lifespan for ourselves is both a sign and a cause of our failure to open ourselves to procreation and to any higher purpose' (2002: 271) overlooks the fact that people can have high purposes for prolonging their own lives and thus their opportunities to do good in the world. And his pronouncement 'The salmon, willingly swimming upstream to spawn and die, makes vivid [the] universal truth' (2002: 271) that to accept reproduction is to accept death, invites two questions. First, what does the word 'willingly' mean in this context? Second, are we humans supposed to model ourselves on salmon?

A final set of objections involves inequality. Easiest to deal with is the concern of Eric Juengst and his co-authors that 'if slower aging extended the years available for productive work, vigorous and expert older workers may become more desirable, [leading to] unfair discrimination against the less experienced young' (Juengst *et al.* 2003: 27). Why suppose this would be worse than the present-day workplace discrimination against those no longer young? As with all workplace discrimination, the solution lies in well-enforced anti-discrimination laws if the target group's qualifications are acceptable. If young and less experienced workers are genuinely inferior, it would hardly be unfair for employers to favor more experienced workers. Extended apprenticeships to help the young get their skills up to par are a more humane solution than condemning the elderly to deterioration and death in order to keep them from 'encroaching on [the] careers' of the young (Nuland 1994: 87). The latter words are Sherwin B. Nuland's, as he excoriates what he calls the 'useless vanity' of 'Those who would live beyond their nature-given span' (Nuland 1994: 87).[34] But the charge of vanity seems more applicable to young people who expect their careers to have priority over the lives and health of the elderly.[35] Moreover,

---

(Kübler-Ross 1974: 150). This suggests she has little to offer old people who are more interested in achieving equal opportunities in life than in learning to accept death.

[32] See also Overall (2003: 52 ff.) and Naam (2005, ch. 6).

[33] See also President's Council on Bioethics (2003a: 188–9).

[34] See also President's Council on Bioethics (2003a: 193–7, 297, 302).

[35] I made this criticism in my review of Nuland's book. See Ackerman (1995). On 2 October 2005, when Nuland was interviewed on C-Span's *In Depth* call-in program, I called in and repeated the criticism. Nuland replied on the air that he had no objection to 90-year-olds who wanted to live to be 100; his opposition was directed at attempts to extend greatly the maximum human lifespan. He suggested that I was taking something out of context, misinterpreting him, or being a kind person and

such young people would be short-sighted to overlook the fact that they themselves would eventually reap the benefit of greatly extended life.

A more serious equity problem is that of access to life-extension. What if not everyone has equal opportunity to opt for greatly extended life? This is one question I consider in my final section.

Should Resources Be Allocated to Attempts to Extend Greatly the Maximum Human Lifespan?

As Harris points out, 'Most people fear death, and the prospect of personal extended life-span is likely to be welcomed' (Harris 2000: 59). Harris's observation provides prima facie reason for supporting attempts to extend greatly the maximum human lifespan, although it obviously leaves open the issue of where this should rank among other priorities. Rather than attempting to settle this extraordinarily complex issue, I will focus on rebutting some recent objections to allocating significant resources in this direction at all. Overall mentions that 'most of the modern philosophical discussion . . . along with a great deal of . . . extra-academic cultural commentary, seems weighted against the prolongation of human life' (2003: 15–16). I have already considered various reasons for this, but surely some of the most important have to do with expense and inequity. For example, Ronald Dworkin says,

Science . . . promises—or threatens—new medical and surgical techniques of increasing life expectancy, in some accounts to expand it to biblical magnitudes, but at such enormous cost that developing and testing these technologies, let alone making them available to more than a tiny minority, would drain away the resources needed to make people's lives good as well as long. (Dworkin 1994: 240)

Overall says that 'the main emphasis in longevity programs ought to be placed on those who have been disadvantaged rather than on expensive and risky[36] technologies available only to those who already enjoy life-expectancy advantages' (2003: 200).

These claims cry out for critical examination. More than one type of inequality is at issue here. There are two distinct ways in which life-extension technology

introducing some controversy. Since I was criticizing his opposition to attempts to extend greatly the human lifespan, his reply is surprising. Also surprising is his mention of his age—74—as a defense against the charge of ageism, unless Phyllis Schlafly's gender would likewise count as a defense against the charge that she is sexist.

[36] A discussion of the biological risks of such technology and how they might be minimized or regulated is beyond the scope of this chapter. But see President's Council on Bioethics (2003a: 279–80, 287); Garreau (2005); Kurzweil (2005: 66–7); Naam (2005).

is open to the objection that it would favor the privileged. First is the obvious objection that only the rich may be able to afford it. In principle entirely distinct is the objection that long-lived people are privileged in virtue of their longevity; so it is more egalitarian to direct resources toward bringing short-lived people's longevity up to par than toward extending the lives of the old. In practice, of course, economic inequality is relevant to the second objection, as many causes of early death are related to poverty.

I will consider the second objection first. Battin, drawing upon work of Norman Daniels (1983; see also Daniels 1982, 1988), has endorsed an approach to health care allocation that could also apply to allocation of resources for medical research. This approach relies on the view that rational self-interest maximizers behind a veil of ignorance[37] that made them 'unable to know their own medical conditions, genetic predispositions, physical susceptibilities, environmental situations, health maintenance habits, or ages' (Battin 1987: 322) would, in a condition of scarcity, choose 'to ration health care to the elderly (in order to enhance health care available to younger ... people and, thus, maximize the possibility of each person's reaching a normal life span at all)' (Battin 1987: 324).[38] More recently, she has embraced a global perspective relying on an idealized hypothesis that 'The savings from our earlier deaths ... in the first world [could be directly] translated into resources in the third world' (Battin 2000: 16). After all, behind the stipulated veil of ignorance, people also would not know whether they are Japanese, with a life expectancy (as of 2000) of nearly 80, or Burundian, with a life expectancy (as of 2000) of under 45. Note that the view that rational self-interest maximizers behind the stipulated veil of ignorance would seek to maximize the possibility of each person's reaching a *normal lifespan* is already a departure from the Rawlsian position of maximizing the minimum, i.e. making the worst outcome as good as can be. If (as on Battin's approach) we think in terms of people's complete lives, a maximin rule, on the above idealized hypothesis, would not only ration health care to the elderly, but would deny a 45-year-old in the developed world antibiotics for pneumonia until Burundians' life expectancies had been brought up to par. In fact, such a rule might not allocate any medical resources to adults (except to maintain the minimum number of adults necessary to keep society functioning) until every child who could be saved from death had been. Battin repeatedly refers to deaths in the developed world as occurring 'a little' earlier on her veil-of-ignorance approach (Battin 2000: 12, 13, 16). This would quite likely be a great understatement on a maximin rule.[39]

---

[37] The idea of a veil of ignorance is adapted from Rawls (1991).

[38] Battin mentions another consideration: rational self-interest maximizers would know, behind the stipulated veil, that 'by and large, a unit of medical care consumed late in life will [be much less efficient] than a unit of medical care consumed at a younger age' (Battin 1987: 324). For a related consideration, see Daniels (1988: 88–91).

[39] Daniels (1988: 88–91) discusses his reason for not using a maximin rule for allocation of health care resources. Also see Daniels (2002). Note also that the question of who is worst off is relative to

Overall has offered objections to Battin's approach. One is that 'the first cohort of midlife and elderly people would literally sacrifice a portion of their lives for the sake of this reallotment, without profiting personally from it. [They] would be too old to have benefited from the redistribution of savings to younger people' (Overall 2003: 212).[40] Overall further criticizes Battin on the grounds that 'self-interest ordinarily has a wider purview than merely one's own survival ... even from a Rawlsian veil-of-ignorance perspective, it would be unreasonable to assume that there are no elderly people or potential elderly people who might play key roles in our life' (Overall 2003: 212). But would self-interest incline us to trade our own survival for the survival of these people? That would be expecting quite a lot.

Battin's approach faces other problems. She says that decisions behind the stipulated veil of ignorance parallel those of people who are actually considering health care policy in our ordinary life, because 'ordinary persons who have not yet reached old age or death', i.e. 'those of us who are considering this issue—who would be prepared to develop policy requirements on the basis of these considerations and who would be governed by whatever policies might be devised—are effectively behind the "veil of ignorance" with respect to the specific events of our own aging and death' (Battin 1987: 324, 323). Here she overlooks her own stipulation that rational self-interest maximizers behind the veil would not know their ages (and hence would not know that they have not yet reached old age). She also disenfranchises the actual elderly as policy-makers in the real world and disregards their status as people who will be governed by 'whatever policies might be devised'.

This raises the question of just what is meant by the stipulation that behind the veil of ignorance people would not know their ages. The most natural interpretation seems to be that these people would have particular ages that they realized they simply did not know. But this would threaten the claim that rational self-interest maximizers behind the veil would choose to skew resources toward the young and 'not to underwrite treatment which would prolong life beyond its normal span', where the ' "normal life span" [has] to do with the rough boundary between middle and old age or between early old age and late old age' (Battin 1987: 322, 326 n. 29). After all, the rational self-interest maximizer would realize that, for all he knows behind the veil, he might in fact be old at the very time he is making the decision that is about to go into effect. If we accept Battin's supposition that rational self-interest maximization here involves a highly conservative risk-reduction strategy, wouldn't it be more rational for a self-interest maximizer to maximize his chances of staying

whether the comparison is made in terms of people's complete lives or in terms of current stages of people's lives. See the discussion in Ch. 8, by McKerlie, in this volume. (I thank Ketchum for help formulating the paragraph leading up to this note.)

[40] Battin (1987: 334; 2000: 6) acknowledges this problem. For a response, see Daniels (1982: 535; 1983: 516; 1988: 129–30).

alive, whatever age he actually is, 'even' if, unknown to him, he is presently at or beyond the end of a normal lifespan?[41]

Another interpretation, suggested by Battin's remark that rational self-interest maximizers behind the veil 'must decide *in advance* on a spending plan, budgeting a fixed amount of medical care across their whole lives' (Battin 1987: 322; italics added), is that behind the veil people are allocating resources from the standpoint of someone who envisions his entire life stretching before him, yet to be lived and unknown in its medical specifics. But although Daniels repeatedly insists that age-ignorance prevents biasing the choices in favor of the interests of a particular age group (for example, see Daniels 1988: 64 n. 8, 75), this construal yields a standpoint biased in favor of the young, as it is the standpoint of someone so 'young' that his life has not yet even begun.

A related objection applies to Dworkin's claim that 'The choices Americans of average income make about their employee insurance package in wage negotiations... can offer some guidance' about appropriate priorities for health coverage (Dworkin 2000: 217). The problem arises from his view that

we should aim to make collective, social decisions about the quantity and distribution of health care so as to match, as closely as possible, the decisions that people in the community would make for themselves, one by one, in the appropriate circumstances, if they were looking *from youth* down the course of their lives and trying to decide what risks were worth running in return for not running other kinds of risks.   (Dworkin 2000: 208–9; italics added)

This openly biases priorities in favor of the interests of the young.[42] Looking at choices people actually make about their employee insurance packages also biases priorities in favor of the interests of people healthy enough to be employed.

A third interpretation of Battin's age-ignorance stipulation, suggested by James Dreier in conversation, is as follows. Rational self-interest maximizers behind this veil of ignorance have an atemporal perspective in the sense of having no ages but just comparing different lives atemporally, rather than having ages they realize they do not know. To the extent that I understand this interpretation, it does not seem to be the natural interpretation of the stipulation that decision-makers behind the veil do not know their ages. Moreover, it is clearly out of line with Battin's parallel between these decision-makers and ordinary persons who are aware that they have not yet reached old age.

A further objection to Battin's approach is independent of which, if any, of these interpretations is used. This objection, arising from a basic problem with the

---

[41] Battin stipulates that rational self-interest maximizers behind the veil of ignorance have some general information about health and health care in their society, including the knowledge, cited in n. 38, above, that medical care is much less efficient in old age. But this hardly seems adequate to lead a rational and risk-averse self-interest maximizer to deny all life-prolonging care for people beyond an age he realizes that, for all he knows, he may already have reached.

[42] Overall recognizes this sort of problem; see Overall (2003: 238 n. 13).

veil-of-ignorance technique, is so well known as to have worked its way into introductory philosophy texts. The objection is that it is mistaken to suppose that rational
self-interest maximizers behind the veil of ignorance would all adopt the same risk-
management strategy, let alone that they would all adopt a very conservative one. As
John Hospers puts it, 'unanimity [or even widespread non-unanimous agreement]
even from behind the veil of ignorance would seem unlikely because of the diversity
of human temperaments. Some people are more risk-oriented than others; to some
a risk is a challenge, to others a source of dread' (1988: 400).[43] Hospers is discussing
the maximin rule, but the objection applies as well to the conservative (although
not maximin) rule Battin ascribes to rational self-interest maximizers behind the
stipulated veil. Accordingly, an argument for social policies that aid the disadvantaged should rest squarely on ethical principles rather than on claims about what
rational self-interest maximizers would choose behind a veil of ignorance.

One such argument for age-rationing is the 'fair innings' argument. Thus, Battin
says that 'it is often held' that medical resources should be skewed toward the
young, partly because the elderly 'have already lived full life spans and had claim to
a fair share of societal resources' (1987: 321). Gems says, 'It is generally held that
death is more tragic when it occurs in the young, since it is premature, coming
before its victims have had the opportunity fully to live out their lives' (2003a: 37).
James Lindemann Nelson effectively criticizes the view of age as what he calls a
'superfact', i.e. 'a fact that characterizes a set of people in a manner so relevant to
distribution of goods or assignment of duties that [nothing can] defeat its depositive
relevance' (1999: 116). As Overall points out, there are many ways of being denied
opportunities, and 'Not all older people have received or experienced the things for
which we automatically believe young people should have the opportunity' (Overall
2003: 110) or have had a fair share of social resources.

Hilde Lindemann Nelson and James Lindemann Nelson have argued that 'in
deference to women's greater longevity and the need to correct for the sexism that
has trammeled their opportunities for self-development, women should be eligible
for lifesaving interventions for a longer period than are men' (Nelson and Nelson
1996: 362). But the difference in opportunities for self-development is arguably
much greater within the genders than between them.[44] While there is some intuitive
attraction to the idea that the most 'unfair' death is that of 'someone [who not
only died young but] who wanted to [live] a lot, even though he never had much
happiness or success' (Ackerman 1983: 233),[45] this is not a workable basis for public

---

[43] For Rawls's response to this sort of objection, see Rawls (2000). Rawls seems to me to be the loser
in this controversy, but I cannot go into the details of this here.

[44] Another problem with the Nelsons' proposal is that it is hard to see the relevance of women's
greater longevity. Why should membership in a generally shorter-lived group make an atypically
long-lived person less entitled to life-saving treatment?

[45] This statement comes from the protagonist of my short story 'Not This Time' (Ackerman 1983).
See also the discussion in McMahan (2002, ch. 2).

policy. Rather, in deference to Harris's observation that respecting the desire to stay alive is 'the most important part of what is involved in valuing the lives of others' (Harris 1996: 440), we should accord people equal value by not eschewing attempts to extend greatly the maximum human lifespan and not taking age or 'desert' into account in allocating the life-saving resources that already exist.

I now turn to the more familiar problem of economic inequality. Will anti-aging technology benefit only the rich? The answer depends on the society itself. Egalitarian objections to the gap between rich and poor are a reason for making anti-aging technology available to the poor, rather than for refusing to fund it. They should be seen as objections to economic inequality, not to allocating resources for greatly extended life. To take the most extreme case, suppose immortality is achievable but the resource limits of our planet restrict the number of people to whom it can be offered. Rather than being auctioned off to the highest bidders, it should, as I suggested earlier, be offered by lottery. Similar considerations apply to the more realistic case of anti-aging technology that greatly extends life without making it eternal. The moral imperative is not to eschew funding research into such technology but to ensure that its fruits are available to the poor as well as to the rich. As for the claim that such technology would be very expensive to develop, test, and distribute, thereby deflecting huge sums from poor people's urgent needs that we already know how to meet, we should consider whether this is correct and, if so, whether it could be changed. Such a discussion lies beyond the scope of this chapter, but see Kurzweil (2005: 66), Naam (2005), and Sawyer (2005: 87) for a more optimistic view of the economics involved.

But suppose anti-aging technology is not equitably distributed. Which would be worse: greatly extended life for only the economically privileged (which may well include not only 'the rich', but also the insured middle class) or greatly extended life for no one? In a different context, Claudia Card says envy in the sense of ' "wishing others to be no better off than oneself" . . . is a form of malice' (Card 1972: 199).[46] Can objections to greatly extended life for only the economically privileged be condemned on these grounds? Certainly not in a country that funds anti-aging research even partly through general taxation, especially in the absence of any sort of guaranteed health care for that country's poor. What if the research is privately funded? This ties in with a larger issue about health care. Some people favor a kind of enforced medical egalitarianism in the form of a single payer system with a proviso that would preclude health care (in the country in question) outside of that system. Such a system, of course, would prevent private interests in that country from developing anti-aging technology and making it available in that country only to the economically privileged. As I have argued elsewhere,

---

[46] Also see Rawls (1991). There is also a literature, which I cannot discuss further here, on what Derek Parfit (2000: 98; see also Temkin 2000) calls 'the Levelling Down Objection', i.e. the view carrying egalitarianism to the extent of holding that it would be desirable that 'those who are better off suffer some misfortune, so that they become as badly off as everyone else'.

Perhaps such a prohibition would be appropriate in a society [that] prohibit[s] private education, private housing, and fax machines. But a society that does not outlaw these private alternatives to public education, public housing, and mail service will have a hard time justifying a prohibition against obtaining medical care outside a public system. Such a prohibition would send a brutal message to people with extremely expensive illnesses: if you cost too much, you have no business staying alive, even if you can pay for it yourself or can obtain private donations or private insurance. (Ackerman 1996: 428–9)[47]

The same point applies to people who want anti-aging technology that is extremely expensive. Rather than restricting the amount the rich may spend on health care, we should, as Dworkin suggests, 'put an excise tax on special health care, and use the proceeds . . . in . . . ways that would make the community distinctly more egalitarian' (Dworkin 2000: 220–1). Furthermore, medical technology is an area where the 'trickle down' effect actually seems to occur—nowhere near enough, in my view, but somewhat.[40] Heart transplants, for example, once available in America only to the rich, are now covered by Medicare. A final point is that economic class is not entirely static. Economic mobility is limited—far too limited—but it sometimes occurs, making it not always unrealistic for the poor to aspire to move up.

This is not to endorse having anti-aging technology be available only to the economically privileged. That situation is better than having no such technology at all, but it is far, far worse than having the technology available to all who desire it. I believe that people's rational interest in greatly increased longevity justifies funding research into attempts to extend greatly the maximum human lifespan and having the fruits of that research be available to all who desire it, poor as well as rich, incurably ill and disabled as well as healthy (if the research does not also bring about cures). Overall's insistence that 'it is worthwhile to employ social and medical means to lengthen the lives of human beings *whose capacities for emotion, perception, thought, and action are at least to some degree intact*' (2003: 191; italics added) is, by current standards, extraordinarily generous. But the qualification I have italicized is problematic. For one thing, unless the standard of intactness is flexible enough to include the ability simply to give consistent responses to such questions as 'Do you want to die?' and 'Do you want to be kept alive?', the qualification shortchanges people who have (whatever would count as) inadequate capacity for action but much rational desire to live. Moreover, the qualification seems odd in view of Overall's enlightened awareness that it is 'an error, of the most presumptuous and

---

[47] A general discussion of what sorts of inequalities a democracy should allow is, of course, far beyond the scope of this chapter. But Alan Wertheimer (1988: 314) offers two reasons for holding that a stronger justification for equalization applies to legal resources of adversaries in a civil case than to health care. First, 'a major purpose of the state is to monopolize binding resolutions to certain sorts of controversies'. Second, 'an improvement in the legal resources available to one party [to a conflict] has a direct negative effect on the interests of [the other]'.

[48] See President's Council on Bioethics (2003a: 282); Garreau (2005); Kurzweil (2005); Naam (2005); Sawyer (2005).

high-handed sort, to assume that changed or reduced abilities necessarily constitute a good reason for refusing to prolong life' (2003: 205).[49]

Some statistics suggest an appropriate ending here. The American life expectancy in 2001 was 77.2 years, in contrast with 1900, when it was 48.3 years for women and 46.3 years for men.[50] As Singer has remarked, 'We are seeing a phenomenon that the world has never seen before: the fit and active over-eighties, who continue to play golf, swim, travel the world, develop new relationships, and generally enjoy life, in a way that would have been thought impossible—and if possible, scandalous—twenty years ago' (1991: 132). Imagine sages of the past shuddering over such a prospect. Imagine a 300-year-old, several centuries hence, reading some of our present-day bioethicists on the folly or inequity of life-extension. Imagine applying to greatly extended human life these words of William Blake on love:

> Children of the future Age,
> Reading this indignant page;
> Know that in a former time,
> Love! sweet Love! was thought a crime.

(Blake 1967)

REFERENCES

ACKERMAN, F. (1983), 'Not This Time', *Arizona Quarterly*, 39/1: 223–34; to be repr. in Ackerman (forthcoming).

—— (1990), 'The Forecasting Game', in W. Abrahams (ed.), *Prize Stories 1990: The O. Henry Awards* (New York: Doubleday); to be repr. in Ackerman (forthcoming), 315–35.

—— (1995), 'No Exit', *American Scholar*, 64/1: 131–5.

—— (1996), 'What Is the Proper Role for Charity in Healthcare?', *Cambridge Quarterly of Healthcare Ethics*, 5: 425–9.

[49] Overall's views further differ from mine in that while she favors 'directing resources, research, and services toward boosting life expectancy, ultimately so that it approaches that of the maximum human life span'; 'in the short term' she is 'not ready to argue that it is . . . desirable to direct resources toward *increasing* the maximum human life span' (Overall 2003: 194, 198; italics added). Moreover, I take issue with her statement 'If people want to live longer, they have to . . . not rely on medical engineering to ensure their longevity. They also have to question and possibly reject [such] key features of dominant Western culture [as its] deprecation of vegetarianism [and] its reliance on prescription and nonprescription drugs' (Overall 2003: 196). Rather than being monolithic enough to have a single set of key features, Western culture is a conglomerate of subcultures. One is the academic subculture, whose key features include great respect for vegetarianism—more respect, frequently, than that subculture gives the chronically ill. (Thus, American academic conferences that include meals virtually always have a special menu option for vegetarians and virtually never have one for diabetics or others on medically restricted diets.) As for decisions about medical engineering and drugs, these should be made on a pragmatic case-by-case basis rather than on an ideological one. For example, many people find anti-cholesterol drugs far more effective and far more agreeable than a stringently restricted diet.

[50] See Tennen (2004).

ACKERMAN, F. (1998a), 'Assisted Suicide, Terminal Illness, Severe Disability, and the Double Standard', in M. P. Battin, R. Rhodes, and A. Silvers (eds.), *Physician-Assisted Suicide: Expanding the Debate* (New York: Routledge), 149–61.

—— (1998b), 'Flourish Your Heart in This World', in M. C. Nussbaum and C. R. Sunstein (eds.), *Clones and Clones: Facts and Fantasies About Human Cloning* (New York: Norton), 310–31; to be repr. in Ackerman (forthcoming).

—— (1999), Letter to the Editor, *Lingua Franca*, 9/1: 7.

—— (2002), Letter to the Editor, Arts and Leisure Section, *New York Times*, 20 Oct., 4.

ACKERMAN, F. N. (2003), 'More about More Life', *Hastings Center Report*, 33/6: 5.

—— (2005a), Letter to the Editor, *The Progressive* (July), 6.

—— (2005b), 'Rose and Blue', *Ragged Edge Online*, <http://www.raggededgemagazine.com /poetry/ackermanpoem0805.html>, accessed 12 July 2006.

—— (2005c), 'We Gather Together', *East Side Monthly* (May), 42–3; to be repr. in Ackerman (forthcoming).

—— (forthcoming), *Bioethics Through Fiction* (Lanham, Md · Rowman & Littlefield).

BATTIN, M. P. (1980), 'Suicide: A Fundamental Human Right?', in M. P. Battin and D. Mayo (eds.), *Suicide: The Philosophical Issues* (New York: St Martin's Press), 267–85.

—— (1987), 'Age Rationing and the Just Distribution of Health Care: Is There a Duty to Die?', *Ethics*, 97/2: 317–40.

—— (2000), 'Global Life Expectancies and the Duty to Die', in J. M. Humber and R. F. Almeder (eds.), *Is There a Duty to Die?* (Totowa, NJ: Humana Press), 3–21.

BLACKBURN, E., and ROWLEY, J. (2004), 'Reason as Our Guide', *Public Library of Science Biology*, 2/4: 0420–2.

BLAKE, W. (1967), 'A Little Girl Lost', in Blake, *Songs of Innocence and of Experience* (New York: Orion Press), 51.

BOSTROM, N. (2003), 'Human Genetic Enhancements: A Transhumanist Perspective', *Journal of Value Inquiry*, 37/4: 493–506.

—— (2005),' 'In Defense of Posthuman Dignity', *Bioethics*, 19/3: 202–14.

BUCHWALD, EPHRAIM (n.d.), 'The Holocaust Is Killing America's Jews', <http://www.njop .org/html/Newslettersandarticles.html#a1>, accessed 12 July 2006, repr. updated from *Los Angeles Times*, 28 Apr. 1992.

CALLAHAN, D. (2002), 'Slippery Slope: Medical Technology and the Human Future', *Christian Century*, 119/19: 30–4.

CARD, C. (1972), 'On Mercy', *Philosophical Review*, 81/2: 182–207.

DANIELS, N. (1982), 'Am I My Parents' Keeper?', in P. A. French, T. E. Uehling, and H. K. Wettstein (eds.), *Midwest Studies in Philosophy*, vii: *Social and Political Philosophy* (Minneapolis: University of Minnesota Press), 517–40.

—— (1983), 'Justice Between Age Groups: Am I My Parents' Keeper?', *Milbank Memorial Fund Quarterly*, 61/3: 489–522.

—— (1988), *Am I My Parents' Keeper? An Essay on Justice Between the Young and the Old* (New York: Oxford University Press).

—— (2002), 'Justice, Health, and Health Care', in R. Rhodes, M. P. Battin, and A. Silvers (eds.), *Medicine and Social Justice: Essays on the Distribution of Health Care* (New York: Oxford University Press), 6–23.

DANIS, M., et al. (1996), 'A Prospective Study of the Impact of Patient Preferences on Life-Sustaining Treatment and Hospital Cost', *Critical Care Medicine*, 24/11: 1811–18.

DWORKIN, R. (1994), *Life's Dominion: An Argument About Abortion, Euthanasia, and Individual Freedom* (New York: Vintage).

—— (2000), 'Justice in the Distribution of Health Care', in M. Clayton and A. Williams (eds.), *The Ideal of Equality* (New York: Macmillan and St Martin's Press), 203–22.

GARREAU, J. (2005), *Radical Evolution: The Promise and Peril of Enhancing Our Minds, Our Bodies—And What It Means To Be Human* (New York: Doubleday).

GEMS, D. (2003*a*), 'Is More Life Always Better? The New Biology of Aging and the Meaning of Life', *Hastings Center Report*, 33/4: 31–9.

—— (2003*b*), 'More about More Life', *Hastings Center Report*, 33/6: 5–6.

GUTMAN, R. A. (1988), 'High-Cost Life Prolongation: The National Kidney Dialysis and Kidney Transplantation Study', *Annals of Internal Medicine*, 108/6: 898–9.

HARRIS, J. (1996), 'The Value of Life', in T. L. Beauchamp and R. M. Veatch (eds.), *Ethical Issues in Death and Dying*, 2nd edn. (Upper Saddle River, NJ: Prentice-Hall), 435–40.

—— (2000), 'Intimations of Immortality', *Science*, 288/5463: 59.

HENIG, R. M. (2005), 'Will We Ever Arrive at the Good Death?', *New York Times Magazine*, 7 Aug., 26–35, 40, 68.

HOSPERS, J. (1988), *An Introduction to Philosophical Analysis*, 3rd edn. (Englewood Cliffs, NJ: Prentice-Hall).

ICHIKAWA, J. (2004), <http://www.brown.edu/Departments/Philosophy/Blog/Archives/002777.html>, accessed 16 July 2006.

JUENGST, E., BINSTOCK, R. H., MEHLMAN, M., POST, S. G., and WHITEHOUSE, P. (2003), 'Biogerontology, "Anti-Aging Medicine", and the Challenges of Human Enhancement', *Hastings Center Report*, 33/4: 21–30.

KASS, L. (2002), *Life, Liberty and the Defense of Dignity: The Challenge for Bioethics* (San Francisco: Encounter).

KOLATA, G. (1997), 'Living Wills Aside, Dying Cling to Hope', *New York Times*, 15 Jan., C10.

KÜBLER-ROSS, E. (1974), *Questions and Answers About Death and Dying* (New York: Macmillan).

KURZWEIL, R. (2005), 'Chasing Immortality: The Technology of Eternal Life', interview by Craig Hamilton, *'What Is Enlightenment?'*, 30 (Sept.–Nov.), 58–69.

LARKIN, P. (1999), 'Aubade', in L. R. Spaar (ed.), *Acquainted with the Night* (New York: Columbia University Press), 84–6.

LIBERT, A. (2005), Letter to the Editor, *New York Times Magazine*, 21 Aug., 8.

MCGEE, G. (2003), 'The Wisdom of Leon the Professional [Ethicist]', *American Journal of Bioethics*, 3/3: vii–viii.

MCKERLIE, D. (2007), 'Justice and the Elderly', in B. Steinbock (ed.), *The Oxford Handbook of Bioethics*. (Oxford: Oxford University Press), 190–208.

MCMAHAN, J. (2002), *The Ethics of Killing: Problems at the Margins of Life* (Oxford: Oxford University Press).

MALORY, SIR THOMAS (1969), *Le Morte D'Arthur*, ii (London: Penguin).

MILL, J. S. (1970), *The Subjection of Women* (Cambridge, Mass.: MIT Press).

MOMEYER, R. (1988), *Confronting Death* (Bloomington: Indiana University Press).

MOONEY, C. (2001), 'Irrationalist in Chief', *American Prospect*, 12/17: 10–13.

NAAM, R. (2005), *More Than Human* (New York: Broadway).

NAGEL, T. (1971), 'The Absurd', *Journal of Philosophy*, 68/20: 716–27.

—— (1979), 'Death', in Nagel, *Mortal Questions* (Cambridge: Cambridge University Press), 1–10.

NELSON, H. L., and NELSON, J. L. (1996), 'Justice in the Allocation of Health Care Resources: A Feminist Account', in S. M. Wolf (ed.), *Feminism and Bioethics: Beyond Reproduction* (New York: Oxford University Press), 351–70.

NELSON, J. L. (1999), 'Death's Gender', in M. Walker (ed.), *Mother Time: Women, Aging, and Ethics* (Lanham, Md.: Rowman & Littlefield), 113–29.

NULAND, S. B. (1994), *How We Die* (New York: Knopf).

—— (2002), 'Send in No Clones', *New York Times Book Review*, 17 Nov., 49.

OVERALL, C. (2003), *Aging, Death, and Human Longevity: A Philosophical Inquiry* (Berkeley: University of California Press).

PARFIT, D. (2000), 'Equality or Priority?', in M. Clayton and A. Williams (eds.), *The Ideal of Equality* (New York: Macmillan and St Martin's Press), 80–125.

PRESIDENT'S COUNCIL ON BIOETHICS (2003a), *Beyond Therapy: Biotechnology and the Pursuit of Happiness* (New York: Regan).

—— (2003b), 'Session 3: Beyond Therapy: Biotechnology and the Pursuit of Human Improvement', <http://www.bioethics.gov>, accessed 12 July 2006.

PUCCETTI, R. (1978), 'The Conquest of Death', in J. Donnelly (ed.), *Language, Metaphysics, and Death* (New York: Fordham University Press), 163–75.

RAWLS, J. (1991), *A Theory of Justice*, rev. edn. (Cambridge, Mass.: Harvard University Press).

—— (2000), 'Reply to Alexander and Musgrave', in M. Clayton and A. Williams (eds.), *The Ideal of Equality* (New York: Macmillan and St Martin's Press), 25–40.

ROGATZ, P. (2005), Letter to the Editor, *New York Times Magazine*, 21 Aug., 8.

ROSEN, J. (2004), 'The Final Stage', *New York Times Magazine*, 26 Dec., 14.

SAWYER, R. J. (2005), 'We Will Be the Lords of Creation: Envisioning Our Immortal Future', interview by Tom Huston, *'What Is Enlightenment?'*, 30 (Sept.–Nov.), 82–90.

SINGER, P. (1991), 'Research into Aging: Should it Be Guided by the Interests of Present Individuals, Future Individuals, or the Species?', in F. Ludwig (ed.), *Life Span Extension: Consequences and Open Questions* (New York: Springer), 132–45.

SLEVIN, M., *et al.* (1990), 'Attitudes to Chemotherapy: Comparing Views of Patients with Cancer with Those of Doctors, Nurses, and General Public', *British Medical Journal*, 300: 1458–60.

STEELE, H. (1976), 'Could Body-Bound Immortality Be Liveable?', *Mind*, 85/339: 424–7.

TEMKIN, L. (2000), 'Equality, Priority, and the Levelling Down Objection', in M. Clayton and A. Williams (eds.), *The Ideal of Equality* (New York: Macmillan and St Martin's Press), 126–61.

TENNEN, M. (2004), 'Gift Keeps Giving: Longer Life', 31 Jan. 2005, <http://www.healthatoz .com/healthatoz/Atoz/hc/wom/life/alert06132003.jsp>, accessed 12 July 2006.

WENDELL, S. (1996), *The Rejected Body: Feminist Philosophical Reflections on Disability* (New York: Routledge).

WERTHEIMER, A. (1988), 'The Equalization of Legal Resources', *Philosophy and Public Affairs*, 17/4: 303–22.

WILLIAMS, B. (1975), 'The Makropulos Case: Reflections on the Tedium of Immortality', in J. Rachels (ed.), *Moral Problems: A Collection of Philosophical Essays* (New York: Harper & Row), 410–28.

WOODS, J. (1978), *Engineered Death: Abortion, Suicide, Euthanasia and Senecide* (Ottawa: University of Ottawa Press).

CHAPTER 15

PRECEDENT AUTONOMY, ADVANCE DIRECTIVES, AND END-OF-LIFE CARE

JOHN K. DAVIS

1. INTRODUCTION

BIOETHICISTS are widely agreed that patients have a right of self-determination over how they are treated. Our duty to respect this is said to be based on the principle of respect for autonomy.[1] In end-of-life care the patient may be incompetent and unable to exercise that right.[2] One solution is to exercise it in advance. Advance

[1] The nature and importance of personal autonomy in bioethics is a disputed topic of late. It has most often been understood along the lines laid out by John Stuart Mill in *On Liberty* as a right of self-determination. However, Onora O'Neill (2002) has proposed to redefine it along Kantian lines and deemphasize it in relation to the importance of trust, while Carl Schneider (1998) argues that many patients do not want as much autonomy as current bioethics declares they need. Because even revisionists like O'Neill and Schneider do not dispense with self-determination altogether, I feel safe in assuming a fairly schematic duty to respect a patient's treatment decisions, and leave the details, weight, and argument behind this duty for others.

[2] It is often said that 'competency' is a legal concept, while 'capacity' is a related concept used in clinical and ethical deliberation. This is not quite correct. Mental capacity is a function of one's

directives, which include living wills and powers of attorney for health care, enable people to decide (or least influence) what medical treatment they will receive later, when they become incompetent.

Advance directives have been criticized in two general ways. First, many critics contend that advance directives fail on a *practical* level to effect a patient's autonomous choices because, for example, people cannot foresee their futures well enough to make informed decisions in advance. Second, many critics contend that, practical problems aside, there is no *moral authority* for exercising control over one's incompetent future self. This second kind of objection tends to work from the premise that, if a patient has lost the mental capacity to understand and mentally reaffirm the interests, preferences, or values expressed in the advance directive, then those interests, preferences, or values can no longer be attributed to that patient; therefore we have no moral reason to respect them, and we should instead promote the patient's current best interests (which are usually welfare interests in avoiding pain, enjoying simple pleasures, and the like). I will briefly mention the practical concerns, but this chapter focuses on the 'Moral Authority Objection', partly because it is more complex, and partly because, if advance directives lack moral authority, there is no reason to work on solving the practical problems, while if the objection fails, there is no reason to give up.

According to a conception of personal autonomy that goes back to John Stuart Mill, a person has something like a jurisdictional right to determine what happens to the things in which he or she has interests. According to what I will call the 'Extension View', people have the same moral authority over their future affairs that they have over their current affairs—it is simply extended forward. The President's Commission for the Study of Ethical Problems in Medicine and Biomedical and Behavioral Research, Allen E. Buchanan, Dan W. Brock, Nancy Rhoden, and Ronald Dworkin have all defended versions of the Extension View. Just as the Mill–Feinberg picture of conventional autonomy has two elements—preferences[3] and interests—so does the Extension View:

1. Preferences concerning one's future—comprised by 'precedent autonomy'.
2. Interests in one's future—aka, 'surviving interests'.

For reasons that will be clear later, the interests in question are investment interests in such things as personal dignity or religious commitments, rather than welfare interests in such things as enjoying simple pleasures and avoiding pain. All but

psychological abilities; to be 'competent' is to have sufficient mental capacity for a given task. However, competence is not a strictly legal concept. Courts consider competence a question of fact, not of law. For this reason (and because I refuse to say 'capacitated' instead of 'competent') I follow Beauchamp and Childress (2001: 69) and Buchanan and Brock (1990: 18) in speaking of both 'capacity' and 'competence' as appropriate, without limiting the latter concept to legal contexts.

[3] By 'preference' I also mean decisions, intentions, willings, and all other mental states arguably covered by the principle of respect for autonomy.

unconscious patients have at least some simple welfare interests, but the Extension View requires surviving *investment* interests.

Critics argue that advance directives lack moral authority for reasons pertaining to both elements:

1. If the patient lacks the competence to comprehend his or her earlier preferences regarding the future, those preferences are not still attributable to that patient, and therefore we have no moral reason to respect them.

2. If the patient lacks the competence to comprehend the things in which he or she earlier took an interest, he or she has 'lost interest' in those things, and therefore his or her right of self-determination does not extend to them.

John A. Robertson and Rebecca S. Dresser are the best-known critics of advance directives. The Moral Authority Objection is an idealized version of their main criticisms of the Extension View, and will help organize the discussion. Having rejected the Extension View, Dresser and Robertson contend that medical professionals should do what is in the current best interests of a now-incompetent patient when the patient's earlier wishes conflict with those interests. A large portion of the medical profession shares their concerns about advance directives.

Narrative theorists, such as Howard Brody, Mark G. Kuczewski, Ben A. Rich, and Jeffrey Blustein, agree with Dresser and Robertson in rejecting the Extension View account of the moral authority of advance directives, but they do not reject advance medical decision-making itself. Instead, they seek to replace the Extension View with a different account of why and how we should respect the earlier values and preferences of a now-incompetent patient.

I explain advance directives in Section 2, present the Extension View and the Moral Authority Objection in Section 3, discuss precedent autonomy and former preferences in Section 4, and discuss surviving interests in Section 5. After reviewing other positions, I will argue that:

- The preferences in question become *former* preferences once the agent becomes too incompetent to comprehend his or her earlier preferences (subsection 4.1).
- The principle of respect for autonomy sometimes requires that we respect former preferences (subsection 4.4).
- The interests in question can survive incompetence (subsection 5.2).

2. BACKGROUND

There are two kinds of advance directives: living wills, and health care powers of attorney (often known as a 'durable power of attorney for health care').[4] Because

---

[4] Although I will not discuss episodic mental disorders, psychiatric Ulysses contracts (often called 'advance directives for mental health treatment' or something similar) are also forms of advance

advance directives are much more common in the United States (and first developed there), my legal points are drawn from American law, but the ethical issues are universal.

Living wills. People use living wills to say how they want to be treated if they later become incompetent. Some living wills are informal documents circulated by religious or right-to-die groups. For example, the one circulated by Concern for Dying, a large right-to-die organization, directs that 'I be allowed to die and not be kept alive by medications, artificial means or "heroic measures"', with spaces to fill in more information. Other living wills use boilerplate language set forth in statutes, and require more detail about what treatments the patient wants under what circumstances. Within the last twenty-five years, virtually all American states extended legal recognition to living wills, and they are beginning to get legal recognition in Germany, Japan, and Great Britain (Sass *et al.* 1998), among other countries. In most American states, living wills become effective immediately upon execution, can be revoked so long as the patient is capable of communicating a revocation, and typically apply in cases of 'terminal illness'.[5] In some states they apply only to life support, and in some states they do not apply to nutrition and hydration.[6]

Surrogates appointed under a health care power of attorney. People use a health care power of attorney to select someone to make decisions for them during later incompetence. That person may be called an 'agent', 'proxy', or 'surrogate decision maker'. The scope of the surrogate's powers can be as broad or narrow as the person executing the power of attorney likes. A health care power of attorney is often combined with a living will.

Surrogates appointed without a power of attorney. Surrogates can also be appointed without a health care power of attorney or living will, for many states have 'family consent' statutes, which specify a relative or relatives to act as surrogate decision maker. Although these surrogates are not appointed under advance directives, their role is much the same as surrogates appointed under a health care power of attorney.

Surrogate decision making. Although American law varies on this point, in general the surrogate decision maker must decide according to the substituted judgment principle, which tells the surrogate to decide as the patient would if he or she were now competent.[7] Evidence of what the patient would want can consist of

medical decision making, for they enable patients to commit themselves voluntarily to psychiatric treatment for their next psychotic episode.

[5] There may now be a movement toward authorizing living wills for less severe conditions. In any case, as discussed below, health care powers of attorney tend not to be so limited in scope.

[6] Furrow *et al.* (2000: 840–59) provides an excellent overview of American law concerning living wills, health care powers of attorney, and surrogate decision making.

[7] Some state courts have restricted substituted judgment to 'clear and convincing' evidence of what the patient would want, usually in the form of very clear, specific past statements about future medical care, effectively making substituted judgment impossible in many cases.

informal statements or comments made earlier, such as remarks to friends and relatives that he 'never wanted to be kept alive as a human vegetable' and similar comments. Such comments may not rise to the level of an actual decision, but do suggest a hypothetical decision, which the substituted judgment principle directs the surrogate to put into effect. In both law and ethics, it is generally agreed that, if there are neither express decisions nor sufficient evidence to know what the patient would decide if he or she were competent, the surrogate should protect the patient's best interest (for respecting the patient's autonomy is impossible).

A spectrum of autonomy. In general, this three-tiered approach to surrogate decision making—express preferences (including living wills), substituted judgment, and best interests, in that order—is endorsed both by ethicists (Buchanan and Brock 1990: 87–126) and by the law. Notice the order of priority: Ideally, we respect the current express preferences of a competent patient (informed consent), but if that is not possible because the patient is no longer competent, then we respect his or her past express preferences (living wills). When there are no express past preferences, then we are restricted to respecting what the patient would now want if he or she were competent (substituted judgment). When we lack even that information (or the patient was never competent), we promote his or her best interests. As we move down this list, the patient's autonomous choices become less clear and more hypothetical. Because surrogate decision making often involves less clearly formulated autonomous choices than living wills, most of the controversy over advance directives concerns living wills, though the same issues can arise with substituted judgment as well.

Practical problems with advance directives. Living wills and (to a lesser extent) substituted judgment extend a patient's autonomous choices into the future. This extension runs into several practical problems. It may be hard to know what medical issues the patient will later face. Many advance directives are vaguely worded, speaking in terms of 'heroic measures' and the like, and require interpretation. One may sign an advance directive prepared by someone else without giving it sufficient thought, or without fully appreciating what it may be like to become demented and severely incompetent. Treatment options might change between the time the directive was executed and the time it must be followed. A person's values and treatment preferences can change over time, and advance directives are not always updated to reflect such changes. Surrogate decision makers may not be well informed about what the patient would want, or may disregard instructions in the living will or power of attorney.[8]

Although much bioethics literature on advance directives concerns these practical issues, I will not explore such issues or their possible solutions. Instead, I will focus

---

[8] The SUPPORT study ('Study to Understand Prognoses and Preferences for Outcomes and Risks of Treatments') suggests that, despite living wills and other forms of end-of-life care planning, many patients do not get the care they want, even when concerted efforts are made to improve doctor–patient communication on this issue (SUPPORT Principal Investigators 1995).

on the *moral authority* of efforts to decide one's future treatment—however well informed, clearly stated, and legally enforceable those efforts may be. If advance directives lack moral authority, then there is no reason to focus on the practical problems, while if they have moral authority, there is all the more reason to strive to solve the problems.

3. THE MORAL AUTHORITY OF ADVANCE DIRECTIVES

Practical problems aside, there are theoretical problems with extending the right of self-determination into an incompetent future. In this section we will look at the Extension View, which attempts to do just that, and review the Moral Authority Objection to that attempt.

3.1. The Extension View

According to the earliest and still standard way to characterize the moral authority of advance directives, they have the same kind of moral authority as autonomous decisions in general—just extended into the future. We can call this the 'Extension View, for, as Buchanan and Brock explain, 'The dominant tendency, both in recent legal doctrine and in the bioethics literature, has been to view the rights of incompetent individuals as an *extension* of the rights of competent individuals, through arrangements by which these rights are exercised for the incompetent by others' (Buchanan and Brock 1990: 90; emphasis added). The Extension View was articulated in a 1983 report on advance directives by the President's Commission for the Study of Ethical Problems in Medicine and Biomedical and Behavioral Research (1983: 182), and later defended by Buchanan and Brock, Nancy Rhoden, and Ronald Dworkin, among others.

On the Extension View, the right of self-determination may be qualified by circumstances peculiar to advance decision making: Just as a patient's current choice has less moral weight when the patient is uninformed about the issue in question, so the moral authority of an advance directive is weakened to the extent that the patient did not understand or foresee the medical issues that would later arise (President's Commission 1983: 182–3; Buchanan and Brock 1990: 101, 105–7). However, while this may happen more often with advance directives than with other kinds of self-determination, that fact does not lessen their moral authority when the patient *is* sufficiently informed about his or her future. Buchanan and Brock appeal to the Extension View to explain the moral authority not only of living wills but of substituted judgment decision making as well (1990: 99).

Buchanan and Brock, former staff philosophers for the President's Commission who contributed to the 1983 report, stress that advance directives are not merely evidence of what will be good for the later incompetent patient (which may be rejected when better evidence comes along), but are *acts of self-determination* (Buchanan and Brock 1990: 99, 116).[9] Buchanan and Brock filled out the President's Commission's account by noting that, just as ordinary autonomy extends over the person's own interests, so the moral authority of advance directives extends over a certain kind of interest in the future, which they call a 'surviving interest'. For example, 'One may have an interest in how one's family will fare after one's death, and that interest survives one in the sense that whether or not it is satisfied will depend upon events that occur after one is gone' (Buchanan and Brock 1990: 100). This fits a common picture of the right of autonomy as a kind of authority over a sphere of interests—as Joel Feinberg puts it, somewhat like the sovereignty of a nation over its territory (Feinberg 1986: 47–51). John Stuart Mill, too, spoke of personal liberty as coextensive with 'a sphere of action in which society, as distinguished from the individual, has, if any, only an indirect interest' (Mill 1986: 18).

Thus, the Extension View can be stated this way: Just as we have a moral right of autonomy to effect our preferences over our interests in the present, so we have a moral right of *precedent* autonomy to effect (in advance) our preferences over our *surviving* interests (with a few caveats about the difficulty of foreseeing one's future and anticipating all contingencies).[10]

3.2. The Moral Authority Objection

Critics of the Extension View are motivated in part by a well-known kind of case sometimes referred to (a bit flippantly) as the Happy Alzheimer's Patient. In one of the earliest such cases, a 65-year-old woman was admitted for surgery to correct a clogged artery. She knew this could lead to a disabling stroke, and her living will said: 'If . . . there is no reasonable expectation of my recovery from physical or mental disability, I request that I be allowed to die and not be kept alive by artificial means or heroic measures. I do not fear death itself as much as the indignities of deterioration, dependence, and hopeless pain' (Eisendrath and Jonsen 1983). The day before surgery, she told her surgeon she wanted the living will followed if she had a stroke, and said 'she felt life was worth living only if she could be healthy and independent'. Soon after surgery, a stroke left her with a 'profound neurological

---

[9] Buchanan and Brock also believe the moral authority of advance directives rests in part on the value of protecting people from unwanted, virtually futile interventions, and of enabling people to save their relatives from emotional and financial burdens (Buchanan and Brock 1990: 100).

[10] For a recent, clear, and succinct statement of this view, see Joanne Lynn *et al.* (1999). Many of Lynn's co-authors disagree with this view, of course.

deficit', and a few days later she developed a breathing problem. Her doctors had to decide whether to follow her living will and let her die. Such cases are a mainstay of the advance directives literature.[11]

Do such patients still have the preferences and interests they had when the living will was executed, and if not, why should we respect living wills? Once they become permanently incompetent and unable to comprehend their earlier preferences and interests, it is hard to say that they still have those preferences and interests. If we cannot attribute those preferences and interests to the patient at the time a living will takes effect, how are we respecting the patient's autonomy, or promoting his or her interests, by following the living will? The same questions arise with substituted judgment: If the patient no longer has the preferences that support that judgment, why should we treat the patient as he or she would want if he or she were competent?

Rebecca S. Dresser and John A. Robertson argue that preferences and interests do not survive a loss of the mental capacity necessary to comprehend them, and that respecting those preferences and interests does not constitute respect for that person's autonomy. Robertson:

Unless we are to view competently held values and interests as extending even to situations in which, because of incompetency, they can no longer have meaning, it matters not that as a competent person the individual would not wish to be maintained in a debilitated or disabled state . . . Yet the premise of the prior directive is that patient interests and values remain significantly the same, so that those interests are best served by following the directive issued when competent . . . we should focus on [incompetent patients'] needs and interests as they now exist and not view them as retaining interests and values which, because of their incompetency, no longer apply.   (Robertson 1991: 7)

The problem is not simply that earlier preferences and interests may not survive, but also that following the earlier preferences, or promoting the earlier interests, may harm the now-incompetent patient (Robertson 1991: 7).[12] In most medical cases, when a patient's treatment preference conflicts with his or her current welfare interests, medical ethics tells us to respect the preference—so long as the patient is choosing autonomously. However, in most cases the patient has that preference when the treatment is given; this may not be true when the preference was formed before the patient became incompetent and unable to comprehend that preference. The same point applies to surviving interests.

3.3. Personal Identity

Many bioethicists discuss these issues in terms of personal identity, invoking a theory of personal identity of the kind proposed by John Locke, Derek Parfit, and

[11] Similar cases, some real and some fictional, are discussed by Allen E. Buchanan and Dan W. Brock (1990: 108), Ronald Dworkin (1993: 221, 226), Norman Cantor (1993: 101), and Dresser and Astrow (1998).

[12] See also Lynn et al. (1999: 274); Wolf et al. (1991: 1668–9).

others. Parfit's version involves continuity and connectedness: A given person at time T_1 is the same person as a given person at time T_2 only if the T_2 person has some minimum quotient of the memories and psychological properties of the T_1 person (connectedness), or some minimum quotient of overlapping chains of memories and psychological properties (continuity) (Parfit 1984: 204–9). These bioethicists question whether a patient who suffers severe, permanent mental incompetence has lost the properties necessary for retaining personal identity over time, thereby becoming a different moral person (King 1996: 76–7, 84). If the patient is no longer the same person, treating the patient in accord with earlier choices seems to impose someone else's will on that new person.[13]

Allen E. Buchanan has defended the Extension View against this objection by arguing that the degree of psychological continuity and connectedness necessary for remaining the same person over time is a moral question, not a metaphysical one, and that we have moral reasons to set that degree fairly low—otherwise we would lose useful social institutions and practices such as contracts, promises, civil and criminal liability, and the assignment of moral praise and blame. In fact, the proper degree of continuity necessary is sufficiently low that in any case where the patient has ceased to be the *same* person, he or she has ceased to be a *person* altogether, for personhood should be understood as requiring the ability to be conscious of oneself as existing over time, to appreciate reasons for or against acting, and the ability to engage in purposive sequences of actions, and deeply incapacitated people cannot do these things. Because such a patient is no longer a person, no harm is done by imposing the earlier person's wishes upon that former person's still-living body. Buchanan qualifies his conclusion, however, by noting what he regards as very rare cases where the now-incompetent patient, though not a person, nonetheless feels pleasure and pain, and where honoring a living will can mean ending the apparently worthwhile life of such a non-person. In some of these cases, he believes, paternalism may be justified (Buchanan 1988).

Narrative theorist Mark G. Kuczewski goes further than Buchanan, arguing that personal identity is not lost even in cases where Buchanan would say the patient is no longer a moral person. Kuczewski argues that a person's identity is part of the narrative identity of the group to which that person belongs: 'I conceive of myself objectively as part of a larger group that contains a "part" of me that transcends my individual consciousness and psychological continuity' (Kuczewski 1997: 135). Therefore, if the group survives, so does that person—or at least his or her interests (more of this later). Some non-narrative theorists reach a similar conclusion. Newton (1999) favors a 'bodily continuity' view of personal identity, such that persons can survive so long as their bodies do, while DeGrazia (1999) argues that we are not essentially persons, but essentially animals, and thus survive considerable disruption of psychological continuity.

[13] See also Quante (1999).

As popular as the Personal Identity Objection has been, however, it is not likely that most of its proponents truly believe that even profoundly demented or changed patients are really new persons (Kuczewski 1999: 33). Most of us judge that Grandmother, there in the ICU, is still Grandmother, even if she cannot recognize her family and her temperament and cognitive abilities are drastically different. We say that Grandmother has changed, not died—otherwise the person in the ICU would be only months or weeks old, and Grandmother's estate would be in probate (Rich 1997: 139).

The Personal Identity Objection is motivated by the fact that a patient can lose so much mental capacity that the patient's past preferences and interests seem no longer attributable to the patient. It is easy to conclude that the patient has lost those preferences and interests because he or she is now a new person, and we should not dismiss the possibility that in some unusual cases that could be true. However, in most or all actual cases it is better to say that the patient is the same person but seems to have lost his or her earlier preferences and interests by losing the capacity to understand and reaffirm them, rather than losing his or her entire identity. When one loses the capacity to comprehend one's preferences and interests, one loses the disposition to reaffirm them—and arguably thereby loses the preferences and interests themselves.[14]

4. Precedent Autonomy and Former Preferences

The Moral Authority Objection includes the claim that, when a patient is sufficiently and permanently incompetent, the patient loses his or her earlier preferences and interests. This section concerns preferences; Section 5 concerns interests.

4.1. Former Preferences

There are two questions about preferences: (1) Do advance directives express former preferences? (2) If so, how can we respect autonomy by respecting former preferences? This subsection addresses the first question; the remaining three subsections address the second.

Typically, a former preference is a preference a person once had but has since renounced. However, advance medical decision making does not easily fit this definition, for incompetent patients who made decisions in advance have not

---

[14] Dresser and Robertson effectively acknowledge this when they note that, even if personal identity persists over time, 'a person's interests may change dramatically once incompetence develops' (1989: 237 n. 1).

changed their mind—they have simply lost the mental capacity to comprehend and reaffirm their earlier preferences. If the preference has never been renounced but cannot be reaffirmed, does she still have that preference?

One can argue that the patient still has the preference provided that the patient would reaffirm if he or she could (see Savulescu and Dickenson 1998: 234; May 1997; cf. Ryle 1949). However, this move does not work in our cases, which concern permanently incompetent patients. To be *disposed* to do X, one must be *capable* of doing X. A patient who is permanently incompetent is incapable of reaffirming her earlier preference, and therefore cannot be disposed to reaffirm it. One might reply that there is a sense in which even permanently incompetent patients can regain competence, given some imaginable medical breakthrough, and therefore they retain their dispositions. However, to say that someone has a disposition to do X is to say that he or she is disposed to do so in his or her actual circumstances, not in other possible world. There is, for example, a possible world where I was raised as a devout Muslim who intends to make a pilgrimage to Mecca, but I do not have that intention—or the accompanying disposition—in this, the *actual* world. Of course, this reply requires the premise that restoring a permanently incompetent patient to competence is so radically unlikely that it cannot happen in the actual world, and this premise may be questioned: how infeasible must something be before we say it *cannot* happen in the actual world? Still, while it may be hard to say when something is effectively impossible in the actual world, we do tend to classify some incompetencies as permanent, and in the cases where we do, we must conclude that the patient lacks the disposition to reaffirm earlier preferences.

Thus, when a patient becomes permanently incompetent (to a sufficient degree), he or she loses some or all preferences. Because cases of permanent incompetence feature *former* preferences, bioethicists speak of a special kind of autonomy, called 'prospective', 'future-oriented', or 'precedent' autonomy.[15] I define 'precedent autonomy' to comprise acts of self-determination under conditions where the agent's earlier preference becomes a former preference, during at least part of the time for which it was meant to be satisfied, because the patient has lost the competence to reaffirm it.[16]

The answer to the first question about precedent autonomy is that it comprises former preferences. This brings us to the second question: Does the principle of respect for autonomy require that we respect former preferences? At first glance, it

---

[15] Some writers have spoken of 'self-paternalism' (Dresser 1982: 789), but that term is a misnomer in such cases. Paternalism involves interfering with someone's freedom for her own good; to act paternalistically toward yourself requires (among other things) doing something to yourself for your own good. However, autonomy is not necessarily about promoting one's own good; autonomous choices might promote family welfare, or religious commitments, at the expense of one's personal welfare.

[16] For an earlier, longer discussion of this issue, see Davis (2002). My arguments for this position have changed a little since then.

seems not (Savulescu and Dickenson 1998: 230); we respect someone's autonomy by respecting what that person wants, not what he or she *used* to want.

4.2. Extension View Treatments of Precedent Autonomy

Should we respect former preferences? Buchanan and Brock write as if this is not a problem:

A person can exercise self-determination not only by accepting or rejecting treatment that is now offered, but also by making decisions that will influence what is to happen in the future, when the person becomes incompetent. Consequently, following an advance directive can be viewed as a case of respecting self-determination, even if the individual has no self-determination to respect at the time the advance directive is carried out.   (Buchanan and Brock 1990: 98–9)

It is true that trying to influence one's future is an attempt at self-determination, but does it follow that respecting such earlier efforts amounts to respecting that person's autonomy *now*, after he or she 'has no self-determination to respect'? The question is not whether, at T_1, that person is attempting to exercise self-determination, but whether, at T_2, when we try to respect those earlier wishes, we thereby respect his or her self-determination—not at T_1, before we act, but at T_2, when we do act.

Nancy Rhoden

Nancy Rhoden rejects what she calls the 'objective standard', according to which we should treat the formerly competent in accord with their present welfare interests (Rhoden 1990: 846). One of Rhoden's reasons for rejecting the objective standard is that it disregards the moral authority of earlier medical treatment decisions by patients who have become permanently incompetent (to the point of having no current preferences which might compete with the earlier preferences).[17] Rhoden contends that 'Actual prior choices are an exercise of autonomy and hence deserve far more weight than informally expressed preferences... because a person who makes a living will has exercised her right to decide' (Rhoden 1990: 860).

However, according to the Moral Authority Objection, when someone is irreversibly incompetent, and therefore permanently unable to comprehend his or her earlier preferences, those preferences can no longer be attributed to that person,

---

[17]   Rhoden also rejects the objective standard on the grounds that, as a standard for withdrawing or withholding treatment, it can almost never be met except in cases of severe pain, and not every case where terminating life support is warranted fits this description. However, her main argument that some cases call for terminating life support even in the absence of severe pain is that prior preferences command respect, so I will concentrate on her positive arguments for respecting precedent autonomy, rather than her criticisms of the objective standard.

and thus we have no moral reason to respect those preferences—even if the patient has no current preferences to compete with the earlier ones. Although Rhoden does not articulate this objection, one of her arguments seems directly relevant to it. She contends that 'rejecting future-oriented choices threatens present ones' (Rhoden 1990: 856). If we reject every future-oriented choice once a patient becomes incompetent, then we will reject such choices even when they were made immediately before the patient became incompetent, and in anticipation of the incompetence itself. This means that, in cases where the patient's incompetence is reversible, we end up rejecting a person's *current* preferences, for if the incompetence is reversible, the preferences are not former ones. For example, 'a Jehovah's Witness could refuse a blood transfusion until he "bled out" and became incompetent, after which he could be transfused' (Rhoden 1990: 857). The Witness is incompetent, and according to the Moral Authority Objection the refusal should be ignored, yet the refusal seems clearly to be one we should respect. Therefore, becoming incompetent does not invalidate one's earlier preferences.

Rhoden argues that the only difference between such cases and other cases of advance medical decision making is that the preference was expressed immediately before competence was lost and treatment was indicated. However, the passage of time is irrelevant (assuming no other factors alter with time). Therefore, the treatment preferences expressed in living wills should be respected. Rhoden concludes that 'present autonomy and precedent autonomy are simply two ends of a continuum', and that 'rejecting precedent autonomy threatens a fairly broad spectrum of present, prior, and mixed present/prior choices' (Rhoden 1990: 857). Let us call this the Continuum Argument.

However, to refute the Moral Authority Objection, this case would have to involve former preferences, not current ones—and that requires *ir*reversible incompetence. If the Witness's incompetence were medically irreversible, then the preference announced in his living will would be a former one. Here, the Witness's incompetence *is* reversible, so he retains both the capacity and the disposition to refuse blood transfusions.[18] Therefore, his preference against being transfused is not a former preference even when he is unconscious. Proponents of the Moral Authority Objection do not deny that current preferences should be respected, and would doubtless agree that the Witness's refusal should be respected even while he is unconscious. Because the case which supports the Continuum Argument does not concern former preferences, it does not refute the Moral Authority Objection.

---

[18] The Jehovah's Witness's incompetence can be reversed only if he is transfused. If we honor his wishes and do not transfuse him, he will never regain competence. However, this does not make his incompetence irreversible. The fact that regaining competence requires acting against the patient's preference does not mean that he cannot regain competence—only that it is not possible to honor his wishes and simultaneously restore him to competence. *His incompetence is reversible even if it is never reversed.* Thus, this is not a case of permanent incompetence and former preferences.

Soft Paternalism

Understanding that precedent autonomy involves former preferences also under-mines the possibility of defending the Extension View on soft paternalist grounds. Although not prominently discussed in bioethics writings on precedent autonomy, a soft paternalist strategy is worth considering. Soft paternalism consists of inter-fering with someone's liberty either to ascertain whether he or she is informed and rational, or on the ground that he or she is not both informed and rational, and that we are doing what that person would want if he or she *were* informed and rational. One could argue that, even if a patient does not currently have the preference expressed in his or her advance directive, we should treat the patient in accord with the advance directive on the grounds that the patient really does want what he or she earlier wanted, but does not realize it because his or her mental capacity is impaired. However, a soft paternalist defense of the Extension View runs into the same problem that confronts Rhoden. An agent does not 'truly' want a thing if he or she no longer wants it at all. If he or she truly wants that thing, the preference is not a former one (Just not fully understood right now).

Ronald Dworkin

Dworkin, another proponent of the Extension View, coined the phrase 'precedent autonomy' for cases where the patient is incompetent 'in the general, overall sense' and 'lacks the necessary capacity for a fresh exercise of autonomy' (Dworkin 1993: 226–7). To show why we should respect precedent autonomy, Dworkin poses another Jehovah's Witness case. This time the Witness suffers a medical crisis which impairs his competence, and he asks to be transfused. His earlier preference not to be transfused is a former preference, and he acquired his current preference in a state of incompetence. Which preference should we respect? 'Suppose we were confident that the deranged Witness, were he to receive the transfusion and live, would become competent again and be appalled . . . In those circumstances, I believe, we would violate his autonomy by giving him the transfusion.' Presumably most of us agree, and, according to Dworkin, this judgment implies that we believe some former preferences should be respected, so long as no current preference, formed while competent, overrules the former preference (Dworkin 1993: 227).

However, Dworkin runs into the same problem as Rhoden and the soft paternalist approach, for, despite his disclaimer, his case involves a current preference, not a former one. He declares that 'this is not like a case in which someone who objects to a given treatment is unconscious when he needs it', but also stipulates that the Witness will regain competence once he is transfused (1993: 227). In fact, this *is* like a case where the patient is temporarily unconscious, for this patient will recover once transfused. The only difference is that, unlike an unconscious patient, Dworkin's Witness now has a current incompetent preference to be transfused. Because Dworkin's Witness is temporarily incompetent, he has not lost his earlier preference against being transfused, any more than a temporarily unconscious patient would. Most advance directive cases, however, involve permanent incompetence. Dworkin's argument works only if one makes the same judgment in an altered version of his case where the Witness *is* permanently 'deranged', and he will *never* be 'appalled' at what we have done. That is quite a different case, and exactly the kind of case where Dresser, Robertson, and many medical professionals are inclined to say we should *not* respect the patient's former preferences, but should promote his or her current welfare instead.

4.3. Narrative Approaches to Precedent Autonomy

Many bioethicists reject the Extension View in favor of a narrative approach to understanding end-of-life decision making. This approach fits less easily with the two questions about precedent autonomy raised above, but we can use those questions to highlight how the narrative approach differs from other approaches.

Although proponents of the narrative approach trace it to chapter 15 of Alasdair MacIntyre's *After Virtue*, Howard Brody is probably its best-known bioethics advocate.[19] The basic idea is that lives can be seen as stories, with story-like structures. The metaphor of life as a narrative fits nicely with the substituted judgment principle of surrogate decision making, for, according to the narrative approach, the surrogate is to make the decision that best continues the themes of the patient's life narrative (Brody 2003: 254; Blustein 1999: 20). If, for example, the patient was always a strong-willed, independent individual who valued a physically active life, then her life story is better concluded by a chapter in which she dies of natural causes without delay, than by a chapter in which she is kept alive for years in a state of deep incompetence on a ventilator and feeding tube.

However, proponents of this approach believe it does more than explicate substituted judgment. They believe it highlights features of end-of-life decision making that tend to be obscured by a more simplistic picture of well-informed, decisive, self-reliant agents planning their own future care. Mark G. Kuczewski (1999) cites studies that suggest that surrogates are not very good at discerning what people would want when they are incompetent, and argues that surrogates should try instead to determine what decision best fits the themes, values, and overall direction of a patient's life (Kuczewski 1999: 34). Brody argues that people do not always want to be sole authors of their own life stories, or at least not the final chapter. Brody claims (citing other studies) that people want close relatives to make end-of-life decisions for them as seems best when the time comes, and

---

[19] Outside the bioethics and narrative literature, David Velleman (1991) has developed a rigorous account of how the narrative structure of a life contributes to its overall value, using a series of thought-experiments to demonstrate that we tend to believe that how much value a given episode contributes to a life depends in part on when that episode occurs within that life (Velleman 1991).

that the narrative approach better accommodates this (Brody 2003: 257). Jeffrey Blustein believes that the narrative approach shows how to respect the autonomy of someone who never worked out a clear plan for his future: continue the story, even if that person never expressly decided how this should be done (Blustein 1999: 24).

The narrative approach is an important reminder that not everyone exercises precedent autonomy over his or her future. For the many who do not—who prefer instead that close family members make the decision for them, or that the surrogate simply decide in accord with the spirit of their life, or who have not considered end-of-life issues at all—the narrative approach provides a more sophisticated model for surrogate decision making than simply asking what the patient would now want if he or she could tell us.

However, for patients who *do* try to control their own future medical treatment, the narrative approach seems less of a fit. Such agents are their own authors, and when they succeed in clearly stating preferences that are relevant to their later circumstances, they leave little discretion to end-of-life editors. For this reason, the narrative approach simply does not address whether an earlier preference is still attributable to a now-incompetent patient, or whether former preferences command our respect just as current preferences do. As discussed earlier, Kuczewski has argued, on narrative grounds, that a permanently incompetent patient is the same person as his earlier self, but again, personal identity is not the real issue here: the real issue is the persistence of preferences.

Nor is it clear what moral reason we have to treat an incompetent patient so as to best continue and finish the themes of his or her life story. If the reason is to respect the patient's autonomous wishes that his or her life story be continued in that manner, then we are back to respect for precedent autonomy and the questions it raises: Is the patient's preference to live according to those themes and patterns still attributable to him or her, and if not, why should we respect it? If the moral reason for continuing (or ending) that life story so as to achieve good narrative fit has nothing to do with respecting the patient's autonomy, what *is* the moral reason for doing so?

One could argue that the narrative approach is a way of promoting the patient's best interest. If so, then the narrative approach might be paired with the Moral Authority Objection, and offered as a sophisticated best interests alternative to the Extension View. This requires the claim that what continues the narrative themes and patterns of a life coincides with what is best for a patient. However, that may not always be true. Some people live self-destructive or careless lives, or live to promote causes other than their own welfare.

One could also argue that narratively well-structured lives have a kind of aesthetic or moral value in their own right (as any good narrative does), and that that value gives us reason to be careful how we finish those narratives. However, if that is the moral reason to make end-of-life decisions in a narratively inspired way, then more needs to be said about the moral value of such life narratives—especially lives that are poorly written, leaving them disjointed or directionless. Some lives, after all, lack significant meaning, or are self-destructive. A life may be a tragedy, or a farce. The best ending to a life may be redemptive precisely by *not* continuing its themes.

4.4. An Argument for Respecting Former Preferences

In this subsection I offer an argument that, under the right circumstances, we *do* have a moral duty to give people what they *used* to want.[20]

The expressions of autonomy we must respect are not just *any* desires or leanings, but those the agent decides or prefers to see fulfilled. This is an issue when someone has two or more conflicting preferences on a given issue. When that happens, what that person prefers, all things considered, is the preference he or she prefers to satisfy above others it conflicts with. I call the preferences which cannot be jointly satisfied 'conflicting preferences', and the preference for resolving the conflict by satisfying one of them at the expense of the other a 'resolution preference'. To respect that person's autonomy, we must respect his or her resolution preference. That person formed the resolution preference by considering his or her other preferences on that issue. Therefore, that person's resolution preference is a choice among conflicting preferences, and to respect his or her autonomy, we must respect the resolution preference.

If resolution preferences were always current preferences, we would have no reason to believe that former preferences should ever be respected. It may seem that resolution preferences *are* always current preferences. After all, to form a resolution preference, one must be aware of two conflicting preferences. For one to be aware of both conflicting preferences, those preferences must exist before or at the time one is aware of them, and thus a resolution preference must exist simultaneously with or later than the conflicting preferences it adjudicates among. Therefore, it seems that resolution preferences must always be among one's current preferences, and can never be former preferences. When the conflicting preferences exist at different times, typically a resolution preference exists at the same time as the later conflicting preference (how else would one know about both conflicting preferences?), and favors the later one over the earlier one.

However, in some cases where the conflicting preferences exist at different times, the resolution preference is not a current preference, but another former preference, usually contemporary with the former conflicting preference. This will happen when the patient's competence declines substantially over time, and later in life he or she lacks the competence to comprehend both conflicting preferences, and at that time cannot form a resolution preference concerning their conflict. Earlier, however, the patient could comprehend both conflicting preferences, and

----

[20] For a longer exposition of this argument, see Davis (2004).

choose between them. Precedent autonomy cases concern people with declining competence—their decreased competence prevents them from having a later resolution preference to conflict with their former resolution preference; what they prefer, all things considered, is satisfaction of the former conflicting preference. This account of conflicting and resolution preferences fits a hierarchical theory of the will (Frankfurt 1971),[21] as well as nonhierarchical theories of the will, such as Gary Watson's discussion of an agent's judgment about whether a desire should be satisfied (Watson 1975: 217).

One might object that we cannot respect a former preference any more than we can vote in an election after the polls have closed. However, it is easy to respect an agent's former preference; we do it the same way we respect or have relations with other things that exist only in the past. Every February we celebrate Abraham Lincoln's birthday. To respect a former preference we simply stay out of the way when it is being fulfilled, or help to fulfill it if we have a duty to do so. The fulfillment or assistance occurs after that preference has become a former preference. The fact that the former preference is no longer attributable to someone does not mean that respecting that preference does not constitute respecting his or her autonomy.

The reason why it seems that we do not respect an agent's autonomy by respecting his or her former preference is that, in most cases involving a former preference, the agent also has a current preference that conflicts with the former one, and a tacit resolution preference favoring satisfaction of the current preference over any conflicting former preferences. If we respect the former preference, we thereby disrespect the current preference and violate the agent's right of autonomy. However, what violates the agent's autonomy is not that we respected a former preference, but that we failed to respect a current preference. The reason why failing to respect the current preference violates the agent's right of autonomy is that a current preference is usually coupled with awareness of the former preference, and is therefore accompanied by a tacit resolution preference favoring satisfaction of the current preference over the former preference. However, this is not true in cases of a permanent, substantial decline in competence.

This argument also provides a way to respond to Derek Parfit's objection that it is absurd to give the satisfaction of past desires equal weight with the satisfaction of present desires: 'When I was young, I most wanted to be a poet... Now that I am older, I have lost this desire... [The proponent of temporal neutrality] must... claim that I have a strong reason to try to write poems now, because this was what I most wanted for so many years... Most of us would find this claim

---

[21] There is some controversy over whether hierarchical models of the will can explain free will or personhood, as they are meant to. However, the moral authority of advance directives does not require an explanation of these topics; for our purposes any model of conflicting desires will do, provided it allows us to say that, when someone has two or more conflicting preferences, and that person autonomously prefers to resolve that conflict in a particular way, we respect his or her autonomy by not interfering with (or assisting, if duty-bound to do so) his or her efforts to resolve that conflict.

hard to believe' (Parfit 1984: 157). It is absurd only if there is a current desire (or preference) which conflicts with the past desire (or preference) and there is no resolution preference to select between them. That is the usual case, but not always. In the poet case, the older man has no current preference to write poems, and thus has a current preference to use his time in other ways. Moreover, he is aware of both his past and his current preferences on this issue, and has a resolution preference favoring the current preference. In the cases I have in mind, the patient had an earlier resolution preference favoring his or her earlier treatment preference.

Here is the argument that the principle of respect for autonomy sometimes applies to former preferences:

(1) When a person has conflicting preferences on an issue, and a third, resolution preference favoring one conflicting preference over the other, respect for autonomy requires respecting the resolution preference.

(2) In cases where the person's competence declines over time, sometimes the resolution preference is a former preference, existing at the same time as the conflicting former preference.

(3) It is possible to respect a person's autonomy by respecting his or her former preferences.

(4) Therefore, when there is a former resolution preference favoring an earlier conflicting preference over a later conflicting preference, respecting autonomy requires respecting the former resolution preference and the conflicting former preference it favors.

5. SURVIVING INTERESTS

The Mill–Feinberg picture of autonomy includes both preferences and interests. In Section 4 we discussed whether patients retain their preferences after they become too incompetent to comprehend them, and whether we should respect former preferences. This section concerns the other half of the Extension View: the claim that the interests over which people have a right of self-determination survive into the future. If such interests do not survive, then precedent autonomy does not command respect, for we have no right of self-determination over things in which we lack the appropriate interest.

5.1. Why Investment Interests Might Not Survive

We must be clear about what kinds of interests are said to survive. Although the terminology varies, many philosophers distinguish between what we may call 'investment interests' and 'welfare interests' (Regan 1983: 87–8). You have welfare interests in things that are good for you whether or not you value them, like good vision, a healthy diet, or avoiding pain. Because these interests do not depend on the holder valuing their objects, losing the capacity to care about them should not affect their survival; even severely incompetent patients retain such interests. 'Investment interests', by contrast, are created when a person invests effort and concern in something—for example, affirming and living in accord with a conception of personal dignity that requires independence and activity—and cease to exist when he or she ceases to care about that thing. Advance directives typically concern investment interests in things like personal dignity, religious commitments, the welfare of one's family, and the like. A surviving interest—if such things exist—is an investment interest that requires a certain psychological capacity to create, which the holder never renounced, and which survives a loss of the capacity to care about it.

Rebecca Dresser and John Robertson question the existence of surviving interests in such things as dignity and privacy. Dresser contends that 'the interests of demented patients might differ from those they had as competent persons . . . when people become demented and physically debilitated, what was once important to them often is forgotten, while physical comfort and what we might view as low-level interactions with people and their environments often become vitally significant' (Dresser 1992: 75–6; see also Robertson 1991: 7).

Dresser's argument is highly elliptical, but we can reconstruct it by noting that an investment interest might cease to affect your well-being because you cease to care about its object. We lose investment interests when we cease to care about them, and if an interest cannot survive a loss of *concern*, then it cannot survive a loss of the *capacity* for concern. Therefore, an investment interest cannot survive a loss of the mental capacity necessary for creating that interest and continuing to care about its object. Call this the Argument from Loss of Concern.

There is an argument for surviving interests that begins with the premise that many of us believe some interests survive death. As Joel Feinberg puts it, 'we can think of some of a person's interests as surviving his death, just as some of the debts and claims of his estate do' (1986: 83). Allen Buchanan and Dan Brock argue that, if interests can survive death, surely they can survive lesser losses, like dementia or permanent unconsciousness (Buchanan and Brock 1990: 162–3). Let us call this the Argument from Interests that Survive Death.[22]

Both the Argument from Loss of Concern and the Argument from Interests that Survive Death trade on the relations between three things: loss of *concern* about the interest, loss of *capacity* for concern about the interest, and loss of life. According to the Argument from Loss of Concern, a loss of capacity for concern is relevantly similar to loss of concern itself, so that if interests cannot survive a loss of concern,

---

[22] Ronald Dworkin believes that investment interests can survive incompetence, but provides no argument for this claim (1993: 222–37).

they cannot survive a loss of capacity. According to the Argument from Interests that Survive Death, a loss of capacity for concern is relevantly similar to death, and if interests can survive death, they can survive a loss of capacity. In the next subsection I present a different argument for surviving interests.[23]

5.2. How Investment Interests Can Survive

The first step in arguing for surviving interests is to understand that investment interests are not metaphysical entities that exist independently of our moral judgments. They are simply a figure of speech used to say that we believe that a certain state of affairs has a certain moral valence because of its relation to what someone has cared about. Having an investment interest does involve psychological states which we often express by saying that someone is 'interested' in such and such, but the investment interest itself is not a psychological state, but a way of summarizing our moral judgments about how we should behave concerning the objects of such states. Therefore, our moral judgments about states of affairs where someone has cared in a certain way about something is a good test of whether his or her investment interest in that thing has survived.

So consider this case: A patient suffers some condition that leaves her permanently unconscious but without brain damage, and current medical science cannot cure this condition. Suppose further that she is (yet) another Jehovah's Witness, and that her doctor gives her a blood transfusion even though he knows she opposed them on religious grounds. A year later a cure is discovered and she wakes up—outraged at what he did.

Most readers probably share the judgment that it was wrong to transfuse her. There are many plausible judgments of this kind; for example, it seems a wrong—to *her*— to slander her even though her unconsciousness is permanent in light of current medical science. But what feature of this case makes the transfusion wrong? The doctor made no promise, nor (as I tell the story) assumed any contractual or other duty not to transfuse her. Her later outrage did not make his action wrong, for several reasons. First, the judgment is that, at the time of acting, it *is* wrong, not that there is a slim chance that it might later *become* (retroactively) wrong. Second, she was outraged because she was wronged; it was not wrong because she was outraged, otherwise her outrage would be justified by her outrage (a strange sort of wrong). Third, if it was wrong because she later recovered and became outraged, then it would be ethical for doctors to transfuse Jehovah's Witnesses provided the Witnesses never find out. The fact that her condition later became curable and she recovered makes it easier to see that her doctor's action was wrong, but if it was wrong when he did it, it would have been wrong even if medicine had

---

[23] There is a longer version of this argument in Davis (2006).

never discovered a cure for her disease. The best explanation of why it was wrong to transfuse her is that her interest in avoiding transfusions survived her sleeping disease, for again, saying that someone has an investment interest in something is simply a way of summarizing the moral judgment that it would be wrong to treat that thing in a way that would bother that person if he or she knew we did it.

The sleeping disease case reveals something important about the conditions for investment interest survival: It *is* possible, in a certain sense of possibility, for permanent conditions to change, no matter how unlikely that may be. The kind of possibility involved in suggesting that a permanent condition might not be permanent after all is very loose; 'medical' possibility will not do. There are two suitable kinds of possibility in this case. First, it is 'logically' possible for her to recover from permanent unconsciousness, for regaining competence would not violate the constraints of formal logic or other metaphysical limits on how the universe can be. Second, it is 'nomologically' possible, for regaining competence would not violate the laws of the natural world or the constraints science tells us govern the universe. Because both kinds of possibility are present in cases of permanent incompetence, and because logical possibility is broader than needed for an argument that interests can survive, let us say that an interest can survive provided it is nomologically possible for the person who holds that interest to recover the mental capacity necessary to care about the object of that interest. Moreover, it does survive if, were he or she to recover the necessary capacity, he or she would care about it. Thus, it would be wrong to transfuse (or slander, etc.) this person even if medical science never discovers a cure for her sleeping disease. I call this the Argument from Sleep.

This case differs from Dworkin's case in two ways. First, our Witness is permanently incompetent, or as permanently as anyone can be without massive brain damage (more of this later). Second, this case has a different argumentative purpose. Dworkin's case was meant to show that we should respect former preferences—a conclusion I have argued for on very different grounds. This case is used, instead, to show that we believe that investment interests survive so long as it is still nomologically possible for the interest holder to regain competence.

Both interests and preferences are dispositional in nature. However, whether one has a given preference in one's actual circumstances depends on one's disposition in one's actual circumstances, not in some other possible world; this is why permanent incompetence creates *former* preferences. Interests, by contrast, depend on one's dispositions in the nomologically possible world where regaining the capacity to care is possible. The argument for interest survival is not that people retain their dispositions to care in their actual circumstances, but that it is nomologically possible for their circumstances to change such that they *could* be so disposed.

(Defining the relevant counterfactual is a task beyond this chapter, but, roughly speaking, it will be the *closest* possible world in which competence can be regained.) It is not surprising that preferences and interests differ on these points, for preferences are psychological entities, while investment interests are moral entities whose survival turns on moral judgments.

How the Argument from Sleep Relates to Loss of Concern and Interests that Survive Death

The Argument from Interests that Survive Death requires the premise that interests survive death while my argument does not. As for the Argument from Loss of Concern, my argument enables us to draw a convincing distinction between loss of concern and loss of capacity for concern. My argument shows that interests survive if, assuming it is nomologically possible, the holder would affirm the interest if he or she regained the capacity to do so. This is how to distinguish between loss of concern and loss of capacity: When the holder loses concern, the holder will not affirm the former interest even though he or she has the capacity to do so, whereas when the holder loses capacity, the holder may or may not affirm the former interest if he or she regains capacity. That is why an interest can survive a loss of capacity even though it cannot survive a loss of concern.

6. CONCLUSION

Like ordinary personal autonomy, the autonomy expressed in advance directives is grounded in suitable preferences and interests. Most defenders of the moral authority of advance directives have claimed or assumed that the preferences expressed in advance directives are still attributable to the now-incompetent patient, or that the patient is still the same person (and therefore, presumably, has the same preferences). This defense fails, however, for even if the patient is the same person, a sufficient loss of mental capacity transforms the patient's earlier preferences into former preferences. After reviewing arguments that overlook this fact, and assessing Dworkin's argument that we should respect former preferences, I have offered a different argument that sometimes we have a moral duty to respect former preferences. As for interests, critics of advance directives have often viewed investment interests the same way they view preferences. After reviewing arguments for and against surviving interests, I have offered an argument that some investment interests, unlike preferences, *can* survive a loss of mental capacity.

I have not addressed the practical problems facing advance directives or the substituted judgment principle. I have tried, however, to show that the Moral Authority Objection to the Extension View is no reason to give up on those problems.

References

BEAUCHAMP, T. L., and CHILDRESS, J. F. (2001), *Principles of Biomedical Ethics*, 5th edn. (New York: Oxford University Press).

BLUSTEIN, J. (1999), 'Choosing for Others as Continuing a Life Story: The Problem of Personal Identity Revisited', *Journal of Law, Medicine and Ethics*, 27: 20–31.

BRODY, H. (2003), *Stories of Sickness*, 2nd edn. (New York: Oxford University Press).

BUCHANAN, A. E. (1988), 'Advance Directives and the Personal Identity Problem', *Philosophy and Public Affairs*, 17/4: 277–302.

―― and BROCK, D. W. (1990), *Deciding for Others: The Ethics of Surrogate Decision Making* (Cambridge: Cambridge University Press).

CANTOR, N. L. (1993), *Advance Directives and the Pursuit of Death with Dignity* (Bloomington: Indiana University Press).

DAVIS, J. K. (2002), 'The Concept of Precedent Autonomy', *Bioethics*, 16/2: 114–33.

―― (2004), 'Precedent Autonomy and Subsequent Consent', *Ethical Theory and Moral Practice*, 7/3: 267–91.

―― (2006), 'Surviving Interests and Living Wills', *Public Affairs Quarterly*, 20/1: 17–30.

DEGRAZIA, D. (1999), 'Advance Directives, Dementia, and "the Someone Else Problem"', *Bioethics*, 13/5: 373–91.

DRESSER, R. S. (1982), 'Ulysses and the Psychiatrists: A Legal and Policy Analysis of the Voluntary Commitment Contract', *Harvard Civil Liberties Law Review* (Winter), 789.

―― (1986), 'Life, Death, and Incompetent Patients: Conceptual Infirmities and Hidden Values in the Law', *Arizona Law Review*, 28: 373–405.

―― (1992), 'Autonomy Revisited: The Limits of Anticipatory Choices', in R. H. Binstock, S. G. Post, and P. J. Whitehouse (eds.), *Dementia and Aging: Ethics, Values, and Policy Choices* (Baltimore: Johns Hopkins University Press), 71–85.

―― and ASTROW, A. B. (1998), 'An Alert and Incompetent Self: The Irrelevance of Advance Directives, Commentaries', *Hastings Center Report*, 28/1: 28–30.

―― and ROBERTSON, J. A. (1989), 'Quality of Life and Non-Treatment Decisions for Incompetent Patients: A Critique of the Orthodox Approach', *Law, Medicine and Health Care*, 17/3: 234–44.

DWORKIN, R. (1993), *Life's Dominion* (New York: Knopf).

EISENDRATH, S. J., and JONSEN, A. R. (1983), 'The Living Will: Help or Hindrance?', *Journal of the American Medical Association*, 249/15: 2055–6.

FEINBERG, J. (1986), *Harm to Self* (Oxford: Oxford University Press).

FRANKFURT, H. G. (1971), 'Freedom of the Will and the Concept of a Person', *Journal of Philosophy*, 68/1: 5–20.

FURROW, B. R., *et al.* (2000), *Health Law*, 2nd edn. (St Paul, Minn.: West Group).

JONSEN, A. R., VEATCH, R. M., and WALTERS, L. (eds.) (1998), *Source Book in Bioethics* (Washington, DC: Georgetown University Press).

KING, N. M. P. (1996), *Making Sense of Advance Directives*, rev. edn. (Washington, DC: Georgetown University Press).

KUCZEWSKI, M. G. (1994), 'Whose Will Is It Anyway? A Discussion of Advance Directives, Personal Identity, and Consensus in Medical Ethics', *Bioethics*, 8/1: 27–48.

—— (1997), *Fragmentation and Consensus: Communitarian and Casuist Bioethics* (Washington, DC: Georgetown University Press).

—— (1999), 'Commentary: Narrative Views of Personal Identity and Substituted Judgment in Surrogate Decision Making', *Journal of Law, Medicine and Ethics*, 27/1: 32–6.

LYNN, J., *et al.* (1999), 'Dementia and Advance-Care Planning: Perspectives from Three Countries on Ethics and Epidemiology', *Journal of Clinical Ethics*, 10/4: 271–85.

MacINTYRE, A. (1984), *After Virtue: A Study in Moral Theory*, 2nd edn. (Notre Dame, Ind.: University of Notre Dame Press).

MAY, T. (1997), 'Reassessing the Reliability of Advance Directives', *Cambridge Healthcare Quarterly*, 6/3: 325–38.

MILL, J. S. (1986), *On Liberty* (Buffalo, NY: Prometheus Books).

NEWTON, M. J. (1999), 'Precedent Autonomy: Life-Sustaining Intervention and the Demented Patient', *Cambridge Healthcare Quarterly*, 8/2: 189–99.

O'NEILL, O. (2002), *Autonomy and Trust in Bioethics* (Cambridge: Cambridge University Press).

PARFIT, D. (1984), *Reasons and Persons* (Oxford: Oxford University Press).

PRESIDENT'S COMMISSION FOR THE STUDY OF ETHICAL PROBLEMS IN MEDICINE AND BIOMEDICAL AND BEHAVIORAL RESEARCH (1983), 'Deciding to Forgo Life-Sustaining Treatment: A Report on the Ethical, Medical, and Legal Issues in Treatment Decisions', repr. in Jonsen (1998: 159–219).

QUANTE, M. (1999), 'Precedent Autonomy and Personal Identity', *Kennedy Institute of Ethics Journal*, 9/4: 365–81.

REGAN, T. (1983), *The Case for Animal Rights* (Berkeley: University of California Press).

RHODEN, N. K. (1990), 'The Limits of Legal Objectivity', *North Carolina Law Review*, 68: 845–65.

RICH, B. A. (1997), 'Prospective Autonomy and Critical Interests: A Narrative Defense of the Moral Authority of Advance Directives', *Cambridge Quarterly of Healthcare Ethics*, 6/2: 138–47.

ROBERTSON, J. A. (1991), 'Second Thoughts on Living Wills', *Hastings Center Report*, 21/6: 6–9.

RYLE, G. (1949), *The Concept of Mind* (London: Hutchinson).

SASS, H., VEATCH, R. M., and KIMURA, R. (1998), *Advance Directives and Surrogate Decision Making in Health Care* (Baltimore: Johns Hopkins University Press).

SAVULESCU, J., and DICKENSON, D. (1998), 'The Time Frame of Preferences, Dispositions, and the Validity of Advance Directives for the Mentally Ill', *Philosophy, Psychiatry and Psychology*, 5/3: 225–46.

SCHNEIDER, C. (1998), *The Practice of Autonomy: Patients, Doctors, and Medical Decisions* (Oxford: Oxford University Press).

SUPPORT PRINCIPAL INVESTIGATORS (1995), 'A Controlled Trial to Improve Care for Seriously Ill Hospitalized Patients: The Study to Understand Prognoses and Preferences for Outcomes and Risks of Treatments (SUPPORT)', *JAMA* 274/20: 1591–8.

VEATCH, R. M. (1993), 'The Impending Collapse of the Whole-Brain Definition of Death', *Hastings Center Report*, 23/4: 18–24.

VELLEMAN, J. D. (1991), 'Well-Being and Time', *Pacific Philosophical Quarterly*, 72/1: 48–77.
WATSON, G. (1975), 'Free Agency', *Journal of Philosophy*, 72/8: 205–20.
WOLF, S. M., *et al.* (1991), 'Sources of Concern About the Patient Self-Determination Act', *New England Journal of Medicine*, 325/23: 1666–71.

CHAPTER 16

PHYSICIAN-ASSISTED DEATH: THE STATE OF THE DEBATE

GERALD DWORKIN

When I first began writing on the topic of physician-assisted suicide and active voluntary euthanasia it seemed to me that the philosophical literature was unlike that of most other controversial topics, e.g. abortion, cloning, etc. On those topics there was much debate about the moral status of individual acts, as well as discussion of the social policy issues that tended to rely on predictions about future consequences. But as regards physician-assisted suicide there seemed to be general consensus that at least with respect to individual acts of physician-assisted suicide there could be occasions on which it was morally permissible. I am aware, of course, of the existence of a large non-philosophical literature that argued that all killing of innocent persons (whether consensual or not) is wrong. But among philosophers writing from a secular perspective that conclusion seemed not to be accepted.

Almost all of the discussion centered on the policy and institutional issues. Should physician-assisted suicide and/or active voluntary euthanasia be legalized? Should codes of conduct allow physician-assisted suicide? And the discussion of these issues was largely consequentialist in nature. People's views differed according to whether they believed that things would be horrible or not if we legalized physician-assisted suicide. Much was made of the only data we had, which was from the Netherlands, and that data was read in optimistic or pessimistic ways. Why nobody paid attention to the Swiss, who had legalized physician-assisted suicide for some time, is a mystery.

It also seemed to be an issue that promised little new by way of theoretical issues. The themes of intended versus foreseen consequences, killing versus letting die, the principle of double effect, had been pretty well worked over. There were still epicycles that could be introduced, as Frances Kamm has done with respect to both double effect (her idea of triple effect) and the significance of cases where everything is held constant and we judge that killing is no worse than letting die.

It was not simply that it was very unlikely that introducing some new way of looking at the problem (comparable, for example, to Thomson's take on abortion) was going to affect the policy debate. It did not seem that relevant considerations were likely to generate new ideas of intrinsic philosophical interest. This no longer seems to be the case. There are a number of interesting problems and issues that need to be further explored. I shall first set out what I take to be the current state of discussion on the topic and then present a budget of problems that deserve further investigation.

THE CURRENT STATE OF THE DEBATE

The essential outlines of the debate over voluntary euthanasia have not changed very much since Glanville Williams and Yale Kamisar debated the issues almost fifty years ago. On the one hand, an appeal to considerations of autonomy and the relief of suffering: individuals should be able to choose the timing and mode of their dying and they should not have to suffer from pain and other modes of indignity such as incontinence, paralysis, muscular wastage, and mental deterioration. So far these would only generate a right or permission to take one's own life, but when we consider the problems in the context of end-of-life medical care and the uncontroversial duty of physicians to relieve the suffering of their patients we get a claim to assistance in dying. The claim may be only to the assistance of a willing physician with perhaps a derived claim to referral to a willing physician if the physician as a matter of conscience cannot participate. Or it may be to an obligation on the part of the physician if the mode of relief is the administration of pain-relief medication—even if the physician knows that eventually this will result in the death of the patient. (Would we regard it as acceptable for a physician to invoke a 'conscience clause' and refuse to administer morphine under such circumstances?)

Those who opposed physician-assisted suicide do not generally deny the value of autonomy and the relief of suffering. Many, but not all, even concede that in particular cases a physician would be justified in providing a patient with the knowledge or means for them to take their own life. Yale Kamisar, for example, a strong opponent of legalizing physician-assisted suicide, said that if he were convinced that someone was terminally ill, suffering from intolerable pain that could not be relieved, were competent, and requested death, he would 'hate to have to argue that the hand of death should be stayed' (Kamisar 1958: 975). But opponents believe that there are a number of different considerations, usually of a consequentialist nature, that lead to the conclusion that, important as the values of autonomy and relief of suffering are, they cannot justify the institutionalization or legalization of physician-assisted suicide. These considerations include the possibility of discovery of cures, the dangers of mistaken diagnosis, the difficulties of knowing when requesters are rational, the dangers of patients being coerced or pressured by relatives or by their physicians, and the effects of legalization on the doctor–patient relationship. In addition, there are the slippery slope arguments: physician-assisted suicide will lead to active voluntary euthanasia and this in turn to involuntary euthanasia. Physician-assisted suicide for the terminally ill will be extended to those who are suffering whether or not they are terminal. Physician-assisted suicide, which requires contemporaneous consent, will lead to physician-assisted suicide by means of advance directives. Given that the number of patients who need assistance in dying and who meet the usual conditions (terminal, non-relievable suffering, competence, wishing to die) is small, and given the seriousness of the dangers, physician-assisted suicide should not be legalized.

Given the uncontroversial nature of the values invoked by supporters of physician-assisted suicide, their moral arguments are usually attempts to show that the arguments of the opponents are faulty rather than to present positive arguments in favor of physician-assisted suicide. And the attempts to show the inadequacy of the opponent's arguments are usually *ad hominem*. I don't mean any disparagement by that term; much of moral argument is *ad hominem* and no worse for that. I mean that the argument takes the form of claiming that those who oppose physician-assisted suicide are inconsistent. They favor various policies such as the administering of pain medication that leads to the death of the patient, or they favor withdrawing life-support at the (competent) patient's request, or they favor DNR orders, or they favor terminal sedation (putting a patient into a coma and then withdrawing food and water). The proponent of physician-assisted suicide presents arguments that claim to show that there is no way of distinguishing between these (favored) policies and physician-assisted suicide. So one cannot both favor these policies and reject physician-assisted suicide. The opponents of physician-assisted suicide must either accept physician-assisted suicide or reject the favored policies. The argument is *ad hominem* because it does not seek to show that the opponents must accept physician-assisted suicide. They may instead abandon their favored policies. So the arguments do not establish physician-assisted suicide. They merely show that the opponents must give something or other up. That is why the arguments are *ad hominem*; they are addressed only to people who accept certain premises, e.g. that the favored policies are permissible. Someone who starts out by having no views about, for example, terminal sedation, or who actually thinks it impermissible is unaffected by these arguments.

Since it is, as a matter of fact, the case that most physicians favor the policies in question, and indeed the right of a competent patient to decline medical treatment (including food and water), even if death is inevitable as a result, is firmly entrenched in the legal system, the dialectic of the opponents is to dispute the claim that there is no way of distinguishing the favored policies from physician-assisted suicide. This is where the various hoary distinctions of killing versus letting die, intending versus foreseeing, doing versus allowing, make their appearance. The opponents of physician-assisted suicide claim that these distinctions are (1) real distinctions and (2) morally relevant, and that the favored policies fall on one side of the distinction whereas physician-assisted suicide falls on the other. To this the proponents either deny that the distinctions exist, or that they are morally relevant, or that they distinguish physician-assisted suicide from the favored policies.

With respect to the legalization issues, the arguments are, for the most part, questions about the nature and quality of the evidence for the potential dangers and harms. It is, or should be, recognized by all that it is not enough to claim that some danger might come from physician-assisted suicides, or that it could happen. That claim is far too weak to establish that some morally permissible action should not be allowed by the legal system. (Even defenders of what has been called the 'precautionary principle' do not think that the mere logical possibility of some ecological disaster is a reason for not acting in some way.) On the other hand, it is too strong to demand that the dangers are certain or inevitable. After all, a possibility less than a half of a very serious danger may be quite enough to worry about. What has to be argued is not that the disasters are possible, or inevitable, but that their probability (given their degree of harm) is serious enough to justify making an otherwise permissible act illegal. And, of course, it is not their probability given legalization, but their probability given legalization *with* the safeguards proposed by the defenders of legalization.

So the debate has focused on the meager database of the Netherlands and Oregon. The former has played a larger role because of the greater number of cases and the scrutiny to which it has been exposed. If anything is clear from this discussion, it is that the interpretation of the data is highly correlated with the normative position of the investigator. If the investigator is strongly opposed to physician-assisted suicide, it is highly likely that he will think the fact that some 900 persons were killed or allowed to die without explicit request shows that the dangers are not merely possible but real. If the investigator is highly favorable to physician-assisted suicide, then it will be pointed out that in most of these cases the patients would have died very shortly thereafter, that these cases include patients who had made preliminary requests for euthanasia and then gone into comas, or had otherwise become incompetent to renew their request, and that many of these cases involved the withholding or withdrawal of medical care rather than either physician-assisted suicide or active voluntary euthanasia. In any case, as Kuhse and Singer (1988) have pointed out, since we have no reliable statistics for the incidence of physician-assisted suicide or active voluntary euthanasia *prior* to the quasi-legalization of these practices in the Netherlands, we have no idea whether the number of cases of medically assisted dying without full and explicit consent of the patients is greater or less under the existing system than it was before. We do know from a number of surveys in Australia and the United States that many physicians have assisted their patients in dying. One argument for legalization is that it permits this underground, completely unregulated, practice to be scrutinized by official institutions.

None of this is to deny that we have to work with the empirical evidence we have. If it is of poor quality, or quantity, then we should do whatever we can to increase the amount and quality of our database. The experiment currently taking place in Oregon is useful if not decisive. Some critics of the Oregon experiment predicted that the patients most likely to take advantage of the new law would be depressed, socially vulnerable, and without access to good hospice cares. In fact the patients have been mostly middle-class, with 92 per cent of them having access to hospice care.

One possible source of empirical data that has not, to my knowledge, been evaluated is the very large number of patients who have refused life-support such as CPR, who have been allowed to withdraw from life support, who have refused artificial hydration and alimentation, or who have been killed by increasing doses of pain medication. When these practices were proposed by physicians, and when they were sanctioned by the courts, there were the same kinds of prediction made by opponents as are now made about physician-assisted suicide. Patients would be manipulated or coerced into making, or agreeing, to such practices. Patients who might be cured by new discoveries would mistakenly request to be removed from life-support. The slippery slope from voluntarily requesting DNR to having such orders entered on their chart without consent would be traversed. Why haven't studies of the misuse and abuse of the right to refuse medical treatment been made? If the predictions prove, for the most part, to have been false, then, barring some hypothesis as to why the situation is quite different with respect to physician-assisted suicide, we would have plausible reasons to suppose that the worst fears of the critics are groundless.

Now, it might be argued that the two situations—physician-assisted suicide and withholding or withdrawal of treatment—are distinct in the following sense. In the case of the refusal of treatment even if the predicted horrors were likely we cannot cite them in an argument. For patients have a right to refuse treatment and rights trump (at least over some range) bad consequences. It is not merely that it is permissible for patients to refuse treatment. It is impermissible to force them to have treatment against their will. It is an invasion of their bodily autonomy to force them to have feeding tubes, or to undergo CPR. So even if the study I suggested showed that there were many cases of abuse or misuse, we simply have to accept them as the price to be paid for not violating the rights of patients. This leads to the next issue.

IS THERE AN ASYMMETRY BETWEEN DENYING WITHHOLDING/WITHDRAWING REQUESTS AND DENYING ASSISTANCE IN DYING?

This argument is the first one of my budget of problems that deserves further research. It is more or less common ground between the two sides that there is the asymmetry just mentioned. In my book *Euthanasia and Physician-Assisted Suicide: For and Against*, I also assumed that the premises of this claim were correct, i.e. that physician-assisted suicide and withholding or withdrawing treatment were morally distinct because of the right to bodily integrity (Dworkin *et al.* 1998). I argued that, though there was a moral distinction, it was not sufficiently weighty to justify denying physician-assisted suicide to patients who were in otherwise exactly the same condition, i.e. were terminal, wished to die, competent, etc.

In both situations we have patients in identical positions who have to endure further life under circumstances that they find intolerable. In both cases, by denying their respective demands to have medical treatment cease, or to have assistance in dying, we force upon them a continued existence that is incompatible with their fundamental views as to how their life should be led. Even were there an additional right that is violated in one case but not the other (the right to control over what is done to one's body), this might make the refusal to withdraw treatment morally worse than the refusal to allow assistance in dying, but they are both above a threshold that forbids the state to deny the patient's wishes.

I now think that it is not so clear that the claim to withdrawal or withholding of treatment rests on the claim to bodily integrity. Consider the following case. A person has a disease such that any exposure to the sun's rays would be immediately fatal. He is protected from death by an electro-magnetic field, which has no other effect on him than to protect him from exposure to the sun. He discovers that he now has a different, terminal, illness that is causing him great pain. He wishes to end his life. He asks for the field to be turned off so that he can die immediately. It does not seem to me that his request for withdrawal of treatment is any less stringent because refusing to comply with it would not be a violation of his bodily integrity. His claim rests on the fact that his autonomy requires us to respect the fact that he does not want to have medical treatment. And this in turn rests on his right to determine for himself how to lead his life and when to end it. But this is exactly the same basis for the claim to assistance in dying.

There is, moreover, the thought that there are not two independent rights—bodily integrity and autonomy—but one basic right (autonomy) from which both the right to bodily integrity and the right to assistance in dying derive. If, as Dan Brock has argued, it is plausible to argue that the right to bodily integrity is itself ultimately grounded on the right to autonomy, then to argue for the right to withdraw or withhold treatment on the ground of a right to bodily integrity, but to deny that it is grounded in a more fundamental right of self-determination, is inconsistent (Brock 1999).

WHAT IS THE RELEVANCE OF INTENTION AND MOTIVE TO ACT-EVALUATION?

The next issue that I believe needs further exploration is one raised most clearly by Judith Thomson (1999) and James Rachels (1986). Judith Thomson argues that the intention with which the agent acts in a particular situation is not relevant to whether the act is morally permissible, though intentions may be relevant to the evaluation of the person's character.

In her view we are led to very strange consequences if we accept the traditional idea, incorporated into the principle of double effect, that the intention with which the agent acts bears upon the question of whether his act is morally permissible. She gives the following as an example of the absurdity to which this view leads.

According to the PDE [principle of double effect], the question of whether it is morally permissible for the doctor to inject a lethal drug turns on whether the doctor would be doing so intending death or only intending relief from pain. This is just . . . [an] absurd idea. If the only available doctor would inject the pain to cause the patient's death, or is incapable of becoming clear enough about her own intentions to conclude that what she intends is *only* to relieve her patient's pain, then—according to PDE—the doctor must not proceed, and the patient must be therefore allowed to suffer. That cannot be right.   (Thomson 1999: 515–16)

This view, which has important consequences for ethics more generally, is one that deserves a degree of critical scrutiny that so far it has not received. First, with respect to the specific application at hand, there is the issue of how the PDE should be understood. As Thomson understands it, the view applies to the evaluation of moral permissibility of act tokens. It is the specific intention with which this agent acts in this particular set of facts that is supposed to determine moral permissibility. This may have a degree of plausibility as a reading of the doctrine as it has been historically formulated. But those who wish to defend the principle have open to them the idea that what is being evaluated is act types, not tokens. The idea, then, is that an act type is morally permissible if its performance does not necessitate intending what is forbidden (where this has to be specified independently of the principle) either as an end, or as the means to some other end. Thus, in the case at hand, since the doctor can administer the lethal injection without intending either the death of the patient as an end, or the death as the means to ending his suffering, this suffices to show that the act in question is permissible quite independently of the specific intention with which the agent acts.

Second, there is the larger issue of how we are to identify acts. If the intention with which an agent acts is part of how we identify *which* act he is performing, then the idea that the same act can be performed with different intentions is mistaken. So the act is not simply injecting a lethal dose of morphine (which can be performed either with the intention to kill or not), but is rather the act of injecting a lethal dose of morphine as a way of controlling pain, or injecting the lethal dose as a way of killing the patient.

In any case, no matter what view one takes on the matter, it is not going to be settled by means of specific examples. As to the larger issue that Thomson raises—that intention or motive is not relevant to act-evaluation—this is a topic that badly needs further thought. One will need an investigation whose form is: which way of understanding the relation of act and intention leads to results in moral theory that are most satisfactory on the whole. The relation between motive and act-evaluation is not a new one in the history of moral philosophy, but the physician-assisted suicide debate has raised it again in a sharply focused manner.

IF PEOPLE WOULD, IN THE ABSENCE OF OTHERS MISTAKENLY CAUSING HARM, HAVE A RIGHT TO DO X, CAN WE PROHIBIT THEM FROM EXERCISING THEIR RIGHT ON THE GROUNDS OF THE HARM THAT WILL RESULT?

The general issue that is raised is the following: Suppose we have established some normative status for particular acts under certain circumstances. In particular, suppose we have established that some people have a moral right to do X. The right may be *pro tanto* or not. Then what is the relevance of the fact that some set of people are likely either to harm themselves mistakenly, or to be pressured into harming themselves, or some (possibly quite different) set of people are likely to be harmed by those who mistakenly use the right, to the question of whether we should allow doing X to be legally permissible?

It might be useful in thinking about this kind of argument in the context of physician-assisted suicide to compare it to a similar argument that occurs in the context of the prohibition of alcohol or guns. In the case of, say, alcohol the argument takes the following form. Many of us are responsible drinkers. We do not get drunk. We do not drink and drive. We do not drink and operate heavy machinery. But there are some who are not responsible drinkers. These people do a lot of damage, not just to themselves but also to their families. They cause a significant number of injuries and deaths to other drivers and pedestrians. So, on balance, we are entitled to restrict the ability of responsible drinkers to obtain alcohol in order that we reduce the amount of injury and death caused by these irresponsible drinkers. Of course, if we could have a set of policies that distinguished between the responsible and irresponsible drinkers and only denied access to the irresponsible, this is the policy that would be morally required.

But, if that is not feasible, then we are entitled to restrict some individuals from doing what is (otherwise) morally permissible. This argument has both paternalistic and non-paternalistic elements. Part of the harms we seek to avoid are the harms the alcoholic does to himself. These might include cirrhosis, or injuries to himself caused by his bad driving. In addition, there are the harms to others he inflicts. Similarly, in the physician-assisted suicide case the paternalistic argument is that people may quite freely, but mistakenly, avail themselves of the means to death. Perhaps they have been misdiagnosed, or their prognosis is more optimistic than they think. In so far as we are concerned with manipulation or pressure put on people to choose physician-assisted suicide, this is not paternalism; we are seeking to stop others from injuring such patients. The only difference between this form of argument and that which cites, say, the harm done to others by drunken drivers is that the harm is self-inflicted. But, to the extent that the cause of the decision is pressure or manipulation by others, then we are sometimes entitled to cite their actions as the cause of harm.

I am willing to concede that under certain circumstances we are entitled to restrict innocent persons because of the harms by others that are thereby avoided. What are these circumstances? There is no uniform answer to this question. One has to take into account such considerations as how significant the right in question is to the person's leading a meaningful life. What is the mechanism by which harm is produced? Is it that exercising the right allows others to make mistakes? Allows others to deliberately create harms? Provides an opportunity to convince others to cause harms? Makes it more likely that others will reason mistakenly and enlarge the right in harmful ways? What are the alternative ways of seeking to minimize the harms at issue? Do those ways violate rights?

But I also think that, when we are justified in restricting the right, we are obligated to adopt the least restrictive alternatives available. We should first concentrate our restrictions on those who are known or likely to be the direct causes of harms. If we are concerned about drunk drivers, then that is the class we should seek to restrict. We can use random highway stops, ignitions linked to breathalyzers, heavier penalties for those caught driving intoxicated, imposing liability on bartenders who continue to serve intoxicated customers. It is only if such policies fail to do much in the way of reducing injuries to others that we should consider the possibility of prohibition. I am ignoring here all the issues about whether prohibition can work, and its costs in illegal activities, corruption, etc. And in terms of restriction of the responsible, a scheme of licensing would be better than forbidding all access.

It is also more reasonable to forbid activities that do not have a major impact on the meaning or significance of a person's life. I like my wine as much as anybody, but I do not think that not being able to drink it would make anyone's life a less good one—although it might make it less pleasurable. Whereas, say, denying homosexuals the right to the only sexual life available to them is quite a different sacrifice.

To return, then, to the case of the regulation of physician-assisted suicide: since the conduct being regulated is one relevant to a central part of a meaningful life, namely the determination of the mode and timing of the ending of one's life, and since it is aimed at avoiding a great evil, unrelenting pain and suffering, the burden of proof has to be significant for those who favor forbidding the activity.

Since there are both paternalistic and non-paternalistic justifications, let us look at them separately. Assume that the only dangers we were looking at were the dangers of mistake on the part of the patient. Would we be justified in forbidding physician-assisted suicide?

I do not believe so. There are many instances in which people can make mistaken judgments, which can result in their deaths. People who engage in dangerous activities such as mountain climbing or hang-gliding, people who agree to clinical trials of untested therapies, people who work in dangerous occupations such as high iron construction. We do not believe that the fact that some of them will die needlessly is a good reason for forbidding the activities in question. The most relevant comparison is with patients who wish either to withdraw or not to initiate life-saving treatment. They are subject to exactly the same risk of misdiagnosis, new cures discovered, and so forth. But we forbid legal interference with their decisions provided they are competent.

So if we are to forbid physician-assisted suicide it must be on the grounds of the risks of non-paternalistic harms. Again for the sake of argument, and not because I believe the evidence is very strong, let us assume that there are non-negligible risks of harms imposed on patients against their will. In the words of the New York State Task Force, prohibitions on physician-assisted suicide are justified 'by the state's interest in preventing the error and abuse that would inevitably occur if physicians were authorized to . . . aid another person's death' (New York State Task Force on Life and the Law 1994: 68). Note the use of the word 'inevitably' in this concluding judgment. This implies that there is no scheme of regulation that would not keep these harms within some reasonable bounds. Of course, no scheme would reduce the risk to zero, but that is not required in order for legalization to be warranted.

Since we are assuming a right on the part of those who wish physician-assisted suicide, we must look for the least restrictive alternative for regulating the practice given the risk of serious harms. I believe one of the advantages of physician-assisted suicide over active voluntary euthanasia is that many of the risks of harm are sharply reduced. For example, David Velleman claims that

once euthanasia is established as a 'therapeutic' alternative, the line between patients competent to consent and those who are not will seem irrelevant to some doctors... As with other medical decisions, some doctors will feel they can and should make a decision in their patient's best interests, for patients clearly incapable of consenting and for those with marginal or uncertain capacity to consent.   (Velleman 1992: 678)

But how is this supposed to work in the case of physician-assisted suicide? Are these doctors going to forge written documents, procure willing colleagues to give a second opinion, inject a lethal dose and claim the patient took pills himself?

Perhaps what is meant is that the slippery slope will appear. Once we have physician-assisted suicide, active voluntary euthanasia will inevitably follow. But, in addition to the absence of any evidence for this claim (we have no empirical data on a society that has adopted only physician-assisted suicide and then seen active voluntary euthanasia come into effect as well), the moral issue is posed most clearly here. We are denying citizens who have a moral claim to an exercise of their liberty (access to physician-assisted suicide) not because they will misuse the liberty to harm others, not because if they exercised this particular liberty others would misuse that liberty to impose harms on others, but because if they have this liberty then others will press for legislative changes to allow a *different* liberty (active voluntary euthanasia) that will then impose harms on others. I cannot think of another instance in which this argument is justified for imposing legal restrictions on otherwise permissible liberties.

The closest argument that I can think of is that which argues against making some exception to freedom of speech, say by prohibiting hate speech, because of the fear that the relevant authorities, say the administration of a university, will be led to make further (unjustified) exceptions. But in this case what we fear is the abuse of power by authorities over which we have very little power. It is not the fear that legislatures or elected officials will be swayed by their constituents to enact dangerous policies.

David Velleman, who thinks the arguments for legalization must proceed more slowly, recognizes that 'these collateral harms might have to be tolerated if there were a fundamental right to choose between life and death. We can't deprive all people of a choice to which they are morally entitled just because some people would be better off without it' (Velleman 1999: 620). It is only because he thinks there is no such right that he believes the danger of collateral harms have important weight in the argument.

IS PHYSICIAN-ASSISTED SUICIDE REALLY NECESSARY?

An important argument against physician-assisted suicide and euthanasia, which has not received much attention, is that there are alternative ways of achieving the end of control over one's mode and time of dying that avoid some of the problems with physician-assisted suicide. This is not the argument that pain and loss of dignity can be handled by a greatly expanded system of hospice care. Of course everyone agrees that much more attention should be given to the alleviation of suffering at the end of life. It is an empirical question of whether (almost) all forms of pain can be handled by doctors who are trained in pain relief, and are willing to administer whatever it takes to control pain. And much progress has been made in recent years in the training of physicians in palliative care. Ironically, surely some of this is the result of the publicity and attention given to the Oregon experiment, and to the responsibility that physicians who oppose physician-assisted suicide have for doing more for their patients *in extremis*.

It is important, however, to note that pain is not the only issue. Those who are incontinent, or paralyzed, or unable to think clearly, or free from pain but in a mental state that is disconnected from reality, or slowly losing their ability to control their muscles, are not in pain. But they are suffering. And pain medication is not going to help them.

In addition, there is the point that Velleman has stressed, that there are people who because of their suffering have lost their sense of self—of who they are. Again, psychiatric assistance can be useful and ought to be provided. But there comes a point at which the life of the patient (in their eyes) is one of degradation and misery. What they want is to end their life, not to have it extended in a slightly improved fashion. Again, those whose pain would be intolerable without large doses of pain medication can find their pain decreased but at the cost of losing contact with the world around them—in particular with those loved ones with whom they would like to communicate.

The argument that I think is more significant is that there is an alternative say in which patients can retain control over their living or dying. They can always refuse food and water. They will die more slowly than with physician-assisted suicide but die they will. It might be objected that this mode of dying is quite unpleasant and patients should not have to choose this way of dying. The empirical evidence, however, is that provided adequate hydration of the mouth is maintained, this is not a particularly unpleasant way to die. People who are terminally ill generally do not have a good appetite, so that the deprivation of food is not perceived as serious. And at least for a while such patients are able to maintain contact with their friends and loved ones.

Why then, the argument goes, should we institutionalize a practice that at least might have harmful consequences? Why should we take risks when there is a non-risky alternative; one that is simply an extension of the recognized right to refuse medical treatment? There is a further point, which is that the process of assisted suicide is itself not well understood. The dosage, the mode of administration, is quite imperfect. Patients throw up the medication. Others wind up in coma or persistent vegetative state. Indeed some think the Oregon figures are fishy simply because there are no reports of bungled assisted suicide. Although they report cases in which the patient lingers on for substantial periods of time, all the patients did die eventually.

What we ought to do is expand our system of palliative care, at the same time informing patients of their right to refuse food and water and giving them the best evidence we have about what the process would be like. I think this is clearly correct, but what is less clear is whether this is a good reason to continue to keep physician-assisted suicide illegal—except for the state of Oregon.

The first important thing to note is that the argument does not show that refusal of food and water (henceforth rfw) is morally speaking an improvement over physician-assisted suicide. It is not as if in rfw but not physician-assisted suicide the intention of the physician is morally superior. In neither case need the physician intend the death of her patient. In the former case the physician need only intend to follow the wishes of his patient to cease all treatment as well as food and water. But in the latter case the physician may only intend to provide his patient with the security of ultimate control over her living or dying, and may even think that the patient is less likely to end her life prematurely as a result of being so empowered. It is true that in the case of physician-assisted suicide the doctor must prescribe the lethal medication but in the former case the doctor must order nurses and orderlies not to provide the normal food and water.

In neither case is the cause of death the illness of the patient. In one case it is the lethal medication (if the patient chooses to take it) and in the other it is the lack of food and water (if the patient chooses not to take them). So the argument cannot be that rfw is superior to physician-assisted suicide on moral grounds.

The argument might be that there are risks to legalization of physician-assisted suicide that are not present in the current state of legalized rfw. Again the matter is not so clear. In both cases there is a possible danger of manipulation by either patients or family. In both cases the doctor is responsible for taking steps that may lead to the death of his patient and it is possible this might have some effect on the doctor–patient relationship. In both cases there is the issue of whether they should be restricted to the terminally ill or extended to the incurably ill and suffering. Actually it appears as if rfw is already something that the incurably ill have a right to demand, so I suppose the issue would be whether we should require forced nutrition for those not terminally ill. Since the risks seem similar, again this is not reason for relying only on rfw and keeping physician-assisted suicide illegal.

The argument has to be that we should stay with the status quo and not enlarge the options thereby increasing the risks. We should simply concentrate on making sure there are adequate safeguards in place to ensure that rfw is not misused or abused. For those whose pain cannot be controlled sufficiently during the process of dying from lack of nutrition and hydration we can resort to terminal sedation, the administration of sufficient medication to induce unconsciousness.

Whether this argument works is partly a matter of determining whether the additional risks could not be adequately handled by the same kinds of safeguards that we would put in place to limit the risks of rfw, and whether there are benefits to physician-assisted suicide that could not be achieved with only rfw.

There is, however, a further argument that must be considered which weighs in favor of legalizing physician-assisted suicide. We know that physician-assisted suicide and voluntary euthanasia do take place, and in not insignificant numbers. Some even use this fact to argue against legalization by saying that doctors do in fact help patients to die and it is better to let this continue without making this public via legalization. On this view a certain amount of hypocrisy is a desirable feature. But I should think that those who are worried about risks and abuse ought to worry about what is going on in the sub rosa practice of assisted suicide. It seems to me a way of risk-reduction to bring the whole situation out in the open, with public scrutiny as has been done in Oregon.

When, and for What?

The next set of issues I wish to discuss are, first, the question of when persons ought to be eligible for physician-assisted suicide—i.e. should it be limited to those who are competent at the time of death or extended to those who, while competent, agreed, but who are now incompetent—and the question of what conditions ought to be necessary, i.e. are only those suffering from terminal illness to be allowed to request physician-assisted suicide?

Felicia Ackerman raises an interesting question in a provocative article: is the idea that legal physician-assisted suicide should be limited to certain specific conditions, i.e. terminal illness, a consistent one (Ackerman 1998)? Her claim is that, while it may be consistent to argue either for the complete legalization, or the complete prohibition, of physician-assisted suicide, the position that argues for a limited legalization is morally untenable. Her reasons are quite varied: some are supposed counter-examples; some appeal to the underlying rationale for wanting physician-assisted suicide to be available; some involve appeal to empirical factors.

One difficulty in her argument is a failure to distinguish between a general legal right to request assistance in suicide and a specific right to request assistance from physicians. These are logically independent of one another. While it is obvious that one may be in favor of physician-assisted suicide without being in favor of allowing others to assist suicide, it takes a moment's thought to realize that it is also possible to believe that one ought to have a right to request assistance from anyone while thinking it should be illegal for physicians to provide such assistance. One might hold this view because, say, one thought that allowing physicians to use their medical skills to cause death is a perversion of the role of physician. I do not think this is true in general, but there may be specific cases in which it does hold (G. Dworkin 2002).

So an argument for the right to assistance in killing oneself that relies on the value of autonomy may not be inconsistent with an argument for limiting physician-assisted suicide to, say, terminally ill persons—even if the latter argument also relies, in part, on an appeal to the value of autonomy. What is special about physician-assisted suicide is that it is death that takes place in the medical context and in the course of the practice of medicine. One might even think that there ought to be people who are trained in giving advice to others as to how they can commit suicide, and even assisting them to die if for some reason they are unable to kill themselves, say, because they are paralyzed. But one still might restrict physician-assisted suicide to those who are already part of the medical context. One might, for example, believe that lethal injection as a mode of execution ought to be available to those prisoners who prefer to die this way, but that doctors should not be executioners (G. Dworkin 2002).

The question then arises—within the medical context—how broadly should the conditions that warrant physician-assisted suicide be specified? Is there any special reason to focus on terminal illness? After all, if relief of suffering is an important part of the rationale, then it would appear *more* important to relieve the suffering of those who are not terminal and will suffer longer. And while those who are not dying shortly have a longer period in which it is possible that cures for their condition may be discovered, this seems a slim reed upon which to distinguish the cases.

There are certainly pragmatic considerations for limiting the scope of physician-assisted suicide in a period when it is difficult to get any change in the status quo. And it is certainly reasonable to want to try out such reforms on a small scale before widening their scope. But, apart from such pragmatic matters, the arguments for extending physician-assisted suicide at least to those who suffer acutely and whose suffering is not easily remediable seems strong. By 'suffering' I mean more than physical pain. Consider someone with 'locked-in' syndrome—who is totally paralyzed (with perhaps eye blink motion) and completely conscious. Since some patients may experience this not only as mentally torturous but also as a condition that denies them all meaningful life, the case for death seems as secure as that for someone with painful metastasized cancer.

Opponents will immediately raise the issue of where the line should be drawn. Recall the patient in *The Singing Detective* who suffers from a terrible skin affliction that is not only painful but limits his range of motion and the use of his hands. Is he a candidate for physician-assisted suicide? Or what about a person suffering from morbid obesity, weighing 800 pounds, confined to his bed, unable to work. Or consider a person whose face has been eaten away by flesh-eating bacteria and cannot bear to face the world. All of these would meet the criterion proposed by Professor Kluge of the University of Victoria—an incurable, irremediable disease or medical condition that the patient experiences as incompatible with her fundamental values.

My own view is that one should accept something like this condition and that it is a matter of judgment for the physician as to whether the facts of the particular case fall under this criterion or not. If, in his judgment, they do, then the law ought to allow assisted suicide.

Another important issue is whether euthanasia ought to be available by means of advance directives. This question can be put as follows: Given that competent patients have some kind of right based on autonomy to request assisted dying, does such a right extend to their situation when they are no longer competent? This could be because they are in a coma or a persistent vegetative state, or because they are demented. This is a genuinely difficult issue, on which philosophers have come to very different conclusions (R. Dworkin 1993; Shiffrin 2004). On the one hand, if we do not allow advance directives, then we prevent those who wish their life to be ended, rather than living on in a condition which they regard as incompatible with their most basic values, from being able to achieve their wishes. On the other hand, if we carry out such advance directives, then we end the lives of those who do not contemporaneously express a wish to die. Indeed, at the time they may not wish to die. If we think of the person as divided into stages, then the earlier person is clearly the most competent decision-maker, but the later person is the one whose life will be shortened. It is she who bears the consequences of the earlier decision. I believe that becoming clearer about the issue in this case will require further thought about the authority of earlier versus later stages of a person's life, about the significance of the fact that demented or comatose persons do not have the power of autonomy they once possessed, and what respect for the person comes to in situations like this. It is also clear that the issue of dementia is different in important ways from the issue of lack of consciousness. It is crucial in the former case that the person is able to express wishes and desires, including the fact that they do not wish to die.

Is There a Moral Difference, and If So, Ought There to Be a Legal Difference, Between Assisted Suicide and Voluntary Euthanasia?

By definition, there is only one descriptive difference between assisted suicide and euthanasia. It lies in who performs the last causal act leading to death. In the case of assisted suicide it is the patient; in the case of euthanasia it is the physician. This entails that only in the latter case does one person kill another. Many physicians have the visceral feeling that this makes euthanasia morally more problematic, that responsibility for the death lies more heavily on the doctor than in assisted suicide.

But it is hard to see why this should be so. Consider a case where the doctor puts an intravenous line into the patient which is attached to a supply of a lethal drug. All that needs to be done to procure death is to turn the spigot on the line. In one case the patient does so; in another the doctor does. Can this difference in who acts last be a morally relevant difference? Of course, in some circumstances it can: if, for example, the patient has requested that he be allowed to turn the spigot and the doctor ignores his wishes. But, if all other factors are held constant, can this difference matter in and of itself? If a patient asks to be withdrawn from, say, a respirator, would it make a moral difference if the patient, rather than the doctor, pulled the plug? Would the doctor bear more responsibility for the subsequent death of the patient in the latter case?

Still, I think there are various strategic reasons for drawing the line at assisted suicide. The medical profession seems to think that it is worse for doctors to kill than to provide the means for the patient to kill herself. It is plausible to think that a system that works via the doctor giving a lethal injection is more subject to abuse than one in which the patient must take the pills himself. In Oregon the physician need not even be present when the patient takes the pills.

The only drawback to not legalizing euthanasia is that a small number of patients, who are not able to swallow the medication, or even to bring it to their mouth (paralysis), will not be able to be assisted in dying. But, as is always the case, they have the right to refuse food and water. Perhaps that small sacrifice on their part is warranted to bring most of us an important benefit.

References

Ackerman, F. (1998) 'Assisted Suicide, Terminal Illness, Severe Disability, and the Double Standard', in M. Battin, R. Rhodes, and A. Silvers (eds.), *Physician-Assisted Suicide: Expanding the Debate* (New York: Routledge), 149–61.

Brock, D. (1999), 'A Critique of Three Objections to Physician-Assisted Suicide', *Ethics*, 109/3: 519–48.

Dworkin, G. (2002), 'Patients and Prisoners: The Ethics of Lethal Injection', *Analysis*, 62/2: 181–9.

—— Frey, R., and Bok, S. (1998), *Euthanasia and Physician-Assisted Suicide* (Cambridge: Cambridge University Press).

Dworkin, R. (1993), *Life's Dominion* (New York: Knopf).

Kamisar, Y. (1958), 'Some Non-Religious Views Against Proposed "Mercy Killing" Legislation', *Minnesota Law Review*, 42: 969–1042.

Kuhse, H., and Singer, P. (1988), 'Doctors' Practices and Attitudes Regarding Voluntary Euthanasia', *Medical Journal of Australia*, 148: 623–7.

New York State Task Force on Life and the Law (1994), *When Death Is Sought: Assisted Suicide and Euthanasia in the Medical Context* (Albany, NY: New York State Task Force on Life and the Law).

Rachels, J. (1986), *The End of Life: Euthanasia and Morality* (Oxford: Oxford University Press).

Schiffrin, S. (2004), 'Autonomy, Beneficence and the Permanently Demented', in J. Burley (ed.), *Dworkin and His Critics* (Oxford: Blackwell), 195–218.

Thomson, J. (1999), 'Physician-Assisted Suicide: Two Moral Arguments', *Ethics*, 109/3: 297–518.

Velleman, D. (1992), 'Against the Right to Die', *Journal of Medicine and Philosophy*, 17: 665–81.

—— (1999), 'A Right to Self-Termination?', *Ethics*, 109/3: 665–81.

PART V

REPRODUCTION AND CLONING

CHAPTER 17

ABORTION REVISITED

DON MARQUIS

CLASSICAL ARGUMENTS CONCERNING ABORTION

OPPONENTS of abortion choice typically have argued that because (human) foetuses are human, alive, and innocent, and because an abortion ends innocent human life, abortion is, unless special circumstances obtain, immoral. Call this argument 'the human life argument'. Most supporters of abortion choice (in the philosophical world, at any rate) have argued that because (human) foetuses are not yet persons, and because what makes killing wrong is that the victim is a person, abortion is, unless special circumstances obtain, morally permissible. Call this argument 'the personhood argument'. Both of these arguments are based on an understanding of why killing is wrong in cases where a consensus exists. Proponents of each argument argue that their understanding implies a conclusion concerning abortion.

Many discussions of abortion take the human life view of the wrongness of killing for granted and then go on to argue that foetuses either are or are not fully human or that foetuses either are or are not potential, but not actual, life. These issues are easy to resolve. The foetuses in which we are interested are all fully human, of course.

Thanks to Katrina Elliott, Ben Eggleston, and Bonnie Steinbock for helpful comments.

They are not mosquitoes or mice. Because they exhibit growth and metabolism they are actually, not merely potentially, alive. When the argument is conducted within the human life framework those opposed to abortion choice easily win the argument.

Many other discussions of abortion take the personhood view for granted and go on to discuss whether or not foetuses are persons. This issue is also easy to resolve. In the sense of 'person' generally used by personhood proponents, no foetus is a person. When the argument is conducted within the personhood framework, those in favor of abortion choice easily win the argument. Thus, the far more important issue concerns which understanding of the wrongness of killing is correct. This point can be put in another way for readers who know a bit of logic. The syllogisms in terms of which we can understand the abortion debate are not really controversial because of their *minor* premises. The truth of their *major* premises is at the heart of the matter.

The human life and personhood arguments are alike in another respect. Their views of the wrongness of killing are subject to similar criticisms. The human life account is subject both to a theoretical difficulty and to a difficulty concerning cases. The theoretical difficulty concerns the connection between the biological properties of being human and being alive and the moral property of having a right to life. Critics argue that this connection needs to be established, not merely asserted. They argue that the connection is not self-evident, that religious considerations are insufficient to establish it, and that no other argument establishes the connection. The human life account also faces a difficulty concerning cases because it seems to make too much killing wrong. It makes deliberately ending the lives of humans who will never be conscious (such as anencephalic newborns and persons in persistent vegetative state) wrong. It seems to make deliberately ending the life of a sperm or an unfertilized ovum (which are, after all, human and alive and not guilty) wrong. The human life account of the wrongness of killing seems to be both theoretically insufficient and too broad.

The classic personhood account comes in two versions: Mary Anne Warren's version and Michael Tooley's desire version. According to Warren the traits 'most central to the concept of personhood' are (1) consciousness and, in particular, the capacity to feel pain, (2) reasoning, (3) self-motivated activity, (4) the capacity to communicate in a reasonably sophisticated way, and (5) the presence of self-concepts (Warren 1979: 45). According to Warren, an individual need not have all of these traits to be considered a person, or even any particular one of them. However, an individual with none of these traits is plainly not a person. And even if an individual had only the capacity to feel pain, 'it cannot be said to have any more right to life than, let us say, a newborn guppy' (Warren 1979: 47). In Warren's view what makes a killing wrong is that the victim is a person. Since foetuses clearly aren't persons, abortion is morally permissible.

Warren's classic personhood account faces difficulties very much like the diffi-culties that face the human life account. The theoretical problem with Warren's account concerns the connection between the psychological traits in terms of which personhood is defined and the moral property of having the right to life. Neither the mere assertion by Warren that there is such a connection nor the general belief that there is such a connection is enough to establish an actual connection. From a theoretical perspective Warren's personhood view is no more compelling than the human life view.

Warren's classic personhood argument is also plagued by difficulties concerning cases. The claim that foetuses lack the right to life because they are not persons seems to imply that it is permissible to kill a newborn child because she is not a person. It also seems to entail, because being a person involves exhibiting certain psychological traits, that killing someone who is temporarily unconscious is morally permissible. Warren tries to avoid the former conclusion by arguing that infanticide is wrong because of the attitudes that adults have toward newborns (Warren 1979: 50–1). However, this has the consequence that if, for any set of infants, adults did not value those infants, then infanticide would be morally permissible. (Think of the infanticide of females in some cultures.) Thus, Warren's classic defense of abortion choice in terms of personhood suffers from problems that are the mirror image of the human life account's problems. The two accounts suffer from similar theoretical difficulties. Both have problems with cases. The human life account makes *too much* killing wrong; Warren's personhood account makes *too little* killing wrong.

Michael Tooley's personhood account is different from Warren's account. Tooley's account has the great virtue of avoiding the theoretical problem that plagues both the human life argument and Warren's classic personhood argument. Tooley stipulates the truth of 'X is a person if and only if X has a serious moral right to life' (Tooley 1972: 42). He then claims that 'An organism possesses a serious right to life only if it possesses the concept of a self as a continuing subject of experiences and other mental states, and believes that it is itself a continuing entity' (Tooley 1972: 45). Tooley defends this claim by arguing that an organism possesses a serious right to life only if she desires to live and she desires to live only if she possesses a concept of herself as a continuing subject of experience. Thus, the desire to live is basic to Tooley's account of the right to life. Accordingly, I refer to Tooley's personhood account as 'a desire account', both to characterize it and to distinguish it from Warren's account.

Here is how Tooley defends the moral importance of desires.

The basic intuition is that . . . in general, to violate an individual's right to something is to frustrate the corresponding desire. Suppose, for example, that you own a car. Then I am under a *prima facie* obligation not to take it from you. However, the obligation is not unconditional: it depends in part upon the existence of a corresponding desire in you. If you do not care whether I take your car, then I generally do not violate your right by doing so. (Tooley 1973: 60)

From this intuition Tooley generates the following argument. To have the right to life is to have the right to continue to exist. The right to continue to exist presupposes the desire to continue to exist. One has the desire to continue to exist only if one has a concept of oneself as a continuing subject of experience. No foetus has a concept of herself as a continuing subject of experience. Therefore, no foetus has a right to life. So abortion is morally permissible.

Tooley's desire account of the wrongness of killing is not subject to the theoretical difficulties that plague both the human life account and Warren's classic personhood account. Tooley's basic intuition is a plausible attempt to locate his abortion view within a general account of wrong action. However, he has noted that the desire account seems not to explain the wrongness of some cases of killing. Consider the case of an individual suffering from depression who says that she wishes she were dead, or, for that matter, who says sincerely that she sees no point in living. Consider the case of someone who is not a self-conscious being because she is temporarily unconscious and therefore not conscious of anything, including her own self. Consider the case of an individual who 'may permit someone to kill him because he had been convinced that if he allows himself to be sacrificed to the gods he will be gloriously rewarded in a life to come' (Tooley 1972: 47–8). Apparently Tooley's account of the wrongness of killing implies that it is morally permissible to kill all of the above individuals. It is not. Thus, Tooley's account, like Warren's personhood account, permits too much killing.

On more than one occasion Tooley struggled with these apparent problems with his view (Tooley 1972: 48; 1973: 65–6; Purdy and Tooley 1974: 146). Tooley's problem was finding qualifications that rescue the desire account, that do not seem to be merely ad hoc, and that preserve abortion choice. Because of these difficulties Tooley eventually gave up his desire account (Tooley 1983: 109–112).

The three major classical accounts of the morality of abortion are all subject to at least one major problem. Can we do better? The purpose of this chapter is to discuss three accounts that purport to be superior to the classical accounts. First, I shall discuss the future of value argument for the immorality of abortion. I shall defend the claim that the future of value argument is superior to all three of the classical accounts. I shall then go on to discuss Warren's attempt to fix up her personhood account and David Boonin's attempt to fix up Tooley's desire account. Warren claims that her updated version of a personhood account is superior to any potentiality account, such as the future of value account. I shall evaluate her claim. Boonin argues that his improved desire view both deals adequately with the apparent counterexamples to Tooley's original account and also is superior to the future of value account. I shall evaluate his views.

Because of considerations of length, this chapter will not deal with arguments that purport to show that even if foetuses have a full right to life, even if they have the same moral status that we do, abortion is morally permissible because foetuses do not have the right to the life support that women must provide for nine months if foetuses are to survive.

THE FUTURE OF VALUE ACCOUNT

According to the future of value argument for the immorality of abortion the best explanation for the wrongness of killing is that killing deprives us of our futures of value. Our futures of value consist of all of the goods of life we would have experienced had we not been killed. Foetuses have futures like ours, for their futures contain all that ours contain and more. Therefore (given some defensible assumptions and qualifications), abortion is seriously wrong on almost all occasions (Marquis 1989).

What is a future of value? Consider the life of someone who lives to 'a ripe old age'. The value of that life to the person who lives it consists of experiences that, at various times in her life, she values. These are the goods of her life. They are what make her life worth living. The list of these goods will vary somewhat from person to person. The list includes friendships, loves, absorption in various projects, aesthetic experiences, identification with larger causes seen as valuable, such as one's team winning a victory, and physical pleasures. One's future of value is the class of goods in one's future that occur later than a given time in one's life, if one does not die prematurely.

On the future of value account the wrongness of killing is based on the harm of killing. A present action cannot affect one's past. Strictly speaking, a present act of harming does not make another worse off in the present either, for the present is instantaneous, and harm, involving, as it does, causation, requires at least a small temporal interval for its effect to occur. A present act of harm affects the victim's future. It makes someone worse off in the future. To make someone worse off is to reduce that person's welfare, to reduce the quantity or quality of the goods in her future that she would otherwise have possessed. On the future of value account killing is wrong because it harms a victim.

Killing someone deprives her of *all* the goods of her future she otherwise would have experienced. Thus killing is a very serious harm. The future of value view accounts for why we regard killing as one of the worst of crimes. It coheres with why we believe that the premature death of a human being is one of the greatest misfortunes she could suffer. Thus the future of value account is plausible, not only because it coheres with our understanding of killing as a harm, but because it coheres with our understanding of premature death as a great misfortune.

We know that foetuses have futures of value because we were all foetuses once and their futures of value are the goods of our past lives, our present lives, and our future lives. (I am assuming that we are biological organisms. Jeff McMahan has offered interesting and important arguments for the falsity of this assumption; McMahan 2002.) Each of us has had first person experience with the future of value of one (former) foetus. Since we have friends and acquaintances, we know of the futures of value of many (former) foetuses. Since abortion deprives a foetus of a valuable future like ours, and since depriving an individual of a future like ours is what makes killing her seriously presumptively wrong, abortion is seriously presumptively wrong. Because 'like' is a vague predicate the precise scope of the future of value account of the wrongness of killing is indeterminate. Animal rights proponents may want to exploit this vagueness. However, because portions of the future of a foetus are *identical* to ours, human foetuses will clearly be within its scope.

An individual's future of value is based on her present potentiality. We have futures of value in virtue of being individuals who have the present potential to have experiences we will value in the future. This present potential is a function of our present biological nature. (In the case of persons from outer space whom it would be wrong to kill, this might not be so.) The future of value account should be distinguished from other potentiality arguments intended to deal with the morality of abortion. One might claim that what makes it wrong to kill a foetus is that it is a potential human being. This claim is incompatible with the future of value account because, according to the future of value account, what makes it wrong to kill a foetus is *exactly* the same property that makes it wrong to kill you and me. It certainly is not wrong to kill you and me because we are potential human beings. This is because we are *not* potential human beings; we are actual human beings.

One might claim that it is wrong to kill a foetus because it is a potential person. This claim is also incompatible with the future of value account because according to the future of value account what makes it wrong to kill a foetus is exactly what makes it wrong to kill you and me. But it is not wrong to kill you and me because we are potential persons, for the very simple reason that we are not potential persons. We are actual persons.

The future of value account should be thought of in the following way. In this universe there are many individuals. Some of them (such as virtually all other humans) have a present potential to have futures like ours and some of them (such as trees, rocks, and snails) do not. That present potential makes it wrong to kill individuals who are members of the former class.

The future of value account is not subject to the theoretical difficulties of the human life account and Warren's (1979) personhood account. The former account rests on an alleged connection between a biological property and a moral property and the latter account rests on an alleged connection between psychological properties and a moral property. In neither account is there an adequate defense of the connection between a property with value content and a purely natural property. The future of value account, like Tooley's desire account, is based on a connection between two properties with value content. Because the whole account is imbedded in an account of what harm is, the whole account is imbedded in a plausible general account of wrong action. Therefore, in this theoretical respect, the future of value account of the wrongness of killing is superior to those earlier accounts.

The future of value account handles cases better than any of the three classic accounts. Consider the problems that the human life account has with persons in persistent vegetative state and with anencephalic newborns. It is difficult to understand what is wrong with ending the lives of humans in either category. Ending their lives cannot deprive them of anything they would ever value. Accordingly, it is difficult to understand how *they are harmed* by their lives being ended. This being the case, it is difficult to understand how *they are wronged* by their lives being ended. Because of this anencephalic newborns have been intentionally allowed to die for centuries. The human life account cannot account for this. The future of value account easily accounts for this. The same considerations apply to humans who are in persistent vegetative state.

Warren's early account is plagued with the difficulty of accounting for the wrongness of infanticide. By contrast, according to the future of value account of the wrongness of killing, ending the life of a little baby is as obviously wrong as we all think it is. Warren's account also faces problems accounting for the wrongness of killing the temporarily unconscious. Since exhibiting psychological traits is necessary for being a person and since the temporarily unconscious do not exhibit psychological traits, her view apparently entails that killing the temporarily unconscious would not wrong *them*. This is, of course, a disaster for her view.

Strategies for repairing her view do not show promise. One strategy for fixing her view might be to allow that one is a person either in virtue of actually manifesting certain psychological traits or in virtue of being able to manifest certain psychological traits in the future. The trouble with this strategy is that foetuses are able to manifest psychological traits in the future, if allowed to live. The consequence of such an alteration would convert Warren's account to an anti-choice view. No doubt she would not welcome that consequence.

Another strategy for fixing her view might be to allow that one is a person either in virtue of actually manifesting certain psychological traits or in virtue of being able to manifest certain psychological traits now. That move avoids the anti-choice conclusion, but only at the price of not being able to account for the wrongness of killing the temporarily unconscious again. Accordingly this strategy would not work. A third strategy for fixing Warren's view might be to hold that the capacity to manifest psychological traits in the future as long as one has manifested such psychological traits in the past is the basis for the right to life. This move eliminates the unwelcome anti-choice consequence without allowing us to kill the temporarily unconscious. However, *sole* justification for *this* particular wrinkle in her theory is that it both can account for the case of the temporarily unconscious and also can produce the pro-choice conclusion that Warren desires. So such a wrinkle cannot *justify* her abortion view.

The future of value account also handles cases better than Tooley's desire account. In a nutshell, Tooley's desire account does not account for the wrongness of killing many persons who, for one reason or another, do not desire to live. The future of value account handles such cases nicely. Consider two classes of such persons: (1) persons who, perhaps because of a terminal illness, face a future of pain and suffering that cannot be alleviated and (2) persons who, because of depression, can be helped, through the aid of psychotherapy and psychotropic drugs, to live lives that they will later value. On the future of value account it is not wrong to kill persons in the former class, although getting the analysis just right demands some attention to detail. On the future of value account, it is wrong to kill persons in the latter class. This is exactly what most sensible people believe. The future of value account deals with Tooley's problem cases in the correct way. We can conclude, therefore, that the future of value account offers theoretical advantages over two of the three classical accounts and deals with cases better than any of them. Because it fits into a general account of harm, which, in turn, fits into a general account of wrongs, and because it, by comparison with alternative theories, handles cases well, it seems to be the basis for a correct account of the ethics of abortion.

WARREN'S MORAL STATUS ACCOUNT

In 1997 Mary Anne Warren offered an updated personhood defense of abortion choice (Warren 1997). Whereas her earlier view paid little attention to the connection between her psychological account of personhood and the right to life, her later view is anchored in a comprehensive account of moral status. Warren's account contains seven different principles, each of which underwrites some degree of moral status. Fortunately, evaluation of her defense of abortion rights does not require appraisal of her entire theory. Many of her principles do not concern the moral status of humans at all. They underwrite a level of moral status inferior to the status of humans. For our purposes, such principles can be neglected. The abortion issue turns on whether or not foetuses have the same full moral status as you and I. Because women have a strong presumptive right to control their own bodies, if foetuses have some, but less than full, moral status, then their interests would not be sufficiently strong to override the interests of women, who, after all, do have full moral status. The interests of a foetus could trump a pregnant woman's presumptive rights only if foetuses have the same full right to life as you and I have now.

Warren's AGENT'S RIGHTS Principle

In order to defend abortion choice in terms of the lack of full fetal moral status Warren needs some account (1) that explains why those humans whose moral status is not a matter of controversy do indeed have full moral status and (2) that does not include foetuses within the scope of that explanation. Warren's primary full moral status principle is what she calls 'the Agent's Rights principle'. According to this principle

Moral agents have full and equal basic moral rights, including the rights to life and liberty. (Warren 1997: 156)

A moral agent is 'an individual who is capable of using reason to discern and follow universal moral laws'. (Warren 1997: 156)

This principle is not controversial. Because it offers only a sufficient, but not a necessary, condition for the possession of full moral status, it cannot be criticized for excluding humans who are not moral agents. Warren defends this principle by appealing to the moral philosophy of Kant and to the Kantian moral philosophies of John Rawls and Alan Gewirth. It is reasonable to assume that such foundations for the Agent's Rights principle are sufficient to save it from the theoretical difficulties that beset the human life view or Warren's earlier personhood view. Warren's more recent view is a genuine improvement over her earlier view.

Warren's HUMAN RIGHTS Principle

Warren's Agent's Rights principle plainly needs supplementation. It does not underwrite the full moral status of young children and the mentally disabled. Because she is well aware of this, Warren adds to her account what she calls 'the Human Rights principle'. According to this principle:

Within the limits of their own capacities and of [the Agent's Rights principle], human beings who are capable of sentience but not of moral agency have the same moral rights as do moral agents. (Warren 1997: 164)

Although in philosophy it is customary first to determine just what a claim means and then to ask whether or not it is true, this procedure is not apt for analysis of Warren's Human Rights principle. Warren first defends the Human Rights principle as it applies to already born humans and then discusses whether or not the principle should be extended to protect foetuses. Adequate appraisal of her defense of her view requires following the path of her argument. It is also worth noting that Warren does not believe that the Human Rights principle is literally true. It entails that 3-year-olds have the liberty rights of moral agents. This is, as Warren realizes, absurd. Warren actually believes that in the case of children 'their interests carry the same moral weight as do those of other human beings' (Warren 1997: 164). My appraisal of her defense of the Human Rights principle will take this 'moral equality of interests' interpretation for granted.

Because Warren's defense of the Human Rights principle as it applies to children after birth is not extensive it is possible to quote it in full:

in reality human beings become moral agents only through a long period of dependence upon human beings who are moral agents already. During this period of dependency we learn language, and all of the other mental and behavioural capacities that make moral agency possible. In Annette Baier's words, 'A person is best seen as one who was long enough dependent upon other persons to acquire the essential arts of personhood. Persons essentially are second persons, who grow up with other persons.'

For this reason, it is both impractical and emotionally abhorrent to deny full moral status to sentient human beings who have not yet achieved (or who have irreparably lost) the capacity for moral agency. If we want there to be human beings in the world in the future, and if we want them to have any chance to lead good lives, then we must at least value the lives and well-being of infants and young children. Fortunately, instinct, reason, and culture jointly ensure that most of us regard infants and young children as human beings to whom we can have obligations as binding as those we have to human beings who are moral agents. (Warren 1997: 164–5)

Much of Warren's defense of her Human Rights principle seems quite implausible. Is the dependency of children on moral agents sufficient for treating children as the moral equals of moral agents? House plants are dependent on moral agents. We do not think that this implies that we should treat them as our moral equals. Is the education of children by moral agents a good reason for giving children the same rights as moral agents? Adolescents learn to drive from persons who have the right to drive. It does not follow that such adolescents have the right to drive. Is the emotional abhorrence of rejecting the rights of children a good reason for treating them as if they have the same rights as moral agents? Many people in our society find sexual relations between two males emotionally abhorrent. Surely that is not a good reason for being opposed to gay rights. Do instinct and culture constitute solid grounds for the truth of the Human Rights principle? If they do, then the instinct and culture of the Christian conservative opponent of abortion rights constitute solid grounds for outlawing women's right to choose. No doubt Warren would not welcome this conclusion. Thus many of the considerations to which Warren alludes do not support the truth of her Human Rights principle.

I suspect (although I am not sure) that Warren would choose to go to the bank with something like the following argument in defense of her Human Rights principle: It is necessary to award full rights to those humans who will become moral agents or who are mentally disabled in order to respect the rights of the moral agents those humans will become or once were. This is an interesting argument that deserves some analysis. I shall confine my attention to children.

It is worth noting that, strictly speaking, this argument reduces the Human Rights principle to a corollary of the Agent's Rights principle. We are asked to respect the rights of (grant the rights to?) children in order to respect the rights of the moral agents those children will become. So the question becomes: Is Warren's Agent's Rights principle sufficient to underwrite our obligations to children? Warren says little about this. However, it is hard to believe that we should treat any child as having a full right to life *because* the moral agent the child will become has a full right to life. After all, if the child is killed, there is no agent the child will become, and therefore killing the child does not violate the rights of that agent. On Warren's account killing such a child would be a victimless crime. Furthermore, it is certainly reasonable to think that some children are such poor prospects for becoming productive members of society that, if they have no right to life *as children*, it would not be wrong to kill them. The best argument in defense of Warren's Human Rights corollary is implausible.

This failure is fatal to Warren's theory. One typical problem for pro-choice moral status theories, as we have already seen, is that they are too narrow. They make too little killing wrong. In this respect Warren's (1997) theory is no improvement over her earlier theory and over Tooley's desire theory. Indeed, it is a step backward. Warren's (1979) theory could not account for the wrongfulness of infanticide and so she had to offer weak arguments against killing little babies. Warren's (1997) theory, by finding the locus of full moral status *only* in the nature of moral agents, offers us a theory of moral status that seems far more theoretically defensible than her (1979) view. The price that she pays for this advantage is that she has trouble accounting for the wrongness of killing not only infants, but any young children.

The inadequacy of Warren's theory should be judged in the context of the alternatives to it. On the future of value account, killing young children is wrong because it deprives them of the goods of their future. Thus, killing young children is wrong for the same reason that killing adults is wrong. No special explanation is needed to deal with the wrong of killing young children. Warren's account of the wrongness of killing must be judged a failure.

The HUMAN RIGHTS Principle and Non-Sentient Foetuses

There are, however, additional problems with Warren's view. Let us suppose that the argument of the preceding section is entirely wrong and that the Human Rights principle has been justified. The foetuses in which we are interested are, after all, human. Accordingly, there seems to be a reason for extending the Human Rights principle to include the unborn. Warren has arguments for rejecting this extension. Her arguments for not extending the Human Rights principle to foetuses before they are sentient are different from her arguments for not extending the Human Rights principle to foetuses after they are sentient.

Let us consider first her arguments for not extending the Human Rights principle to foetuses before they become sentient. Warren offers two arguments for such a restriction, a direct argument and a *reductio* argument. Her direct argument for the exclusion of non-sentient foetuses is that 'prior to the initial occurrence of conscious experience, there is no being that suffers and enjoys, and thus has needs and interests that matter to it' (Warren 1997: 204). Presumably Warren believes that because non-sentient foetuses have no interests and needs, they fall, like rocks, outside the scope of serious moral concern.

Warren's view that each being that lacks interests and needs falls outside the scope of serious moral concern certainly seems right. What Warren requires for her argument is the claim that if an individual has no interests and needs that matter to it, then she has no interests and needs. Is this true? It all depends upon what counts as mattering. On the one hand, if something can matter to an individual only if she is conscious of it, then no non-sentient foetus can have interests and needs that matter to it. However, on this interpretation of the 'mattering' claim we are not justified in inferring that no non-sentient foetus has interests and needs. Plainly there can be things that a young child needs or that are in her best interest that do not matter to her at all on this interpretation of 'mattering'. On the other hand, if something can matter to an individual whether or not she is conscious of it, then Warren's argument fails to establish that non-sentient foetuses must fall outside the scope of serious moral concern. This difficulty with Warren's view can be seen less abstractly if one considers persons who have been anaesthetized for surgery. In one clear sense nothing matters to them; in another sense, many things matter to them. They certainly have interests and needs.

Warren seems to be aware of this difficulty. She says that persons who are unconscious 'have not lost the capacity for sentience; they are simply not exercising it at present, or not at present able to exercise it'. Surely it is true that in one clear sense of 'capacity', non-sentient foetuses lack the capacity for sentience and anaesthetized persons have the capacity for sentience. The problem is that it does not follow from this that non-sentient foetuses lack interests and needs. Neither does it follow that, in one clear sense of 'mattering', nothing matters either to non-sentient foetuses or to anaesthetized persons. Accordingly, the difficulty with Warren's direct argument for excluding presentient foetuses from the Human Rights principle remains.

Warren also claims that 'that the potential of the presentient foetus to become a human being is enough to give it full moral status is subject to a *reductio* argument'. Her *reductio* is that, if this were so, then an unfertilized ovum (hereafter UFO) would also have full moral status because of its potential to become a human being. This, of course, is absurd (Warren 1997: 206).

One problem with this *reductio* argument is that it is directed against the wrong target. Those who are anti-choice typically do not hold that early abortions are wrong because presentient foetuses are potential human beings. They claim that foetuses before they become sentient *are* human beings, just very young and undeveloped and non-sentient ones. Nevertheless, because the human life account is unsound, the claim that a foetus before it becomes sentient is a human being does not imply that such a foetus has full moral status. The argument that it does have full moral status must be a potentiality argument of some kind. This leaves open the possibility that Warren's argument against attributing moral status on the basis of potentiality may have some force.

The claim that a foetus prior to sentience has a future of value is a claim about that foetus's potential. Is this claim open to the *reductio* that, if it were true, then UFOs would have a future of value? According to the future of value view, that killing you would deprive you of your future of value makes it wrong to kill you. An individual now has that sort of future of value just in case a later phase of that same individual would have a future it would value at later times and it has a future like ours. Accordingly, that earlier phase of that individual and those later phases of that individual must be phases of the *same* individual. That a UFO does not meet this condition can be shown by the following argument. Suppose the UFO that was my precursor was the same individual as I. If this were so, then there is just as good reason to hold that the sperm that was my precursor was the same individual as I. Since identity is transitive, it follows that the UFO that was my precursor and the sperm that was my precursor were the same individual. This is false. Therefore, the supposition is false. Accordingly, Warren's *reductio* argument is unsound (Stone 1987).

If one believes that the issue is whether a foetus prior to sentience is a potential human being, this point might be missed. According to Warren: 'In any case, the identity debate seems irrelevant to whether ova or zygotes are potential human beings. If an entity may develop into a human being, then surely it is a potential human being—even if the developmental process would alter it so greatly that we might reasonably wonder whether it has remained the selfsame entity' (Warren 1997: 207).

The reason the identity debate is entirely relevant is because the argument Warren needs is not about whether an entity can develop into a human being, but rather about whether an individual has a future of value. Thus, both Warren's direct argument and her *reductio* argument for excluding non-sentient foetuses from the scope of the Human Rights principle are flawed.

The HUMAN RIGHTS Principle and Sentient Foetuses

The analysis in the previous section shows that the sentience restriction on the Human Rights principle is unjustified. One might be tempted to conclude that, as a consequence, Warren's Human Rights principle commits her to an anti-choice view through and through. Notice, again, her Human Rights principle:

Within the limits of their own capacities and of [the Agent's Rights principle], human beings who are capable of sentience but not of moral agency have the same moral rights as do moral agents. (Warren 1997: 164)

If the sentience condition is removed, then the Human Rights principle *might be thought* to entail that, because foetuses are human beings, they have the same rights as moral agents. Moral agents have the right to life. Therefore, foetuses have the right to life. The claim that foetuses have the right to life implies (given some defensible assumptions) that killing them is wrong. So apparently Warren's Human Rights principle corrected for her error concerning non-sentient foetuses supports an anti-choice view. Is this correct?

Warren rejects the above line of reasoning. According to her the Agent's Rights principle limits the Human Rights principle. She says:

Unlike presentient foetuses, women are moral agents, with the rights to life, liberty, and the responsible exercise of moral agency. These rights are undermined when women are denied the freedom to decide whether and when to have children, and how many of them to have. (Warren 1997: 210)

Thus:

Birth . . . ends the infant's complete and necessary dependence upon the woman's body, thus removing the potential conflict between her moral rights and the infant's rights under the Human Rights principle, and bringing the latter principle fully into play for the first time. For these reasons, birth is still the most appropriate point at which to begin fully to enforce the moral rights that the Human Rights principle accords to sentient human beings. (Warren 1997: 218)

Therefore, even with the sentience condition removed, Warren's argument, if sound, would justify abortion at any time during pregnancy.

Is Warren's argument sound? Warren argues that foetuses don't have the right to life because, if they did, their right to life would conflict with the liberty rights of moral agents. The trouble with this view is that virtually no one has thought that liberty rights have such a broad scope that they include the liberty right to kill other human beings. Indeed, even libertarians believe that a moral agent's liberty rights are limited by the rights of other human beings not to be harmed. But if this is so, then there could be no conflict between a moral agent's liberty rights and the human rights of foetuses. Hence, Warren's argument fails.

Warren's argument won't do for another reason. The claim that the liberty rights of moral agents always trump the alleged rights of humans who are not yet moral agents is incompatible with parenting as we know it. This is the deep truth behind the remark attributed to the rabbi who claimed that life begins not at conception, and not at birth, but when the kids leave home and the dog dies. Warren is fond of claiming that while, one is pregnant, one is not free to hand off one's child to another, but after birth, it is possible for someone else to raise it. However, social attitudes being what they are, we are not free to hand off our children after birth. There are strong reasons having to do with social stability why this is so.

Accordingly, we may conclude that although Warren's updated (1997) person-hood defense of abortion choice is more elaborate than her earlier account, it is even less successful. This is because her view does not adequately meet the challenge that anti-choice moral status views must face. She has failed to show that her account of moral status is sufficiently broad to account for the wrongness of killing in those cases in which there is a consensus that it is wrong. Worse, even if we suppose (falsely) that she *had* shown that her view is not too narrow, she would not have shown that either non-sentient foetuses or sentient foetuses lack full moral status. Thus, her account would fail to support the abortion choice position that she plainly wishes to defend. Her updated personhood view is doubly unjustified.

DAVID BOONIN'S IMPROVED DESIRE ACCOUNT

Michael Tooley's desire based abortion choice view has been updated by David Boonin. Boonin has recently developed a sophisticated version of a desire account of the wrongness of killing that, he claims, (1) deals in a satisfactory way with the difficulties to which Tooley's (1972) desire account is subject and (2) is superior to the future of value account (Boonin 2003). Boonin calls the desire account a *present* desire account. He characterizes the future of value account as a *present or future* desire account, as follows:

If an individual P has a future-like-ours F *and* if either (a) P now desires that F be preserved, *or* (b) P will later desire to continue having the experiences contained in F (if P is not killed), then P is an individual with the same right to life as you or I. (Boonin 2003: 63)

Boonin's *present* desire account drops clause (b) from the antecedent of the above conditional thus:

If an individual P has a future-like-ours *and* if P now desires that F be preserved, then P is an individual with the same right to life as you or I. (Boonin 2003: 64)

Plainly the present desire account allows for abortion choice (unless there is another sufficient condition for having the same right to life as you or I), while the present or future desire account does not.

Boonin proposes two strategies for dealing with Tooley's apparent counter-examples to the present desire account. Consider, first, the temporarily comatose adult whom we believe it is wrong to kill, but who, because of lack of awareness, not only does not desire to continue to exist, but is incapable of desiring to continue to exist. Boonin argues that, although such an adult lacks an occurrent desire to live, she continues (under ordinary circumstances) to have a dispositional desire to continue to live. He goes on to argue for the continued existence of beliefs and desires while one is comatose on the grounds that such beliefs and desires do not have to be reacquired when one becomes conscious. Furthermore, it is reasonable to believe that a woman desires that her husband not commit adultery even when she is thinking of an issue associated with her profession. Accordingly, we have good reasons for accepting the reality of dispositional desires. Boonin's account of and defense of a dispositional desire strategy for dealing with the alleged temporarily unconscious adult counterexample to the present desire view seems reasonable (Boonin 2003: 64–70).

Consider now persons who lack a present occurrent or dispositional desire to live, but who would have, in the future, a desire to live. Boonin notes that a person's actual desires may be formed 'in conditions of great emotional distress' or when there is 'a lack of full and accurate information' (Boonin 2003: 70, 71). In these cases the *present* desire one '*would* have had if the actual desire had been formed under more ideal circumstances' is morally important (Boonin 2003: 70). Boonin calls such desires 'ideal desires'. The person who is depressed because of mental illness or because of great emotional trauma or who wants to die because of misinformation concerning her future will (typically) have an ideal desire to live, even though she lacks an actual desire to live. Accordingly, a *present ideal dispositional desire* version of a desire account of the wrongness of killing is not vulnerable to any of the Tooleyan counterexamples. Because foetuses have no desires at all, whether occurrent, dispositional, or ideal, abortion choice is morally permissible (Boonin 2003: 73). Boonin offers three arguments for his view that his present ideal dispositional desire account of the wrongness of killing is superior to the present or future desire, that is, the future of value, account.

Boonin's Parsimony Argument

According to Boonin his present ideal dispositional desire account is preferable to the present or future desire account because it is more parsimonious. On the present desire account we need to appeal only to one property of an individual to explain the wrongness of killing; on the present or future desire view, an appeal to two properties is required (Boonin 2003: 66–7, 73).

Boonin's argument is successful only if the future of value argument's lack of parsimony is due to the nature of the future of value account itself rather than to Boonin's rendering of it. In short, Boonin's appeal to parsimony would fail if the future of value account can be stated in a way that is as parsimonious as Boonin's account.

It usually is stated in just such a fashion. It makes reference only to the value of one's future, not to the value of one's present or past. Accordingly, the lack of parsimony that Boonin finds in the future of value account is really a function only of Boonin's statement of that account of the wrongness of killing, not of the account itself. Because there is no good reason to include present desires in the statement of the future of value account, other than for the purpose of rejecting the account on grounds of parsimony, I shall discard the unwieldy locution of present or future desires and refer to the account Boonin rejects as a future of value account.

Boonin's Salience Argument

Boonin claims that his present ideal dispositional desire account of the wrongness of killing is more 'salient' than a future of value account. He means that his account of the wrongness of killing 'enables us to account for the prima facie wrongness of killing by understanding killing as one instance of a more general category of acts that are prima facie wrong: acts that fail to respect the desires of others' (Boonin 2003: 74). The future of value account, by contrast, makes the wrongness of killing the suicidal 'an anomaly' (Boonin 2003: 76).

There are reasons for thinking that neither of Boonin's claims is true. Consider the second. Let us, following Boonin, discuss the case of Hans, who 'has been dumped by his girlfriend and has plunged into a deep depression. He can think about nothing else and has no desire to go on living' (Boonin 2003: 70). The future of value account makes killing Hans wrong for the same reason it is wrong to kill almost all other human beings. To kill Hans is to make him worse off than he otherwise would have been. To make him worse off than he otherwise would have been is to harm him. To harm him greatly is prima facie wrong. Boonin's claim that the future of value account makes the wrongness of killing the suicidal anomalous is plainly false.

Now consider Boonin's first claim. Boonin seems to be committed to the view that an account of wronging others in terms of failing to respect their desires is salient. There is something to be said for such a view. Of course, it is presumptively wrong to fail to respect the desires of others. The desires we should respect are the *actual* desires of others. In the case of Hans, Boonin holds that we should *not* respect his *actual* desires. Therefore, Boonin's account of the wrongness of killing Hans is anomalous with respect to the actual desire account of wrongness that meets his test of salience. Boonin has the matter of anomalies and the contrast between his present desire view and the future of value view exactly backwards.

Worse is to come. According to Boonin it is wrong to kill Hans because killing him fails to respect his ideal desires. A nice feature of a present *actual* desire view is that it is not difficult to determine what the actual desires of others are. One just asks them. Ideal desires are harder, because they are hypothetical. We cannot determine what they are by asking the relevant other. How then does one determine their content?

On this score Boonin is not especially helpful. He says, 'I am no more prepared to offer a full-blown theory of ideal desires than I am to offer a full-blown theory of dispositional desires. But again I do not believe that anything like this is necessary' (Boonin 2003: 78). Boonin justifies this lack of an account of the central notion in his theory of the wrongness of killing by noting that it is as difficult to determine that Hans would have a future of value as it is to determine what Hans's ideal desire concerning his future would be (Boonin 2003: 78).

It is not, of course, difficult to have good reasons for believing that certain persons who are suicidal have futures of value. Such persons are like other persons who have been suicidal and who have been treated with psychotropic drugs or with psychotherapy, and whose lives have improved. Psychiatrists have a great deal of data concerning such persons. To the extent that they are committed to scientific medicine, they will regard gathering such data as one of their professional responsibilities. Our judgment that many persons who are suicidal have a future of value has a sound empirical basis. It is indeed no more difficult to determine what a person's present ideal desire is in these cases than it is to determine whether or not such a person has a future of value. This is because someone's present ideal desire is nothing more than the desire of a rational and fully informed individual in that individual's situation, and a rational, fully informed desire about one's own future is based on the judgment that a rational and prudent individual would make about the value of her future. (Tricky issues arise in contexts in which duties to others are involved, of course.) Therefore, Hans will have an ideal desire to live just in case a rationally, fully informed individual in Hans's situation will judge that his future life has positive value as compared with death. A rationally, fully informed individual in Hans's situation will judge that Hans's life has positive value as compared with death just in case Hans has a future of value. Boonin's claim that the present ideal desire view and the future of value view will pick out (with one rare exception) the same range of (postnatal) cases is quite true. It is true because the present ideal desire view, when explicated in an obvious way, is *parasitic upon* the future of value view! The present ideal desire view turns out to be concerned, in the final analysis, neither with one's desires, as contrasted with one's future welfare, nor with one's present as compared to one's future. Thus, although Boonin's claim that the future of value view fails the salience test is incorrect, his claim that the present ideal desire view is salient is correct. It is salient *because* it *is* the future of value account stated in the language of desires.

Boonin's Counterexample Argument

Boonin believes that there is a counterexample to the future of value view that is not a counterexample to the present ideal desire view. He asks us to imagine a case of a person whose future will contain many of the sorts of experiences other humans take to be valuable, but, because of an irreversible chemical imbalance in her brain, does not now and never will value any of those experiences. Boonin claims that the future of value theory implies that it would not be wrong to kill this person. He is correct. Boonin claims that the present ideal desire view entails that this person 'has the same right to life as you and I'. Is this true?

The ideal desire view asks us to imagine what a fully informed rational person would *presently* desire in this chemical imbalance case. So let us imagine that we ourselves are in this chemical imbalance situation, but that there is a drug that can relieve us of the imbalance only temporarily, only briefly, and only once so that we can survey our future rationally and with full information. It is hard to imagine why such a person would have the present desire to live after the drug was no longer effective. Boonin's analysis of this alleged counterexample is incorrect.

Boonin's argument fails in another respect. Suppose his analysis were correct and our chemically imbalanced individual did have the ideal desire to live. Why should this show that the future of value theory is false? Because, says Boonin, 'virtually every critic of abortion will agree that [this individual] has a right to life' (Boonin 2003: 77). Boonin's criterion of truth is not correct. If it were, then we would have a (too easy) proof for the existence of God! We may conclude that none of Boonin's arguments for the superiority of the ideal desire account over the future of value account of the wrongness of killing is successful.

Why Boonin's Account Is Arbitrary

Boonin's ideal desire account of the wrongness of killing suffers from another problem. At least two versions of an ideal desire account are possible. On Boonin's version, having an ideal desire at a time requires having some actual desire at that time. An ideal desire is an actual desire that is corrected, when necessary, to account for imperfect information and imperfect rationality. Because no preconscious foetus has an actual desire, no preconscious foetus has an ideal desire to live, and because no preconscious foetus has an ideal desire to live, no preconscious foetus has the right to life. However, the Boonin version of the ideal desire account could be altered so that the actual desire requirement is dropped. Then foetuses could have ideal desires also. So just as Hans, were he fully rational and fully informed, would have the desire to continue to exist, a preconscious foetus, were she rational and fully informed, would have (because she, like Hans, has a future of value) the desire to continue to exist. Why prefer Boonin's version of the ideal desire account to the 'Marquis version' of the ideal desire account? The characterization of the second version is apt because, of course, such a version of the ideal desire account is just the future of value account in ideal desire clothing.

Boonin emphasizes that his preferred account is the Boonin, not the Marquis, version. That is no argument. Boonin notes the differences between the Boonin and the Marquis versions of the ideal desire account (Boonin 2003: 80–3). That is no argument either. Perhaps Boonin regards the following as an argument: 'There is no desire that a rock would have under more ideal circumstances, for example, because a rock does not have any desires to begin with. But it follows from this that a particular ideal desire can meaningfully be attributed only to someone who has at least some other actual desires' (Boonin 2003: 80). If this is a claim about Boonin's version of the ideal desire theory, this is true, but does not establish the superiority of Boonin's version. One would not attribute even ideal desires to rocks because there is no present or future stage of the rock that it would later value or disvalue. Foetuses are quite different. Hypothetical desires can be attributed as easily to foetuses as to Hans. There are reasonably clear criteria for the attribution in both cases. Accordingly, even if Boonin had shown that an ideal desire account of the wrongness of killing were superior to the future of value account, he still would not have established that *his* ideal desire account of the wrongness of killing should be accepted. Hence, he would not have adequately defended abortion choice.

We may safely conclude that, although Boonin's ideal desire version of Tooley's desire account of the wrongness of killing is not vulnerable to counterexamples, Boonin fails to show that his theory is better than the future of value theory. Indeed, if we eliminate an arbitrary feature of Boonin's theory, Boonin *could* not have shown that the ideal desire theory is preferable to the future of value theory. With this elimination, the ideal desire theory *is the same as* the future of value theory.

Summary and Conclusion

A brief survey of the analysis of this chapter will be useful. Think of individuals whom we all agree it is presumptively seriously wrong to kill. If pressed, we might say that it is wrong to kill them because they are human beings or because they are persons. Each reason has different implications for the ethics of abortion. There are difficulties, as we have seen, with each reason. A number of philosophers have attempted to resolve the abortion controversy by finding reasons for the wrongness of killing embedded in broader, and clearly relevant, moral considerations. There are at least three such accounts. The desire account is based on the moral truth that, in general, impeding the self-regarding desires of others is wrong. The future of value account is based on the moral truth that, in general, inflicting harm on others is wrong when we would regard it as wrong to inflict a harm of that sort on us. The moral agency account is based on the moral truth that, in general, failing to respect the will of rational moral agents is wrong. The purpose of this chapter was to appraise these three accounts, all of which are intended to support particular views of the ethics of abortion.

The future of value account seems to deal adequately with cases in which there is a consensus that killing is wrong and also with cases in which few object to ending intentionally a life. It supports the view that abortion is immoral. Is there an account that is at least as plausible that underwrites abortion choice? According to the desire account, because foetuses do not desire to live, they lack the right to life. The desire argument strategy fails because many adults who do not desire to live plainly do have the right to life. David Boonin has attempted to plug the holes in this Tooleyan actual desire account by proposing to replace it with an ideal desire account. However, Boonin's strategy faces, as we have seen, many difficulties. In general, our duty not to interfere with the desires of others is a duty not to impede their actual desires, not their ideal desires when those ideal desires are different. Furthermore, the ideal desire view, in order to deal adequately with consensus cases, turns out to be parasitic on the future of value view. In addition, Boonin preserves abortion choice only by adopting an ad hoc restriction to avoid attributing ideal desires to foetuses.

Mary Anne Warren's (1997) defense of abortion choice shares a difficulty with the actual desire account: Her Agent's Rights principle, although it clearly embodies a generally acknowledged principle of respect, fails to account for the wrongness of killing many individuals whom we all believe it is wrong to kill. Warren attempts to deal with this gap by adding a Human Rights principle to her account. Because her Human Rights principle does not fit easily into a general theory of wrong action her defense of this principle is inadequate. It seems more like an ad hoc attempt to deal with the problems with her view. Worse, without utterly arbitrary restrictions to the Human Rights principle, the principle supports the claim that abortion is immoral.

Interestingly, Warren's and Boonin's views are similar. Neither a 'bare bones' desire view nor a respect for moral agency view account for the wrongness of killing all those who clearly have the right to life. Hence, strategies must be found for expanding both views. Unless arbitrary restrictions are placed on both expansions, both views will support the view that abortion is immoral. Hence, both Warren and Boonin, in the final analysis, must restrict their accounts in arbitrary ways.

The analysis of this chapter supports the conclusion that, of the alternatives considered in this chapter, the future of value view is superior and abortion is immoral. There are, of course, other alternatives to, and objections to, the future of value view that have not been discussed in this chapter. Furthermore, the important view that, even if foetuses have the right to life, women do not have the obligation to provide them with uterine life support also has not been considered.

REFERENCES

BOONIN, D. (2003), *A Defense of Abortion* (Cambridge: Cambridge University Press).

MCMAHAN, J. (2002), *The Ethics of Killing: Problems at the Margins of Life* (New York: Oxford University Press).

MARQUIS, D. (1989), 'Why Abortion Is Immoral', *Journal of Philosophy*, 89: 183–202.

PURDY, L., and TOOLEY, M. (1974), 'Is Abortion Murder?', in R. Perkins (ed.), *Abortion: Pro and Con* (Cambridge, Mass.: Schenkman).

STONE, J. (1987), 'Why Potentiality Matters', *Canadian Journal of Philosophy*, 17: 815–30.

TOOLEY, M. (1972), 'Abortion and Infanticide', *Philosophy and Public Affairs*, 2: 37–65.

——— (1973), 'A Defense of Abortion and Infanticide', in J. Feinberg (ed.), *The Problem of Abortion*, 1st edn. (Belmont, Calif.: Wadsworth), 51–91.

——— (1983), *Abortion and Infanticide* (Oxford: Clarendon Press).

WARREN, M. A. (1979), 'On the Moral and Legal Status of Abortion', repr. in R. A. Wasserstrom (ed.), *Today's Moral Problems*, 2nd edn. (New York: Macmillan), 35–51.

——— (1997), *Moral Status: Obligations to Persons and Other Living Things* (Oxford: Clarendon Press).

···

CHAPTER 18

MORAL STATUS, MORAL VALUE, AND HUMAN EMBRYOS: IMPLICATIONS FOR STEM CELL RESEARCH

··

BONNIE STEINBOCK

INTRODUCTION

···

HUMAN embryonic stem cells (ES cells) are of scientific and medical interest because of their ability to develop into different tissue types and because of their ability to be propagated for many generations in laboratory culture. Grown in a laboratory,

The first version of this chapter was given at the 24th Annual Philosophy Conference on moral status, held at the University of Santa Clara in 2002. I owe thanks to its organizer, Larry Nelson, for inviting me to write on the topic, and to the participants for helpful and searching comments. Versions were also presented to the Philosophy Departments at Utah University, Syracuse University, and Carnegie Mellon, where the discussions were extremely helpful. Finally, I owe a large debt to Alex John London and David DeGrazia for very helpful comments on an earlier draft.

they might one day be used in the treatment of degenerative diseases such as Parkinson's and Alzheimer's. They could provide bone cells for the treatment of osteoporosis, eye cells for macular degeneration, blood cells for cancer, insulin-producing cells for diabetes, heart muscle cells for heart disease, nerve cells for spinal cord injury. The potential for benefit to so many people is a strong argument for doing—and funding—embryonic stem cell (ESC) research. Yet ESC research is very controversial because the derivation of ES cells—at least at the present time—destroys the embryo. Thus, the morality of ESC research depends primarily on the morality of destroying human embryos, raising the question of the moral status of the human embryo.[1]

This chapter begins with an introduction to the biology behind ESC research. Next I present briefly four views of moral status, based on four different criteria: biological humanity, personhood, possession of interests, and having a future-like-ours (FLO). On two of these views (the person view and the interest view), embryos clearly lack moral status, but they most likely do not have moral status on the FLO account either. Only the biological humanity criterion *combined with* the view that life begins at conception results in the conclusion that very early extracorporeal embryos have full moral status, making ESC research that destroys embryos morally wrong. This explains why even some who are anti-abortion are not against ESC research: they do not view the very early, extracorporeal embryo as having the same moral status as the fetus. However, the morality of stem cell research is not completely determined by the question of moral status, for that issue, I argue, is not exhaustive of morality. Some entities, including human embryos, that do not have moral status nevertheless have *moral value*, and are entitled to respect. In the last section of the chapter, I give an account of what this respect requires and how it differs from Kantian respect. I conclude that the respect due to embryos is consistent with ESC research; that it is ethically acceptable to use either cloned embryos or spare IVF (*in vitro* fertilization) embryos; and that there are no ethical (as opposed to political) reasons that demand the development of alternative sources of human pluripotent stem cells.

EMBRYOS AND ES CELLS

In the normal course of events, an embryo is the product of fertilization, the union of male and female gametes.[2] Once fertilization is completed, the resulting

---

[1] Paul Lauritzen (2005) disagrees. He thinks that the real concern is not the status of the embryo but that stem cell therapies, including both adult and embryonic stem cells, may erode the notion of human nature by undermining the notion of a natural human lifespan, or by blurring species boundaries.s

[2] Embryos can also be created without fertilization via cloning or parthenogenesis.

single-cell zygote divides to produce two cells; these two divide to produce four; four divide to produce eight, to form a blastocyst. The cells of the blastocyst, known as blastomeres, are separated into two parts: an outer layer, called the trophoblast, that eventually becomes the placenta, and an inner cell mass that contributes to the future embryo. Each blastomere is *totipotent*—this means that each individual cell has the ability to form a complete human being. ES cells are derived from the inner cell mass at roughly five to nine days after fertilization, when the blastocyst is comprised of between 100 and 200 cells. Scientists used to distinguish between totipotency—the capacity to become a complete human organism—and pluripotency—the capacity to develop into certain cells. ES cells were held to be merely pluripotent, not totipotent. However, the distinction between blastomeres and ES cells is no longer so clear. Single ES cells have been used to create whole mice, and perhaps could be used to create whole human beings. (We do not know if this can be done, since no one is currently doing the research, owing to the widespread opposition to reproductive cloning.) In today's laboratories, the distinction between totipotency and pluripotency is relatively meaningless.[3]

Sources of Embryos

Where do the extracorporeal embryos from which ES cells can be derived come from? One source is the creation of embryos by IVF in the course of infertility treatment. Since many more embryos are created than are likely to be needed for reproductive purposes, couples may donate their 'spare' or 'surplus' or 'discarded' embryos for research purposes. The main advantage to using spare embryos to derive ES cells is that the vast majority will be discarded (or perpetually frozen) in any event. This makes a very strong intuitive case for allowing couples who desire to do so to donate their left-over embryos to medical research, including ESC research. Embryos can also be created via IVF specifically for research purposes, using donated gametes. Embryos can also be cloned for research purposes, using the same technique that created the cloned lamb Dolly, namely, somatic cell nuclear transfer (SCNT). Although many mammals, including sheep, goats, and cats, have been cloned, until relatively recently it was thought that it would be impossible to clone a human embryo. Then, in February 2004, a team of scientists in South Korea, led by Dr Woo Suk Hwang and Dr Shin Yong Moon of Seoul National University, announced that, using SCNT, they had cloned a human blastocyst and derived a pluripotent embryonic stem cell line from it (Hwang et al. 2004). The following year they announced that they had developed a faster and more efficient method of cloning embryos and deriving human ES cell lines (Hwang et al. 2005).

---

[3] I thank Lee Silver and the late Lorraine Flaherty for helping to clear this up for me.

While it took them 200 tries to derive just one cell line in 2004, they reported in 2005 that they were able consistently to derive a cell line in fewer than twenty tries. Unfortunately, it was later discovered that Dr Hwang had fabricated evidence for all of that research. This was a sharp set-back for therapeutic cloning, 'forcing cloning researchers back to square one' (Wade and Sang-Hun 2006: A12). At the time of this writing, no one has managed to clone a human embryo, although several laboratories are pursuing this goal. The advantage of cloned over fertilized embryos is that the derived stem cells will have the same genome as the donor. If it becomes possible to create tissue for replacement purposes, the fact that the tissue is genetically identical to the donor should, in theory, avoid problems of rejection.

A similar advantage might be obtained using parthenogenesis, a process by which an unfertilized egg is chemically stimulated to divide into what scientists call 'parthenotes'—embryo-like products from which stem cells may be extracted. Tissue from stem cells derived from parthenogenesis would be easier to match with patients and less likely to be rejected because the parthenote would contain the DNA of only one person. Moreover, because a parthenote is assumed to lack entirely the potential for development as a human being, it is therefore, arguably, not a true embryo. Its creation and destruction might, therefore, raise fewer ethical concerns than those raised by embryos.

Other Kinds of Stem Cells

Embryonic stem cells are not the only kind of stem cells. Another kind of stem cell is embryonic germ (EG) cells, which are isolated from the gonadal ridges of 5- to 9-week-old fetuses donated after induced abortions. Although there are fewer data from animal EG cell experiments than from ES cell experiments, it is assumed that EG cells have less plasticity, that is, less ability to become different kinds of cells than ES cells, because the EG cells are much further along in development (five to nine weeks as opposed to five to nine days).There are also adult stem (AS) cells, which have been found in many different kinds of tissue, including bone marrow and heart muscle, as well as umbilical cord blood and the placenta. Although the term 'adult stem cells' is widely used, it is slightly misleading, as AS cells are not found only in adults; they are found in children and even in fetuses. A more accurate, though less commonly used, term is 'non-embryonic stem cell'. The primary function of AS cells is to maintain and repair the tissue or cells in which they are found. Research into AS cells does not raise any special ethical issues (beyond the usual ones involved in any research using human subjects) because AS cells can be collected without lasting harm to the donor. However, many scientists believe that AS cells have less clinical promise than ES cells precisely because they are more differentiated and therefore likely to give rise only to a limited number of tissues. For this reason, they are sometimes described as *multipotent*, rather than pluripotent (Chapman et al. 1999). However, other scientists argue that, unlike ES cells, AS cells have already proved successful in the treatment of disease, for example, in bone marrow transplants, which have been done for the past thirty years. In November 2004 two studies in the *New England Journal of Medicine* (Laughlin et al.; Rocha et al.) concluded that umbilical cord blood works nearly as well as bone marrow transplanted from unrelated donors for leukemia patients. Another potential substitute for ethically controversial ES cells is multipotent cells derived from post-birth human placentas. Such cells could be derived without killing embryos, and might prove to have greater potential than AS cells (Yen et al. 2005). However, it could be a decade before the required tests and clinical trials to determine the viability of placenta-derived multipotent cells (PDMCs) are completed.

Admittedly, no one can know at this point whether ES cells will live up to their therapeutic promise, or if they will prove more successful than AS cells or PDMCs in the treatment of disease (Schwartz 2006). AS cells might prove better for some diseases than ES cells, despite the greater plasticity of ES cells. At the same time, the fact that no therapies have yet been developed using ES cells is surely no reason not to engage in ESC research. From a *scientific* perspective, it makes sense to do research on all of these alternatives. The real objection to ESC research is moral, not scientific. It is based on the opposition to the destruction of human embryos in biomedical research. 'At the heart of the debates over stem cells and cloning are questions that politicians cannot settle: When does human life begin, and what is the moral status of the human embryo?' (Stolberg 2001). To decide how we should think about human embryos, we need an account of moral status.

THE BIOLOGICAL HUMANITY VIEW

In the Western moral and legal tradition, it is often taken for granted that what gives someone (full) moral status and moral rights is *biological humanity*. All and only members of the species *Homo sapiens* have full moral status and moral rights. This view of moral status is derived from the Judeo-Christian tradition, which teaches, first, that human beings *alone* of creation are created in God's image, which gives human beings a status far superior to the rest of creation, and second, that *all* human beings are created in God's image, which makes us all God's children. The Judeo-Christian approach is clearly a moral advance over earlier views that limited moral status to members of one's own group or tribe. Theoretically (though often not in reality), it prohibited the enslaving or killing of other human beings simply because they were outsiders. On the traditional view of moral status, *all* human beings count, regardless of race, ethnicity, nationality, or gender.

When Does Human Life Begin? The Conception View

The biological humanity view holds that it is *human beings* who have moral status. But what is a human being? 'Human being' cannot be defined as any entity with a human genetic code, because *every* cell in a human body has a human genetic code. The biological humanity criterion must be understood as according moral status to the human *organism*: an integrated whole with the capacity for self-directed development. Otherwise, there is no way to distinguish human cells, which are merely parts of a human organism, from the organism itself. The next question is 'When is there a human organism?' or 'When does the human organism begin to exist?' One answer is that a human organism comes into existence at conception or fertilization (let us call this the 'conception view'). If we combine the biological humanity criterion of moral status with the conception view about when a human organism begins, we get the view that a fertilized human egg, or human zygote, is a human being with the same moral status as any other human being, such as you or I.

Proponents of the conception view usually hold it to be a matter of 'plain biological fact' that a human organism begins at conception. However, the biological facts are not so simple, owing to the complexities of conception. Contrary to much of the anti-abortion literature, there is no 'moment of conception'. The uniting of sperm and egg—fertilization—is a process that occurs over many hours. Understanding the biology of conception presents complications to the simple picture of the uniting of sperm and egg as the beginning of human life.

During the first hours after penetration, the genetic material provided by the male and female remain segregated. The chromosomes of the egg and sperm remain in their own nuclear envelopes, known as pronuclei, because each contains only half the genetic material found in the normal nuclei of somatic cells. The chromosomes in the two pronuclei duplicate themselves separately, as they migrate toward each other. Once the single-cell zygote divides, the envelopes surrounding the two pronuclei dissolve, and the condensed chromosomes of both paternal and maternal origin align on a common spindle. This merging of chromosomes, known as syngamy, does not occur until the two-cell stage. Now each of the two nuclei of the two-cell embryo contains a complete set of forty-six chromosomes, and fertilization is complete (Silver 1998: 45). This occurs about thirty hours after initial contact of sperm and egg (Mauron 2004: 708). However, it is not clear that there is a uniquely individuated organism even at the two-cell stage, because of what is known as the twinning argument. The blastocyst contains inner mass cells (blastomeres), which are totipotent. Each is capable, if properly manipulated, of developing into a full human being (Green 2001: 48). Embryo splitting occurs naturally in the case of identical twins (or triplets or even quadruplets or quintuplets). Mary Warnock, Chair of the Warnock Committee in Great Britain, alluded to the possibility of twinning by saying, 'Before fourteen days the embryo hasn't yet decided how many people it is going to be' (Lockwood 1988: 190). This fact has ontological implications. If the blastocyst can become more than one person, then the relationship between the blastocyst and its later stages is not the same one-to-one relationship that exists between the later embryo and the fetus or born human being (Mauron 2004: 710). The activation of the diploid genome may begin at the blastocyst stage, but because twinning can still occur, that diploid genome is not the genome of one and only one individual. As Green (2001: 29) expresses the point, 'If biological humanness starts with the appearance of a unique diploid genome, twins and triplets are living evidence that the early embryo is not yet one human being, but a community of possibly different individuals held together by a gelatinous membrane.' It is only when twinning is no longer possible that there is a unique human organism. This happens when the primitive streak, the precursor of the nervous system, begins to form. This process, called gastrulation, occurs at about fourteen days after fertilization. This is why the Warnock Committee, as well as the Human Embryo Research Panel in the United States, recommended that research on human embryos should be limited to the first fourteen days of development.

It may be asked, what difference does it make whether the embryo could develop into one human being or two (or three or even more)? Why should the fact that it might become more than one human being deprive the early embryo of moral status? Indeed, if it might become two people, does not that give us twice as much reason to protect it? This question misses the point, which is whether the embryo, which is still capable of becoming two or more people, can be said to be a *unique* individual, for either biological or moral purposes (Green 2001: 31).

We have seen that the line marking the beginning of the new human organism can be drawn at different stages: the very beginning (the penetration of the egg by the sperm); a day or so later, when the chromosomes of the mother and father merge (syngamy); or about two weeks after fertilization begins, when the primitive streak appears (gastrulation), after which twinning is no longer possible. Which of these stages correctly marks the beginning of the new human being? There is no definite, scientific answer to this question, because it depends on one's conception of an organism. One might hold that the cluster of undifferentiated cells within the zona pellucida is sufficiently integrated to constitute an organism, but one might also plausibly maintain that the organism begins to exist only later, when the cells become differentiated and lose their totipotency. Neither view is obviously wrong, and neither is rationally required of us (McMahan 2002: 28).

This indeterminacy regarding the beginning of the human organism may help to explain why adherents of the biological humanity criterion can differ in their views about the moral status of early human embryos, and why many opponents of abortion are not opposed to ESC research.

Abortion and Embryo Research

'In recent polls, 57 percent of abortion opponents have said they support embryonic stem-cell research. So have 72 percent of Roman Catholics. Senator Orrin Hatch, as anti-abortion as they come, argues that "a frozen embryo stored in a refrigerator in a clinic" just isn't the same as "a fetus developing in a mother's womb"' (Begley 2001: 24). In a letter to Tommy G. Thompson, the Secretary of the United States Department of Health and Human Services, Senator Hatch wrote, 'To me a frozen embryo is more akin to a fertilized egg or frozen sperm than to a fetus naturally developing in the body of a mother' (Wade 2001: 20). For Hatch, then, pregnancy, not conception, marks the beginning of the life of a human being.[4] The fetus growing and developing in its mother's body is a much more developed and complex entity than a pre-implantation blastocyst, and one with which we can more easily identify. As one columnist (Kinsley 2001) expressed it, 'These [blastocysts] are not fetuses with tiny, waving hands and feet. These are microscopic grouping of a few undifferentiated cells.'

Another explanation for support for ESC research on the part of opponents of abortion is that abortion is morally charged in a way that embryo research is not. How one thinks about abortion depends at least as much on one's views about sexuality, motherhood, and the proper role of women as it does on abstract views about the moral status of the embryo (Luker 1984). For many pro-lifers, abortion is equated with loose morals and the absence of sexual responsibility. By contrast, embryo research is devoid of any sexual connotations, and, moreover, is potentially life-saving, something that is not literally true of the vast majority of abortions.

Even if ESC research is regarded as morally different from abortion, many people remain troubled by the destruction of embryonic life. ESC research would be more acceptable to them if there were a way to derive ES cells (or their equivalent) without killing embryos. This might be achieved by deriving ES cells from no-longer living embryos or from a biological entity that is not a true embryo. Both of these ideas were presented to the President's Council on Bioethics and discussed in its White Paper (2005).[5]

---

[4] A similar view is reflected in Jewish Law. Genetic materials outside the uterus have no moral or legal status since they are not part of a human being until implanted in the womb. 'Even in the uterus, the embryo is considered a "formed" human fetus only after the first forty days. And as the commandment to save lives is central to Judaism, the creation of embryos by cloning for therapeutic purposes is justifiable' (Neiger 2005). In an interesting parallel, Aquinas also regards forty days after conception as having moral significance, for it is only then that the (male) embryo is supposed to acquire a human form, and thus can have a human soul. Female fetuses do not become ensouled until ninety days after conception (Cole-Turner 2004: 735).

[5] For a discussion of all four proposals considered by the President's Council on Bioethics, see Steinbock (2005).

Alternative Sources of ES Cells

Don Landry and Howard Zucker, both from the College of Physicians and Surgeons at Columbia University, propose to derive stem cells from no longer living embryos. Their proposal is based on a close analogy with the use of human cadavers for biomedical research or as sources of organs. If it is acceptable to remove organs from no longer living developed human beings, it should be equally acceptable (and consistent with the Dickey Amendment, which prohibits the use of federal funds for research in which human embryos are destroyed or harmed) to remove stem cells from no longer living human embryos. To be considered for use, embryos would have to be originally created with reproductive intent, healthy enough to be cryopreserved for future reproduction, and, after thawing, turn out to be dead.

Landry and Zucker apply the traditional concept of death—the irreversible loss of the integrated functioning of an organism as a whole—and apply it to the embryo, using the notion of 'organismic death'. They write:

For a developed human organism, brain death marks the irreversible loss of the capacity for all ongoing and integrated organic functioning. We propose that the defining capacity of a 4- or 8-cell human embryo is continued and integrated cellular division, growth, and differentiation. We further propose that an embryo that has irreversibly lost this capacity, even as its individual cells are alive, is properly considered organismically dead (Landry and Zucker 2004).

A significant fraction of embryos created *in vitro* simply stop dividing after the four- to eight-cell stage. Most of these spontaneous 'cleavage arrests' are associated with chromosomal abnormalities, preventing the embryos from being a good source for stem cells. However, some turn out to be 'mosaic', that is, they contain some normal blastomeres as well as cells with chromosomal abnormalities. The normal blastomeres could be a source of ES cells.

The proposal raises questions about both the definition of death and the criteria for determining it. The arrested embryos must contain at least some viable cells that retain normal developmental potential; otherwise they will not be a source of stem cells. Placed in the proper milieu, some of these cells might resume dividing. The President's Council on Bioethics asked, 'How, then, can we be sure that such an embryo is really dead? More generally, can we confidently declare that an embryo is dead just because all its cells have stopped dividing? What exactly do we mean by the "organismic death" of an embryo?' (2005: 12).

Part of the problem is that the concept of organismic death—the death of an organism *as a whole*—has not been commonly applied to an embryo, that is, to any largely undifferentiated organism so close to the beginning of its life. A further question is how to determine its death. This is more difficult than for an adult because the embryo has no integrating vital organs: no brain to be considered 'brain dead', no heart that has ceased to beat and pump blood (President's Council 2005: 12). Is spontaneous cleavage arrest the same as death? Some might view this question as sophistical. It might be argued that the point is not whether death has occurred. Rather, it is that embryos that have stopped dividing lack the potential for further development. Without the potential for further development, they are not genuine human organisms, and so do not have human moral status.

If, however, the potential for further development is a sine qua non of moral status, then non-viable embryos—embryos that are living but cannot develop further, and therefore are not candidates for transplantation into a uterus—are not human beings. This interpretation is rejected by, for example, the Roman Catholic Church. When Richard Doerflinger, Deputy Director of the Secretariat for Pro-Life Activities, United States Conference of Catholic Bishops, was asked in his testimony before the Human Embryo Research Panel (HERP) in 1994 whether it would be permissible to use in research non-viable embryos created during infertility treatment, he gave a categorical 'no'. Their lack of developmental potential does not deprive them of their humanity. Non-viable embryos are dying human subjects, he said, and to use them in research would be just like using a dying AIDS patient in an experiment without that individual's consent (Green 2001: 18). One question, then, about the Landry–Zucker proposal is whether it can persuasively draw a sharp distinction between a dead embryo and a non-viable embryo.

Another proposal comes from Dr William Hurlbut, who is himself a member of the President's Council. Rather than redefining embryo death, Hurlbut proposes a technique that would create a biological artifact, lacking the moral status of a human embryo, from which pluripotent stem cells could then be derived (President's Council 2005: 36). According to Dr Hurlbut, what differentiates a human embryo from other human cells is that it contains within itself the organizing principle for the self-development and self-maintenance of the full human organism. An entity that lacked this intrinsic potential for development would not be a true embryo. This can happen in natural reproduction, when an embryo lacks certain essential elements, making it impossible for the embryo to develop. For example, research in mice has demonstrated that mutations in the Cdx2 gene cause death at the blastocyst stage because the embryos fail to form a trophectoderm, which normally gives rise to the placenta. Hurlbut's proposal attempts to mimic these natural examples, using a technique he calls altered nuclear transfer (ANT). ANT is based on the SCNT technique, with one modification. Particular developmental genes in the somatic cell nucleus would be silenced prior to transfer to the enucleated oocyte. 'Removal of cells from, or even disaggregation of, this artifact would not be killing or harming, for there is no living being here to be killed or harmed' (President's Council 2005: 37). To ensure that the stem cells taken from the artifact were usable, the missing genes would be reinserted after the cells were extracted.

Since ANT is as yet untested experimentally (even in animals), it is not known whether it would work in humans. SCNT, which inserts a normal nucleus into the enucleated egg cell, has proven difficult enough; some commentators are highly skeptical that ANT, which inserts a defective nucleus into the egg cell, would work (President's Council 2005: 90). Another source of opposition comes from those who think it is unethical to create embryo-like entities and then intentionally modify them to prevent them from developing into human embryos. Robert Lanza of Advanced Cell Technologies says, 'I think this is an abuse of cloning technology. It will be a sad day when scientists use genetic manipulation to deliberately create crippled embryos to please the Church' (Holden and Vogel 2004: 2175).[6]

The Hurlbut proposal is based on the idea that human pluripotent cells might be derived from something that is not an embryo, not an organism, not a 'living being'. However, as we saw earlier, some maintain that a distinctive human organism appears only at gastrulation, when twinning is no longer possible. If blastocysts are not uniquely distinctive human organisms, it is not clear why ANT is superior to SCNT, or the use of spare IVF embryos. Moreover, ANT is complex, technically challenging, and not even testable without time-consuming experiments involving substantial investment of precious resources (President's Council 2005: 47), and so could set back the progress of ESC research considerably. As Michael Gazzaniga, a member of the President's Council, expressed it in an appendix to the White Paper: 'Why delay what we know works with this sideshow?' (2005: 77).

The motivation for finding alternative sources of human pluripotent cells is the conviction that the destruction of human embryos is morally wrong. This is in turn based on acceptance of the biological humanity criterion. But is this the correct criterion of moral status? In the following sections I will argue that it is not, that species membership by itself does not endow or deprive a being of moral status. I begin with the critique of the biological humanity criterion of moral status presented in Mary Anne Warren's classic article on abortion (1973).

THE PERSON VIEW

Warren argues that the conservative[7] on abortion confuses two distinct senses of the word 'human being': a biological or genetic sense which means 'member of the species homo sapiens' and a moral sense which means 'full-fledged member of the moral community'. Unquestionably, the human fetus is human in the biological sense (what else could it be?), but it does not follow that it is human in the moral sense. Indeed, this is exactly what is at issue in the abortion debate. It needs to be

---

[6] In their White Paper, the President's Council on Bioethics (2005: 69) makes the following observation: 'Curiously, in September 2002, Advanced Cell Technology, the company for which Dr. Lanza works, filed a patent for producing genetically altered artificial embryo-like entities, partly for the same purposes.'

[7] The terms 'conservative' and 'liberal' are terms of art, standard in the abortion literature, and are not intended to convey general political positions.

argued (not simply assumed) that biological humanity endows a being with moral humanity. And this, Warren maintains, cannot be done.

To show the irrelevance of species membership to moral status, Warren gives the following thought experiment: Imagine we came into contact with non-humans who were sentient, rational, and capable of moral agency (for example, intelligent aliens, like ET). Surely the fact that they were not genetically human, not members of our species, would not determine, or even be relevant to, their moral status. We would not be justified in eating them, or enslaving them, or putting them in zoos, or using them (without their consent) in scientific research. This shows that being biologically human is not a necessary condition of moral status. Nor is it a sufficient condition, according to Warren, for some genetic human beings lack full moral status, for example, irreversibly unconscious human beings, such as those in a persistent vegetative state (PVS) or anencephalic infants, who are born without a cerebral cortex. Someone in PVS is alive, but, as it might be expressed, the person is no longer there. Anencephalic infants are biologically human, but without a cerebral cortex, they lack the capacity to become persons. According to Warren, it is persons who have moral status, and genetic humanity is only an imprecise marker for personhood. Warren then goes on to suggest that the traits that are most central to the concept of personhood are sentience (the capacity to experience pleasure and pain), consciousness, self-consciousness, the capacity for reasoning, self-motivated activity, and the capacity to use language. Warren does not give an account of why these traits have moral significance, but rather suggests that if we were trying to decide whether an alien life form has 'human rights' or whether it may be used, for example, as a source of food, it would be the presence or absence of these traits that would settle the question.

The implication for the moral status of embryos is clear. Embryos have none of the person-making characteristics Warren enumerates. As we have seen, whether very early embryos are human organisms, and thus qualify as human beings in the genetic sense, can be debated, but ultimately it does not matter on the person view, since it is persons, not genetic human beings or human organisms, who have moral status.

Warren's claim is not that moral status is contingent on possession of *all* the person-making characteristics she lists. It is rather that beings that have *none* of these characteristics cannot be persons, or human beings in the moral sense. Since embryos have none of these characteristics, they cannot be members of the moral community. Moreover, even late-gestation fetuses have fewer person-making characteristics than most adult mammals, or even adult fish. If fish do not have a right to life, neither do fetuses.

One obvious difficulty with the person view is that it appears to exclude many individuals who most of us think are members of the moral community, such as elderly people with advanced dementia, individuals with severe developmental disabilities, and even normal newborns. (Their potential to become persons cannot be a basis for ascribing moral status to them without being a basis for ascribing moral status to fetuses and embryos.) Advocates of the genetic humanity criterion maintain that any criterion other than genetic humanity will have this fatal flaw. However, it may be possible to modify the person view so that it does not exclude so many human beings from the moral community. Instead of basing moral status on fairly high level abilities, such as the capacity for abstract thought or self-consciousness, it can be argued that the important characteristic is *sentience*, or the capacity to feel pain (and pleasure). An advantage of sentience-based views is that they are more inclusive, and thus less counter-intuitive, than views based on personhood.

Another defect of the person view is its failure to explain *why* certain psychological abilities, such as the ability to use language or to reason, are relevant to moral status, treatment, and rights. By contrast, the moral relevance of sentience is clear: the fact that a being can suffer gives us a reason to treat it in certain ways and not in other ways. To take a homely example, it is morally permissible for a child to pluck the petals off a daisy, while saying 'He loves me, he loves me not'. It is not permissible for the child to pull the legs off an insect, or the feathers off a (trapped) bird. It *matters* to sentient beings what one does to them; they have a stake in their own lives and how their lives go. This insight is central to what I call 'the interest view'.[8]

THE INTEREST VIEW

The interest view of moral status derives from Joel Feinberg's 'interest principle', which was intended to answer the question, What kinds of beings logically can have rights? Feinberg (1974) suggests that the answer comes from the purpose or function of rights, which is to protect interests. The interest principle states that rights-holders must be capable of having interests of their own, which rights are intended to protect. Feinberg's insight about the logical conditions of having rights can be applied more generally to having moral status. For what is it to have moral status? As noted earlier, an entity has moral status if it counts or matters, from 'the moral point of view' (Baier 1965). And this in turn means that when we moral agents are deciding what we ought to do, we are required to take its interests seriously. Obviously, if a being does not have interests, its interests cannot be considered.

Next, Feinberg makes a conceptual connection between interests and sentience. In general, to have an interest in something is to have a stake in it. Interests are connected to what we care about or want, to our concerns and goals, to what

---

[8] This section summarizes the main arguments in Steinbock (1992, ch. 1).

is important or matters to us. If we think of interests as stakes in things, and understand what we have a stake in as defined by our concerns, by what matters to us, then the connection between interests and sentience becomes clear. Sentience, narrowly conceived as the ability to feel pleasure and pain, can be thought of more broadly as the capacity for having experiences of any kind, for awareness of our surroundings. Sentience, broadly conceived, is a necessary condition for having interests, for beings that completely lack awareness or experiences cannot care about anything.[9] Nothing matters to non-sentient, non-conscious beings.

One question raised by sentience-based views is, which living organisms are sentient? Surely all mammals are sentient (though Descartes, justifying vivisection, notoriously denied this), but what about clams or insects? Ants sprayed with insecticide will scurry away, and if directly hit, will writhe. If lemon juice is dropped on a clam, its muscles contract. Are these pain behaviors, or mere reflexes, analogous to heliotropism in plants? To some extent, this is an empirical question. We ascribe sentience to mammals, but not to plants, because plants do not have a nervous system. Whether insects or mollusks can feel pain depends, in part, on the kind of nervous system, if any, they have. But in part this is a conceptual question about what sentience, or consciousness generally, is. We have an intuitive notion of what it is to be 'awake and aware', but the analysis of consciousness is difficult, controversial, and (obviously) not something to be attempted here. Suffice it to say that if the bar is set too low, then any living creatures that react to their surroundings, e.g. bacteria, will be said to be sentient. Set the bar too high, and beings that lack self-consciousness, e.g. dogs and human babies, will be said not to be sentient. What is needed, for moral purposes, is a notion of sentience that is connected with feelings. Babies can experience pain, loneliness, and fear, and they can be comforted and soothed. Bacteria cannot.

To understand the importance of sentience to moral status, consider something that is undoubtedly non-sentient: an ordinary rock, say. It is impossible to think of a rock as having interests. This is because it does not matter to the rock what is done to it. A rock has no interests of its own, and so no welfare that is compounded out of its interests. Nothing can be done for *its* sake. Thus, sentience appears to be both a necessary and a sufficient condition for having interests. Necessary, because unless a being is sentient, it does not matter to it how it is treated. Sufficient, because if a being is sentient, it does matter to it how it is treated. Thus, *all* sentient beings

---

[9] There are some human beings who lack the capacity to feel physical pain. It is sometimes claimed that such people are a counter-example to the claim that only sentient beings have interests. However, I would say that while it is true that they are not sentient in the extremely narrow sense of being able to feel physical pain, they are sentient in the sense of having sensory experiences, such as vision and hearing, and presumably are capable of experiencing physical pleasure. They are also sentient in the broader sense of having the capacity for conscious experiences. Admittedly, they do not have an interest in not experiencing physical pain (since they cannot feel it), but this does not mean that they do not have other interests, including an interest in continued existence.

have moral status. And *only* sentient beings have moral status because without the capacity for sentience—or, more broadly, experiences and emotional states that accompany them—a being cannot have interests and a welfare of its own, making it impossible to consider its interests and welfare from the moral point of view.

The implication of the interest view for embryos is exactly the same as the implication of the person view: embryos have no moral status. They are not sentient beings; they are not even close. A blastocyst, lacking even the very beginnings of a nervous system, has about as much consciousness as a plank of wood. And even after the primitive streak forms, at around fourteen days after fertilization, the nervous system is too undeveloped to make possible any experiences, even the most rudimentary ones, such as the experience of pain. Without experiences of any kind, embryos cannot have wants. Without wants, they cannot have a stake in anything, including their health or continued existence. I am certainly not denying that embryos can be healthy or deformed, or that they can live or die. My claim is rather that they do not have an interest in being healthy or in continuing to exist.

Some people think this is because I have confused two senses of 'interest'. In the first sense, which we may call interest$_1$, to have an interest is to *take* an interest in something, or to be interested in it. Another sense of 'interest', which we may call interest$_2$, refers to things that are *in* someone's interest. Taken together, a being's interests$_2$—all those things that are in its interest—constitute its welfare. The two senses do not always or necessarily coincide. I can *take* an interest in something (e.g. eating rich desserts) without its being *in* my interest; equally, something can be *in* my interest, or promote my welfare (e.g. refraining from rich desserts) even though I do not *take* any interest in it. Lacking any form of consciousness, embryos clearly cannot have interests$_1$, but does that mean that they cannot have interests$_2$? Don Marquis thinks they can. He writes, 'The plant world appears to provide counter-examples to this assertion. Plants can flourish or wither. Therefore, they seem to have a welfare of their own' (Marquis 1994: 73).

But this is exactly what I wish to deny. From the fact that plants can flourish or wither, I do not think it follows that they have a welfare of their own. To say that a being has a welfare of its own suggests that one can act on its behalf, or for its sake. Clearly, one can do this for sentient beings, to whom it matters how their lives go. It does not matter to mere things, or to living non-sentient beings, like plants. For this reason, I do not think that they have a welfare or sake of their own, at least not in the sense in which sentient beings do. *We* may have reasons to make sure plants do not die, but the reasons do not refer to *their* welfare. In seeking to preserve them, we are not acting on their behalf.

However, even if this is right about plants, it may be objected that it is not right about embryos, because of an important difference between plants and embryos, namely, that embryos can, and plants cannot, become conscious beings with interests and a welfare of their own. This insight is the basis of Don Marquis's 'future-like-ours' (FLO) account of the wrongness of abortion (Marquis 1989).

MARQUIS AND THE FLO ACCOUNT

Marquis begins by asking why it is prima facie wrong to kill an adult human being, and answers that killing inflicts on the victim one of the greatest losses one can suffer: the loss of one's life. 'The loss of one's life deprives one of all the experiences, activities, projects, and enjoyments that would otherwise have constituted one's future.... Inflicting this loss on me is ultimately what makes killing me wrong' (Marquis 1989: 189–90). But exactly the same loss is inflicted on a fetus[10] when it is aborted. If it were not aborted, it would come to have a life it would value and enjoy, just as you and I value and enjoy our lives. Therefore, abortion is seriously wrong for the same reason that killing an innocent adult human being is seriously wrong: it deprives the victim of his or her valuable future. Although admittedly an early-gestation fetus has no desires now, and thus cannot *take* an interest in anything, Marquis insists that the early fetus nevertheless has an interest$_2$ in its future; a valuable future is *in* its interest. Just as we can attribute interests to a presently insentient being (someone in a temporary coma, for example) in virtue of desires it had when it was formerly sentient, we can 'attribute interests to a presently insentient being in virtue of its well-being at some future sentient stage of its natural history' (Marquis 1994: 72).

One of the defects of the interest view, according to Marquis, is that it cannot explain the wrongness of killing a temporarily comatose individual. For if sentience is a condition of having interests, then someone in a coma has no interests, including the interest in continued existence. Since everyone agrees that it would be wrong to kill someone in a temporary coma, the explanation has to be in terms of the value of his future existence. But exactly the same future of value applies to the presently non-sentient fetus.

This is a mistaken representation of the interest view. On the interest view, a temporarily comatose person *does* have an interest in continued existence based on the desire to go on living. Admittedly, while comatose, he does not have that or any other *conscious* desire. But he still *has* desires, in a dispositional sense. This is persuasively argued by David Boonin (2003), who draws an analogy between desires and beliefs. Not all of our beliefs are ones of which we are consciously aware. They are not all *occurrent* beliefs. Many of our beliefs are *dispositional*. For example, it is unlikely that ten minutes ago you were consciously aware of believing that a

---

[10] Marquis (1989) refers to fetuses, not embryos. However, it is clear that what he has to say applies as much to the implanted embryo as it does to the fetus.

triangle has three sides; it was not an occurrent belief. Yet it is one of your beliefs, a belief you already have. It would be implausible to think that it goes out of existence when you go to sleep and is created again when you wake up.

The same is true in the case of desires. My desire to go on living is not one I consciously entertain very often, but it is one of my desires, and remains so when I am asleep or temporarily comatose. Thus, contrary to Marquis, the example of a temporarily comatose adult does not expose a deficiency in the interest view. The interest view does not (implausibly) require permanent wakefulness as a condition of moral status. However, it does limit moral status to beings that have been at some time conscious and sentient, for this is a condition of acquiring interests. To be precise, then, we should say that sentience is a condition, not of *having* interests, since temporarily non-sentient beings can continue to have interests in the dispositional sense, but of *acquiring* interests. By contrast, non-sentient beings like embryos cannot acquire interests in the first place, because they have no desires, occurrent or dispositional, that could be the basis for these interests.

The interest view and the FLO account disagree sharply about the moral status of the fetus. However, the implication of the FLO account for the moral status of the pre-implantation embryo is less clear. For, as we saw earlier, the twinning argument casts doubt on the identity of the pre-implantation blastocyst with one specific individual. If this identification is not possible at the blastocyst stage, then the blastocyst presumably does not have FLO, since the valuable future the blastocyst has is the future of the specific adult it would become. (If FLO were not constrained in this way, sperm and ova could also have FLO, and contraception would be as seriously wrong as abortion.) And if a blastocyst does not have FLO, then killing it is not wrong, or at least not wrong for the same reason as it would be wrong to kill you or me. *Non-viable* blastocysts certainly lack FLO, but whether they would yield usable stem cell lines remains unclear.

To recap: On views of moral status that are not based on biological humanity, such as the person view, the interest view, and arguably the FLO approach, very early human embryos do not have moral status, or at least not the same moral status as you or I. Only on one view of moral status—the conception view—does the very early human embryo have full moral status. However, the conception view is rejected even by many who accept the biological humanity criterion. Is there any reason to accept the conception view, and accord full moral status to blastocysts?

The following example (ascribed to Leonard Glantz) shows, I think, that no one really does think that blastocysts have full moral status. Suppose a fire broke out in an infertility clinic where 100 frozen embryos were stored. Imagine that a 2-month-old baby was trapped in the clinic and you could either save one baby or 100 embryos, but not both. Would anyone hesitate for a second before saving the baby? Surely not, but if embryos were really morally equivalent to babies, the fact that there were many embryos and only one baby would be a decisive reason for saving the embryos (Annas 1989: 22).

RESPECT FOR EMBRYOS

I have been arguing that very early, extracorporeal embryos do not have moral status, and that this is reflected not only in most theories of moral status, but also in ordinary intuitions (as the fire in the clinic example shows). Should we conclude that blastocysts are just 'stuff', of no moral significance? In other words, if embryos lack moral status, can they be treated like any other bodily tissue? Such a conclusion, while intellectually tidy, is likely to make many people profoundly uncomfortable. Many people, even those who support ESC research because of the potential benefits to humanity, share the intuition that there should be limits to the uses of human embryos.

This compromise position, between those who think that human embryos are human subjects with all the rights of any other human subjects, and those who think that human embryos are disposable tissue, has been taken by several important official bodies, including the Warnock Committee in Great Britain and HERP in the United States. The HERP report concluded that, while the pre-implantation human embryo 'does not have the same moral status as infants and children', it 'deserves special respect' and 'serious moral consideration as a developing form of human life' (Green 2001: 92). Critics of HERP have called its compromise position incoherent. Dan Callahan, for example, wrote, 'An odd form of esteem—at once high-minded and altogether lethal. What in the world can that kind of respect mean?' (Callahan 1995: 39). Callahan concludes that offering 'respect to embryos' is really just a way to feel less uncomfortable while preparing to kill them.

The challenge, then, is to give content to the notion of respect for embryos: the basis of such respect and what restrictions it imposes on us. In the next section I will argue that although the interest view gives the correct account of *moral status*, we need another category to adequately explain our moral judgments. I call this category 'moral value'.

MORAL VALUE

The interest view limits *moral status* to beings with interests, and I have argued that only sentient beings have interests. However, this is consistent with recognizing that non-sentient beings can have *moral value*. A being has moral value if there are moral reasons to treat it in certain ways and not in others. Some of those reasons may concern the interests of people or animals, bringing the matter within the morality of interests, but not all of them do. The distinction between moral status and moral value concerns the kinds of reasons that are invoked. Whatever our reasons for protecting works of art, ancient oaks, wilderness areas, and entire species of plants or animals, these reasons do not stem from *their* interests or *their* welfare, because they do not have any. There are moral reasons for protecting non-sentient beings, but they are importantly different from the reasons provided by sentient beings. The motivation for distinguishing between moral status and moral value is that this avoids conflating very different kinds of moral reasons.[11]

In order to show that there is this category of moral value, distinct from moral status, I offer the following examples.

The Flag

Consider the American flag, the proper display and disposal of which (especially after 11 September 2001) has received a great deal of attention. A flag that is torn and tattered is supposed to be ceremonially burned and the ashes discarded properly, either by being buried or by being scattered over veterans' graves. Here are some typical comments taken from an article about the proper disposal of the American flag: 'Many people will take them and just throw them in the garbage. It just isn't right.' 'The most important thing is do not throw it in the garbage. It deserves more respect than that.' I take it these are not simply statements about flag etiquette; they are moral claims. However, such moral claims are not supported by golden-rule-type reasons, such as 'How would you like it if you were a flag and someone tossed you in the trash?'

It might be objected that, while appeal to the interests of the flag is absurd, nevertheless the wrongness of improper disposal of the flags belongs within the morality of interests, namely, the interests of those who are offended by such treatment. In other words, to say that the flag has moral value is just to say that it has symbolic value for most Americans, and that their feelings about the flag should be respected. It seems to me that this is partly right and partly wrong, depending on whether one is inside or outside the group to which the object in question has symbolic value. An object can have symbolic value only for those within a particular group: a nation, a culture, a religion. For those outside the group, a flag is just a piece of cloth, although a piece of cloth that has significance for others. Similarly, the Koran is sacred to Muslims, but not to Christians or Jews. It is wrong for Christians or Jews to treat the Koran disrespectfully, not because the Koran has or ought to have symbolic value for them, but because such handling is deeply offensive to Muslims, and causing such offense is prima facie wrong, for golden-rule-type reasons. However, from an internal perspective, reference solely to the feelings of members of the group is not an adequate explanation of why it is wrong to toss a flag in the garbage or flush the Koran down the toilet. The claim

---

[11] This explains the difference between the view I am proposing and Mary Anne Warren's (1997) multi-criterial view of moral status. She accords moral status to the beings I claim have only moral value.

made by the speakers quoted above is not (or not merely) that throwing the flag in the garbage offends *them*, or that the wrong consists in the hurt to *their* feelings. Their claim is rather that the flag, as a symbol of America, is owed respect. They would regard throwing it in the garbage as wrong even if it was done in secret, so that no one knew about it and could be offended. Equally, it would be wrong even if no one cared. Part of what is claimed is that people *ought* to care.

Of course, one might deny that the American flag deserves respect. The burning of the flag might be intended to show disrespect for the country for which it stands, and specifically for certain of its policies. Still, such a protest is possible only because the flag has symbolic value. One could not—logically could not—make a political protest by burning an old T-shirt.

The flag is an example of something that has moral value, even though it is not itself a moral subject or rights-bearer, and does not belong within the morality of interests. At the same time, the symbolic significance of a flag is entirely conventional and cultural. It is certainly possible to imagine human groups that do not have flags at all, and some nations (the United Kingdom, for example) do not take their flags quite as seriously as Americans do. Presumably, the claim that embryos deserve special respect is not intended to be culturally specific in this way. Let us turn, then, to a different example, one with a more universal appeal.

Human Remains

Respect for a flag is culturally specific in a way that respect for human remains is not. That is, although societies differ in their views about *how* to treat the dead, with some insisting that bodies must be buried and never burned, and others insisting that they must be burned and never buried, every human society has rituals and ceremonies for the disposal of dead bodies. Rituals for disposing of dead bodies are so much a part of human history and culture that they are part of what it means to be human. Indeed, debates over whether a particular group can be seen as 'human' or 'pre-human' often turn on whether they had burial customs. These rituals are intended to assuage the grief of the living, but also to pay respect to the dead. (We see this when, for example, an unknown infant is found dead in a trash can, and given a decent burial, even when there are no family members to mourn.)

The moral importance of showing respect for the dead becomes evident when dead bodies are treated inappropriately. When it was discovered some years ago that a crematorium in Georgia had not cremated bodies, but rather scattered the remains over the crematory property, people were outraged, and this too is a moral emotion. Yet dead bodies are inanimate corpses, decaying pieces of organic matter, without feelings or awareness. How are we to understand the idea that the dead are entitled to respect?

It might be claimed that 'respect for the dead' can be accounted for within the morality of interests. Many people have an interest in what happens to them after they die. They want to be buried in a particular spot or not to be buried at all, but cremated. If someone has asked to be cremated, and others agree to carry out this plan, then it is a wrong to that person, and a violation of his rights, to fail to carry out the promised cremation (much less to scatter the remains about). In addition, the morality of interests requires us to consider the feelings of survivors. People want their loved ones put to rest, not treated like trash. Both of these reasons—the prior wishes of the deceased and the feelings of the survivors—play a role in explaining the moral wrong of the action of the Georgian crematorium, but they are not the whole story. There would be something missing in a society that simply dumped human remains without ceremony. As a story in the *New York Times* expressed it, 'A funeral, like ceremonies of birth and marriage, signifies that a person belongs somewhere, which is a kind of definition of being human' (Sengupta 2002).

Dead bodies are owed respect both because of what they are—the remains of the once-living human organism—and because of what they symbolize   the human person who is no more. Human embryos deserve respect for similar reasons: they are a developing form of human life, and also a symbol of human existence. John Robertson puts the point this way:

> Treating the early embryo with special respect as a thing of unique value does not depend on metaphysical assumption or religious belief, though it does depend on openness to the meanings that the early embryo stimulates. Precisely because the early embryo is genetically unique and has the potential to be more, it operates as a powerful symbol or reminder of the unique gift of human existence . . . . The flag, the Torah, certain works of art, religious relics, and human remains are examples of other objects that are revered and respected because of their symbolic import, even though they are not themselves moral subjects or rights-bearers.   (Robertson 1990: 447)

A human embryo is something special, and a source of awe, precisely because it contains within itself the capacity to develop into a complete human being.[12] Moreover, human embryos are part of the human story, because every living human person began life as an embryo. If the entire life of a human being has intrinsic value, then it is reasonable to accord value to the very beginning stages of that life. This does not require us to treat human embryos as if they had interests, much less as if they were autonomous beings worthy of Kantian respect. But neither are they nothing. Michael Sandel, a member of the President's Council, expresses this view when he says, 'As one who supports embryonic stem cell research, I do not regard the early embryo as inviolable. But neither do I regard it as disposable, open to any use we may desire or devise' (President's Council 2005: 91).

The claim here is not the strong claim that a human embryo is sacred or inviolable, which suggests something like a right to life, but the weaker claim that

---

[12] Actually, no one knows if cloned human embryos have the potential to develop into fetuses and babies, and some scientists think that they could never become 'normal' organisms (Jaenisch 2004: 2787). One might think this would be a reason in favor of using cloned embryos, as opposed to spare IVF embryos, in ESC research, but, to my knowledge, no one has made this argument.

human life in all its stages is worthy of respect. Some have thought that such respect is incompatible with research that destroys the embryo. In the next section I will argue that this is a mistake that equates respect with Kantian respect.

Respect for Human Embryos

I have been arguing that embryos do not have moral status because they do not have interests. However, as McMahan points out, the morality of interests does not exhaust all of morality, but only that aspect which is concerned with the effect our action has on the interests or well-being of others (2002: 245). Morality includes also the 'morality of respect', which is 'made up of constraints on our behavior toward others that spring from our recognition of others as mature agents on an equal moral footing with ourselves' (Quinn 1984: 39). Let us call this kind of respect 'Kantian respect'.

According to Kant, persons (autonomous agents) have a special moral worth or dignity, which is the basis for the respect that is owed to them. Respect for *persons,* as Kant (1959: 46) instructs us, means never using persons merely as means to our ends, but always treating them also as ends in themselves. This rather obscure phrase means that we are required to act on principles that 'sustain and extend one another's capacities for autonomous action. A central requirement for doing so is to share and support one another's ends and activities at least to some extent' (O'Neill 1986: 323–4). To treat others as ends in themselves, we must take seriously their ends—their interests, projects, and goals—and not just our own. Since pre-implantation embryos do not have interests, projects, or goals, they are not 'ends in themselves'. For this reason, the notion of Kantian respect cannot be intelligibly applied to embryos.

Should we conclude that embryos are mere things, and that we can do whatever we want with them? Surely not. As Michael Sandel has said in an interview, 'It's a mistake to claim respect is all or nothing, on or off' (Meckler 2002). We demonstrate respect for embryos as a form of human life, not by treating them as inviolable and prohibiting embryo research, but by placing restrictions on their use. Respect for embryos rules out frivolous or trivial uses, such as using human embryos to create jewelry or cosmetics. These are situations in which there is no need to use human embryos and their use displays contempt rather than respect for human life. However, respect for human life does not rule out significant research that could cure devastating diseases or save lives—indeed, quite the contrary.

The Discarded–Created Distinction

Some think that it is permissible to use embryos left over from infertility treatment in research, since they would be otherwise be discarded, but that embryos may not be created for research. This position was taken by the National Bioethics Advisory Commission, on the grounds that there is an important difference between creating embryos for reproductive purposes, and then discarding those no longer needed, and creating embryos solely for the purpose of research, and destroying them in the process. The difference is that creating embryos for research treats the embryo as a mere object. Doing this 'may increasingly lead us to think of embryos generally as means to our ends rather than as ends in themselves' (National Bioethics Advisory Commission 1999: 56).

But this justification, I submit, confuses respect for embryos with Kantian respect. We *cannot* treat embryos as ends in themselves; they are not that kind of thing. However, we can and should use them only for morally significant purposes. The creation of IVF embryos to enable infertile people to become parents is a morally significant purpose, and therefore consistent with respect for embryos. However, many of the embryos that are created arc not used to establish a pregnancy, but are frozen and ultimately discarded. The justification for the creation of excess embryos is to spare the woman several rounds of superovulatory drugs, which is both physically burdensome and expensive. Thus, the destruction of embryos is as much a part of IVF as the creation of embryos. This is justified by the value of reproduction. However, medical research that has the potential to prolong and improve people's lives is at least as valuable as enabling infertile people to become parents. Therefore, the creation and destruction of human embryos in important scientific research is as justified as it is in the treatment of infertility. Neither contravenes the principle of respect for embryos as a form of human life. The search for new ways to derive ES cells without creating embryos is unnecessary and, in so far as it inhibits the discovery of cures, morally wrong.

References

ANNAS, G. (1989), 'A French Homunculus in a Tennessee Court', *Hastings Center Report*, 29/6: 20–2.

BAIER, K. (1965), *The Moral Point of View* (New York: Random House).

BEGLEY, S. (2001), 'Cellular Divide', *Newsweek*, 9 July, <http://www.keepmedia.com/pubs/ Newsweek/2001/07/09/314856?extID=10026>, accessed 6 July 2006.

BOONIN, D. (2003), *A Defense of Abortion* (Cambridge: Cambridge University Press).

CALLAHAN, D. (1995), 'The Puzzle of Profound Respect', *Hastings Center Report*, 25: 39–40.

CHAPMAN, A. R., FRANKEL, M. S., and GARFINKEL, M. S. (1999), *Stem Cell Research and Applications: Monitoring the Frontiers of Biomedical Research*, Report from the American Association for the Advancement of Science and the Institute for Civil Society, <http://www.aaas.org>, accessed 6 July 2006.

COLE-TURNER, R. (2004), 'Embryo and Fetus: Religious Perspectives', in S. G. Post (ed.), *Encyclopedia of Bioethics*, 3rd edn. (New York: Macmillan Reference USA), 732–40.

FEINBERG, J. (1974), 'The Rights of Animals and Unborn Generations', in W. T. Blackstone (ed.), *Philosophy and Environmental Crisis* (Athens: University of Georgia Press).

GREEN, R. M. (2001), *The Human Embryo Research Debates: Bioethics in the Vortex of Controversy* (Oxford: Oxford University Press).

HOLDEN, C., and VOGEL, G. (2004), 'Cell Biology: A Technical Fix for an Ethical Bind?', *Science*, 306: 2174–6.

HWANG, W. S., RYU, Y. J., PARK, J. H., and PARK, E. S., et al. (2004), 'Evidence of a Pluripotent Human Embryonic Stem Cell Line Derived from a Cloned Blastocyst', *Science*, 303: 1669–74.

_____ et al. (2005), 'Patient-Specific Embryonic Stem Cells Derived from Human SCNT Blastocysts', *Science*, 308: 1777–83.

JAENISCH, R. (2004), 'Human Cloning: The Science and Ethics of Nuclear Transplantation', *New England Journal of Medicine*, 351/27: 2787–91.

KANT, I. (1959), *Foundations of the Metaphysics of Morals*, trans. Lewis White Beck (Indianapolis: Bobbs-Merrill).

KINSLEY, M. (2001), 'If You Believe Embryos Are Humans . . . ', *Time*, 25 June, 80.

LANDRY, D. W., and ZUCKER, H. A. (2004), 'Embryonic Death and the Creation of Human Embryonic Stem Cells', *Journal of Clinical Investigation*, 114/9: 1184–6.

LAUGHLIN, M. J., et al. (2004), 'Outcomes After Transplantation of Cord Blood or Bone Marrow from Unrelated Donors in Adults with Leukemia', *New England Journal of Medicine*, 351: 2265–75.

LAURITZEN, P. (2005), 'Stem Cells, Biotechnology, and Human Rights: Implications for a Posthuman Future', *Hastings Center Report*, 35/2: 25–33.

LOCKWOOD, M. (1988), 'Warnock Versus Powell (and Harradine): When Does Potentiality Count?', *Bioethics*, 2/3: 187–213.

LUKER, K. (1984), *Abortion and the Politics of Motherhood* (Berkeley: University of California Press).

MCMAHAN, J. (2002), *The Ethics of Killing: Problems at the Margins of Life* (Oxford: Oxford University Press).

MARQUIS, D. (1989), 'Why Abortion Is Immoral', *Journal of Philosophy*, 76: 183–202.

_____ (1994), 'Justifying the Rights of Pregnancy: The Interest View', *Criminal Justice Ethics* (Winter–Spring), 67–81.

MAURON, A. (2004), 'Embryo and Fetus: Development from Fertilization to Birth', in S. G. Post (ed.), *Encyclopedia of Bioethics*, 3rd edn. (New York: Macmillan Reference USA), 707–12.

NATIONAL BIOETHICS ADVISORY COMMISSION (1999), *Ethical Issues in Human Stem Cell Research*, i (Rockville, Md.: NBAC).

NEIGER, R. (2005), 'Pushing the Boundaries of Stem Cell Research', <http://www.israel21c.com>.

O'NEILL, O. (1986), 'The Moral Perplexities of Famine and World Hunger', in T. Regan (ed.), *Matters of Life and Death: New Introductory Essays in Moral Philosophy* (New York: Random House).

PETERS, P. (2005), 'The Meaning of Human Conception', unpub. MS.

PRESIDENT'S COUNCIL ON BIOETHICS (2005), *Alternative Sources of Human Pluripotent Stem Cells* (Washington, DC: President's Council on Bioethics).

QUINN, W. (1984), 'Abortion, Identity and Loss', *Philosophy and Public Affairs*, 13: 24–54.

ROBERTSON, J. A. (1990), 'In the Beginning: The Legal Status of Early Embryos', *Virginia Law Review*, 76/3: 437–517.

ROCHA, V., et al. (2004), 'Transplants of Umbilical-Cord Blood or Bone Marrow from Unrelated Donors in Adults with Acute Leukemia', *New England Journal of Medicine*, 351: 2276–85.

SCHWARTZ, R. S. (2006), 'The Politics and Promise of Stem Cell Research', New England Journal of Medicine, 355: 1189–91.

SENGUPTA, S. (2002), 'Why Disposing of the Dead Matters to the Living', *New York Times*, Week in Review Desk, 24 Feb., sect. 4, 5.

SILVER, L. M. (1998), *Remaking Eden: How Genetic Engineering and Cloning Will Transform the American Family* (New York: Avon).

STEINBOCK, B. (1992), *Life Before Birth: The Moral and Legal Status of Embryos and Fetuses* (New York: Oxford University Press).

——— (2005), 'Alternative Sources of Stem Cells', *Hastings Center Report*, 35/4: 24–6.

STOLBERG, S. G. (2001), 'Controversy Reignites Over Stem Cells and Clones', *New York Times*, 18 Dec., F1.

WADE, N. (2001), 'An Old Question Becomes New Again: Stem Cell Issue Causes Debate Over the Exact Moment Life Begins', *New York Times*, 15 Aug., 20.

——— and SANG-HUN, C. (2006), 'Human Cloning Was All Faked, Koreans Report', *New York Times*, 10 Jan., A1, A12.

WARREN, M. A. (1973), 'On the Moral and Legal Status of Abortion', *The Monist*, 57: 43–61.

——— (1997), *Moral Status: Obligations to Persons and Other Living Things* (New York: Oxford University Press).

YEN, B. L., et al. (2005), 'Isolation of Multipotent Cells from Human Term Placenta', *Stem Cells*, 23: 3–9.

CHAPTER 19

....

THERAPEUTIC CLONING: POLITICS AND POLICY

....

ANDREA BONNICKSEN

THERAPEUTIC cloning has been called 'one of the most divisive topics in modern biology' (*Nature* 2004). As envisioned, it would involve transferring a patient's somatic cell to an enucleated egg in order to generate embryonic stem (ES) cells that share the patient's genome and, after differentiation, can be used as therapy without the need for immunosuppressive drugs. This prospect is a highly political matter that is contentious on at least two fronts. It shares a technique—somatic cell nuclear transfer (SCNT)—with reproductive cloning, and therefore provokes concerns that pursuing it will invariably lead to the pursuit of reproductive cloning. In addition, it relies on stem cells extracted from human embryos in a procedure that destroys the embryos. This resurrects sensitive issues about the moral status of human embryos and whether they should be destroyed in pursuit of individual and societal benefit. The concerns it elicits are salient across nations, which have adopted mixed policies about the legality and fundability of therapeutic SCNT (Jones and Cohen 2004: S44–5; Gruss 2003).

In light of the controversy engendered by therapeutic SCNT and the many scientific questions yet to be addressed, the procedure may be expected to proceed slowly. Yet it may be expected to advance nevertheless. The technology is explicitly legal in some nations and implicitly legal in the absence of restrictive laws in others.

Its theoretical supposition is elegant, intriguing to investigators, and inviting to prospective patients. Even if the link to the destruction of embryos becomes moot if investigators learn how to produce genetically compatible ES cells without first having to create a potentially viable embryo, the broader issue of making science policy in the presence of heightened politics will not. Other technologies with problematic connotations and evocative labels, such as animal–human hybrids, parthenotes, or chimeras, are waiting to be vetted in the policy arenas. Therapeutic SCNT, in other words, is a case study of how to incorporate 'new scientific findings . . . into a policy framework that is developing under intense political pressure' (Kennedy 2004).

Academics and policy advisory groups, among others, have contributed to an expansive literature exploring the ethical and moral dimensions of ES cell research and therapeutic SCNT (e.g. American Association for the Advancement of Science/Institute for Civil Society 1999; Committee on the Biological and Biomedical Applications 2002; FitzPatrick 2003; Juengst and Fossel 2000; Holland *et al.* 2001; National Bioethics Advisory Commission 1999; National Institutes of Health 1999; Nuffield Council on Bioethics 2000; President's Council on Bioethics 2002, 2004). Some themes and areas of agreement emerge from the literature. For example, it is widely agreed that matters relating to SCNT are of societal interest, touch on deeply felt values that must be acknowledged, and warrant public deliberation. It is also expected that ethical dimensions should be discussed before rather than in reaction to scientific developments (Parens and Knowles 2003; Cohen 2001). This includes ethical issues raised by ES cell clinical trials and eventual medical therapies (Faden *et al.* 2003; Dawson *et al.* 2003). There is some agreement that discussion should be comprehensive (President's Council on Bioethics 2002) and include a range of reprogenetic techniques, defined as 'all interventions involved in the creation, use, manipulation, or storage of gametes and embryos'. These techniques raise 'complex and sometimes profound ethical questions that call out for informed policy, publicly and transparently developed' (Parens and Knowles 2003, S4, S6).

A number of commentators in the United States advocate the establishment of a national-level body to deliberate and ensure the responsible development of reprogenetics. Proposals range from a narrow body, such as the Recombinant DNA Advisory Committee (Committee on the Biological and Biomedical Applications 2002) to a more comprehensive body such as the United Kingdom's Human Fertilisation and Embryology Authority (Parens and Knowles 2003). Others believe institutional review boards (IRBs) and local oversight are sufficient (American Medical Association 1999). Commentators also recommend federal funding of the research as a way of securing federal oversight (Committee on the Biological and Biomedical Applications 2002). Yet the distinct possibility exists that no body will be developed, or that the body will be less effective than hoped, or that federal funding will never reach the level needed for thoughtful deliberation and careful oversight.

In the current situation, three things are intersecting at once. First, an area of contentious biomedical research is proceeding, although the scope of that research is difficult to assess. Second, although there is no legal impediment to this research, significant guidance is lacking at the national level given the refusal of the government to fund research in which embryos are injured or destroyed. Third, the issue touches on fundamental values and is highly salient to supporters, who see it as a possible aid to illness and a reflection of scientific liberty, and to opponents, who see it as an immoral act in which human life is destroyed. It is this saliency and intensity of feeling that makes scientific prospects distinct from many other areas of biomedical research. Concern about the societal nature of the issues generates calls for guiding policy, which might include voluntary acceptance of ethical principles and/or legally binding regulations.

Much of the literature on therapeutic SCNT covers the moral arguments for and against proceeding and the policy stall occasioned by conflicts over the moral status of embryos. Yet it is also worthwhile to view policy from the standpoint of the resources available as well as of deficiencies in those resources. This chapter uses the idea of a policy community to examine policy making from a starting point that focuses not on what divides, but rather on the groups and individuals committed to enabling ES cell research and therapeutic SCNT. Although written with international dimensions in mind, the chapter focuses on the United States, where the politics are particularly volatile and the likelihood of policy leadership at the national level is remote.

A policy community is a set of academics, policy analysts, interest group members, and others who share an interest in the same set of policies, although they do not necessarily agree on all matters (Majone 1989: 161; Kingdon 1984: 123). Of interest in this chapter is the narrower policy community of advocates of ES cell research, including therapeutic SCNT. This community of advocates has a distinct bias, to be sure, but its members share a commitment, a sense of mission, and a personal interest in the outcome that positions them to be creative problem solvers. Given the prospect of continued research without governmental guidance at the national level, it is instructive to examine their potential contributions to policy development.

This chapter identifies groups within the community of advocates and discusses roles they might play in policy development. As background, it first reviews reasons for a policy stall over therapeutic SCNT at the national level and suggests roles the US Congress has played short of rule making. It then identifies seven groups or agencies in the community of advocates: national legislature, private funding agencies, state governments, international policy, corporations, professional associations, and policy advisory groups. It pursues the theme that these sources serve as a forum for policy development. While a comprehensive and enforceable policy is unlikely to develop from their activities, members of the community contribute to the lengthy 'softening up' of policy proposals requisite for the emergence of policy (Kingdon 1984: 123).

POLITICAL DIMENSIONS OF THERAPEUTIC SCNT

Politics connotes scarcity, competition, and struggle over desired resources. Within this meaning, in the year or so after the announced birth of Dolly the lamb, reproductive SCNT was not particularly political because desired goals were not highly threatened. On the contrary, a key goal was shared: advisory groups and commissions around the world expressed concerns about cloning's implications for children, family, and society, and surveys revealed widespread consensus about not proceeding with humans (e.g. Eiseman 1997; National Bioethics Advisory Commission 1997). These concerns ranged from the societal level, such as reduced heterogeneity in the gene pool, to the individual level, such as whether women would be exploited in the rush to secure eggs for reproductive SCNT. Most of the commentary was critical, and particular attention centered on the physical and psychological risks cloning might pose to the child. Some commentators challenged unsupported suppositions about the risks of cloning (Brock 1997; Robertson 1998; Steinbock 2000) and others advocated reproductive SCNT (Eibert 2003; Pence 1998). The early sense of urgency by critics to study the issues dissipated as it became clear that low success rates with animal cloning meant reproductive SCNT with humans would not take place in the near future even if the will existed to do so.

Although the debate was not intensely political in the sense of competition over values, it did elicit more intense reactions nationally and internationally than perhaps any scientific biomedical development to date. Reproductive SCNT had a fantastical element to it; it has long provoked creative scenarios among filmmakers (e.g. *The Boys from Brazil* (1978), *Multiplicity* (1996), *Godsend* (2004)), fiction writers (Huxley 1932; Nussbaum 1998); political cartoonists, and essayists. It also tapped an intuitive element, reflected in Kass's admonition to listen to the 'wisdom of repugnance' (Kass 1997). The political struggle over reproductive SCNT revolved more around the means than the end as fault lines arose over what mechanisms could best ensure that no one attempt to clone a human (National Bioethics Advisory Commission 1997). Some nations had already banned it before Dolly's birth and others enacted new prohibitions after her birth. In the United States the National Bioethics Advisory Commission recommended that Congress enact a five-year moratorium on efforts to clone a human. Others advocated postponing decisions until more was known and, in the meantime, relying on voluntary moratoriums urged by professional associations on their members. Numerous bills were introduced to ban reproductive SCNT in the US Congress (Bonnicksen 2002).

An effort to bring to a vote a bill banning reproductive SCNT failed in the US Senate in early 1998, and the issue receded (Bonnicksen 2002). Intense politics through most of 1998 were kept in check by a basic consensus about the folly of pursuing cloning when so many ethical reservations existed, a realization that human reproductive SCNT was remote, and a notice by the Food and Drug Administration (FDA) that it would not let reproductive SCNT proceed. Nevertheless, a precedent for policy in biomedical research had been set by the extensive debate in Congress over whether to ban a particular biomedical technology and, if so, to do so before it was even imminent. Heretofore, Congress had expressed approval or disapproval over developments in biomedical research by its control over appropriations, not by a prior restraint on a whole category of research.

Politics in the US Congress escalated in late 1998 when scientists announced that they had derived and isolated human ES cells from the inner cell mass of seven to nine day embryos (Thomson *et al.* 1998). This announcement fostered visions of a limitless source of versatile cells that could be coaxed to differentiate for medical therapy. For this research, the investigators used embryos that had been donated by patients in fertility programs who no longer needed or wanted the embryos for their reproductive efforts. This had the ethical advantage of avoiding the destruction of embryos beyond those certain to be destroyed anyway, and it gave couples the opportunity to feel they had contributed to the research effort. On the other hand, reliance on donated embryos from persons struggling with infertility could skew research findings if couples had genetic reasons for the infertility, hinder the growth of cell lines from genetically diverse embryos, and deprive investigators of the opportunity to control all aspects of the derivation and return to the original embryo to secure more ES cells if necessary.

To circumvent these problems, investigators proposed creating embryos for ES cell derivation with gametes donated for the purpose. Furthermore, with an eye to eventual medical therapy, researchers proposed creating embryos through SCNT, using the nucleus from a patient's somatic cell and an enucleated donor egg. From the inner cell mass of this embryo, technicians could generate cells for therapy that would carry the 'genetic blueprint' of the intended patient and thereby circumvent the need for immunosuppressive drugs (Daley 2003; Hochedlinger and Jaenisch 2003).

The idea of using SCNT for nonreproductive use generated a distinction for ethical and policy deliberations between reproductive SCNT (creating an embryo for transfer to a uterus for a possible pregnancy) and therapeutic SCNT (creating customized cell lines for medical therapy). These two were linked by technique but distinguished by intended outcome. From one perspective, the intended outcome is determinative, and therapeutic SCNT can be distinguished from reproductive SCNT for policy purposes, with the most likely option of allowing the former while banning the latter. The United Kingdom has adopted this perspective inasmuch as its Human Fertilization and Embryology Authority allows research licenses for therapeutic SCNT but prohibits reproductive SCNT. Similarly, the Republic of South Korea allows therapeutic SCNT under guidelines of its National Ethics

Committee but forbids reproductive SCNT (*Asia* 2004), Singapore permits the first on a case by case basis with approval of the relevant governmental body but forbids the second (*Asia* 2004), and Finland's Medical Research Act No. 488/1999 has been interpreted as allowing therapeutic but forbidding reproductive SCNT (*Europe* 2004).

From another perspective, technique is determinative and both forms of SCNT should be banned. Some nations, such as Italy (*Europe* 2004) and Australia (*Oceania* 2004), forbid both. One survey revealed that approximately seven nations allow therapeutic SCNT in some form, approximately thirty-three do not, and in twelve nations the status is unknown (Jones and Cohen 2004). Different arguments defend the perspective of banning both forms. Among other things, it is argued that the creation of any embryo for research purposes is immoral; the embryo has the moral status of a person, so creating an embryo through SCNT is the same as creating a child through SCNT; if SCNT works to create a dividing embryo for therapy, the temptation to try to create an embryo for reproduction will be too much to resist; and it will be too difficult to police facilities to guard against the one but not the other.

In the US Congress, policy options gravitated to two main possibilities outside of doing nothing: making reproductive SCNT a crime (narrow ban) or making therapeutic and reproductive SCNT criminal (broad ban). It was around this time that the issue of SCNT became highly political, because opponents of SCNT were willing to sacrifice a ban on reproductive SCNT only, a proposal for which there was widespread agreement, in order to hold out for a ban on both reproductive and therapeutic SCNT. The House passed a broad ban on 31 July 2001, by a 265–162 vote, the Human Cloning Prohibition Act of 2001 (H.R. 2505). It passed the same bill, now renumbered, on 27 February 2003, by a 241–155 vote (H.R. 534). The Senate has not at the time of writing voted on the issue, and those holding out for a broad ban cannot gather the requisite sixty votes needed to overcome a motion to close debate. The administration of George W. Bush pursued the same strategy of holding out for a broad ban at the United Nations (Walters 2004).

Human ES cell research (and therapeutic SCNT as a subset) provokes heightened politics for several reasons. First, because it involves the destruction of human embryos it has been swept into the 'intractable', 'vitriolic', and 'polarizing' abortion debate in the United States (Annas *et al.* 1996; Parens and Knowles 2003). As the President's Council on Bioethics observed about the inability to forge a consensus on ES cell research in the United States,

One side believes that what is involved is morally abhorrent in the extreme, while the other believes embryo research is noble or even morally obligatory and worthy of praise and support. It would be very difficult for the government to find a middle ground between these two positions, since the two sides differ not only on what should or should not be done, but also on the moral premises from which the activity should be approached. (President's Council on Bioethics 2004: 39)

Second, ES cell research is highly personal and salient. In contrast to reproductive SCNT, which is abstract and saddled with intuitions, therapeutic SCNT has been paired in the public debate with living people in need of therapy. The number of people with chronic and untreatable conditions who could potentially benefit from ES cell research runs in the millions, but research proponents personalize these numbers by bringing human faces to them. Michael J. Fox and the late Christopher Reeve are two of the celebrities who have promoted the research, and Nancy Reagan and Orrin Hatch are two political figures who moved outside their pro-life positions to advocate federal funding for ES cell research. The research has been recast as regenerative medicine, a category removed from a label of embryos or procreation. Proponents mobilize patient advocacy groups, garner petitions signed by stellar scientists, and bring together coalitions of scientists, health care workers, researchers, and prospective patients and their families.

Third, therapeutic SCNT involves funding, which raises issues about public moneys for activities deemed immoral by some. In the United States this led to months of lobbying President Bush in anticipation of his decision on ES cell funding. A parallel example of the politics of funding comes from the efforts of the European Union (EU) to find common ground for funding research involving human embryos. Members of the EU in 2003 were unable to agree, after months of discussion, on a policy for funding human ES cell research as part of the 6th Framework Program for science funding in 2002 (Vogel 2003).

Fourth, the debate over SCNT is punctuated by colorful and sensational announcements that roil the public. For reproductive SCNT, Richard Seed, a physicist, announced in 1998 that he would open a cloning clinic in Chicago. In 2001 Panos Zavos announced that he and two other physicians would attempt to clone a human in an unnamed country. Also in 2001 Clonaid, through its spokesman, Rael, said that it had fifty women ready to act as surrogates for embryos created through cloning. Each announcement precipitated hearings in Congress and calls for legislation.

An early destabilizing announcement for therapeutic SCNT came in late 2001, when personnel at Advanced Cell Technologies, Inc. (ACT), a Massachusetts-based firm, announced that their scientists had created three early-stage human embryos through SCNT, two of which divided to four cells and one divided to six cells. A triad of press releases announced this: a scientific article in *e-biomed: The Journal of Regenerative Medicine* (Cibelli *et al.* 2001), a cover story in *U.S. News and World Report* entitled 'The First Clone' (Fischer 2001), and a story in *Scientific American* with additional coverage on the magazine's website (Cibelli *et al.* 2002). Special efforts had been taken to ensure a news blackout until all three articles came out at once.

Two years later ACT announced, in a press release that coincided with a cover article entitled 'The Making of a Human Clone' in *WIRED*, that it had created ten human embryos through SCNT and eight parthenotes (Rohm 2004). According to the reporter who had been following the story, five of the cloned embryos reached the four to eight cell stage and one divided to sixteen cells. The investigators planned to save for a scientific publication an answer to whether the sixteen cell embryo divided still further. ACT was criticized for making this announcement before publication of a scientific report (Stolberg 2001).

Scientists affiliated with Seoul National University reported in 2004 that they had generated human embryos through SCNT, and in 2005 that they had derived ES cell lines from SCNT-generated embryos (Hwang *et al*. 2004, 2005). A great amount of media attention accompanied the published reports but the findings were later found to be fabricated (Normile *et al*. 2006). While this set back studies in Korea and showed the temptations that can accompany high publicity research, the revelations arguably did not appreciably limit SCNT research. Among other things, researchers who had moved to other research after supposing the Korean team had locked up the SCNT research now resumed an interest in conducting their own investigations.

In short, therapeutic SCNT has links to both reproductive SCNT and embryo destruction, touches core values that are not easily amenable to negotiation, operates in the absence of the usual methods of oversight, and is characterized by effective advocacy on both sides. Many scientific as well as ethical concerns remain to be addressed before researchers begin clinical trials. In particular, investigators are striving to find alternatives to the mouse feeder cells used to culture ES cells in early studies, such as human cells; culturing ES cells without any feeder cells; or developing ways to ensure that animal cells are safe and will not transmit pathogens (Gearhart 2004; Rosenthal 2003). More study is also needed to understand how to make cells differentiate, control cell proliferation, ensure ES-derived cells do not form tumors after transplantation, isolate cell types, control for the spread of infectious disease, ensure that enough cells integrate into recipients' tissues to take over the functions of the tissues, and direct the cells to the correct organ (Dawson *et al*. 2003; Hwang *et al*. 2004; Phimister and Drazen 2004; Rosenthal 2003; Zerhouni 2003*b*). Despite these 'daunting' scientific challenges, however, none is 'beyond theoretical reach' (Phimister and Drazen 2004: 1351). Ethical issues may dissipate somewhat if researchers learn how to reprogram somatic cells directly without having to create embryos as intermediaries (Daley 2003; Hochedlinger and Jaenisch 2003), and, indeed, direct programming is one of the purposes of basic research (Rosenthal 2003). What, then, is guiding the emergence of ES cell science?

Pluralism and Therapeutic SCNT

Pluralism is the view that many groups compete 'in a reasonably open political system and that policy results from this group competition' (Birkland 2001: 269).

Policy making itself has been described as a long process of 'softening up' in which 'ideas are floated, bills introduced, speeches made; proposals are drafted, then amended in response to reaction and floated again' (Kingdon 1984: 123). Proposals are made and discussed in policy communities comprised of groups and individuals willing to invest 'time, energy, reputation, and sometimes money' in order to meet personal interests and promote policies and values (Kingdon 1984: 129–30).

Among the voices in the policy community of advocates for therapeutic SCNT are scientists, researchers, and a significant grass roots element made up of patient advocacy groups and coalitions. Techniques involving petitions by Nobel laureates, testimony by celebrities, and supportive letters and speeches by persons usually associated with anti-abortion positions are among the methods used to keep proposals to expand funding for ES cell research on the public agenda. Interest in ES cell research has prompted corporations, professional associations, funding agencies, and even state governments to lay out research plans with minimal leadership from the US legislative and executive branches. The following sections identify some players in the policy community of advocates and ask about the capacities of each to contribute to the emergence of guiding policies. It starts with the US Congress, where the pluralist interests honed their voice.

National Legislature

The US Congress is generally viewed as a barrier to reprogenetic policies through its long-standing refusal to authorize federal spending for research that involves injury to or destruction of human embryos. This provision stops policy in its tracks, and it causes observers to look elsewhere for policy direction. Yet Congress's refusal to authorize money for research on reprogenetics does not preclude it from playing a multidimensional role in the matter of SCNT and ES cell research. On the contrary, Congress has asserted influence in its traditional roles of representing constituencies and clarifying policy options. Congress was the place where the struggle over SCNT took shape. The announcements of Dolly's birth and of ES cell derivation provoked Congress between 1997 and 2003 to hold a total of twenty-two hearings on reproductive cloning and/or stem cell research in both chambers: the House of Representatives held eight and the Senate held fourteen. The hearings were held in five different committees in the Senate (Appropriations; Commerce, Science, and Transportation; Judiciary, Health, Education, and Pensions; and Labor and Human Resources) and four in the House (Commerce and Energy; Judiciary Government Reform; and Science). Hearings were the primary avenues for gathering information and educating the public and members of Congress.

Some hearings were convened in response to news headlines. While most were relatively staid, others, as when the Raelians testified, had a more sensational tone. Well over fifty witnesses representing a variety of interests testified in ES cell and/or cloning hearings from 1997 to 2004. A review of witness lists indicates that scientists and physicians testified most frequently; representatives of interest groups and organizations came in second; and ethical, legal, and policy commentators made up the third largest category. As time passed, a policy community took shape, with some legislators more active than others and some witnesses testifying two or more times. These hearings provided a forum for the emergence of repeated themes and arguments. Congress also clarified policy options by the introduction of numerous bills that in the beginning were diverse. Over time, however, key provisions kept reappearing to produce what was like a model narrow ban (to bar the transfer of an embryo created through SCNT to a woman's uterus) and a model broad ban (to bar any creation of an embryo through SCNT). The preambles of the bills revealed ideological underpinnings, as did debate by members of Congress printed in the *Congressional Record*.

While some are critical of Congress for not passing substantive legislation, the merits of a non-lawmaking role can also be argued. Law passed in this area would not necessarily establish a good precedent given the sense of headline-driven impulse that periodically puts SCNT on the Congressional agenda. In addition, political strategy permeates actions. For example, in 1998 Senate proponents of a broad ban attempted to use parliamentary maneuvers to rush the bill to the chamber floor for a vote, bypassing hearings on the bill in the process (Bonnicksen 2002). Later the broad ban bill that passed the House in July 2001 'received little serious debate' (Maienschein 2003: 288). It is not unusual for House members to be 'quick to pass what they see as politically useful legislation that they know the Senate will not support' (Maienschein 2003: 290).

In addition, passing an SCNT law in Congress, even a protective law, would establish precedent by involving Congress substantively in biomedical research and doing so in a technique-specific way. If more contentious techniques are in sight, this could set the stage for future technique-based laws that are brittle and unresponsive to scientific change. More normally, Congress delegates technical policy making to administrative agencies, where administrative discretion allows more flexibility and responsiveness to changing technologies. The absence of a body such as the Office of Technology Assessment, which wrote informative reports for Congress before it was disbanded in 1995, also argues against narrow technique-driven legislation.

Moreover, a disparity exists between the technical nature of science policy and the political needs and interests of members of Congress. Congressional decisions involve 'bargains and compromises and . . . strategies' (Morgan and Peha 2003*a*: 8). This attention to 'synthesis and balancing of interest' is removed from the 'systematic analysis' needed for science and technology (Morgan and Peha 2003*b*: 173). Members of Congress, writes one observer, 'seek agreement, not truth' (Smith and Stine 2003: 25), a goal hampered by deep-seated differences about the moral status of the embryo. Even the President's Council on Bioethics, which identified seven main policy options for ES cell research, produced a divided vote on the question of funding (President's Council on Bioethics 2002). As a consequence, the federal government retreats: it 'does not explicitly prohibit embryo research but also does not officially condone it, encourage it, or support it with public funds' (President's Council on Bioethics 2004: 39).

In summary, it helps to look expansively at Congress's functions when evaluating its impact on the development of cloning policy. Although the body has not, at the time of writing, passed a law directed at reproductive or therapeutic SCNT, it has helped defuse the sense of urgency, gather information, perform representation functions, and clarify policy options. It has also served as a forum in which a policy community of advocates and opponents has emerged. If, indeed, policy options need to be discussed over time in a process of 'softening up', Congress plays a role in keeping deliberation alive.

Funding Agencies

Ideally, the federal government funds promising research, which brings studies to the open, asserts quality control through peer review, enables sustained investment, and invites oversight. After intense lobbying of the executive branch between 1999 and 2001, President Bush presented a compromise agreement to allow funding of a narrow range of studies using ES cell lines derived by 9 August 2001. At the time the administration believed around sixty usable lines existed, but the number turned out to be fewer than twenty. Even with a limited role, however, the National Institutes of Health (NIH) became part of the community of advocates for ES cell research using cell lines derived before 9 August 2001. To spur more research proposals, it set up a Human Embryonic Stem Cell Registry to list (but not distribute) cell lines as they become available, an NIH Stem Cell Task Force to coordinate NIH programs and identify problems in funded research, an NIH Characterization Unit to provide data from assays on ES cell lines, and an award program to train mid-career investigators to use the cells (Zerhouni 2003*a*, *b*). The Department of Health and Human Services also announced an initiative to create a National Embryonic Stem Cell Bank (Holden 2004*a*). In one year of funding, sixty investigators at forty-eight institutions received money, with most (forty-four) receiving supplements to existing research and others (fourteen) receiving funds for newly initiated research (Zerhouni 2003*b*). Research involving therapeutic SCNT is not funded.

The uncertain outlook for expanded federal funding has propelled institutes, foundations, and even state governments to make available alternative sources of support. For example, on the west coast, Stanford University received a $12 million donation to set up a privately funded Institute for Cancer/Stem Cell Biology. Because therapeutic SCNT research is explicitly legal in California, this leaves open the possibility that such studies will be conducted. On the east coast the Howard Hughes

Medical Institute, Juvenile Diabetes Research Foundation, and Harvard University together funded ES cell research conducted by Harvard-affiliated investigators that led to the derivation of seventeen ES cell lines that were made available to researchers for noncommercial studies (Cowan *et al.* 2004; Gearhart 2004). The study was approved by Harvard's IRB, and the investigators' method for deriving the lines was applauded as setting 'a standard for the characterization of embryonic stem-cell lines' and recommended for inclusion in the NIH registry (Phimister and Drazen 2004: 1352).

These and other well-publicized subnational and private funding programs provide a context in which policy and ethical issues can be identified and debated, especially when universities are the recipients. For example, planners of a privately financed stem cell institute at Harvard University announced that they would consider ethical issues with the help of the 'schools of government, law, business, and divinity' at the university (Lawler 2004). Other universities are also using or planning to use private funds for stem cell research, such as the University of California–San Francisco and Johns Hopkins University. These funded studies will, when they reach the clinical stage, presumably bring with them protections for human research participants, including IRB review, and can, with proper leadership, solicit broad deliberation and produce guiding principles and practices.

State Governments

Another avenue for innovative policy and public deliberation arises at the state level. Two states—California and New Jersey—have passed laws authorizing ES cell research, including studies using embryos created through SCNT (Cohen 2004: 113). Although a number of states bar therapeutic SCNT by law, others have introduced bills to allow ES cell research. California, which was the first state to ban reproductive SCNT, was also the first state to endorse therapeutic SCNT. Its law, which went into effect in early 2004, is designed to lessen suffering from diseases in view of the 'immense promise' of stem cell research and to protect against economic losses if research does not proceed. In relevant part, it permits 'research involving the derivation and use of human embryonic stem cells, human embryonic germ cells, and human adult stem cells from any source, *including somatic cell nuclear transplantation*' (California Health and Safety Code 2003; emphasis added). The bill's preface points out that the United States and California 'have historically been a haven for open scientific inquiry and technological innovation'.

New Jersey's governor signed a Stem Cell Research Bill (S1909) into law in 2004. The law is designed to assure researchers that the state will not interfere with ES cell, embryonic germ cell, and adult stem cell research, including cells developed from SCNT (Mansnerus 2004). It regards 'open scientific inquiry and publicly funded research' as the most efficient and responsible way to produce benefits from stem cell research. New Jersey's governor set aside $6.5 million in the state budget to establish a Stem Cell Institute to be administered by Rutgers University and the University of Medicine and Dentistry of New Jersey, funded by state and private money (Kocieniewski 2004; Mansnerus 2004). The governor noted at the bill-signing ceremony that the law would make New Jersey 'a leader in medical research and medical care' (State of New Jersey 2004).

The effort to proceed with ES cell research in states with permissive legislation will be undercut by public misunderstanding of therapeutic SCNT. In addition, political divisions even within supportive states may interfere with well-intentioned policy. This is especially true for issues relating to human embryos, about which the lack of 'societal accord about the moral and legal status of the embryo' makes lawmaking difficult (Andrews 2004: 220). At the least, however, the efforts can, in the presence of committed leadership, encourage discussion of goals and priorities and public participation in the development of science policy (Holman and Dutton 1978: 1524). The California and New Jersey laws have a greater potential for deliberative decision making than exists at the federal level. New Jersey's law, for example, establishes a nine-member IRB to advise the governor and legislature on stem cell issues (State of New Jersey 2004). This body sets up the basis for participatory deliberations about the goals and practice of ES cell research in the state. Or, with attention, commitment, and a sense of mission, it could be a location for thoughtful deliberations. It is, at the least, a point of access for pluralist interests to prompt problem solving to protect research participants, acknowledge the interplay of conflicting values, and weigh the merits of future research and development.

California's law recommends 'full consideration' of the 'ethical and medical implications' of the research and notes that ES cell research raises ethical and policy issues that must be 'carefully considered' even though they are 'not unique' (California Health and Safety Code 2003). The research must be reviewed by an IRB, although this does not appear to be a new state-wide body. Another effort at making stem cell policy democratic was undertaken by citizens in California, who gathered more than the requisite number of needed signatures to place a Stem Cell Research and Cures Initiative on the November 2004 ballot. The measure passed (Knight 2004a). Among other things, this initiative provided for the raising of $3 billion from state-backed funds ($295 million per year for ten years) to fund stem cell research and set up the California Institute of Regenerative Medicine at universities and medical research facilities. These facilities were to be built separately to avoid overlap with research facilities using federal funds (Holden 2004b). The initiative was designed to encourage stem cell research, and specifically ES cell research, which is unlikely to receive federal funds. It permitted funding for therapeutic but not reproductive SCNT. The new law sets up an Independent Citizen's Oversight Committee to issue, among other things, annual reports and to hold at least two public meetings a year. Funded researchers were to follow NIH protections for human research participants. Payments for cells were to be limited and research on embryos could not proceed for more than twelve days after the first cell divisions. Much of the oversight is to be conducted by working groups. The initiative has been criticized on both moral and financial grounds (Knight 2004*b*).

International Policy

An important international element underlines ES cell research as investigators and/or governments in Australia, Singapore, the United Kingdom, and other nations set up centers and cell banks for storing cells and providing products derived from ES cells for further research (National Institute for Biological Standards and Controls 2004; Nelson 2004). Nations operate under a variety of laws (Jones and Cohen 2004), which provides an opportunity to witness deliberations and innovative policies. In the United Kingdom therapeutic SCNT is supported by the government, and this policy brings with it guidelines and a supportive rationale. It is also witnessing plans for a large stem cell institute at the University of Cambridge. Therapeutic SCNT research would be allowed inasmuch as it is permissible under national law. In Canada the government passed in 2004 an Assisted Human Reproduction Law that, in relevant part, allows the derivation of ES cells from donated embryos (but not therapeutic SCNT). The law establishes a body to license the research (Canada/Government 2004). In the Netherlands it is permissible to create embryos for ES cell research (Gruss 2003). Each nation with emerging policy has held meetings and produced advisory group opinions that become part of the advocacy community.

While a review of the policies in these nations is beyond the scope of this chapter, the point is that policy making becomes enriched when perspectives go beyond national borders to examine policy developed through an open and pluralistic process in nations where ES cell research is welcomed. Policy governing therapeutic SCNT in the United Kingdom, for example, is not ethically less persuasive or authoritative than policy in California or New Jersey simply because it lies outside US borders. Taking an international perspective greatly broadens the resources for modeling ethical and policy analysis.

Corporations

The extent to which biotechnology companies conduct research into ES cells is hard to gauge. Corporations follow FDA regulations if they are developing biological products for eventual marketing, but this process is protected by secrecy. Companies may voluntarily follow federal guidelines for protecting research participants even if conducting privately funded research, and some follow or modify guidelines produced by an NIH ad hoc working group that made recommendations for obtaining donated embryos for stem cell research in 1999 (Cohen 2004: 110; National Institutes of Health 1999). Although one would not expect corporations to play a critical role in ES cell policy development, they are part of the community of advocates. In at least two instances corporations have set up ethics advisory boards (EABs) to propose guidelines for ES cell research and they have made public the process.

One, Geron Corporation, the company that funded the 1998 study by Thomson *et al.* in which the researchers first derived human ES cells, set up an EAB in mid-1998 to advise the company on ethical issues raised by ES cell research. After publication of the study, Geron contacted editors of the *Hastings Center Report*, and in spring 1999 the journal published a symposium with a report by Geron's EAB and essays by commentators. The company's EAB reached conclusions similar to those reached in the NIH's 1994 Human Research Policy report (Tauer 1999). Among other things, it advised that researchers should not engage in reproductive SCNT or mix the ES cells of different humans or of humans with a different species to make a chimera. The EAB also spoke of the importance of securing informed consent from egg donors. It advised that all research on human ES cells be approved by the EAB as well as an IRB (Geron Ethics Advisory Board 1999).

A second company, ACT, initiated an EAB in 1999 with a bioethicist as chair, to 'weigh the moral implications of therapeutic cloning research' (Green 2001). The EAB published the guidelines on the magazine's website, which included the restriction that research on embryos created through SCNT could continue for no more than fourteen days after fertilization. In regard to egg donation, the EAB advised that donors be limited to women aged 24–32 who had at least one child. Donors were required to undergo psychological and physical tests and could be compensated no more than $4,000 (Green 2001). Investigators aimed to secure approximately ten eggs from each donor. The researchers used anonymous somatic cell donors for fibroblasts. Some were healthy and others had conditions potentially helped by SCNT research (Cibelli *et al.* 2002). Somatic cell donors were warned about media attention and were told that their identity would be kept secret. Embryos were kept in a secure location, and measures were initiated to ensure that the embryos were not used for procreation (Saletan 2001).

In an example of clinic-based ethics review, the Jones Institute for Reproductive Medicine published guidelines for obtaining eggs from women to create embryos (through fertilization) for ES cell research. Clinic personnel did not actively recruit women for donation. Instead, they queried women who had applied to give eggs to help others conceive but were turned down because of problems with their medical background or because no recipients were available. They also used as donors women who had heard of the research and contacted the program (Lanzendorf *et al.* 2001).

Corporate EABs have obvious limits as conduits of ethics deliberations and as sources of policy. Open discussion is difficult in the context of corporate secrecy.

Corporations are also geared more to product development than to basic research, where ethical questions about whether one should proceed are appropriately raised. As entities set up by companies, corporate EABs may be insufficiently independent or critical and they may be set up after research has commenced rather than before (Hall 2000). Given their scarcity, they have minimal impact. As one analyst noted, 'the work of a small advisory board convened by one private company in no way measures up to the task of exercising oversight of human stem cell research or other types of research that the company invests in and investigators may choose to pursue' (White 1999: 41; emphasis omitted). In addition, there is 'no real motive to share guidelines across companies' (White 1999: 41). Even if corporations mutually sponsor an EAB, they will lack an incentive to enforce guidelines.

Corporate EABs are also criticized for their narrow focus on procedures rather than broader ethical issues (Fischer 2001; Saletan 2001). Questions about payment for EAB members and conflict of interest also dog these committees (Saletan 2001). One bioethicist notes that as of 2004 'no common ethical standards for conducting embryonic stem cell research have been developed in the private sector' (Cohen 2004: 111). In addition, the guidelines do not cover embryos created by SCNT or studies on parthenogenesis or other studies involving embryos created outside of fertilization (Cohen 2004: 111). Furthermore, the private sector has not produced 'commonly accepted ethical guidelines' for the range of issues arising from ES cell research that might, for example, involve the derivation of gametes from stem cells (Cohen 2004: 112). The paucity of national ethical standards evokes concerns that privately funded researchers will 'wing it' ethically (Cohen 2004: 111).

While such criticisms identify flaws in corporate ethics oversight, they need not foreclose an interest in corporate policy. The corporate EAB makes an interesting case study. Corporations are under no obligation to develop guidelines beyond IRB or equivalent review or FDA standards, much less to publish them. Thus, an examination of the motivating forces for doing so might encourage others to follow suit. Moreover, the content of the guidelines and deliberations is noteworthy and may be added to a meta-analysis of guidelines. The corporate world, in a nation with limited federal funding, is an early place for indicating issues and directions in research and development. Certainly an expectation that they will consider issues in the public interest and pledge not to undertake some forms of research is preferable to no pledge. Geron's EAB arranged to publish its guidelines, according to its members, to 'contribute to and invite . . . public discourse' stemming from the 'complex ethical issues emerging from ES cell research' (Geron Ethics Advisory Board 1999: 32). Also, it contributed specific recommendations, such as warnings to include explicit provisions about financial disclosure when securing consent from couples donating embryos. One commentator has observed that Geron's EAB 'provides an example of private–public ethical collaboration through the board's acknowledgement and application of previously developed federal guidelines' (Tauer 1999: 45).

Professional Associations

Professional associations, made up of professionals in science and medicine, have issued statements related to both reproductive and therapeutic SCNT. After Dolly's birth, the three main associations with members who could theoretically be involved in reproductive SCNT research—American Society for Reproductive Medicine (ASRM), the Biotechnology Industry Organization, and the Federation of American Societies for Experimental Biology (FASEB)—all called on their members to observe a moratorium on reproductive SCNT. After scenarios of therapeutic SCNT emerged, numerous groups recommended that it proceed, including the Institute of Medicine, the American Medical Association, FASEB, the American Association for the Advancement of Science, and the ASRM in the United States. Internationally, supportive groups include the European Society of Human Reproduction and Embryology and the Australian Academy of Science (ESHRE Task Force 2002; Australian Academy of Science 1999).

These and other organizations can be expected to take part in developing guidelines for therapeutic SCNT as questions arise in research and later practice. They provide a forum, through journals, conventions, ethics committee statements, and press releases, for mobilizing discussion. For example, professional associations proposed a somewhat more stringent process for securing consent from couples to donate spare embryos for ES cell than for other types of research using embryos. It is reasoned that ES cell research is different because the cell lines can exist indefinitely, potentially be traced to donors, and may hold considerable commercial value (ESHRE Task Force 2002). Among other things, groups recommend giving detailed information to potential donors about the specific research protocol and erecting a 'solid wall' in the consent process between the person seeking to help the patient become pregnant and the person seeking ES cells for research (American Association for the Advancement of Science 1999). The Ethics Committee of the ASRM in 1997 issued a statement for donating embryos for research and in 2002 issued a second statement directed to donating embryos for ES cell research (Ethics Committee, ASRM 1997, 2002). The latter was more explicit in what should be conveyed to potential donors in the consent process inasmuch as ES cell lines may have 'considerable commercial value' and can potentially be traceable.

Concern has been expressed about egg donors in therapeutic SCNT research and practice (European Group on Ethics in Science and New Technologies 2000). The need to secure human eggs is a limiting factor in this research because eggs are scarce and are secured at some risk to the donor. Investigators in South Korea used 2,061 eggs from 129 women in research to derive ES cells from embryos created through SCNT (Steinbrook 2006). Ethical questions were raised early on about the way the volunteers were recruited, however, and critics were later vindicated when it turned out that junior members of the research team were, indeed, among those who gave eggs. This development suggests the possibility of subtle if not explicit pressure placed upon the women to participate (Normile *et al.* 2006). Although it is not unusual for researchers to involve themselves in their investigations, the alleged lack of transparency in this case led the government to place a hold on further studies until a licensing system for using human eggs could go into effect (Cyranoski 2004). Irregularities in the recruitment of donors had taken place before the policy changes.

On the matter of recruiting egg donors, the ASRM Ethics Committee said that paying women who donate eggs for reproduction over $5,000 would 'require justification' and payments above $10,000 'go beyond what is appropriate' (Ethics Committee, ASRM 2000: 219). According to the committee, sums above this might cause donors to minimize physical and psychological risks and convey the message that eggs are commercial products. In addition, high sums might make donation too costly for all but wealthy recipients and, if given to donors with particularly desirable traits, might have eugenic overtones (Ethics Committee, ASRM 2000: 217).

With therapeutic SCNT, medical therapy, not reproduction, is the end. Some might argue that higher payment is justified here because the taint of 'buying' gametes for reproduction does not apply and because the potential benefit reaches more people. On the other hand, the same arguments that urge caution for reproductive donation arguably apply for research donation. Donors may, if offered high sums for their time and effort, be more likely to discount risks. In addition, high payments for medical therapy might again make treatments too costly for all but the wealthiest patients.

Another issue relates to women who donate repeatedly. The number of donations for reproduction that lead to births can justifiably be limited by concerns of inadvertent consanguinity of offspring. In donation for research, however, this restriction does not inhere. Should women willing to accept the risks of donation be limited in the number of times they donate for research as well as for reproduction, albeit for different reasons? In addition, if donors are scarce, what is the impact on fertility programs if women donate instead to research programs? The impact could be significant if the price is higher for regenerative medicine than for fertility purposes. It is not unreasonable to assume that wealthier citizens will have access to cell therapies made possible from therapeutic SCNT, especially if insurance companies are reluctant to reimburse for procedures using cells derived from human embryos.

In another aspect of egg donation, if therapeutic SCNT were to proceed and eggs were still needed, would it be ethical for patients to recruit their own egg donors? Would special protections be needed in this situation to ensure donors are not pressured to donate? Presumably donors would also be given a background check for mitochondrial disease and would need to be apprised of that. In a related scenario, what guidance would be needed if female patients wanted to use their own eggs for tailor-made ES cell lines? All donors would have to be told of commercial potential resulting from research and development and whether they would share in the profits. As developed by those in the field, consent by egg donors must enable them to 'understand how exactly the gametes, embryos, and cell lines will be used in the future and the possible financial benefits the institution may receive as a result of any ESC lines the donor's gametes produce' (Lanzendorf *et al.* 2001: 136).

Somatic cell donors provide another topic that invites voices from the field. For example, ACT used 'several . . . anonymous individuals' to donate fibroblasts. Some were healthy and some had disorders that therapeutic SCNT might one day address (Cibelli 2002). Somatic cell donation would not be physically risky, as it would pose only a 'remote possibility of an infection at the site of the skin biopsy' (Green 2001). In might, however, draw negative publicity, so the EAB of the ACT recommended confidentiality (Green 2001). In addition, if the SCNT process worked, the embryo potentially could be transferred for a pregnancy. Thus the investigators would be obligated to undertake restrictions to ensure that this did not happen. This might involve not freezing embryos created through SCNT, for example. Investigators would also need to make clear to somatic cell donors that the embryos would not be used for procreation even if the donors wanted to use them for procreation. In case donors had moral reservations about embryo research, they must be told in the consent process 'that ES cell research typically involves deriving cells from the inner cell mass of an embryo at the blastocyst stage, which leads to the embryo's destruction' (Ethics Committee, ASRM 2002).

Professional associations are not neutral but neither are they one-dimensional. They are pluralistic and they represent differing perspectives. Not all members should be regarded as supporting therapeutic SCNT even if the official position is supportive. Yet they are part of the community of advocates who can be expected to play a role in developing guidelines and who provide a forum, albeit one with borders, for ethics deliberation and guidance.

Policy Advisory Groups

Policy advisory groups refer to groups that are governmental or nongovernmental and permanent (e.g. the Institute of Medicine) or temporary (e.g. the National Bioethics Advisory Commission). An example of a nongovernmental group is the eighteen-member interdisciplinary body initiated by the Program in Cell Engineering, Ethics, and Public Policy at Johns Hopkins University and funded by the Greenwall Foundation to 'discuss novel ethical and policy challenges in stem cell research' (the JHU group) (Dawson *et al.* 2003: 1077). The JHU group started with the assumption that ES cell research will proceed and it asked what should be done to prepare. Its members identified ethical and policy issues arising from basic research, clinical trials, and human therapies. It did not review issues relating to SCNT, although it provided a model for how therapeutic SCNT could be studied. The group published one report exploring the preconditions for ethically proceeding with clinical trials (Dawson *et al.* 2003) and a second report raising questions about the ethical allocation of benefits after therapies are available (Faden *et al.* 2003).

In its first report, the group warned that several preconditions were necessary for clinical trials. First, new cell lines must be developed; clinical trials should not commence using ES cells derived prior to 9 August 2001 because these lines were cultured on animal feeder cells that risk the spread of infectious disease. Developing new lines means more human embryos will be destroyed, but this is justified by the need to protect human subjects by producing stem cell lines not exposed to mouse cells. In a second precondition, ES cell lines require quality control and standards and assays for making sure the lines are stable. If the lines do not meet the standards, investigators must not use the cells in clinical studies even if it means a delay in research. Third, investigators must consider the genetic risks posed by using cells derived from donated embryos. Existing cell lines are problematic because investigators do not know what genetic mutations to screen for in the lines. Therapeutic SCNT would mitigate this concern; for political and ethical reasons, however, this option may not be available. Fourth, investigators must be able to monitor cells so they will not go to the wrong target or de-differentiate, ensure that the cells will not form tumors, and develop methods to prevent immune rejection. Sponsors, researchers, and regulators must interact and develop criteria for testing.

The group also urged not proceeding without advance thinking about how to select participants for clinical trials and adequately protect participants. Federal funding is essential for protecting the safety of research participants, but funding restrictions mean the science is attracting insufficient federal oversight of ethics. It is important regularly to 'engage in serious discussions about the next generation of ethical and policy issues' for stem cell research before rather than after scientific developments (Dawson *et al.* 2003: 1077). In preparation for clinical trials, health care professionals should set up patient advisory boards, specify people to monitor the consent process, appoint patient advocates, and enact procedures to protect earliest human subjects. The group was not persuaded that a body such as the Recombinant DNA Advisory Committee would be helpful for protecting human subjects, owing in part to the lack of federal funding.

In a second report, the JHU group asked how 'equitable biological access' to cell lines can be secured for research and therapy (Faden *et al.* 2003). The group posited that some people will have greater biological access to banks of stem cell lines than others. The members were concerned that the banks will not adequately reflect the country's ethnic and racial biological diversity. The group advised preemptive planning and envisioned a stem cell bank in the United States that 'would be composed of the fewest number of cell lines that would reflect the ancestral backgrounds of all of the major ethnic groups in the United States' (Cohen 2004: 109). Among other things, this would draw attention to diseases that are not limited to occurrences primarily among Caucasians. Therapeutic SCNT would address the access problem because it would allow transplantation using a patient's own cells. But this technique is 'not practical at present' because of the costs of developing individualized therapies and the political barriers wrought by the 'political and moral controversy' of therapeutic SCNT (Faden *et al.* 2003: 15).

The difficulty in securing eggs, especially from minority populations, further burdens the creation of stem cell banks, at least with current technologies. So too do moral controversies about using embryos, although these could be lessened by waiting until there is 'solid evidence' that ES cell therapies will work before building stem cell banks. Still, to get to that stage, more embryos will need to be used. For this reason, private funds presumably will be needed to develop the bank. In short, the group confronted some of the decisions that must be made for ES cell benefits to be realized. This will involve calculations about whether ensuring equitable benefit from ES cell research or protecting embryos is more valuable. It will also involve revisiting federal funding policy, financial incentives, and patent protections to address justice concerns.

CONCLUSION

One observer has said that 'the prospect of a patchwork approach to human stem cell research is not encouraging' (White 1999: 42). If a policy patchwork holds for ES cell research in general, it does even more so for research into therapeutic SCNT as a subtype of ES cell research. Whereas ES cell research is burdened by conflicts over the status of the embryo, therapeutic SCNT shares a technique with reproductive SCNT, which makes it doubly contentious. Yet research is proceeding, however slowly, and few signs of national oversight are in view.

In an effort to seek alternative policy sources and suggest new directions for academic commentary, this chapter directs attention to what might be called a policy community of advocates—the advisory groups, experts, interest group members, and others who share an interest in ES cell research, including therapeutic SCNT. This community, loosely defined, took form in debates in the US Congress. Because it is not neutral, it must not be the only voice in deliberations. Still, its biased voice can play a role in policy making in that its members presumably have a sense of mission that can be marshaled to promote research and development under guiding principles. This community exists in the public sector (states and other nations) as well as the private sector (corporations and professional associations). It is a source of oversight generated by those eager for research and clinical application to succeed and to be practiced ethically. The community is a case study in policy development where federal oversight is minimal, and it opens the door to policy leadership.

To look at the community of advocates is to identify alternatives to federal policy when national-level guidance beyond existing regulations is not forthcoming. Identifying the components is only an initial step, however, to be followed by evaluation of the integrity of the emerging expectations and practices and of the deliberations that preceded them. In addition, the enforceability of this decentralized policy is open to question. As a result, more than anything else, this community is a place of 'softening' of later more authoritative policy through open discussion and forums for learning and talking about policy proposals. The targets of these repeated deliberations are the general public, the specialized public, and the policy community itself (Kingdon 1984: 135). In this process norms and expectations evolve. As one analyst put it, 'the more a proposal is discussed, the more seriously it is taken' (Kingdon 1984: 148).

Several points can be made about future inquiry by policy analysts and commentators. First, a mindset is in order that begins with the assumption that the research will proceed. This shifts what is often a defensive posture about why research should proceed to a more pragmatic orientation about how to proceed ethically. This includes studies that anticipate issues and prepare for their management. Deliberations by the JHU group illustrate this mindset. Looking at ES cell research in general, the members anticipated issues such as justice questions in stem cell banks, discussed them, weighed values, and reached conclusions based in ethical analysis. While this may not please those who prefer not to proceed with ES cell research at all, it is realistic in view of ES cell studies underway.

Second, the 'patchwork approach' to stem cell oversight may not be as inchoate as first appears. An important contribution to the literature could be made by conducting a meta-analysis to create the equivalent of a data bank for guidelines. This helps to identify principles of agreement, treat these principles as a policy base, focus on how they can be implemented, and look to other problematic issues. A policy meta-analysis should include position statements and informal policies from the private sector as well as legally binding regulations. The policies should be critically examined for empty verbiage and bland acceptance as well as for creativity and anticipatory problem-solving. The need exists, in short, for an empirical dimension to inquiry to help consolidate and examine the array of commentaries already available.

Third, a meta-analysis should be undertaken with a cosmopolitan perspective. ES cell research is anchored in centers across nations, and it is here where practices can be examined to identify issues and methods of problem solving. The United Kingdom stands out, where ethical principles and codes of practice can guide policy even in nations that do not and never will have a central licensing system for research involving embryos. In addition, the international feature of trade in ES cells raises issues about oversight, conflicting pharmacologic guidelines, and transparency. An international perspective would be a welcome contribution to the literature; it depends on a willingness to go beyond national borders to seek policy leadership.

Fourth, given that additional politically volatile technologies are on the horizon, it makes sense to consider science under intense politics as a topic of inquiry in its own right. The usual truisms about science policy do not necessarily apply in the context of heightened politics. How, then, can policy be developed that allows for political intensity, which is a barometer of public values, and also enable effective guidance? In the case of SCNT, Congress provided a forum for political arguments and, in so doing, helped defuse sensationalism and avoid premature legislation. Yet this was a messy process that resulted in stalemate. The experience suggests that attention can be paid to improving the way Congress can deliberate in a reassuring way when new technologies evoke concern. Among the reforms might be to institute a consultative body for Congress to provide reliable and impartial analysis of issues in science and technology (Morgan and Peha 2003b). While the Congressional Research Service provides immediate technical information and the National Research Council is one of several sources for long-term analysis, no body under Congressional auspices provides mid-range studies of approximately a year (Morgan and Peha 2003b). If an office equivalent to the disbanded Office of Technology Assessment were held to be a priority by members of Congress and were instituted and consulted, it would provide an analytic alternative to the information-oriented and sometimes repetitive hearings.

In conclusion, therapeutic SCNT invites innovative analysis about managing science policy in a setting of heightened politics. This case suggests that a step in the analysis is to look critically and with a problem-solving mindset at resources promoted by those who are want to proceed in an ethical and responsible way.

REFERENCES

AMERICAN ASSOCIATION FOR THE ADVANCEMENT OF SCIENCE/INSTITUTE FOR CIVIL SOCIETY (1999), *Stem Cell Research and Applications: Monitoring the Frontiers of Biomedical Research* (Washington, DC: American Association for the Advancement of Science), <http://www.aaas.org/spp/dspp/sfrl/projects/stem/report.pdf>, accessed 2 Jan. 2004.

AMERICAN MEDICAL ASSOCIATION (1999), 'H-140.890: Cloning for Biomedical Research', <http://www.ama/pub/category/11964.html>, accessed 6 Nov. 2003.

ANDREWS, L. B. (2004), 'Appendix E. Legislators as Lobbyists: Proposed State Regulation of Embryonic Stem Cell Research, Therapeutic Cloning and Reproductive Cloning', in President's Council on Bioethics, *Monitoring Stem Cell Research* (Washington, DC: President's Council on Bioethics), 199–224, <http://www.bioethics.gov/reports/stemcell/appendix_e.html>, accessed 1 June 2005.

ANNAS, G. J., CAPLAN, A., ELIAS, S. (1996), 'The Politics of Human–Embryo: Avoiding Ethical Gridlock', *New England Journal of Medicine*, 334: 1329–32.

Asia (2004), <http://www.glphr.org/genetic/asia2–07.htm>, accessed 28 May 2004.

AUSTRALIAN ACADEMY OF SCIENCE (1999), *On Human Cloning: A Position Statement* (Canberra: Australian Academy of Science).

BIRKLAND, T. A. (2001), *An Introduction to the Policy Process* (Armonk, NY: M. E. Sharpe).

BONNICKSEN, A. L. (2002), *Crafting a Cloning Policy: From Dolly to Stem Cells* (Washington, DC: Georgetown University Press).

BROCK, D. W. (1997), 'An Assessment of the Ethical Issues Pro and Con', in National Bioethics Advisory Commission, *Cloning Human Beings*, ii: *Commissioned Papers* (Rockville, Md.: National Bioethics Advisory Commission), E1–23.

California Health and Safety Code (2003), sect. 125115.

CANADA/GOVERNMENT (2004), 'An Act Respecting Human Reproduction and Related Research (Bill C-6)', Ottawa, 29 Mar., <http://laws.justice.gc.ca/en/a-13.4/218740.html>, accessed 20 June 2006.

CIBELLI, J. B., KIESSLING, A. A., CUNNIFF, K., RICHARDS, C., LANZA, R. P., and WEST, M. D. (2001), 'Somatic Cell Nuclear Transfer in Humans: Pronuclear and Early Embryonic Development', *e-biomed: The Journal of Regenerative Medicine*, 2: 25–31.

—— LANZA, R. P., and WEST, M. D., with EZZELL, C. (2002), 'The First Human Cloned Embryo ', *Scientific American*, <http://www.sciam.com/search/index.cfm>, accessed 8 Dec. 2001.

COHEN, C. (2001), 'Leaps and Boundaries: Expanding Oversight of Human Stem Cell Research', in S. Holland, K. Lebacqz, and L. Zoloth (eds.), *The Human Embryonic Stem Cell Debate: Science, Ethics, and Public Policy* (Cambridge, Mass.: MIT Press), 209–22.

—— (2004), 'Stem Cell Research in the U.S. After the President's Speech of August 2001', *Kennedy Institute of Ethics Journal*, 14/1 (Mar.), 97–114.

COMMITTEE ON THE BIOLOGICAL AND BIOMEDICAL APPLICATIONS OF STEM CELL RESEARCH; BOARD ON LIFE SCIENCES, NATIONAL RESEARCH COUNCIL; BOARD ON NEUROSCIENCE AND BEHAVIORAL HEALTH, INSTITUTE OF MEDICINE (2002), *Stem Cells and the Future of Regenerative Medicine* (Washington, DC: National Academy Press).

COWAN, C. A., KLIMANSKAYA, I., MCMAHON, J., ATIENZA, J., *et al.* (2004), 'Derivation of Embryonic Stem-Cell Lines from Human Blastocysts', *New England Journal of Medicine*, 350: 1353–6.

CYRANOSKI, D. (2004), 'Crunch Time for Korea's Cloners', *Nature*, 429: 12–14.

DALEY, G. Q. (2003), 'Cloning and Stem Cells: Handicapping the Political and Scientific Debates', *New England Journal of Medicine*, 349: 211–12.

DAWSON, L., BATEMAN-HOUSE, A. S., AGNEW, D. M., BOK, H., *et al.* (2003), 'Safety Issues in Cell-Based Intervention Trials', *Fertility and Sterility*, 80: 1077–85.

DEPARTMENT OF HEALTH (2000), *A Report from the Chief Medical Officer's Expert Group Reviewing the Potential of Developments in Stem Cell Research and Cell Nuclear Replacement to Benefit Human Health. Stem Cell Research: Medical Progress and Responsibility* (London: Department of Health).

DRAZEN, J. M. (2003), 'Legislative Myopia on Stem Cells', *New England Journal of Medicine*, 349: 300.

EIBERT, M. (2003), 'Human Cloning: Myths, Medical Benefits, and Constitutional Rights', in B. Steinbock, J. Arras, and A. London (eds.), *Ethical Issues in Modern Medicine*, 6th edn. (New York: McGraw-Hill).

EISEMAN, E. (1997), 'Views of Scientific Societies and Professional Associations on Human Nuclear Transfer Cloning Research', in National Bioethics Advisory Commission, *Cloning*

Human Beings: Report and Recommendations of the National Bioethics Advisory Commission, ii: *Commissioned Papers* (Rockville, Md.: National Bioethics Advisory Commission), C1–31.

ESHRE [European Society of Human Reproduction and Embryology] Task Force on Ethics and Law (2002), 'Stem Cells: Ethical Issues', Considerations No. 4, *Human Reproduction*, 17: 1409–10.

Ethics Committee, ASRM (American Society for Reproductive Medicine) (1997), 'Informed Consent and the Use of Gametes and Embryos for Research', *Fertility and Sterility*, 68: 780–1.

—— (2000), 'Financial Incentives in Recruitment of Oocyte Donors', *Fertility and Sterility*, 74: 216–20.

—— (2002), 'Donating Spare Embryos for Embryonic Stem-Cell Research', *Fertility and Sterility*, 78: 957–60.

Europe (2004), <http://www.glphr.org/genetic/europe2–7.htm>, accessed 20 June 2006.

European Group on Ethics in Science and New Technologies (2000), *Opinion of the European Group on Ethics in Science and New Technologies: Ethical Aspects of Human Stem Cell Research and Use*, 14 Nov., <http://ec.europa.eu/european_group_ethics/docs/avis15_en.pdf>, accessed 20 June 2006.

Faden, R. R., Dawson, L., Bateman-House, A. S., Agnew, D. M., *et al.* (2003), 'Public Stem Cell Banks: Considerations of Justice in Stem Cell Research and Therapy', *Hastings Center Report*, 33: 13–27.

Fischer, J. (2001), 'The First Clone', *U.S. News and World Report*, 3 Dec., 51–63.

FitzPatrick, W. (2003), 'Surplus Embryos, Nonreproductive Cloning, and the Intend/Foresee Distinction', *Hastings Center Report*, 33: 29–36.

Gearhart, J. (2004), 'New Human Embryonic Stem-Cell Lines: More Is Better', *New England Journal of Medicine*, 350: 1275–6.

Geron Ethics Advisory Board (1999), 'Research with Human Embryonic Stem Cells: Ethical Considerations', *Hastings Center Report*, 29: 31–6.

Green, R. M. (2001), 'The Ethical Considerations', 24 Nov., <http://www.sciam.com/article.cfm>, accessed 20 June 2006.

Gruss, P. (2003), 'Human ES Cells in Europe', *Science*, 301: 1017.

Hall, S. S. (2000), 'The Recycled Generation', *New York Times Magazine*, 30 Jan., 30–5, 46, 74, 78–9.

Hochedlinger, K., and Jaenisch, R. (2003), 'Nuclear Transplantation, Embryonic Stem Cells, and the Potential for Cell Therapy', *New England Journal of Medicine*, 349: 275–86.

Holden, C. (2004*a*), 'Advocates Keep Pot Boiling as Bush Plans New Centers', *Science*, 305: 461.

—— (2004*b*), 'Stem Cell Research Could Be a Ballot Issue', *Science*, 303: 293.

Holland, S., Lebacqz, K., and Zoloth, L. (eds.) (2001), *The Human Embryonic Stem Cell Debate: Science, Ethics, and Public Policy* (Cambridge, Mass.: MIT Press).

Holman, H. R., and Dutton, D. B. (1978), 'A Case for Public Participation in Science Policy Formation and Practice', *Southern California Law Review*, 51: 1505–34.

Huxley, A. (1932), *Brave New World* (New York: Harper & Row).

Hwang, W. S., Ryu, Y. J., Park, J. H., Park, E. S., *et al.* (2004), 'Evidence of a Pluripotent Human Embryonic Stem Cell Line Derived from a Cloned Blastocyst', *Science*, 303: 1669–74.

_____ Roh, S. I., Lee, B.C., et al. (2005), 'Patient-Specific Embryonic Stem Cells Derived from Human SNCT Blastocysts', *Science*, 308: 1777–83.

Jones, H. W., Jr., and Cohen, J. (2004), 'IFFS Surveillance 04', *Fertility and Sterility*, 81 (suppl. 4), S1–54.

Juengst, E., and Fossel, M. (2000), 'The Ethics of Embryonic Stem Cells: Now and Forever, Cells Without End', *JAMA* 284: 3180–4.

Kass, L. (1997), 'The Wisdom of Repugnance', *New Republic*, 2 (June), 17–26.

Kennedy, D. (2004), 'Stem Cells, Redux', *Science*, 303: 1581.

Kingdon, J. W. (1984), *Agendas, Alternatives, and Public Policies* (Boston: Little, Brown).

Knight, J. (2004a), 'Joys Match Fears as California Agrees to Stem-Cell Proposal', *Nature*, 432: 135.

_____ (2004b), 'War of Words Escalates in Run-Up to California's Vote on Stem Cells', *Nature*, 430: 125.

Kocieniewski, D. (2004), 'McGreevey Signs Bill Creating Stem Cell Research Institute', *New York Times*, 13 May, A23.

Lanzendorf, S. E., Boyd, C. A., Wright, D. L., Muasher, S., Ohehinger, S., and Hodgen, G. D. (2001), 'Use of Human Gametes Obtained from Anonymous Donors for the Production of Human Embryonic Stem Cell Lines ', *Fertility and Sterility*, 76: 132–7.

Lawler, A. (2004), 'Harvard Enters Stem Cell Fray', *Science*, 303: 1453.

Maienschein, J. (2003), *Whose View of Life? Embryos, Cloning and Stem Cells* (Cambridge, Mass.: Harvard University Press).

Majone, G. (1989), *Evidence, Argument and Persuasion in the Policy Process* (New Haven: Yale University Press).

Mansnerus, L. (2004), 'In Stem-Cell Law, Supporters See Opportunity for New Jersey', *New York Times*, 6 Jan., A24.

Marshall, E., and Vogel, G. (2001), 'Cloning Announcement Sparks Debate and Scientific Skepticism', *Science*, 294: 1802–3.

Morgan, M. G., and Peha, J. M. (2003a), 'Analysis, Governance, and the Need for Better Institutional Arrangements', in M. G. Morgan and J. M. Peha (eds.), *Science and Technology Advice for Congress* (Washington, DC: Resources for the Future), 3–20.

_____ (2003b), 'Where Do We Go From Here'?, in M. G. Morgan and J. M. Peha (eds.), *Science and Technology Advice for Congress* (Washington, DC: Resources for the Future), 173–81.

National Bioethics Advisory Commission (1997), *Cloning Human Beings: Report and Recommendations of the National Bioethics Advisory Commission* (Rockville, Md.: National Bioethics Advisory Commission).

_____ (1999), *Ethical Issues in Human Stem Cell Research: Report and Recommendations of the National Bioethics Advisory Commission* (Rockville, Md.: National Bioethics Advisory Commission).

National Institute for Biological Standards and Controls (2004), 'UK Stem Cell Bank', <http://www.ukstemcellbank.org.uk>, accessed 20 June 2006.

National Institutes of Health (1999), 'Draft National Institutes of Health Guidelines for Research Involving Human Pluripotent Stem Cells', *Federal Register*, 64: 67576–9.

Nature (2004), 'Ethics of Therapeutic Cloning', 429: 1.

Nelson, L. (2004), 'Britain Opens First Repository to Speed Work on Stem Cells', *Nature*, 429: 333.

NORMILE, D., VOGEL, G., and COZIN, J. (2006), 'South Korean Team's Remaining Human Stem Cell Claim Demolished', *Science*, 311: 156–7.

NUFFIELD COUNCIL ON BIOETHICS (2000), *Stem Cell Therapy: The Ethical Issues. A Discussion Paper* (London: Nuffield Council on Bioethics).

NUSSBAUM, M. C. (1998), 'Little C', in M. C. Nussbaum and C. R. Sunstein (eds.), *Clones and Clones: Facts and Fantasies About Human Cloning* (New York: Norton), 338–46.

Oceania (2004), <http://www.glphr.org/genetic/oceania.htm>,.

OKARMA, T. B. (1999), 'Human Primordial Stem Cells', *Hastings Center Report*, 29: 30.

PARENS, E., and KNOWLES, L.P. (2003), 'Reprogenetics and Public Policy: Reflections and Recommendations', *Hastings Center Report* (July–Aug.), special suppl., S1–24.

PENCE, G. E. (1998), *Who's Afraid of Human Cloning?* (Boulder, Col.: Rowman & Littlefield).

PHIMISTER, E. G., and DRAZEN, J. M. (2004), 'Two Fillips for Human Embryonic Stem Cells', *New England Journal of Medicine*, 350: 1351–2.

PRESIDENT'S COUNCIL ON BIOETHICS (2002), *Human Cloning and Human Dignity: An Ethical Inquiry* (Washington, DC: President's Council on Bioethics), <http://www.bioethics. gov>.

—— (2004), *Monitoring Stem Cell Research* (Washington, DC: President's Council on Bioethics), <http://www.bioethics.gov>.

ROBERTSON, J. A. (1998), 'Human Cloning and the Challenge of Regulation', *New England Journal of Medicine*, 339/2: 119–21.

ROHM, W. G. (2004), 'Seven Days of Creation: The Inside Story of a Human Cloning Experiment', *WIRED* (Jan.), 120–9.

ROSENTHAL, N. (2003), 'Prometheus's Vulture and the Stem-Cell Promise', *New England Journal of Medicine*, 349: 267–74.

SALETAN, W. (2001), 'The Ethicist's New Clothes', *Slate Magazine*, 17 Aug., <http://www. slate.com/id/113959>, accessed 20 June 2006.

SMITH, B. L. R., and STINE, J. K. (2003), 'Technical Advice for Congress: Past Trends and Present Obstacles', in M. G. Morgan and J. M. Peha (eds.), *Science and Technology Advice for Congress* (Washington, DC: Resources for the Future), 23–52.

STATE OF NEW JERSEY (2004), 'McGreevey Signs Landmark Stem Cell Research Act', press release, 4 Jan., <http://www.state.nj.us/cgi-bin/governor/njnewsline/default_full_listing. pl>, accessed 20 June 2006.

STEINBOCK, B. (2000), 'Cloning Human Beings: Sorting Through the Ethical Issues', in B. McKinnon (ed.), *Human Cloning: Science, Ethics, and Public Policy* (Urbana: University of Illinois Press), 68–84.

STEINBROOK, R. (2006), 'Egg Donation and Human Embryonic Stem-Cell Research', *New England Journal of Medicine*, 354: 324–6.

STOLBERG, S. G. (2001), 'Cloning Executive Presses Senate', *New York Times*, 5 Dec., A22.

TAUER, C. A. (1999), 'Private Ethics Boards and Public Debate', *Hastings Center Report*, 29: 43–5.

THOMSON, J. A., ITSKOVITZ-ELDOR, J., SHAPIRO, S. S., WAKNITZ, M. A., SWIERGIEL, J. J., MARSHALL, V. S., and JONES, J. M. (1998), 'Embryonic Stem Cell Lines Derived from Human Blastocysts', *Science*, 282: 1145–7.

VOGEL, G. (2003), 'E.U. Stem Cell Debate Ends in a Draw', *Science*, 302: 1872–3.

WALTERS, L. (2004), 'The United Nations and Human Cloning: A Debate on Hold', *Hastings Center Report*, 34: 5–6.

WHITE, G. B. (1999), 'Foresight, Insight, Oversight', *Hastings Center Report*, 29: 41–2.

ZERHOUNI, E. A. (2003*a*), 'Stem Cell Programs', *Science*, 300: 911–12.

—— (2003*b*), 'Stem Cell Research', Testimony to 108th Congress, 22 May, Session 1, <http://olpa.od.nih.gov/hearings/108/session1/summaries/stemcell.asp>, accessed 20 June 2006.

PART VI

GENETICS AND ENHANCEMENT

CHAPTER 20

....

POPULATION GENETIC RESEARCH AND SCREENING: CONCEPTUAL AND ETHICAL ISSUES

....

ERIC T. JUENGST

IN 2003 victory was declared by the scientists pursuing the Human Genome Project (Collins *et al.* 2003). This declaration marked the realization of three scientific goals: (1) the generation of genetic landmark maps of all the human chromosomes; (2) the production of an ordered, overlapping collection of DNA fragments covering the entire human genome; (3) the chemical sequencing of the DNA across the complete collection. Along the way, genome researchers had been identifying the functional coding regions within the genome, and describing an increasing number of correlations between the variant forms of these genes and other human biological traits. With the achievement of what some have called the 'Holy Grail' of human biology (Gilbert 1992), genomic science now prepares itself

This chapter was prepared with support from National Institutes of Health grant P50-HG03390 and the Center for Genetic Research Ethics and Law (CGREAL; as in 'See... Grail'!) that it makes possible at Case Western Reserve University.

to found a new future for medicine, as rich as the Kingdom of the Grail to which Parzival is transported after the completion of his quest (Barber 2004).

Unlike Parzival's discovery, however, the achievement of the Human Genome Project does not offer immediate access to the Grail Kingdom, or to the Grail's reputed other benefits of health, longevity, and abundance. In fact, the Holy Grail of human biology is simply a set of tools for the further questing that must be done before the Fisher King can be cured of his reproductive wound and the Wasteland can be reclaimed. Armed with improved genomic maps and DNA sequencing technologies, the goal now is to pursue a new generation of projects *comparing* human genomes to better understand our similarities, differences, and patterns of relationship at the molecular level. These comparative quests are critical to the development of successful medical applications of genomic research but they also take our genomic knights down some particularly perilous roads. This chapter is the tale of two such perils, concerning first how best to pursue such comparisons and then how best to use their results, when they are made at the level of human populations. The dangers in both adventures are the risks of social harms that might come to people as a consequence of being members of those populations, if the groups are socially defined and the scientific stories told about them undermine their social interests. If genetic populations become identified with both political communities and stigmatizing biological claims, they can tap into our oldest social tensions—tribalism, racism, and suspicion of the 'other'—to open the door to volatile new forms of genetic discrimination. In the end, the ethical challenge for both research and practice in comparative genomics is a fundamental one: how can we preserve our commitment to human moral equality in the face of our growing understanding of human biological diversity?

POPULATION GENOMIC RESEARCH

Since the beginning of the Human Genome Project, there have been calls to map the genetic variation within our species (Cavalli-Sforza *et al.* 1991). The initial interest was primarily genealogical: physical anthropologists and population geneticists would use comparative genotyping to produce the molecular clues they need to reconstruct more completely the global history of human migration and differentiation. But interest in the ways in which human groups vary at different genetic loci has grown much broader within biomedicine, as scientists apply the fruits of genome research to their work in epidemiology, molecular diagnostics, pharmacogenetics, and the analysis of complex genetic traits (Collins *et al.* 1997; Risch and Merikingas 1996). Much of this interest is driven by the prospect of a 'genomic medicine', in which diagnostic protocols, therapeutic interventions, and preventive measures could be tailored to each patient's genetic profile (Guttmacher and Collins 2004). This prospect attracts clinicians concerned about adverse patient reactions to medications, public health officials interested in preventing disease through public risk education and behavior change, and health policy-makers concerned with the persistent health disparities between different population groups.

Whatever its focus, all population genomic research involves collecting DNA samples from individual members of different human groups, genotyping them (through marker mapping or DNA sequencing) at one or more loci, and comparing the results. This immediately raises an important conceptual question for this research: how should scientists define and identify the relevant comparison groups within our species? The initial attempt to use genomic tools in a large-scale study of human variation, the so-called Human Genome Diversity Project, followed the accepted practice of physical anthropologists and epidemiologists of describing its target groups in ethnic, linguistic, and geographical terms, and was called to task by both biologists and social scientists for using socially constructed categories that would obfuscate rather than illuminate underlying patterns of gene flow within our species (Gannet 2001; Reardon 2005). Rather than reifying various human political histories by looking for 'ethnic-affiliation markers' in human DNA, some suggested a random global sampling strategy blinded to social identifiers (National Research Council 1998). The US National Institutes of Health (NIH) followed this approach in developing a major genetic variation research resource—a databank of known single nucleotide variants in human DNA—and was in turn called to task by public health and pharmacogenomic researchers for omitting 'phenotypic data' about the distribution of the DNA variants across different populations (Altshuler and Clark 2005). As a result, the subsequent international effort to produce a variation-measuring 'haplotype map' of the human genome intentionally collected samples from groups defined by their 'continents of origin' (International Hapmap Consortium 2003). Critics charge that this strategy returns population genomics to a set of outmoded racial categories that human scientists of all stripes have repudiated as biomedically meaningless and socially pernicious (Duster 2005). Counterclaims that, nevertheless, research framed in this way has identified patterns of genetic variation that cluster along racial lines, and that these variations may be the key to 'population specific' public health interventions or even 'race-based medicine', have only lent fuel to this conceptual debate (Kahn 2004).

As a result, genetic research has an increasingly complicated message for our inclinations to identify ourselves in terms of larger human populations and ethnic groups. At the same time that we are learning just what a relatively young and genetically homogenous animal species we are, health disparities researchers, physical anthropologists, and forensic scientists continue to bear down on the rare genetic differences that seem to differentiate the social categories of race, ethnicity, people, and nationality (Burchard et al. 2003). Social categories, by definition, provide identities by segregating their members from other people. It is not surprising that research that threatens to drive scientific wedges into the social cracks that already divide people from their neighbors should carry very high moral stakes. Thus, comparative human genetic variation research which continues to use these categories or their proxies (i.e. 'continents of origin' for race) continues to be ethically and scientifically controversial (Cooper *et al.* 2003). On the one hand, no one wants to reify categories that were created and used in contexts of social oppression. Yet for those who have been marginalized and oppressed by the categories in the past, justice seems to demand increased access to whatever benefits genetic research might yield their group when it is framed in terms of this ascriptive identity (Zilinkas and Balint 2001). The need to recognize these categories in redressing injustice becomes particularly acute where health disparities are part of their legacies. At the same time, the claim that those disparities are also genetic—that racism has helped exacerbate genetic differences between specific human superfamilies—have to be very carefully made and evaluated, if they are not to fuel the very social problem they are intended to address.

The second challenge facing population genomic research follows from the first. Assuming that, for the foreseeable future, the definition of comparison groups in population genomics will be informed by socially constructed criteria at some level of resolution (either familial, tribal, ethnic, racial, or regional), how should the interests of group members be protected?

Almost by definition, a complicating feature of many population genomic studies is the fact that this research is increasingly cross-cultural and international. Large genetic variation studies like the Haplotype Mapping Project are increasingly collaborative efforts between scientists in different countries who collect and compare DNA from populations chosen for their phenotypic diversity. Even genetic studies that involve mainstream American immigrant communities, such as African Americans or the Ashkenazim can quickly take investigators all across the globe. As a result, cultural, linguistic, and socioeconomic factors complicate population genetics research in much the same way they complicate international epidemiological research, raising questions about the collective interests of the human groups being studied, and their decision-making role in this context.

Outside of groups with clear political sovereignty, like Native American nations, most targets of genetic analysis have ambiguous moral standing. Is it ethically important for scientists to attempt to discuss their plans with groups at the collective level before recruiting individual group members into genetic variation studies? Some argue strongly that a principle of 'respect for community' needs to supplement our traditionally individualistic principles of research ethics in these contexts, if only because individuals gain so much of their identity through their community memberships and their genetic lineages (Weijer 1999). Others argue that, at least for genetic studies, extensive efforts at community engagement are disingenuous and guaranteed to fail, given the mismatch between genetic populations and the politically defined communities available for consultation (Juengst 1998).

At the crux of this debate is the role of community membership in the personal identity of individuals who participate in genome research. Common bonds of religion, culture, or history can create defining identities for members of groups ranging from global diasporas to nations to local voluntary organizations and support groups. Unlike families or clans, however, genetic relationships are not the basis for the vast majority of these human communities. Despite the interests of population geneticists in identifying human examples of the 'founder effect', human communities that can count as 'genetic isolates' like the Galapagos finches are exceedingly rare. This means that for the fluxuating memberships of human communities like nations, cities, religions, political movements, and social classes, the 'gene pool' does not provide a commons that can be effectively exploited for the good of those communities. Despite the local appeal of promoting the 'unique genomic research resources' of communities like Iceland, Newfoundland, Estonia, the Han Chinese, or the castes of India, members of those communities should not expect research results that differentially benefit their own health.

Since no human communities define unique human genetic populations, moreover, the legitimacy of identifying socially defined communities with genetic populations and the propriety of giving community leaders this gate-keeping role becomes controversial, and complicated questions of loyalty arise for members of those communities (Marshall and Rotimi 2001). Any biomedical research that seeks to recruit research participants through the communities in which they live must always walk a tightrope between the values of group solidarity and individual autonomy. For genetic research, however, the local trust-building virtues of community gate-keeping are offset by a serious hazard: the danger of reinforcing the ultimately vicious impression that the communities being consulted are coincident with the genetic populations under study and therefore biologically distinct from their neighbors.

The discussion of how best to protect communities has moved through several stages. Most regulatory bodies have recognized that since genetic populations are not the sorts of groups that can claim autonomy as moral communities, it makes no sense to hinge the recruitment of their members on some corporate permission. Thus, for example, the 'Points to Consider for Population-Based Genetic Research' developed by the NIH stresses that: 'community consultation is not the same as consent . . . . community consultation is a vehicle for hearing about the community's interests and concerns, addressing ethical issues and communicating information about the research to the community' (NIH 2002).

This interpretation of community engagement places much more emphasis on preserving the special values and cultural lifeways of a given population than on treating the population as a politically autonomous entity. The purpose of this interchange, NIH says, is to solicit the study population's help in identifying any 'intra-community or 'culturally specific' risks and potential benefits, so that the research can be designed in ways that best protect the group's interests (Foster *et al.* 1999). As Marshall and Rotimi point out, this can be difficult:

Despite the obvious benefits of community advisory boards, there are limits and constraints on their ability to represent the values of diverse community members. . . . In some cases community leaders on advisory boards may be politicians. Community activists represent another powerful group who might serve on such boards. Religious leaders or local celebrities also might be asked to participate on the boards. Investigators must be sensitive to the social and political agendas of members on community advisory boards and try to minimize the potential for addressing priorities that may be relevant to only a minority of the local population   (Marshall and Rotimi 2001: 261).

Of course, the increasing dispersion of human populations around the world means that in fact most human superfamilies no longer share common 'culturally specific risks' and benefits. This leads even the staunchest advocates of community engagement to the counterintuitive point of arguing that, for study populations like 'general ethnic, racial or national populations, e.g. Ashkenazi Jews, American Indians, Puerto Ricans, etc.', the lack of distinctive common interests and structured social interaction means that 'community review may not be required' and even for geographically dispersed populations that share distinctive beliefs and practices, like the Amish or the Hmong, 'limited social interactions between members of the study population make intra-community risks unlikely' (Sharp and Foster 2000).

Diverse, dispersed genetic superfamilies of the sort useful to genetic variation studies will not often enjoy the level of organization that can make representative consultations possible. For these cases, Sharp and Foster suggest that all that may be required is the form of community engagement they call 'community dialogue': "an effort to interact with the local communities and institutions at the specific site from which members of a given genetic population will be recruited, in order to acquaint them with the investigators' mission in advance of individual subject enrollment" (Sharp and Foster 2000).

The key move in this interpretation is to acknowledge the complexity of human population structure by sacrificing the ambition to protect all members of a genetic population from the potential harms of the research, and to refocus on the particular families and locale from which investigators hope to solicit DNA samples. Instead of attempting to respect the genetic population as a moral community, or attempting to protect all its individual members from potential harm, the practice of community engagement is reinterpreted to be simply a matter of establishing a viable political collaboration with the local community in which the recruitment of individuals for DNA sampling is to take place.

Narrowing the focus from broad study populations to localized communities does make the prospect of community engagement more plausible. Localized communities will be able to produce representatives authorized to speak for their membership more easily than unorganized populations. Local communities are more likely to face common 'intra-community risks' and needs that might be usefully communicated in designing the research at that site. And to build trust and negotiate access to community members, it will be much more effective to work at the local level.

Nevertheless, it remains important to appreciate the limits of this approach. The study populations of the kinds that are of most interest to genetic variation researchers, the international human population groups whose genetic variations disclose the patterns of disease susceptibilities within the species, will be those least well served by the practice of community engagement. If the concern was to give those larger population groups some involvement in research that may affect them, even negotiating a full-blown 'community partnership' with one localized subset of the population is as likely to be an example of the problem rather than a step toward justice: to the extent that the researcher does not confine his or her scientific claims to the local community at hand, that community's decisions about participation have preempted the interests of the rest of the population.

Moreover, for these same reasons, investigators cannot honestly let local communities speak for the population, and cannot promise that local research designs will protect the communities from population-related harms incurred by studies at other locales. Thus, in this most attenuated model of community engagement, even the local communities to whom the principle of 'respect for community' might apply cannot be afforded the level of involvement in the research decision-making that the principle's proponents advocate.

Finally, there is the interesting twist that the idea of community genetic identity gives the discussion of the commercialization of genetic information. While the first wave of contemporary literature on this topic portrayed genetic information as 'the common heritage of humankind' (Ossario 1999) and thus unsuited to ownership and exploitation by subsets of the species, the organization of genetic research in terms of community membership is shifting the tone of the ownership debate dramatically. While the ownership framework continues to be debated in international policy circles (Thorsteindottir *et al.* 2003), as human communities have come to be (mistakenly) identified with unique human superfamilies they seem to have begun to accept the idea that their genes are akin to the natural resources under their local control (Merz *et al.* 2004). Complaints of 'bio-piracy', and pleas for 'benefit sharing' and 'reciprocity' on behalf of communities under genetic study, as well as charges of unfairness and neglect by those left out of genetic diversity research, all suggest a rising sense that, in fact, subsets of the species do have claims on the genetic information that distinguishes them, and should be compensated appropriately for its use by others (Christie 1996).

The idea that populations are materially invested in their genetic information in economic ways is actually one with a long history in the science of human genetics. It is, however, a conceptually mistaken idea, and one with dangerous political implications. Despite the pleas for justice on the parts of exploited research participants, it is important to look down the road of this line of thinking at the pitfalls it faces. Since we have been down this road before, a digression into that history is instructive.

The scientific term in English for the collection of human alleles and genetic variants is the 'gene pool'. The concept of the 'gene pool' comes to us from population genetics and evolutionary theory. It was introduced surprisingly late, in 1950, by Theodosius Dobzhansky, who used it to help establish a Mendelian definition of 'species' as 'a reproductive community of sexual and cross-fertilizing individuals which share in a common gene pool' (Adams 1979). Dobzhansky seems to have coined the term by translating loosely from the Russian *genofond*, or gene fund, a term used in the 1920s by his mentor in Soviet population genetics, Serebrovsky. In fact, the gene pool is sometimes still referred to as 'the aggregate genetic resources available to the population, its genetic reserves, on which it may draw in undergoing genetic change' (Adams 1979). This fits with the popular idea that humans have, thanks to investments made on our behalf through the 'wisdom of evolution', accumulated a 'genetic endowment' on which we might draw to meet new challenges, and over which we now have stewardship, to manage as a common inheritance.

Adams points out that, as central as it has become as a concept of population genetics, the 'gene pool' has its origins in an effort to help reconcile the science of genetics with the Marxist ideology of the Soviet Union in the 1920s. Against those who argued that Mendelian genetics suffered an inherent social Darwinist bias in favor of the capitalist elite, Serebrovsky argued that:

If we consider our population, the citizens of our Union, we can regard them from one point of view as a group of subjects with full rights who exercise their right to create their own happiness on earth, and from another point of view, we can look at their totality as our social treasure, just exactly as we look upon the total amount of wheat, milk cows, and horses which create the economic power of our country. Our country prospers not only because wheat grows and cows give milk, but also because it has people who produce work of a certain level of quality. This question is especially important when we move to the 'higher' levels of human creativity, to artistic, scholarly, and scientific activity, to administrative work and a whole series of other manifestations of human nature. And if these elements actually rest on a basis of heredity, then we have every right to look upon the totality of such genes which create in human society talented outstanding individuals, or to the contrary idiots, as national wealth, a gene fund, from which society draws its people. It is clear that, not only can we not close our eyes to our gene fund, but to the contrary, we must see if there are processes operating within the gene fund which are changing it, and if there are, to what extent it is for the better or worse.... In order for the reserves of various genes in a given locality to be properly managed, we must look upon this stock as a kind of natural resource, similar to reserves of oil, gold, or coal, for example. (Adams 1979: 257)

This language is still echoed today in the rhetoric of the new national genomic biobanks in Iceland, Estonia, and the United Kingdom, and in the claims of patient groups and health voluntary organizations to 'benefit sharing' in genetic research. But Serebrovosky then went on to advocate a series of eugenic proposals to preserve and improve the glorious Soviet gene pool. The centerpiece to his scheme of 'Soviet Eugenics' was a plan to regulate human reproduction for the benefit of future generations. He argued that:

Children are necessary to support and develop society, children must be healthy, able and active, and society has the right to ask questions about the quality of the output in this area of production. We propose that the solution to the question of the organization of selection in humans will be the widespread induction of conception by means of artificial insemination using recommended sperm, and not at all necessarily from a 'beloved spouse'. (Adams 1979: 265)

Unfortunately, in the context of Germany's reviving power and militant eugenic policies, these proposals did not help Serebrovosky's career in Stalinist Russia, and Adams reports that the term 'geno-fund' disappeared for almost two decades before being revived, shorn of its explicitly eugenic associations, as 'the gene pool'.

Meanwhile, of course, much the same kind of language was used by eugenicists all over the world to help advance political policies of social exclusion. Although these eugenic efforts did not have the benefit of Serebrovksy's 'the gene fund' (they used 'the germ-plasm' instead), they were often much more successful. In the United States immigration restrictions against people from the Mediterranean, prohibitions on interracial marriage, and the involuntary sterilization of 60,000 'feeble-minded' people were all justified in terms of protecting the integrity of the genetic stock on behalf of future generations (Reilly 1991). In some circles today one can still find people decrying the long-term 'dysgenic' effects of modern medicine in just the same way, and advocating the use of population genetic screening tools to reduce a community's genetic liabilities (Cziezel 1988). One arena that is especially susceptible to such proposals is public health, where efforts to reduce disease incidence and save health costs are already accepted as natural and legitimate goals. As population genetic research becomes increasingly designed and conducted in terms of the communal interests of specific human groups, the temptation to use what we learn to improve the stock of those groups by preventing the propagation of their deficits will also have to be addressed.

Public Health Genetics and Population Screening

The emergence of group-based genetic variation research in the wake of the Human Genome Project has already provoked a resurgence of interest in using clinical genetic testing tools at the population level to promote public health goals

(Coughlin 1999). This resurgence raises a number of bioethical issues for public health policy-makers and the health professionals involved in delivering genetic services: questions about the limits of public health authority in this domain, the justice of population-based genetic interventions, the social costs of such screening, and the ethical allegiances of the clinicians involved. All of these issues are animated by the same conceptual issue that lay behind the eugenicists' efforts to purify the human gene pool: the problem of defining 'prevention' for the purposes of a 'public health genetics'.

Mass genetic screening programs have a relatively long history amongst modern genetic services, starting with the screening of newborns for prophylactic therapy against metabolic disorders in the 1960s and continuing into adult carrier testing programs for recessive genetic diseases such as Tay-Sachs (Blitzer and McDowell 1992), sickle cell disease (Bowman 1977), and the thalassemias (Angastiniotis et al. 1986) in specific at-risk populations in the 1970s. The early adult screening programs shared two features that warranted, and garnered, significant attention within bioethics and health policy (National Academy of Sciences 1975; President's Commission 1983). First, they targeted specific socially defined populations, which raised issues of group-specific stigmatization and discrimination (Kenan and Schmidt 1987; Markel 1992). Second, the information about carrier status the screens provided was primarily useful for reproductive rather than therapeutic decision-making, raising issues of parental autonomy, paternalism, and procreative choice (Thomson et al. 1993).

The 1980s witnessed a second wave of adult genetic screening programs, aimed at detecting pregnant women at risk of delivering children with genetic birth defects and chromosomal abnormalities (Cunningham and Kizer 1990; Haddow et al. 1992; Palomaki 1994). These programs are intended to have universal application within populations, and have been routinized into the obstetrical care of pregnant women in many countries, raising issues of voluntariness and informed consent (Press and Browner 1995; Marteau 1995). They have also provoked an outspoken reaction from the community of people with disabilities, who argue that such programs work against attempts to reform social attitudes about disability (Parens and Asch 2000).

Today these three 'traditional' forms of population genetic screening—newborn screening, risk-group carrier testing, and pregnancy screening—continue to make up the vast bulk of population genetic screening activities that are funded and evaluated as state public health initiatives. At the same time, the disease targets of these screening efforts have changed, as public health programs see rationales for shifting specific tests from one form of testing to another. Thus, many states have added sickle cell testing to their universal newborn screening panels (Olney 1999), and calls have been made for universal screening of pregnant women for maternal phenylketonuria (Kaye et al. 2001) and fetal hemoglobinopathies (Cuckle 2001). Moreover, genetic tests originally reserved for clinical use in families at risk of diseases such as cystic fibrosis or fragile-X syndrome have also begun to be used as population screens, both as part of newborn screening panels and as prenatal testing programs (Caskey 1993). In all such shifts, the tests have moved in the direction of earlier and more universal screening.

The new wave of interest in 'public health genetics' generated by advances in genomic science focuses on tests that would have universal application within multi-ethnic populations, like pregnancy testing, but, like newborn screening, would measure the tested individuals' personal risk for disease, with an eye toward prophylactic action. Moreover, in addition to screening for signs of rare 'genetic diseases', like all the traditional forms of screening, the emphasis is now on the detection of molecular markers that confer statistically increased risks for more complex, and more common, chronic diseases of adulthood, like coronary artery disease, cancer, or diabetes (Khoury et al. 2000).

The discussion over using these new tests as public health tools has been dominated by questions of feasibility and utility (Omenn 1996; Holtzman and Marteau 2000). As one review concludes:

Several issues must be addressed, however, before such tests can be recommended for population-based prevention programs. These issues include the adequacy of the scientific evidence, the balance of risks and benefits, the need for counseling and informed consent, and the costs and resources required. Ongoing assessment of the screening program and quality assurance of laboratory testing are also needed.   (Burke et al. 2001: 201)

These concerns mirror those expressed in the literature on using predictive genetic risk assessments as a part of medical care in clinical settings (Geller et al. 1997). The use of these same tests as population screening tools would place them in the larger context of the existing population genetic screening programs, however, and it is in that context that they become most bioethically challenging. As these tests become integrated into the shifting mix of existing 'population-based prevention programs', they expose fundamental questions about the goals of the enterprise that have not been so apparent in the past. What should population-based genetic screening strive to accomplish, and by what criteria should one measure success?

The ubiquitous answer to these questions in the literature of public health genetics is 'the prevention of disease', a classic public health goal. This goal is operationalized as the reduction over time in measures of the morbidity and mortality caused by the target disease within the screened population. To flesh out the kinds of intervention that should be counted in those measures, most authors appeal to the public health field's traditional lexically ordered scheme of primary, secondary, and tertiary 'levels of prevention', and attempt to categorize population genetic screening tests accordingly. Thus, for example, one public health guidance document states:

Primary prevention genetic services are services intended to prevent a birth defect, genetic disorder, or disease before it occurs. Genetic counseling is a form of primary prevention.

Genetic counseling provides couples with information about their pregnancy, and reproductive risks and pregnancy options. Secondary prevention genetic services are services intended to prevent the unfavorable sequelae of an existing disorder or genotype. Newborn screening is a classic example of secondary prevention. Tertiary prevention genetic services are services aimed at ameliorating the unfavorable consequences of existing disorders, through enabling services such as parent-to-parent support and empowerment.   (Kaye *et al.* 2001: 188)

Using this scheme provides a logic for shifting tests into the newborn, prenatal, and preconception stages, because traditionally 'primary prevention' has been considered the ultimate goal of public health interventions.

Unfortunately, this scheme also introduces an important equivocation into public health discourse between two different ways in which genetic screening might be thought to be 'preventive': genetic screening as a technique for *preventing the expression of a genetic disease in an individual* and genetic screening as a technique for *preventing the intergenerational transmission of disease genes*. For convenience, I have called the first kind of prevention 'phenotypic prevention' since its goal is to prevent the manifestation of a particular clinical phenotype. Similarly, I call the second sort of prevention 'genotypic prevention' (or 'geno-prevention') because its goal is to prevent the birth of people with particular genotypes (Juengst 1995). These two senses of prevention reflect quite distinct concepts of disease prevention, with different histories within health care, different philosophical assumptions, and different degrees of moral authority. Both have a role within genetic medicine, but not as equal professional goals. Equivocating between these two senses of prevention in discussions of population screening results in the attribution of genotypic preventive goals to public health genetics. That, in turn, generates the deeper questions of public authority, social justice, and professional allegiance that animate bioethical concern in this area.

Phenotypic prevention is a straightforward medical pursuit which few would criticize: it is designed to further the health interests of individual patients by allowing them to avoid foreseeable medical problems. It encompasses, for genetic medicine, all three of the lexically ordered levels of prevention (primary, secondary, and tertiary) that traditionally define the domain of preventive medicine. Thus, it is illustrated by efforts to monitor and reduce levels of mutagens in the workplace (primary pheno-prevention), newborn screening and dietary prophylaxis for phenylketonuria (secondary pheno-prevention), and somatic cell gene therapy for the respiratory symptoms of cystic fibrosis (tertiary pheno-prevention) (Holtzman 1989).

The concept of pheno-prevention rests on several assumptions: (1) It assumes that there are living individuals who remain around to benefit from having their foreseeable health problems forestalled. Thus, for example, proposals to 'prevent' occupational disease by firing all susceptible employees instead of cleaning up the workplace seem inherently wrongheaded. (2) It assumes that diseases are best defined at the level of the actual health problems that they occasion for individual people, rather than in terms of their preclinical etiology. Otherwise, preclinical interventions like dietary changes would be directly curative, not prophylactic. (3) It assumes that diseases are distinct from the people they burden, so that it becomes appropriate to use metaphors of external defense to describe the beneficiaries as 'vulnerable' to 'attack' by disease without the 'protection' of prevention.

Along with these assumptions, the concept of phenotypic prevention enjoys a high degree of moral authority as an imperative for medicine and society. In fact, the promise of pheno-preventive measures to 'protect the helpless from harm' has been compelling enough in our society to allow both primary and secondary forms of pheno-prevention to become established in effectively mandatory programs as a matter of public policy (President's Commission 1983).

Of course, if primary prevention is the prevention of the onset of a genetic disease in an at-risk patient, then most of the preconception, preimplantation, and prenatal genetic screening interventions usually classified as 'primary prevention strategies' cannot, in fact, qualify for that status. Neither preimplantation embryo screening nor selective termination can serve to prevent the onset of a heritable disease in affected patients. At most, they are capable of preventing *cases* of a disease within a family (or a population) by allowing parents (or a society) to avoid the birth of at-risk individuals.

This conceptual confusion does lead to some cognitive dissonance in the literature. The Centers for Disease Control and Prevention, for example, illustrates the concept of 'primary prevention' in genetics by listing 'medical and community-based interventions focused on carrier detection and premarital counseling as well as on prenatal diagnosis and pregnancy termination', but then adds the confusing parenthetical remark that '(This last may not be considered primary prevention)' (Khoury and the Genetics Working Group 1996: 1718). It is also telling that one can find carrier screening, intrauterine diagnosis, and selective termination classified in the literature as examples of primary prevention (Kaye *et al.* 2001), secondary prevention (Wertz *et al.* 1995), and even tertiary prevention (Porter 1982). An example of a clearer thinker is Holtzman (1989), who sets carrier screening, amniocentesis, and selective termination outside of preventive medicine's traditional trichotomy, by labeling them as a form of genetic disease 'avoidance'.

In fact, when they incorporate reproductive genetic screening programs into their menu of preventive interventions, public health geneticists have been forced to slip between two very different senses of 'prevention'. They have conflated screening to prevent the phenotypic expression of a genotype in a particular patient ('phenotypic prevention') with screening to prevent the birth of individuals with a particular genotype ('genotypic prevention').

Most genetic risk assessments for late-onset disorders are justified solely in terms of their potential for phenotypic prevention in particular patients. However, it is possible that they could also be embraced as mass screening tools for programs aimed at reducing the incidence of particular genotypes within a population. Genotypic prevention, however, is a pursuit that is much more controversial. That is understandable, for several reasons:

First, it is often hard to know what ends genotypic preventive measures are intended to serve. Genotypic preventive measures are usually described as a way of furthering the procreative interests of prospective parents, by allowing them to avoid the birth of individuals with foreseeable health problems (like artificial insemination by donor following adult carrier testing for cystic fibrosis mutations, or selective termination following intrauterine diagnosis of Down syndrome). At the same time, these same interventions are often evaluated in terms of the economic and public health interests of society, according to their ability to reduce the incidence of genetic disease in a population (Caskey 1993). Thus, the famous 'success stories' of genetic screening (like the Mediterranean carrier screening programs for beta-thalassemia, or Tay-Sachs screening in the Ashkenazi American population) most often counted as successful in terms of these societal criteria (cf. Cao et al. 1991; Blitzer and McDowell 1992). In those stories, in fact, the commitment to channeling screening efforts through the individual's voluntary reproductive choices is itself portrayed as simply a savvy strategy for achieving the profession's underlying goal of reducing society's health care costs (Caskey 1993). Second, whether geno-prevention is pursued in the cause of family planning or the public health (or both), it must make two sets of related assumptions. First, it assumes that the diseases it prevents are best understood at the level of the genotype, rather than through the pathophysiology of their expression, just as AIDS is now understood in terms of its causal HIV infection rather than the infection's clinical sequelae. Understanding genetic disease through the lens of the germ theory in this way means that the language of 'molecular disease' and 'DNA-based diagnosis' seems apt, and it makes sense to contrast preventing the 'vertical transmission' of pathogenic 'disease genes' with 'palliative' or 'symptomatic' interventions like low phenylalanine diets.

Third, proponents of geno-preventive efforts must assume important personal (or social) value judgments about the burden of the cases of disease being prevented. Genes are not, like germs, external infectious agents that can be kept (or cleaned) out of a living person's body. Instead, genotypic prevention has to involve avoiding the birth of individuals conceived with the pathological genotype. In most cases, the beneficiaries of such an intervention cannot be the individuals whose births are avoided: if the genotypic transmission has been successfully prevented, there can be no such individuals. That means that to justify geno-prevention someone (parents or society) must make the judgment that the burden of coping with cases of a disease outweighs any other value that individuals with a given genotype might bring to a family or community, and warrants action to exclude individuals with those mutations from the lives of the wild type (Parens and Asch 2000).

Finally, genotypic prevention already has a bad track record as a social and professional goal. It has been accepted before as a societal imperative, on the coattails of the public health movement's successes with the primary prevention of infectious disease (Kevles 1985). Today the eugenics movement of the first half of the twentieth century is remembered primarily for the discriminatory immigration restrictions and coercive sterilization laws it produced (Reilly 1991), and the ease with which it was appropriated to support genocide (Muller-Hill 1988). The horrific consequences of ranking geno-preventive goals over individual interests still effectively undermine any claims to moral authority these goals might make. Against this background, the current professional confusion over the true goals of contemporary geno-prevention services, and the fact that all geno-preventive services require the judgment that some genotypes are predictably burdensome enough to others to outweigh any other potential their bearers might have, make it easy for critics of new approaches to genotypic prevention to remind the public of the excesses of the historical eugenics movement, and label any new efforts accordingly, with powerful political effect (Hubbard 1986).

Of course, it is possible for genetic medicine to eschew genotypic prevention as a professional goal and still support the choices of prospective parents who pursue it for their own reasons: the field of reproductive genetics has successfully subscribed to such a view for decades (Botkin 1990). What will become important as genetic testing diffuses into other specialties is for its practitioners to be reminded of that tradition and to be able to articulate their goals equally clearly. In contemporary political argot, genetic testing should continue to be an empowering, not an exclusionary, service. It should continue to be about helping living people address their individual health problems, and not about protecting society from the ebb and flow of human alleles in populations.

CONCLUSION

Some argue that, as our knowledge of the human genetic variation increases, the practical significance of group identities at this level will diminish. In theory, as full-genome scanning and sequencing capabilities improve, 'group-specific' medicine should fragment into personalized medicine, with risk assessments and interventions tailored to individual genomes without regard to their genealogy. But health policy-making, pharmaceutical development, and genetic variation research itself are all practices that operate within strong economies of scale that keep their focus on large groups of people—constituencies, markets, and populations—rather than on individual patients. As a result, even if personalized medicine becomes an option for some at the clinical level, issues related to group identity will continue to haunt genomic health care in the future.

The most obvious of these issues is the tension between an individual's personal interests and the interests of the larger community. Like all community-based public health campaigns, proposals to use genetic information to improve the health and welfare of communities, whether the old eugenic sterilization campaigns or the routinized population screening programs of today's 'public health genetics', can involve asking affected individuals to make special sacrifices or assume special responsibilities on behalf of the community's welfare. Moreover, unlike public health interventions that restrict individual liberties in order to prevent health problems which all community members risk more or less equally, genetic prevention strategies always require sacrifices on the part of the community who face the genetic risks in question on behalf of those who do not. The irony of 'community genetics' is that most human communities are much too heterogenous to face universal gene pool disasters. Thus, the public welfare problems that are addressed through genetic screening so often boil down to fiscal burdens that those at genetic risk place on the community, and the relative obligations of the genetic 'haves' and the 'have-nots' to shoulder those burdens (cf. Miringoff 1991).

Genome scientists have a wry fondness for Walter Gilbert's depiction of their field as the quest for the Holy Grail. The covers of the proceedings of the annual meetings of this research community at Cold Spring Harbor Laboratories during the Human Genome Project were cartoons depicting leading scientists as characters from Monty Python's *Holy Grail* movie, and the original artwork of these covers decorates a conference room at the National Human Genome Research Institute at NIH. One of the most apt allegorical moments from the original medieval Grail romances, however, has yet to be fully appreciated. In the version of the story attributed to William von Eschenbach, the quest's challenge does not end with Parzival's achievement in finding the Grail. Before he can return with the Grail to the Grail Kingdom, Parzival must come to terms with a 'piebald' knight, Sir Fierfiz, who is its guardian. This knight's skin is alternately black and white in a 'parti-colored' pattern like medieval clothing: the very image of human genetic diversity. Moreover, Sir Fierfiz turns out to be Parzival's half-brother, born of a Moorish queen whom his father married (briefly) while on crusade: a living symbol of the social potency of our group identities and the way our genetic connections can complicate them. Sir Fierfiz is an obstacle to the ultimate completion of the Grail quest, just as the challenges and pitfalls of population genomics are for genetic medicine. In von Eschenbach's tale, Parzival is able to succeed in winning Sir Fierfiz's allegiance and, once they achieve the Grail Kingdom, even (as a token of 'reciprocity'?) gives him the hand of one of the Grail Maidens in marriage (Barber 2004). How he did that is a legend that may now repay rereading, in seeking to negotiate our way to the genomic era in biomedicine.

REFERENCES

ADAMS, M. (1979), 'From "Gene Fund" to "Gene Pool": On the Evolution of Evolutionary Language', *Studies in History of Biology*, 3: 241–85.

ALTSHULER, D., and CLARK, A. (2005), 'Harvesting Medical Information from the Human Family Tree', *Science*, 307: 1052–3.

ANGASTINIOTIS, M., KYRIADOU, S., and HADJIMINAS, M. (1986), 'How Thalassemia Was Controlled in Cyprus', *World Health Forum*, 7: 291–7.

BARBER, R. (2004), *The Holy Grail: Imagination and Belief* (Cambridge, Mass.: Harvard University Press).

BLITZER, M. G., and MCDOWELL, G. A. (1992), 'Tay-Sachs Disease as a Model for Screening In-Born Errors', *Clinical Laboratory Medicine*, 12: 463–80.

BOTKIN, J. (1990), 'Prenatal Screening: Professional Standards and the Limits of Parental Choice', *Obstetrics and Gynecology*, 75: 875–80.

BOWMAN, J. (1977), 'Genetic Screening Programs and Public Policy', *Phylon*, 38: 117–42.

BURCHARD, E., *et al.* (2003), 'The Importance of Race and Ethnic Background in Biomedical Research and Clinical Practice', *New England Journal of Medicine*, 348: 1170–5.

BURKE, W., COUGHLIN, S., LEE, N., *et al.* (2001), 'Application of Population Screening Principles to Genetic Screening for Adult-Onset Conditions', *Genetic Testing*, 5: 201–11.

CAO, A., ROSATELLI, M. C., and GALANELLO, R. (1991), 'Population-Based Genetic Screening', *Current Opinion in Genetic Development*, 1: 48–53.

CASKEY, T. (1993), 'Presymptomatic Diagnosis: A First Step Toward Genetic Health Care', *Science*, 262: 48–9.

CAVALLI-SFORZA, L., WILSON, A., CANTOR, C., COOK-DEEGAN, B., and KING, M. C. (1991), 'Call for a Worldwide Survey of Human Genetic Diversity: A Vanishing Opportunity for the Human Genome Project', *Genomics*, 11: 490–1.

CHRISTIE, J. (1996), 'Whose Property, Whose Rights?', *Cultural Survival Quarterly*, 20: 34–42.

COLLINS, F., GUYER, M., and CHAKRAVARTI, A. (1997), 'Variations on a Theme: Cataloguing Human DNA Sequence Variation', *Science*, 278: 1580–1.

—— MORGAN, M., and PATRINOS, A. (2003), 'The Human Genome Project: Lessons from Large Scale Biology', *Science*, 300: 286–90.

COOPER, R., KAUFMAN, J., and WARD, R. (2003), 'Race and Genomics', *New England Journal of Medicine*, 348: 1166–70.

COUGHLIN, S. (1999), 'The Intersection of Genetics, Public Health and Preventive Medicine', *American Journal of Preventive Medicine*, 16: 89–91.

CUCKLE, H. (2001), 'Extending Antenatal Screening in the UK to Include Common Mongenic Disorders', *Community Genetics*, 4: 84–6.

CUNNINGHAM, G., and KIZER, K. W. (1990), 'Maternal Serum Alpha-Feto Protein Activities of State Health Agencies: A Survey', *American Journal of Human Genetics*, 47: 899–903.

CZEIZEL, A. (1988), *The Right To Be Born Healthy* (New York: Alan R. Liss).

DUSTER, T. (2005), 'Race and Reification in Science', *Science*, 307: 1050–1.

FOSTER, M., *et al.* (1999), 'The Role of Community Review in Evaluating the Risks of Human Genetic Variation Research', *American Journal of Human Genetics*, 64: 1719–27.

GANNETT, L. (2001), 'Racism and Human Genome Diversity Research: The Ethical Limits of "Population Thinking"', *Philosophy of Science*, 68: S479–92.

GELLER, G., BOTKIN, J., GREEN, M., *et al.* (1997), 'Genetic Testing for Susceptibility to Adult-Onset Cancer', *JAMA* 277: 1467–74.

GILBERT, W. (1992), 'A Vision of the Grail', in D. Kevles and L. Hood (eds.), *The Code of Codes: Scientific and Social Issues in the Human Genome Project* (Cambridge, Mass.: Harvard University Press), 83–98.

GUTTMACHER, A., and COLLINS, F. (2004), 'Welcome to the Genomic Era', in A. Guttmacher, F. Collins, and J. Drazen (eds.), *Genomic Medicine* (Baltimore: Johns Hopkins University Press), 166–71.

HADDOW, J. E., PALOMAKI, G., and KNIGHT, G. J. (1992), 'Prenatal Screening for Down Syndrome with Use of Maternal Serum Markers', *New England Journal of Medicine*, 321: 588–93.

HOLTZMAN, N. A. (1989), *Proceed with Caution: Predicting Genetic Risks in the Recombinant DNA Era* (Baltimore: Johns Hopkins University Press).

—— and MARTEAU, T. (2000), 'Will Genetics Revolutionize Medicine?', *New England Journal of Medicine*, 343: 141–4.

HUBBARD, R. (1986), 'Eugenics and Prenatal Testing', *International Journal of the Health Services*, 16: 227–42.

INTERNATIONAL HAPMAP CONSORTIUM (2003), 'The International Hapmap Project', *Nature*, 426: 789–95.

JUENGST, E. (1995), 'Prevention and the Goals of Genetic Medicine', *Human Gene Therapy*, 6: 1595–1605.

—— (1998), 'Groups as Gatekeepers to Genomic Research: Conceptually Confusing, Morally Hazardous and Practically Useless', *Kennedy Institute of Ethics Journal*, 8: 183–200.

KAHN, J. (2004), 'How a Drug Becomes 'Ethnic': Law, Commerce and the Production of Racial Categories in Medicine', *Yale Journal of Health Policy, Law and Ethics*, 4: 101–27.

KAYE, C., LAXOVA, R., LIVINGSTON, J., *et al.* (2001), 'Integrating Genetic Services into Public Health: Guidance for State and Territorial Programs', *Community Genetics*, 4/3: 175–96.

KENAN, R., and SCHMIDT, R. (1987), 'Social Implications of Screening Programs for Carrier Status: Genetic Diseases in the 1970s and AIDS in the 1980s', in H. Schwartz (ed.), *Dominant Issues in Medical Sociology*, 2nd edn. (New York: Random House), 145–54.

KEVLES, D. (1985), *In the Name of Eugenics: Genetics and the Uses of Human Heredity* (New York: Knopf).

KHOURY, M., and the GENETICS WORKING GROUP (1996), 'From Genes to Public Health: The Applications of Genetic Technology in Disease Prevention', *American Journal of Public Health*, 86: 1717–21.

—— BURKE, W., and THOMPSON, E. (eds.) (2000), *Genetics and Public Health in the Twenty-First Century* (New York: Oxford University Press).

MARKEL, H. (1992), 'The Stigma of Disease: Implications for Carrier Screening', *American Journal of Medicine*, 93: 209–15.

MARSHALL, P., and ROTIMI, C. (2001), 'Ethical Challenges in Community Based Research', *American Journal of the Medical Sciences*, 322/5: 259–63.

MARTEAU, T. (1995), 'Towards Informed Decisions About Prenatal Testing: A Review', *Prenatal Diagnosis*, 15: 1215–26.

MERZ, J., McGEE, G., and SANKAR, P. (2004), 'Iceland, Inc.? On the Ethics of Commercial Population Genomics', *Social Science and Medicine*, 58: 1201–9.

MIRINGOFF, M. L. (1991), *The Social Costs of Genetic Welfare* (New Brunswick, NJ: Rutgers University Press).

MULLER-HILL, B. (1988), *Murderous Science: Elimination by Scientific Selection of Jews, Gypsies, and Others, Germany 1933–1945* (New York: Oxford University Press).

NATIONAL ACADEMY OF SCIENCES (1975), *Genetic Screening: Programs, Principles and Research* (Washington, DC: National Academy Press).

NATIONAL RESEARCH COUNCIL (1998), *Assessing Human Genetic Diversity* (Washington, DC: National Academy Press).

NIH (NATIONAL INSTITUTES OF HEALTH) (2002), 'Points to Consider when Planning a Genetic Study that Involves Members of Named Populations', *Bioethics Resources on the Web*, <http://www.nih.gov/sigs/bioethics/named_populations.html>.

OLNEY, R. (1999), 'Preventing Morbidity and Mortality from Sickle Cell Disease: A Public Health Perspective', *American Journal Preventive Medicine*, 16/2: 116–22.

OMENN, G. (1996), 'Genetics and Public Health', *American Journal of Public Health*, 86: 1701–3.

OSSARIO, P. (1999), 'Common Heritage Arguments and the Patenting of Human DNA', in A. Chapman (ed.), *Perspectives on Genetic Patenting: Religion, Science and Industry in Dialogue* (Washington, DC: American Association for the Advancement of Science), 89–111.

PALOMAKI, G. E. (1994), 'Population Based Prenatal Screening for the Fragile X Syndrome', *Journal of Medical Screening*, 1: 65–72.

PARENS, E., and ASCH, A. (eds.) (2000), *Prenatal Testing and Disability Rights* (Washington, DC: Georgetown University Press).

PORTER, I. (1999), 'The Control of Hereditary Disorders', *Annual Review of Public Health*, 3: 277–319.

PRESIDENT'S COMMISSION (PRESIDENT'S COMMISSION FOR THE STUDY OF ETHICAL PROBLEMS IN MEDICINE AND BIOMEDICAL AND BEHAVIORAL RESEARCH) (1983), *Screening and Counseling for Genetic Conditions* (Washington, DC.: US Government Printing Office).

PRESS, N., and BROWNER, C. (1995), 'Risk, Autonomy and Responsibility: Informed Consent for Prenatal Testing', *Hastings Center Report*, 25/3: S9–12.

REARDON, J. (2005), *Race to the Finish: Identity and Governance in an Age of Genomics* (Princeton: Princeton University Press).

REILLY, P. (1999), *The Surgical Solution: A History of Involuntary Sterilization in the U.S.* (Baltimore: Johns Hopkins University Press).

RISCH, N., and MERIKINGAS, K. (1999), 'The Future of Genetic Studies of Complex Human Diseases', *Science*, 273: 1516–17.

SHARP, R., and FOSTER, M. (1999), 'Involving Study Populations in the Review of Genetic Research', *Journal of Law, Medicine, and Ethics*, 28/1: 41–52.

THOMSON, ELIZABETH, *et al.* (1993), 'National Institutes of Health Workshop Statement on Reproductive Genetic Testing: Impact on Women', *American Journal of Human Genetics*, 51: 1161–3.

THORSTEINDOTTIR, H., DAAR, A., SMITH, R., and SINGER, P. (1999), 'Do Patents Encourage or Inhibit Genomics as a Global Public Good?', in B. Knoppers (ed.), *Populations and Genetics: Legal and Socio-Ethical Perspectives* (Boston: Martinus Nijhoff), 487–504.

WEIJER, C. (1999), 'Protecting Communities in Research: Philosophical and Pragmatic Challenges', *Cambridge Quarterly of Health Care Ethics*, 8: 501–13.

WERTZ, D., and FLETCHER, J. (1999), *Ethics and Human Genetics: A Cross-Cultural Perspective* (Berlin: Springer-Verlag).

—— and BERG, K. (1995), 'Summary Statement on Ethical Issues in Medical Genetics: Report of WHO Temporary Advisers', World Health Organization document WHO/HDP/CONS/95, Geneva.

ZILINKAS, R., and BALINT, P. (eds.) (2001), *The Human Genome Project and Minority Communities: Ethical, Social and Political Dilemmas* (New York: Praeger).

CHAPTER 21

....

ENHANCEMENT

....

THOMAS H. MURRAY

INTRODUCTION

....

WHAT could possibly be wrong with enhancement? The dictionary on my desk defines enhance to mean 'advance, augment, elevate, heighten, increase' as well as 'to increase the worth or value of'. One clue to the ethics of enhancement is to ask precisely what is being advanced, augmented, etc. The guards at the Abu Ghraib prison in Iraq may have found that putting hoods on and sexually humiliating prisoners enhanced their ability to keep the prisoners docile and fearful. But no morally sensible person could judge this an ethically praiseworthy use of enhancement. This example alerts us to ask who is affected by the putative enhancement, as well as what values and ends the enhancement serves.

The idea of enhancement covers a lot of ground. Parents have sought biosynthetic human growth hormone (hGH) for their children who were projected to be of average or above-average height even without it (Benjamin *et al.* 1984). Musicians have used beta blockers to keep performance anxiety in check (Slomka 1992). People take Prozac and other selective serotonin reuptake inhibitors (SSRIs) to make themselves more sociable (Kramer 1993). Cyclists, cross-country skiers, and marathon runners take biosynthetic erythropoietin to improve their endurance. Hammer throwers and weightlifters have taken anabolic steroids to increase strength (Sokolove 2004). And writers, the author of this entry among them, rely at times on caffeine, a well-known stimulant for the central nervous system, to boost their fading alertness.

Consider biosynthetic testosterone. Testosterone is the masculinizing or andro-genic hormone. It can be found in the bodies of women as well, but at much lower levels than in men. A relative abundance of testosterone results in voices with lower pitch, hair on the chest and face (and, in time, less of it on the head), and increased muscle mass among other effects. The so-called anabolic steroids are chemical knock-offs of testosterone. By the 1960s athletes had discovered that by incorporating anabolic steroids into their training routines they could throw objects farther and lift heavier weights. The Olympics banned the use of anabolic steroids along with many other drugs athletes were using to enhance their performance. By the 1990s drug testing of steroids had advanced to the stage where biosynthetic testosterone was the anabolic steroid of choice, because finding testosterone in the human body told the testers nothing about how it got there. In time, testers began looking at the ratio of testosterone to another endogenous hormone, epitestoster-one, which normally exist in roughly a one-to-one ratio in the body. If the so-called T/epi–T ratio was grossly abnormal, that was regarded as evidence that athlete had taken testosterone.

A young man who was a world-class sailor and hoped to qualify for the Olympic Games asked his national organizing committee for permission to take testosterone. Although only in his early twenties, both of his testicles had been removed because of testicular cancer. His body could no longer make a normal male amount of testosterone. Without an external supply, his physique would become increasingly feminine. He sought permission to take testosterone much like people with diabetes take insulin to make up for their pancreas's inability to produce it. Some members of the committee that heard his plea were deeply skeptical, suspecting that he might intentionally overshoot his testosterone dose in order to gain an advantage over his competitors. One committee member suggested that it was absurd to think that any other athlete would intentionally find an excuse to have his testicles removed merely so that he could inject testosterone to gain a competitive edge (Noble 1996). Other committee members, including some with decades of experience working with athletes, were not so sure.

Understanding the ethics of enhancement begins with getting clear about the concept, as well as the factors likely to move people to pursue biomedical enhance-ment. We will consider in the next section the usefulness of the distinction between therapy and enhancement for understanding the ethics of enhancement. Once the conceptual underbrush has been cleared away, we can move on to ethics. The following section will examine critically a number of arguments that have been offered to defend biomedical enhancement, or, at least, to claim that efforts to deter it are either ethically or practically mistaken. Finally, we will consider a set of arguments that take the ethics of enhancement to be a serious matter and that give reasons to question whether some biomedical enhancements, for some purposes, may be ethically suspect.

ENHANCEMENT: CONCEPT AND CONTEXT

A good way to begin the search for clarity is to ask what sort of work the concept does, and how well it performs the tasks for which it is recruited. Eric Juengst, in an excellent discussion of the meaning of enhancement in bioethics, borrows from Erik Parens the notion of two overlapping but distinct conversations: one on the limits of biomedicine, the other on the ethics of self-improvement (Juengst 1998; Parens 1998). He then describes how the concept of enhancement is used in those two conversations: as moral boundary and as signpost, warning us that we've entered a poorly mapped and possibly dangerous moral territory.

Enhancement as Moral Boundary

Enhancement is often used to mark off *moral boundaries* within the realm of biomedicine: enhancement is contrasted with 'medically indicated' treatment. Health professionals may find enhancement to be a useful boundary marker that sets off things health professionals are not ethically obligated to do—enhancements—from what their professional moral obligations to patients require—therapeutic interventions. For example, an internist may have an obligation to offer to prescribe a beta blocker to a patient with heart disease, but not to an athlete, say an archer, who wants the drug in order to increase the interval between heartbeats and thus have a longer time to aim and release the arrow. (Olympic athletes in archery and shooting sports have used beta blockers for just this purpose.)

Enhancement as moral boundary may work in a similar fashion for health care institutions. Juengst notes that enhancement provides a 'conceptual cap for the enterprise in an era when its technological capacities seem to have fewer and fewer upper limits' (Juengst 1998: 30). A hospital may be required to provide a broad variety of treatment services; it is not similarly obliged to set up an 'enhancement' clinic, although it may do so if it wants the profits that can come with enhancement services such as cosmetic surgery or botox injections. The public and private entities that pay for health care may use enhancement as a boundary. Government agencies paying for drugs or for the services of health professionals have obligations to use their funds wisely and not for frivolous purposes. Private insurers seek to maximize profit, which also puts them on guard against paying for things that do not serve the goal of health, however it is defined. Finally, enhancement helps set boundaries on biomedical research. What risks to human subjects of research are permissible if there are no health benefits in the offing?

Juengst suggests a test for distinguishing enhancement from the proper range of medicine's concerns:

if criteria drawn from other spheres of experience seem like better measures of improvement than medical measures, then the intervention in question should probably count as an enhancement that goes beyond medicine's domain of expertise... biomedicine should restrict its ambitions to the sphere of bodily dynamics, which it knows something about, and leave the sphere of social dynamics in the hands of the other human values specialists: Parents, educators, preachers, counselors, accountants, and coaches. (Juengst 1998: 43)

Enhancement, that is, leads us outside the terrain of medicine into the larger world of goals, values, and social institutions.

Enhancement as Moral Signpost

When we look at people contemplating whether to attempt to enhance themselves or their children, the concept of enhancement, Juengst suggests, acts like a moral signpost warning that we are approaching unsettled moral territory (Juengst 1998). Recognizing enhancement as a signpost does not settle moral questions, but it alerts us that important values may be at stake. Good parents seek appropriate medical care for their children to treat or prevent illness. Parents regularly seek non-biomedical means of enhancement for their children such as language or music lessons. But what if the means are biomedical but the end unrelated to health? It is clear that certain 'enhancements'—education, training in the moral virtues, immunization against infectious diseases—are not only good but may be important moral obligations of rearing adults to the children for whom they are responsible (Brock 1998). Calling something an enhancement tells us little about what our moral attitude towards the intervention should be. Furthermore, the intrinsic properties of the intervention—that it is, for example, an injection (as in immunizations, hGH, or biosynthetic erythropoietin, EPO)—don't tell us whether it is ethically wrong, permissible, or required. Our task is more difficult, if also more interesting: to ground our moral judgments in an understanding of the goods sought and the values prized in the sphere of human practices at issue.

Enhancement Versus Therapy

There are at least three difficulties with assuming that for biomedical interventions the key distinction is between enhancement and therapy.

First, in an important sense all therapy can be understood as enhancement. Many wise physicians understand their ministrations as building upon the intrinsic healing processes of the body and mind. Their aim is to aid the body in its effort to restore homeostasis. Antibiotics can be understood as a means to enhance the body's capacity to fight off infection; the anti-statin drugs enhance the body's ability to correct the mismatch between our evolutionary adaptation to a subsistence diet and the abundance of saturated fats in the foods now plentifully available to us.

Second, there are a set of biomedical interventions that aim unequivocally at health, yet are just as clearly a form of enhancement: vaccines. Classical vaccines work by enhancing the immune system's capacity to mount a response against an infectious agent. The usual method of developing a vaccine is to present to the immune system something it will recognize as foreign; in the future, the body will rapidly produce antibodies when it sees this thing again. The capacity to produce such antibodies is latent in the immune system to begin with. The vaccine, which may be a piece of the outer coat of bacteria or virus or perhaps a close relative of the organism, which is not virulent in humans, enhances the body's resistance to infection. Effective vaccine prevents disease in the individual and, if a sufficient proportion of the population at risk is also vaccinated, can prevent epidemics. Vaccines, then, are a form of enhancement clearly directed at the usual aims of therapy: preserving health and preventing disease.

A third difficulty with the enhancement versus therapy distinction is that some biomedical interventions, operating through the same physiological pathways, occupy a continuum between what appears to be a clearly 'therapeutic' application and an outright and unabashed pursuit of enhancement. Human growth hormone, given to children whose long bones are growing, can increase final adult height. For children with little or no biologically active hGH, injections of biosynthetic growth hormone look like a biomedical remedy for a physiological abnormality similar to insulin injections for people with diabetes (Parens 1998). Over time, the 'indications' for giving hGH to children otherwise likely to be short adults have been loosened. And some parents have sought hGH for their children predicted to reach average or above average stature. For drugs like hGH, the line between therapy and enhancement can be difficult to draw.

A further conceptual challenge to thinking clearly about biomedical enhancement is that the same goal may be reached by a variety of means—and not all of those means are biomedical. Consider psychological goals such as peace of mind, buoyant self-confidence, or relief from clinical depression. Many people take a class of drugs known as selective serotonin reuptake inhibitors—SSRIs. A paucity of serotonin in the brain is related to a variety of unpleasant psychological states. A drug that relieves the suffering of people with clinical depression is a valuable therapy. But for at least some of these desired states, there may be other paths to the same end. Someone who lacks self-confidence might enhance their psyche by doing things that build self-confidence. Someone uneasy in mind might find that meditation, prayer, or some other spiritual discipline leads to the inner peace they seek. As we think about biomedical interventions as enhancements, we must bear in mind that similar ends may be reached by quite dissimilar means.

ENDS, MEANS, AND INTERMEDIARY STATES

What makes some alteration of human form or function an enhancement? A clue lies in the definition, which says in part: 'to increase the worth or value of'. Some human end or value must be served for an alteration to be an enhancement. Not all desired, goal-directed changes are best understood as enhancements. Some count as therapies, which are presumptively good because the goal of therapy, restoring health, is itself presumptively good. The goodness of any particular enhancement, on the other hand, depends first of all on the goodness of the goal to which it is directed.

For example, people with chronic anemia seek to increase the number of red blood cells circulating in their bodies because more red cells mean more energy and generally better health. For a world-class athlete in the Tour de France, more red cells enhance performance by increasing the flow of oxygen to muscles working at the limits of human endurance. Athletes have many means at their disposal: relentless preparation; a strategy known as 'Train low, rest high' (train at low altitudes where because oxygen is plentiful one can train hard and long before reaching exhaustion; rest at high altitude so that the body at rest will make more red cells to compensate for the lower concentration of oxygen); sleeping in tents or rooms that simulate high altitude; and EPO, a hormone that increases the production of red cells. People suffering from chronic anemia are more likely simply to use EPO. All of the means go through a similar intermediate state—more red cells. But their ends are distinct: relieving anemia to restore health is therapy; taking EPO to pedal a bicycle at astonishing speeds on the flats and up steep, switchback roads in the Alps and Pyrenees is an ethically contentious enhancement.

Human growth hormone shows the need to think clearly about ends. Here the means are limited—hGH alone or in combination with other hormones that promote growth of the long bones; or limb-lengthening surgeries. If hGH is chosen, there is, as far as is known, one common intermediary state—an increased amount of hGH in the body signaling the tissues in the epiphyses—the zones at the ends of the bone where elongation takes place—to grow. But increased height is not in itself the end; rather, it serves other ends important to persons.

If heightism ceased to exist and height conferred no advantages, what justification could parents give for subjecting their child of normal stature to a thousand injections, the unremitting attention to one dimension of their existence, and the risks that follow years of hGH administration? This looks like a case of child abuse. However, in a world where being tall is advantageous, parents who seek hGH for their children of average stature can recite the benefits that being taller purchases.

What of parents whose children would be very short as adults? If height didn't matter at all, had no influence on a person's education, career, social life, or ability to navigate the world successfully, there would be no reason to use growth hormone and, perhaps, no demand for it. But parents of very short children have reasons to believe that their children's lives may be easier if they were taller. Adults with short stature are looked down upon, metaphorically as well as literally. (Even a cursory reflection on the English language reveals that it is shot through with heightism.) Taller people are more likely to hold prestigious, desirable, high-paying jobs. Parents may worry that their short child may be regarded as a less desirable partner for relationships. (I must note that in my experience height seems to have no correlation with the ability to establish the most important, lasting relationships in people's lives. Tall people can have miserable relationships or wonderful ones. Precisely the same is true of short people.) Parents may also be concerned that their children will have difficulty navigating an adult world constructed for people taller than their child (Murray 1987).

These are not trivial worries for parents who want to prepare their child for adult life. Whether on the whole giving hGH to children of short stature benefits them is not a simple question to answer. On average, such children gain approximately 4 inches in height. But height per se is not the ultimate goal. The goal is to enhance that child's chance for a good and fulfilling life—a life not marred by discrimination or undue difficulty navigating the world; a child whose confidence is not crushed under the oppressive conviction that she or he can never 'measure up'. But is a biomedical intervention the surest and wisest path to a fulfilling life? Here the evidence is equivocal. A child who might have been 10 inches below average adult height is now, after growth hormone injections, 6 inches below average. Meanwhile, a thousand injections and many visits to the pediatric endocrinologist have driven home the message that height is very, very important. Meanwhile, those same resources might have gone into promoting and perfecting that child's talents—those ways the child does not 'come up short'—in music, intellectual pursuits, inventions, fixing things, creating art, or any of the myriad of valued human activities. Perversely, the world being as it is, we tip the balance towards the biomedical intervention. Human growth hormone treatment may be subsidized by health insurance, while parents are likely to bear the full cost of developing their child's talents and interests.

THE DEFENSE OF BIOMEDICAL ENHANCEMENT

Five arguments for embracing or, at least not resisting, biomedical enhancement are commonly advanced. We can call them, respectively, the *incoherency* argument, the *line-drawing* objection, the argument from *liberty*, the '*resistance is futile*' claim, and the heroic, romantic, or Promethean assertion that people *should* shape themselves.

First is the *incoherency* argument, the claim that there is no rational basis for distinguishing between acceptable and unacceptable means of enhancement. One implicit premise in this argument is that no ethical distinction can survive unless it is based upon a coherent conceptual distinction. The incoherency accusation goes on to claim that no such conceptual distinction can be found in the case of biomedical enhancement.

This is a common objection to bans on performance-enhancing drugs in sport (Fost 1986). Steroids, on this view, are no different from improved running shoes. Olympic officials therefore had no more justification for stripping Ben Johnson of his gold medal because he used steroids than for the shoes he wore. This objection also pops up in other spheres, for example, in concerns about technologies to choose or shape the characteristics of our children. What is the difference, skeptics say, between preimplantation genetic diagnosis (PGD) to select genes for musical talent or political success, on the one hand, and buying superb instruments and hiring gifted instructors or sending your child to prestigious prep schools and universities, on the other?

There are problems with this argument. For one thing it implies that all means of reaching a goal—say, a faster time in the 100 meter dash than your competitors—are equivalent. But this is not true. Clearly, some means are ethically prohibited: we are not permitted to threaten or intentionally injure our competitors. Other means alter the practice so radically that it threatens what we value in the practice. (More on this point later.) Finally, some means are entirely praiseworthy. In the Olympic 100 meter dash we admire such factors as intensive training, determination, and dedication to perfecting one's talents.

A second problem with the incoherency complaint is that it forgets that means also matter, not only ends. The means chosen to reach a given end may be themselves a valued part of the activity. The discipline and mastery needed to achieve athletic excellence are morally valuable in themselves—in contrast to pharmacological short cuts. Different means can work on different intermediary states, via different paths, and on different objects. Means, then, can matter morally.

The third problem with this complaint is that it ignores the complexity and multiplicity of ends. Achievement in sport is often measured by a simple quantity: how fast I covered this distance; how far I threw this object; how many points I scored. (Some sports invite immensely more complicated calculations. Baseball, notably, inspires encyclopedias of arcane statistics meant to shed light on the performance of individual players. My brief exposure to cricket fans suggests their preoccupation with equally obscure quantitative analyses.) But life, like much of sport, is far too complex to be reduced to a single criterion, let alone a simple quantity. The slogan 'He who dies with the most toys wins' is an eloquent (one hopes ironic) testimony to the folly of simplistic, shallow, quantitative measures of the value of one's life. Even in sport, reducing the goal to a single measure risks shrinking a rich and complex practice into one bare number. The ends of sport are complex and many; they can include developing physical and psychological abilities as well as moral capacities: fitness, strength, and speed; determination, focus, and mental agility; fortitude, courage, and perseverance. Different means favor different combinations of ends.

There is abundant evidence that we make intelligible, consistent, and coherent conceptual and ethical distinctions among different means to achieve the same ends. But, the skeptic may add, show me where and how you draw the line between the acceptable and the unacceptable. This leads to the second objection, the line-drawing problem.

The *line-drawing* objection must concede that we can see differences between the ends of the spectrum (improved training versus trampolines as ways of improving performance in the high jump, for example), but it insists that drawing a line anywhere on that continuum is unavoidably arbitrary and therefore indefensible (Allen and Fost 1990).

This objection conflates two senses of arbitrariness. In the first sense, we describe something as 'arbitrary' when there is no justification that can be offered other than perhaps sheer power or will: 'You must do this, because I say so'. But there is a second meaning of the term that is not morally offensive. When there is a good reason to draw a line on some continuum, and when good reasons can be offered for drawing a line at a particular point—even if a reasonable case could also be made for drawing the line at a slightly different point—then the point chosen can be described as 'arbitrary' yet be readily defended. An example may help.

The game of basketball is played by five players on a side. This is an arbitrary rule in the sense that the rules could specify four or six per team rather than five. The game would look similar, although strategies would evolve that alter the game somewhat from the game we know. Now imagine that no line were drawn—that each team could send as many players as it wished onto the court. Why would any team stop at five if more players increased its chance to win? A likely outcome is a court with players jammed shoulder to shoulder—say forty to a side—and a contest that looks nothing like the quick, slashing, occasionally elegant game we know. Alternatively we could draw the line at two. Indeed, there is a variant of basketball known as two-on-two. It can be enjoyable to play or watch. But it unfolds as a distinct game from the five-on-five version. There is less opportunity for complex team play, a loss from the more intricate basketball played by a full complement of five.

So, there are reasons to draw a line somewhere—otherwise the game could become a matter of sheer brutal numbers rather than skill, teamwork, and grace. And there are reasons to draw the particular line at five—although one could probably also make a case for four or six. Is the rule arbitrary? Yes: But only in the second, unobjectionable sense. And so the line-drawing complaint loses its moral force. Where one can offer good reasons for drawing a line in the first place, and also good reasons for drawing it at this particular place, calling the line 'arbitrary' makes no important philosophical or ethical point.

The third claim frequently encountered is that people should be free to choose whatever ends they value and whatever means they want to reach those ends. Call this the argument from *liberty* (Murray 1983). Assertions of liberty pop up frequently in discussions of assisted reproductive technologies, or ARTs, that would permit parents to choose or shape the characteristics of their children. Liberty is also cited in response to paternalistic worries about athletes hurting themselves by taking performance-enhancing drugs such as anabolic steroids.

One problem is that liberty tends to be treated as a kind of rhetorical trump card. Liberty comes to be seen as an end in itself, rather than having a complex relationship with the ends we pursue. Liberty is vital to the development of dispositions and virtues such as integrity, dignity, agency, and efficacy; liberty is also instrumental in allowing persons to align the possibilities before them with choices based on their preferences rather than the unfettered will of others. But there are circumstances under which the defense of unaccountable liberty is difficult.

When parents attempt to shape their children's characteristics to match their own preferences and expectations, such an exercise of free choice on the parents' part may harm their child's prospects for flourishing. A common riposte to this argument is that many if not all choices made by parents similarly shape and affect their child's prospects in life. True as far as it goes; but the increasing power and specificity that may come with ARTs to choose or shape our children's characteristics may be so different in their magnitude and precision that they justify the increased ethical concern. And concern about children's well-being is justified even if the actual effectiveness of these technologies is much less than parents believe. The harm to the child's future flourishing flows as readily from narrowed parental expectations, and from the disappointment that follows when the child fails to fulfill parental fantasies, as it does from actual, successful engineering of traits.

Opposition to drug use in sport has often been framed in paternalistic terms. This is unfortunate, because the harms attributed to drugs used in sport have sometimes been exaggerated, and athletes are quick to sniff out hypocrisy. For an adult athlete who engages in a sport that carries a substantial risk of injury, the argument that you shouldn't use a performance-enhancing drug because you might hurt yourself sounds hollow and insincere. A much better response to the argument from liberty in this instance is to point out that the intensely competitive nature of sport means that one person's liberty to use a drug that significantly enhances performance affects the other competitors. Their liberty to compete fairly and equally without using drugs is severely constrained by the drug-using athlete's actions (Murray 1983).

The fourth claim can be put colloquially as *'resistance is futile'*. In its less sophisticated form, the argument for the claim is based on some notion of historical inevitability: boundaries were shattered in the past, therefore boundaries will fall in the future. A more nuanced version of the 'resistance is futile' claim rests on what is deemed to be the ineluctable outcome of values, social forces, and incentives. In athletics people value performance and victory; the stakes are high and there are networks of scientists, coaches, and others more than willing to supply enhancements and help the athlete evade detection. In the quest for the 'perfect' child, the value placed on reproductive autonomy combined with every parent's desire to have a healthy, successful child, and the eagerness of reproductive entrepreneurs to sell their services create a potent mix. In *The Pursuit of Perfection*,

Sheila M. Rothman and David J. Rothman describe how plastic surgery grew into a major industry that paid little attention to risks. Consumers, they observe,

typically focus on the benefits, ignoring risks almost completely . . . From the profession's perspective, plastic surgery demonstrates the extraordinary competition that a new enhancement technology sparks among different specialties. When no one group owns a procedure and when the market for it is lucrative, a variety of specialties try to capture a greater share. In the process, they not only publicize the procedure but also experiment with more powerful and riskier techniques. In the end, patient safety is compromised, although the patient may be the last one to know. (Rothman and Rothman 2003: 103)

The 'resistance is futile' claim has problems. For one thing, it is not, in the first instance, a moral claim. It does not say that all forms of enhancement are morally desirable or defensible. It simply asserts that attempts to restrict access to enhancements will be unsuccessful because people will pursue them anyway. True, some attempts at restriction are widely regarded as miserable failures. Prohibition in the United States is a leading example. Many people did not accept the assumptions underlying Prohibition, flouting of the law was widespread, and it had the perverse effect of allowing organized crime to profit from a monopoly. On the other hand, there are restrictions that we regard as ethically justifiable and even necessary for a civilized community. We prohibit theft, murder, and sexual assault. Some people commit these crimes nevertheless, but we don't rush to repeal the laws on the grounds that 'people will do it anyway'. In the absence of widespread moral opposition, efforts to restrict access to particular enhancements are no more likely to be successful than Prohibition was. But, if communities are convinced that certain enhancements are ethically indefensible, restrictions can be justified. They can never be expected to be perfectly observed and enforceable, any more than laws against theft or violence. But they can make a palpable difference in the community's life nonetheless.

The fifth and last objection to controlling enhancement is the claim that could be dubbed heroic, romantic, or Promethean: that people *should* shape themselves. Willful self-design, from this perspective, is a distinctly human enterprise and therefore to be valued for its own sake. We are meant to be self-makers. The Rothmans report a vivid example of this view among the writings of feminist film critics, some of whom 'scoff . . . at interpretations of the anorexic woman as weak and self-destructive'. What appears to be pathological is really independent behavior. The Rothmans (2003: 129) quote Noelle Casky on anorexia: 'Anorexia', Noelle Casky maintains, 'is the cultivation of a specific image as an *image*— it is a purely artificial creation and that is why it is so admired. Will alone produces it and maintains it against considerable odds.' This romanticizing of anorexia may offend people who have struggled with it or who have loved, and perhaps lost, children with anorexia. It does, though, capture the spirit of the heroic–romantic–Promethean ideal.

Whatever its appeal, the heroic–romantic–Promethean take on enhancement encounters serious difficulties. Anorexia threatens to extinguish the very self that is both agent and object of these impulses towards self-design. There is also a remarkable naivety in the portrayal of such image cultivation as the product of individual will, rather than a complex interaction between social norms, which can be oppressive, and the individual's sometimes desperate search for identity and acceptance by self and the world at large. It is no coincidence that anorexia occurs principally among young women: young because identity is still in formation; women, because of strong cultural preferences for slimness.

What of the link the heroic–romantic–Promethean view makes between the distinctively human quality of self-making and the intrinsic value of such a project? There are many distinctively human things that we value enormously: love, art, poetry, charity, and self-sacrifice to name a few. But other distinctively human capacities are not so honored, among them war, genocide, torture, and other forms of intentional cruelty. There is no necessary link between a project's or capacity's distinctively human character and its moral desirability. Some are good, some wonderful; others are unmitigated and shameful horrors. The bare fact that humans are distinctively capable of something does not tell us whether it is morally good.

The romantic notion that the essence of human nature is its plasticity is itself an affirmation that one's view of human nature can have significant moral content. The romantic view is not, of course, the only possible one. Other commentators have tried to find in human nature sound reasons to limit enhancement. There are a number of arguments for placing limits on efforts to enhance human beings. But because the argument for limiting enhancement based on conceptions of human nature has been so prominent, it will be considered first.

CAN HUMAN NATURE BE OUR GUIDE?

If enhancement of humans, by humans, and for—at least some—humans is the issue, can human nature be our guide through the thickets of the ethics of enhancement? This is the central assumption in a report of the US President's Council on Bioethics, *Beyond Therapy* (2003). Before examining the Council's argument in detail, consider three ways of thinking about the relationship of human nature to the ethics of enhancement: human nature as raw material; human nature as contours of the given; and human nature as normative guide.

Human nature as raw material. On this view, human nature, with one exception, has no moral significance. Our nature is raw material to be molded as we desire. Today we can sculpt our bodies with surgeries and decorate them with tattoos and piercings; we are learning to use drugs to bend our moods to our will; and tomorrow, perhaps, we will alter the genetic structure of our cells to shape ourselves—and our children—into the creatures we imagine we want to be. The exception—the morally singular aspect of human nature—is the ability to intend coupled with the skill to remake ourselves according to our own designs. This is the romantic–Promethean view of humans and their nature. Plasticity is all. Tinkering is celebrated as an affirmation of human will and cleverness (Silver 1998).

Human nature as contours of the given. This view acknowledges that we are creatures of a particular kind—embodied, finite, capable of great courage and abiding love; capable also of cowardice, treachery, and indifference. Our natures, always complex and often morally ambiguous, tell us something about the boundaries of what is possible and desirable. If we are irremediably social creatures, if we rely on one another for our flourishing, then a project to make us all indifferent to the feelings—of love or compassion—to those around us is fatally flawed at its core. Another project, directed, say, at preventing premature death, encourages the formation of vital relationships while reducing the likelihood that they will be suddenly, violently sundered. This, of course, is a description of the project of therapeutic medicine and public health. So, this view has teeth: some supposed 'enhancements' are out of bounds; others fit well within the contours of our given nature.

In contrast to the romantic–Promethean view, a focus on the realities of human nature as given (intimations of mortality, if you like) differs in three ways. First, it does not assume that human nature is limitlessly manipulable. Second, it does not elevate human willfulness and technical skill over all other human capacities. And third, it suggests that modesty is in order both concerning our abilities to alter our natures and concerning our wisdom in deciding which alterations are desirable.

Human nature as normative guide. It is worth quoting at length the assertions made in a crucial passage in *Beyond Therapy* because they provide a concise, current, and widely circulated account of the claim that human nature, properly understood, serves as a normative guide.

For only if there is a *human* 'givenness,' or a given humanness, that is also good and worth respecting, either as we find it or as it could be perfected *without ceasing to be itself*, will the 'given' serve as a *positive* guide for choosing what to alter and what to leave alone. Only if there is something precious in our given human nature—beyond the fact of its giftedness—can what is given guide us in resisting efforts that would degrade it. When it comes to human biotechnical engineering beyond therapy, only if there is something inherently good or dignified about, say, natural procreation, the human life cycle (with its rhythm of rise and fall), and human erotic longing and striving; only if there is something inherently good or dignified about the ways in which we engage the world as spectators and appreciators, as teachers and learners, leaders and followers, agents and makers, lovers and friends, parents and children, citizens and worshippers, and as seekers of our own special excellence and flourishing in whatever arena to which we are called—only then can we begin to see why those aspects of our nature need to be defended against our deliberate redesign. (President's Council on Bioethics 2003: 289–90)

For anyone worried that the romantic–Promethean view will dominate debate over the use—and opposing any constraints—on efforts at human enhancement, this passage has an undeniable appeal. But it is worth attending carefully both to the structure of the argument as well as to where it all too easily leads.

Although the loftiness of the language makes it difficult to sort out precisely what is being claimed, the argument seems to be premised on a series of categorical assertions. Take the first sentence: 'For only if there is a *human* "givenness," or a given humanness, that is also good and worth respecting, either as we find it or as it could be perfected *without ceasing to be itself,* will the "given" serve as a *positive* guide for choosing what to alter and what to leave alone.' The 'given', that is, human nature, can be a 'positive' guide to our choices concerning enhancement if and only if what is given is also 'good and worth respecting'. What then is the relationship between the given and the good? The authors of *Beyond Therapy* have already acknowledged that not all that is given is good—some things, we've been told, should be avoided like the plague—the plague itself, indisputably natural and given, among them. The question has been begged: How among all that is given or natural are we to know which are 'positive' guides and which are to be avoided like the plague? And what does it mean that the guide is 'positive'? The connotation of 'positive' suggests that it does not merely warn us against blundering into dangerous territory, but that it also shows us the correct way, the proper object of our aspirations. But again, how are we to know which aspects of the given are trustworthy guides?

The second sentence does little to clarify matters: 'Only if there is something precious in our given human nature—beyond the fact of its giftedness—can what is given guide us in resisting efforts that would degrade it.' Here the focus has shifted from aspirations to be pursued to degradations to be avoided—if and only if, we are told, 'there is something precious in our given human nature'. We are once again chasing our tails: Does being part of our nature make something indisputably precious? But that cannot be or else we would embrace and celebrate the most extreme forms of human suffering and evil along with all the ills to which the flesh is heir. We need some way to distinguish those aspects of our givenness, our human nature, that have moral meaning and value from those we can and should flee from whenever possible.

The long list that follows in the third sentence shows where the authors are heading. It cites one widely admired human capacity after another. But yet again the question is begged: Surely these capacities are 'given' and natural—otherwise they wouldn't be *human* capacities at all. But the bald fact that they are human doesn't distinguish them from other capacities—astounding cruelty, deception, violence, and betrayal among them—that are just as indisputably human. The problem with the underlying theoretical approach in *Beyond Therapy* is its insistence on looking inward—to some account of our natures rooted, as later passages make clear, in the tension between 'the transcendent longings of the soul and the limited capacities of our bodies and minds' (2003: 299). According to this account, only that which is given and natural can be good, and all that is other than natural and given is suspect.

I introduced the hypothetical case of a drug that steadies the surgeon's hand into the enhancement debate long ago to illustrate that not all forms of drug-induced performance enhancement are obviously wrong. Imagine a drug with no significant side-effects (an admittedly shaky assumption) that neurosurgeons involved in delicate procedures could take that reduces the normal tremor and unsteadiness all humans experience. This drug, let us say, has been shown to lower dramatically the morbidity and mortality that usually accompany these procedures. Suppose further that someone you love is about to undergo precisely one of these operations. Between two otherwise equally adept surgeons, which one would you choose: the surgeon who, citing her commitment to her own flourishing as an active, self-aware, self-directed agent (see President's Council on Bioethics 2003: 131), refuses to take the drug, or the surgeon who, citing the benefit to her patients, affirms that she uses the drug faithfully every time she operates?

I would not wish the first surgeon ill, but this is not a tough choice: I would go with the surgeon most likely not to injure or kill my beloved. The goal, after all, of surgical interventions such as this one is to preserve the life and health of the patient—not to show off the virtuosity of the surgeon, although that may be a secondary effect. Suppose the first surgeon also preferred to use antiquated instruments: 'Oh sure, she says, the new scalpels, retractors, and the like are easier to use and safer for the patient—but the old tools sharpen and display my technical skills much better'. Our response should be: 'That's nuts!' Or, in a more reflective frame of mind, we might explain to her that she is missing the point of her practice. Of course, we want her to flourish—but her professional flourishing comes through placing the patient's welfare first. Pursuing personal excellence follows rather than precedes in importance the social goods we seek—restoring to health, saving life, sparing from injury.

The effort to ground an ethics of enhancement on an inward-looking account of human nature fails. Not all that is natural is good, and not all unnatural enhancements are bad. But between human nature as inferior raw material and human nature as ultimate unambiguous and infallible guide to right living, there remains a third possibility: human nature as a framework for the possibilities of human flourishing. Human nature, understood as the tension between our higher longings and our worldly biology, enfolds the possibilities of such flourishing. Our natures establish the contours within which humans flourish or flounder. But, within the context of their biologically given nature, human beings create relationships, practices, and institutions that give structure to their interactions and meaning to their aspirations. Understanding the relationship between social practices, institutions, and human flourishing allows us to consider other reasons for taking the ethics of enhancement seriously.

REASONS FOR ETHICAL CONCERN ABOUT ENHANCEMENT

We err in lumping together a diverse array of possible uses of biotechnology as 'enhancements', assuming that a single overarching moral analysis will serve equally well for all. Different spheres of human life, different practices with different ends, properly call for analyses responsive to our understandings of them, the means appropriate to pursue the ends valued within each. Similarly, of the reasons for ethical concern described below, some will apply more clearly and forcefully to certain uses of biotechnical enhancement than to other uses.

Undermining human nature. The fear that biotechnologies will rob us of what gives shape and motivation to human lives runs though the work of Leon Kass in general, and the prospect of life extension in *Beyond Therapy* in particular. The Council's report (2003), echoing Kass's long-standing concerns, worries that without the spur of finitude all higher human aspirations will dwindle. Without the prospect of death, he fears that we will become ever more complacent and self-centered. The themes that animate our greatest art will shrink to historical curiosities; the motivation to create will evaporate like steam from an uncapped boiler.

Kass's critique is in the thrall of the same Promethean fantasies being peddled by biotechnology hucksters. We may be on the threshold of learning to manage some of the diseases that cause great sorrow and early death. But we are nowhere near to knocking on the door of eternal life. Rooting our analysis of biotechnological enhancement in a far distant fantasy of unlimited life extension may be visionary. But it may also be a colossal distraction from the actual challenges posed by enhancement technologies. The concern with undermining human nature that runs through *Beyond Therapy* is a provocative framework for thinking about the apotheosis of biotechnological life prolongation. But there are more immediate sources of moral concern.

The denial of giftedness. Michael Sandel is the most prominent recent proponent of the idea that biotechnological enhancement threatens to blind us to the giftedness of life. Sandel, although a member of the President's Council on Bioethics, takes issue with *Beyond Therapy*'s judgment that human agency, rather than respect for the given, for human life as a gift, is at the heart of what is threatened by enhancement. Sandel disagrees with what he describes as *Beyond Therapy*'s assertion that 'the main problem with enhancement and genetic engineering is that they undermine effort and erode human agency'. Instead, he asserts: 'The deeper danger is that they represent a kind of hyperagency—a Promethean aspiration to remake nature, including human nature, to serve our purposes and satisfy our desires. The problem is not the drift to mechanism but the drive to mastery' (2004: 54).

Is human agency the threat or the threatened? Sandel argues: 'If bioengineering made the myth of the "self-made man" come true, it would be difficult to view our talents as gifts for which we are indebted, rather than as achievements for which we are responsible.' What's the problem with that? He argues that such a view would have a baleful impact on 'three key features of our moral landscape: humility, responsibility, and solidarity' (2004: 60). Humility opens to the given and unexpected; it reins in the powerful temptation to try to control, for example, the traits of our children. If nothing is left to chance then we are responsible for everything—including our children's talents and interests. As for solidarity, Sandel argues that health insurance, for example, as a way of sharing the financial burdens of unexpected illness, will wither away as the predictability of medical misfortune increases. Solidarity, in his view, is dependent on human frailty and its unpredictability.

Proponents of the Promethean view of biotechnological enhancement may disagree. If, though, Sandel is correct that a goodly measure of humility, a strong pull towards solidarity, and a nuanced view of responsibility are important to a morally vigorous society, then the overthrow of giftedness in favor of hyperagency is, indeed, reason for worry.

An emphasis on giftedness seems particularly well suited for thinking about applying biotechnological enhancements to athletes and to our children. When we look to athletes for excellence or seek athletic excellence in ourselves, we expect to see natural talents and their virtuous perfection. By undermining the very idea of 'natural' talents, biotechnological enhancement strips athletic excellence of what we value in it. When we aim to design our children, we abet the temptation to tyranny; at the same time, we put at risk what makes the parent–child relationship such a vital path to human flourishing.

The temptation to tyranny. Complaints about overweening efforts to control our children's characteristics are often parried by a menu of things parents do now to shape the course of their children's lives. But that menu, even if it lacks a precise ordering, reveals huge variations in moral digestibility. Giving your child a baseball or violin or enrolling them in Little League or music lessons can enlarge their horizons, sharpen their appetites, and teach the connection between natural talent, virtuous training, and success. Parents who fail to open possibilities for their child risk narrowing the range of their children's hopes and dreams. Parents who insist that their child pursue only those goals that the parents dictate and no others, or who similarly insist that their child be just this sort of person, with precisely these character traits, aspirations, and affections, are narrowing that child's horizons to the point of tyranny. The fact that some parents now behave tyrannically even without the tools of biotechnology is no argument for embracing the new forms of tyranny biotechnology may later offer.

It is worth noting that the concern about temptations to tyranny does not require that the technologies successfully deliver the precise control that their promoters promise. If, on the one hand, the technologies of selection and control are highly effective, then the tyranny is accomplished. But, if parents think that because their child is tall, or musical, or has uncommon curiosity or blue eyes, this will assure the life they envision, they will be sorely disappointed. It is one thing to have perfect pitch, another to have the desire and drive to become a successful musician. Making sure that your child is tall or has blue eyes seems more straightforward. But it would be more than a little odd for parents to want their child to have those anatomical traits just to *have* them. It seems likely that parents see those traits as serving other goals; and if being tall and blue-eyed confers social advantages, for example, our fortunate (and expensive) child had better capitalize on those advantages! Even with highly refined control over traits (a dubious prospect scientifically) the prospects for conflict are rich. Of course, the idea that we soon—or ever—would have such precisely targeted control is improbable. The more we learn about the complexity with which genes interact with one another, about the capacity of a single gene to make multiple proteins with distinct functions, and about the unpredictability of development, the more we undercut the assumption that precise control is possible.

What if parents' aspirations for control are disappointed? If the technologies work less effectively than they hope, does the temptation to tyranny fade as a concern? Unfortunately, no. Frustrated tyrants are no less a danger to the individuals under their thumb than satisfied ones. What will be the impact of selection and enhancement on what is morally vital in the relationship between parent and child?

Undermining the relationship of parents and children. With apologies to Dante, there should be a sign above the gateway to parenthood that reads 'Abandon all hope (of control) you who enter here!' It has never been a good idea for parents to try to design and mold their children to meet their fantasies. For one thing, as I noted above, the quest for control is doomed largely to failure. For another, children are not the mere passive recipients of parental instruction like a statue onto which the shaper can endlessly add gobs of clay until the desired result appears. Children act and react; they may accept one influence but rebel against the next. Finally, and most importantly, unrelenting attempts at control choke off the growth of mutual love and respect. The central point here is that we cannot fully understand the ethics of biomedically enhancing children without understanding what is ethically crucial in the relationship between children and parents.

Sandel argues for the importance of accepting the 'givenness' of our children—as they are, with their appetites and enthusiasms, fears and aspirations, however that personal reality might diverge from our idealized image of the child we dreamt of having. The idea of givenness or giftedness fits well with a conception of the relationship between parents and children that stresses *mutuality*.

The usual distinction between human moral motivations—self-interest and altruism—fails to capture a crucial feature of parents' motivations in caring for their children. Good parents discover that they derive deep satisfaction and great personal growth as their children thrive under their care. Growth and satisfaction come when parents aim not at *their own* well-being but at *their children's* flourishing. By acting to advance another's well-being—the classic paradigm of altruism—parents also further their own—what we would usually think of as self-interest. But in parents' love and care for their children, altruism and self-interest are inextricably intertwined in a way neither label adequately captures: hence the need for the concept of mutualism as a third type of moral motivation. The archetype of mutualism, so common and pervasive, is embodied by parents caring for their children (Murray 1996).

Relationships of mutuality are vitally important to moral and emotional growth and maturity. Erik Erikson, who famously coined the phrase 'identity crisis', refers to the challenge that typically gathers force in adulthood as 'generativity' (Erikson 1964). Do we learn to care for people and projects beyond ourselves? Becoming a caring parent may be the most common way adults grapple with the challenge of generativity, but it is by no means the only path. In parenthood, as in other vital relationships that depend upon mutuality, overweening efforts to control the other are anathema to the flourishing of both. These relationships depend upon respect for the other person's individuality and—in the case of children, slowly evolving capacity for—agency. The over-controlling parent damages the child by constraining the child's horizon of possibilities and impairs the child's emerging sense of agency and efficacy. Tyrannical parents suffer as well when children's love is smothered or withheld and ultimately withdrawn. Love freely returned for love generously given is a far more precious reward. Such love is both the source of and the reward for mutuality. When biomedical enhancement is enlisted in the service of fantasies of parental control, all that is most precious and beautiful in the relationship between parent and child is threatened.

There are other reasons why efforts to alter our children's characteristics in the name of enhancement can be misguided. Enhancement can be a foolish waste of resources; it can become complicit with unjust norms; and it can reinforce patterns of injustice. Human growth hormone illustrates all three.

A foolish waste of resources. Human growth hormone to increase final adult height is an expensive and extended proposition, requiring frequent injections over years costing tens of thousands of dollars. Some parents seek hGH for their children who are projected to be well below average in height. Especially for children with a demonstrated deficiency in biologically active hGH, such measures look very much like therapy for other significant hormonal abnormalities such as diabetes. But other parents seek hGH for their children who would be average or above average in height. No case can be made that administering hGH to such children is treating some underlying disease; this is a straightforward example of enhancement.

What, though, is being enhanced, and to what end? Earlier I distinguished between ends, means, and intermediary states. The means are clear enough: growth hormone injections. But it is important also to discern what counts as an end and what as an intermediary state. Increased height is not an end in itself. The whole point of trying to make one's child taller is to give that child the advantages that height provides. Height, then, is an intermediary means. The ends are whatever competitive social and economic advantages height affords.

Earlier I raised questions about whether hGH for short children was the best means of reaching the reasonable parental goals of trying to build one's child's self-confidence and to avoid discrimination. For very short children, increasing height can also be seen as averting what would otherwise be a disability—albeit a mostly socially constructed one: navigating a world constructed for adults within a certain range of heights. The quest for a few additional inches of height has its costs, not least in giving a message to that child that being short is such a significant problem that it is worth all this money, time, and attention. For a child who will nevertheless end up much shorter than average, this is not an entirely supportive message. But, all things considered, the parents of such children are the appropriate agents to weigh advantages and disadvantages and decide on their child's behalf. What about children who are not short?

Years ago I learned of a case in which the parents of a tall young woman sought hGH for her because her high school volleyball coach told them that if she were 4 inches taller he could assure her a full scholarship to any university in her country with a women's volleyball program. That case may be exceptional in its promise of immediate and tangible rewards for a successful course of hGH injections. More common is the general desire to capture for one's child the advantages of heightism. Suppose that all parents thought the same. Imagine that all children were given hGH and that all children ended up on average a few inches taller than they would have been otherwise. Who is better off?

Among those most likely to benefit are the companies that manufacture hGH, the physicians and others who monitor its effects, and fabric manufacturers—because we will all need to wear larger sizes. Your child, however, will not be any better off. He or she will still be in roughly the same percentile of height as before; the entire curve will have shifted to the right, but there will still be the shorter-than-average and the taller-than-average. Children as a group will surely be worse off: having to endure a thousand or more injections, running the risks that accompany long-term administration of hGH, becoming more conscious than ever about the social advantages of being tall and the disadvantages of being short.

Universal administration of hGH to make children taller would be a foolish waste of social resources. No valuable social good would be advanced. Massive resources would be squandered. This example underscores the need to think beyond the isolated individual case and ask what good such an 'enhancement' would do if in good Kantian style we universalized that action or judgment. To an individual parent, hGH might look like a reasonable investment in one's child's future. But that investment creates no increase in social good: no improvement in the available stock of virtue, no progress in the pursuit of justice. And if all other parents did the same it would entail risks and the pain of injections while offering nothing positive even to your own child. For hGH and height, the means are now available, the intermediary state (being a few inches taller) achievable, but the ends—a comparative advantage for my child rooted in a social prejudice—remain ignoble, carrying no intrinsic value and promising no increase in social good, and, if other parents do the same, are ultimately futile.

Enhancement via hGH teaches us to look beyond the individual case and to consider carefully what social value or good is being advanced. Some other enhancement, say of cognitive functioning, general health, or resistance to disease, might add materially to the stock of human well-being. As vaccines enhance the immune system and diminish the misery and premature death wrought by infectious diseases, so certain other instances of biomedical enhancements may do good on the whole. Each proposed 'enhancement' must be evaluated in its full social context.

Complicity with unjust norms. Sometimes a supposed enhancement becomes complicit with and reinforces unjust norms. Cosmetic surgery is often accused of just this offense, and often with good reason. Surgically sculpting one's body to resemble more closely idealized images of youthful slenderness and firmness may help an individual to feel good, and may make that person a hotter property in the dating market. One might argue that it also results in a more comely and attractive world for all of us. But there is no doubt that enhancing one's appearance with cosmetic surgery or botox injections underscores the power of norms of physical appearance that most aging bodies cannot meet without assistance—and that most youthful bodies fall short of as well.

Margaret Olivia Little (1998: 170) proposes that complicity exists 'when one endorses, promotes, or unduly benefits from norms and practices that are morally suspect'. So, for example, surgically reshaping women's bodies to resemble Barbie dolls would make surgeons complicit along with the women whose bodies are being altered. Overseeing a course of hGH injections for a child slightly shorter than average would also count as complicity with unjust norms—given that height should not be a measure of a person's worth.

Little recognizes the quandary surgeons and others are thrown into when we accuse them of complicity with unjust norms: sometimes patients *are suffering*, *are seriously disadvantaged* because these norms, however unjust, weigh down their lives. For a woman deeply unhappy with her body, convinced—perhaps with good reason—that her life would be better with a smaller waist and larger breasts, it seems harsh to say that she should stop complaining and just accept the body she was born with. It feels even crueler to insist that a child cease whining and resign himself to the social disadvantages that come with short stature. Physicians' and surgeons' duties are to their individual patients first of all. If an intervention can alleviate suffering—even if that suffering comes about only because of oppressive and unjust social norms—why should not clinicians do what helps their patients?

As Little recognizes, this is a genuine quandary. She argues that surgeons, for example, should not reinforce or profit unduly from Barbie doll fantasies. The line, though, between being attentive to patients' desires and making a tidy living from indulging anatomical fantasies can be hard to locate. She ends up suggesting that professionals should protest against and avoid promoting or profiteering from unjust norms, even as they assist their patients in pursuing them.

Whatever one thinks about the moral obligations of professionals and those who seek their services in the quest for enhancement, it is important to acknowledge that when professionals give in to patients' pleas for enhancement, unjust norms may be strengthened, however honorable and compassionate one's intentions may be.

Justice and equal access. Of course one way to remedy injustices caused by unequal access is to provide access for everyone. Not all potential enhancements are certain to be like hGH, where no net good is added. (If all children were given hGH the problem would not be injustice but rather colossal waste and universal stupidity.) Distributive justice attends to the balance of burdens and benefits. Imagine some biomedical means to enhance empathy: as with vaccines, the world might well be better off if everyone's capacity for empathy were enhanced; also as with vaccines, some people might reap the benefits of a more empathic world without having to undergo the enhancement themselves—free riders on the empathy train. Indeed, the less empathic might have an advantage in certain spheres—business, politics, and sport come to mind.

We need to distinguish between the persons undergoing enhancement and the persons benefiting from the enhancement. Discussions of enhancement often assume that they are one and the same. Often they will be, but whenever social value is added by enhancement, persons other than those being enhanced may benefit. The neurosurgeon whose steadiness is enhanced may benefit from lower malpractice premiums and peace of mind that comes from causing fewer surgical errors. But that surgeon's patients are the principal beneficiaries.

The question of equal access to enhancements can be recast into the usual mold of distributive justice: the fair allocation of burdens and benefits. Providing enhancements that confer significant competitive advantages to the already powerful and privileged threatens justice. But equal shares to all may not always be the wisest policy either. What will foster justice and at the same time serve important human goods? That question must be asked; but it will have different answers for different enhancement technologies used for different purposes.

The meaning of the practice. Athletes ask to be allowed to compete on a level playing field—the common metaphor for sport untainted by performance-enhancing drugs. This is a plea for justice. It embodies a recognition that drug use by one athlete can affect adversely all other athletes in the event; such use pressures other competitors to use similar performance-enhancing drugs. But since sport honors maximum performance, and since many means of enhancement, like improved equipment, are tolerated, and others, like perseverance and dedication, are celebrated, why are drugs like anabolic steroids and EPO dishonored?

Sport is not just any set of activities; sport is a form—many forms, actually, depending on the particular sport—of *social practice*. Those social practices have particular meanings embedded within them. Whether the sport is the 100 meter dash, the marathon, throwing the discus, or playing basketball or ice hockey, what we look for in athletes is a combination of *natural talents* and the *virtuous perfection* of those talents. The notion of virtuous perfection captures two important insights: first, not all forms of enhancement are regarded as admirable or even permissible; and second, we expect that virtues, such as hard work, dedication, and the willingness to suffer for a purpose, should, along with natural talents, determine athletic success.

There is an alternative to insisting that talent and virtue are central to the meaning of sport. There is another world of competition—I am loath to call it sport—where the performance principle dominates (Todd and Todd forthcoming). The performance principle says roughly that maximum performance is all that counts, and competitors may use any and all means available to achieve that end. Certain power lifting competitions have embraced the performance principle. We shall have to see whether such competitions are likewise embraced by people who love sport.

I believe that the main lesson here is that, along with their broader social consequences, our moral evaluation of putative biomedical enhancements must grapple with the meaning and value of the social practices and institutions affected by them. Genuflecting in the direction of unfettered individual choice will not be an ethically adequate or wise response.

CONCLUDING OBSERVATIONS

Perhaps the most important conclusion of this analysis of the ethics of biomedical enhancement is the moral diversity of enhancements. There are many different means of enhancement, working through a variety of intermediary states, towards a multiplicity of ends. No single ethical principal or distinction will be a reliable guide through this complex thicket.

In particular, the concept of the *natural* takes us only so far. Accounts of the ethics of enhancement that rely on human nature as a positive guide either encounter unsolvable puzzles or else dissolve into incomprehensible vagueness. We see this quandary in *Beyond Therapy*. Consider eyeglasses and anabolic steroids. Both are certainly unnatural. Yet who objects to eyeglasses as an aid to reading or driving on the basis that they are 'unnatural'? The goal of reading or driving is a valued one. If eyeglasses make it easier or safer, that is all to the good. Whether it is natural or unnatural is of no importance. Anabolic steroids used by an Olympic weightlifter are no more unnatural, yet they are almost universally abhorred. The difference lies in the meaning of the activity and the place the idea of the natural plays in it. Excellence in sport is meant to be the product of natural talents and their perfection by hard work and other virtuous activities. The idea of the natural here is integral to the shared social meaning of the practice itself. This is why we disapprove of performance-enhancing drugs in sport. Further, because sport is a rule-governed activity and because we prize fairness in competition so highly, athletes who use banned performance-enhancing technologies are condemned as cheats and as people who compete unfairly and therefore behave unjustly towards their fellow athletes.

There is a very important distinction here between relying on the idea of the natural as the fundamental basis for an ethics of enhancement—a project unlikely to succeed—and understanding that our nature shapes the contours of our moral world. Our possibilities for flourishing are not as unfettered willful agents, but as embodied creatures whose lives and flourishing are deeply intertwined with one another. A thoughtful understanding of the ethics of enhancement must take into account the meaning and purpose of the activities being enhanced, their social context, and the other persons and institutions affected by them. There will be no single ethics of biomedical enhancement. What we need now is a clear conceptual map of the possible types of enhancement coupled with a nuanced understanding of the goods sought, the dangers encountered, and the social and institutional context into which each putative enhancement will be thrust. It will be in the end, as it was in the beginning, about meanings and human flourishing.

REFERENCES

ALLEN, D. B., and FOST, N. C. (1990), 'Growth Hormone Therapy for Short Stature: Panacea or Pandora's Box?', *Journal of Pediatrics*, 117/1: 16–21.

BENJAMIN, M., MUYSKENS, J., and SAENGER, P. (1984), 'Short Children, Anxious Parents: Is Growth Hormone the Answer?', *Hastings Center Report*, 14/2: 5–9.

BROCK, D. W. (1998), 'Enhancements of Human Function: Some Distinctions for Policymakers', in E. Parens (ed.), *Enhancing Human Traits: Ethical and Social Implications* (Washington, DC: Georgetown University Press), 48–69.

ERIKSON, E. H. (1964), *Insight and Responsibility* (New York: W. W. Norton).

FOST, N. (1986), 'Banning Drugs in Sports: A Skeptical View', *Hastings Center Report*, 16/4: 5–10.

JUENGST, E. T. (1998), 'What Does Enhancement Mean?', in E. Parens (ed.), *Enhancing Human Traits: Ethical and Social Implications* (Washington, DC: Georgetown University Press), 29–47.

KRAMER, P. (1993), *Listening to Prozac* (New York: Viking Press).

LITTLE, M. O. (1998), 'Cosmetic Surgery, Suspect Norms, and the Ethics of Complicity', in E. Parens (ed.), *Enhancing Human Traits: Ethical and Social Implications* (Washington, DC: Georgetown University Press), 162–75.

MURRAY, T. (1983), 'The Coercive Power of Drugs in Sports', *Hastings Center Report*, 13/4: 24–30.

—— (1987), 'The Growing Danger from Gene-Spliced Hormones', *Discover*, 8/2: 88–92.

—— (1996), *The Worth of a Child* (Berkeley: University of California Press).

NOBLE, K. B. (1996), 'After Cancer Struggle, Olympic Nightmare', *New York Times*, 15 Feb., A14.

PARENS, E. (1998), 'Is Better Always Good?', in E. Parens (ed.), *Enhancing Human Traits: Ethical and Social Implications* (Washington, DC: Georgetown University Press), 1–28.

PRESIDENT'S COUNCIL ON BIOETHICS (2003), *Beyond Therapy: Biotechnology and the Pursuit of Happiness* (Washington, DC: President's Council on Bioethics).

ROTHMAN, S. M., and ROTHMAN, D. J. (2003), *The Pursuit of Perfection* (New York: Pantheon).

SANDEL, M. (2004), 'The Case Against Perfection', *Atlantic Monthly*, 3/293: 51–60.

SILVER, L. (1998), *Remaking Eden: Cloning and Beyond in a Brave New World* (New York: Avon).

SLOMKA, J. (1992), 'Playing with Propanolol', *Hastings Center Report*, 22/4: 13–17.

SOKOLOVE, M. (2004), 'The Lab Animal', *New York Times Magazine*, 18 Jan., 28–33, 48, 54, 58.

TODD, J., and TODD, T. (forthcoming), 'Reflections on the "Parallel Federation Solution" to the Problem of Drug Use in Sport: The Cautionary Tale of Powerlifting', in T. Murray, E. Parens, K. Maschke, and A. Wasunna (eds.), *Ethical Conceptual and Scientific Issues in the Use of Performance Enhancing Technologies in Sports* (Baltimore: Johns Hopkins University Press).

CHAPTER 22

GENETIC INTERVENTIONS AND THE ETHICS OF ENHANCEMENT OF HUMAN BEINGS

JULIAN SAVULESCU

SHOULD we use science and medical technology not just to prevent or treat disease, but to intervene at the most basic biological levels to improve biology and enhance people's lives? By 'enhance', I mean help them to live a longer and/or better life than normal. There are various ways in which we can enhance people but I want to focus on biological enhancement, especially genetic enhancement.

There has been considerable recent debate on the ethics of human enhancement. A number of prominent authors have been concerned about or critical of the use of technology to alter or enhance human beings (Annas 2000: 753–82; Elliott 2003), citing threats to human nature and dignity as one basis for these concerns (Fukuyama 2003; Kass 2002; Habermas 2003). The President's Council Report entitled *Beyond Therapy* was strongly critical of human enhancement (President's Council on Bioethics 2003). Michael Sandel, in a widely discussed article, has suggested that the problem with genetic enhancement:

is in the hubris of the designing parents, in their drive to master the mystery of birth . . . it would disfigure the relation between parent and child, and deprive the parent of the humility and enlarged human sympathies that an openness to the unbidden can cultivate . . . the promise of mastery is flawed. It threatens to banish our appreciation of life as a gift, and to leave us with nothing to affirm or behold outside our own will. (Sandel 2004)

Frances Kamm has given a detailed rebuttal of Sandel's arguments, arguing that human enhancement is permissible (Kamm 2005). Nicholas Agar, in his book *Liberal Eugenics* (Agar 2003), argues that enhancement should be permissible but not obligatory. He argues that what distinguishes liberal eugenics from the objectionable eugenic practices of the Nazis is that it is not based on a single conception of a desirable genome and that it is voluntary and not obligatory.

In this chapter I will take a more provocative position. I want to argue that, far from its being merely permissible, we have a moral obligation or moral reason to enhance ourselves and our children. Indeed, we have the same kind of obligation as we have to treat and prevent disease. Not only *can* we enhance, we *should* enhance.

I will begin by considering the current interests in and possibilities of enhancement. I will then offer three arguments that we have very strong reasons to seek to enhance.

Tom Murray concludes his thoughtful and wide-ranging treatment of enhancement in this volume by arguing that 'the ethics of enhancement must take into account the meaning and purpose of the activities being enhanced, their social context, and the other persons and institutions affected by them' (Murray, Chapter 21 in this volume). Such caution is no doubt well grounded. But it should not blind us to the very large array of cases in which biological modification will improve the opportunities of an individual to lead a better life. In such cases, we have strong reasons to modify ourselves and our children. Indeed, to fail to do so would be wrong. Discussion of enhancement can be muddied by groundless fears and excessive caution and qualification. I will outline some ethical constraints on the pursuit of enhancement.

CURRENT INTEREST IN ENHANCEMENT

There is great public interest in enhancement of people. Women employ cosmetic surgery to make their noses smaller, their breasts larger, their teeth straighter and whiter, to make their cheekbones higher, their lips fuller, and to remove wrinkles and fat. Men, too, employ many of these measures, as well as pumping their bodies with steroids to increase muscle bulk. The beauty industry is testimony to the attraction of enhancement. Body art, such as painting and tattooing, and body modification, such as piercing, have, since time began, represented ways in which humans have attempted to express their creativity, values, and symbolic attachments through changing their bodies.

Modern professional sport is often said to be corrupted by widespread use of performance-enhancing drugs, such as human erythropoietin, anabolic steroids, and growth hormone. However, some effective performance enhancements are permitted in sport, such as the use of caffeine, glutamine, and creatine in diets, salbutamol, hypoxic air tents, and altitude training. Many people attempt to improve their cognitive powers through the use of nicotine, caffeine, and drugs like Ritalin and Modavigil.

Mood enhancement typifies modern society. People use psychological 'self-help', Prozac, recreational drugs, and alcohol to feel more relaxed, socialize better, and feel happier.

Even in the most private area of sexual relations, many want to be better. Around 34 per cent of all men aged 40–70—around 20 million in the United States—have some erectile dysfunction, which is a part of normal ageing. There is a 12 per cent decline in erectile function every decade normally. As a result, 20 million men worldwide use Viagra (Cheitlin *et al.* 1999).

More radical forms of biological enhancement appear possible. Even if all disease (heart disease, cancer, etc.) were cured, the average human lifespan would only be extended by twelve years (Sarah Harper, personal communication). However, stem cell science has the potential to extend human lifespan radically further than this, by replacing ageing tissue with healthy tissue (Harris 2000, 2002, 2004). We could live longer than the current maximum of 120 years.

But instead of the radical prolongation of length of life, I want to focus on the radical improvement in quality of life through biological manipulation. Some sceptics believe that this is not possible. They claim that it is our environment, or culture, that defines us, not genetics. But a quiet walk in the park demonstrates the power of a great genetic experiment: dog-breeding. It is obvious that different breeds of dog differ in temperament, intelligence, physical ability, and appearance. No matter what the turf, a Dobermann will tear a corgi to pieces. You can debilitate a Dobermann through neglect and abuse. And you can make him prettier with a bow. But you will never turn a chihuahua into a Dobermann through grooming, training, and affection. Dog breeds are all genetic—for over 10,000 years we have bred some 300–400 breeds of dog from early canids and wolves. The St Bernard is known for its size, the greyhound for its speed, the bloodhound for its sense of smell. There are freaks, hard workers, vicious aggressors, docile pets, and ornamental varieties. These characteristics have been developed by a crude form of genetic selection—selective mating or breeding.

Today we have powerful scientific tools in animal husbandry: genetic testing, artificial reproduction, and cloning are all routinely used in the farming industry to create the best stock. Scientists are now starting to look at a wider range of complex behaviours. Changing the brain's reward centre genetically may be the key to changing behaviour.

Gene therapy has been used to turn lazy monkeys into workaholics by altering the reward centre in the brain (Liu *et al.* 2004). In another experiment, researchers used gene therapy to introduce a gene from the monogamous male prairie vole, a rodent that forms lifelong bonds with one mate, into the brain of the closely related but polygamous meadow vole (Lim 2004). Genetically modified meadow voles became monogamous, behaving like prairie voles. This gene, which controls a part of the brain's reward centre different from that altered in the monkeys, is known as the vasopressin receptor gene. It may also be involved in human drug addiction.

Radical enhancements may come on the back of very respected research to prevent and treat disease. Scientists have created a rat model of the genetic disease Huntington's Chorea. This disease results in progressive rapid dementia at the age of about 40. Scientists found that rats engineered to develop Huntington's Chorea who were placed in a highly stimulating environment (of mazes, coloured rings, and balls) did not go on to develop the disease—their neurons remained intact (van Dellen *et al.* 2000; Spires *et al.* 2004). Remotivation therapy improves functioning in humans, suggesting that environmental stimulation in this genetic disease may affect brain biology at the molecular level (by altering neurotrophins) (Sullivan *et al.* 2001). Prozac has also been shown to produce a beneficial effect in humans suffering from Huntington's Chorea (De Marchi *et al.* 2001). Neural stem cells have also been identified that could potentially be induced to proliferate and differentiate (Rietze *et al.* 2001), mediated through nerve growth factors and other factors (Palma *et al.* 2005). We now know that a stimulating environment, drugs like Prozac, and nerve growth factors can affect nerve proliferation and connections—that is our brain's biology. These same interventions could, at least in theory, be used to increase the neuronal complement of normal brains and increase cognitive performance in normal individuals.

IQ has been steadily increasing since first measured, about twenty points per decade. This has been called the Flynn effect (Holloway 1999). Large environmental effects have been postulated to account for this effect (Dickens and Flynn 2001). The capacity to increase IQ is significant. Direct biological enhancement could have an equal if not greater effect on increase in IQ.

But could biological enhancement of human beings really be possible? Selective mating has been occurring in humans ever since time began. Facial asymmetry can reflect genetic disorder. Smell can tell us whether our mate will produce the child with the best resistance to disease. We compete for partners in elaborate mating games and rituals of display that sort the best matches from the worst. As products of evolution, we select our mates, both rationally and instinctively, on the basis of their genetic fitness—their ability to survive and reproduce. Our (subconscious) goal is the success of our offspring.

With the tools of genetics, we can select offspring in a more reliable way. The power of genetics is growing. Embryos can now be tested not only for the presence of genetic disorder (including some forms of bowel and breast cancer), but also for less serious genetic abnormalities, such as dental abnormalities. Sex can be tested for too. Adult athletes have been genetically tested for the presence of the ACTN3 gene to identify potential for either sprint or endurance events. Research is going on in the field of behavioural genetics to understand the genetic basis of aggression and criminal behaviour, alcoholism, anxiety, antisocial personality disorder, maternal behaviour, homosexuality, and neuroticism.

While at present there are no genetic tests for these complex behaviours, if the results of recent animal studies into hard work and monogamy apply to humans, it may be possible in the future to change genetically how we are predisposed to behave. This raises a new question: Should we try to engineer better, happier people? While at present genetic technology is most efficient at selecting among different embryos, in the future it will be possible to genetically alter existing embryos, with considerable progress already being made to the use of this technology for permanent gene therapy for disease (Urnov 2005). There is no reason why such technology could not be used to alter non-disease genes in the future.

The Ethics of Enhancement

We want to be happy people, not just healthy people.

I will now give three arguments in favour of enhancement and then consider several objections.

First Argument for Enhancement: Choosing Not to Enhance Is Wrong

Consider the case of the Neglectful Parents. The Neglectful Parents give birth to a child with a special condition. The child has a stunning intellect but requires a simple, readily available, cheap dietary supplement to sustain his intellect. But they neglect the diet of this child and this results in a child with a stunning intellect becoming normal. This is clearly wrong.

But now consider the case of the Lazy Parents. They have a child who has a normal intellect but if they introduced the same dietary supplement, the child's intellect would rise to the same level as the child of the Neglectful Parent. They can't be bothered with improving the child's diet so the child remains with a normal intellect. Failure to institute dietary supplementation means a normal child fails to achieve a stunning intellect. The inaction of the Lazy Parents is as wrong as the inaction of the Neglectful Parents. It has exactly the same consequence: a child exists who could have had a stunning intellect but is instead normal.

Some argue that it is not wrong to fail to bring about the best state of affairs. This may or may not be the case. But in these kinds of case, when there are no other relevant moral considerations, the failure to introduce a diet that sustains a more desirable state is as wrong as the failure to introduce a diet that brings about a more desirable state. The costs of inaction are the same, as are the parental obligations.

If we substitute 'biological intervention' for 'diet', we see that in order not to wrong our children, we should enhance them. Unless there is something special and optimal about our children's physical, psychological, or cognitive abilities, or something different about other biological interventions, it would be wrong not to enhance them.

Second Argument: Consistency

Some will object that, while we do have an obligation to institute better diets, biological interventions like genetic interventions are different from dietary supplementation. I will argue that there is no difference between these interventions.

In general, we accept environmental interventions to improve our children. Education, diet, and training are all used to make our children better people and increase their opportunities in life. We train children to be well behaved, cooperative, and intelligent. Indeed, researchers are looking at ways to make the environment more stimulating for young children to maximize their intellectual development. But in the study of the rat model of Huntington's Chorea, the stimulating environment acted to change the brain structure of the rats. The drug Prozac acted in just the same way. These environmental manipulations do not act mysteriously. They alter our biology.

The most striking example of this is a study of rats that were extensively mothered and rats that were not mothered. The mothered rats showed genetic changes (changes in the methylation of the DNA) that were passed on to the next generation. As Michael Meaney has observed, 'Early experience can actually modify protein–DNA interactions that regulate gene expression' (Society for Neuroscience 2004). More generally, environmental manipulations can profoundly affect biology. Maternal care and stress have been associated with abnormal brain (hippocampal) development, involving altered nerve growth factors and cognitive, psychological, and immune deficits later in life.

Some argue that genetic manipulations are different because they are irreversible. But environmental interventions can equally be irreversible. Child neglect or abuse can scar a person for life. It may be impossible to unlearn the skill of playing the piano or riding a bike, once learnt. One may be wobbly, but one is a novice only once. Just as the example of mothering of rats shows that environmental interventions can cause biological changes that are passed onto the next generation, so too can environmental interventions be irreversible, or very difficult to reverse, within one generation.

Why should we allow environmental manipulations that alter our biology but not direct biological manipulations? What is the moral difference between producing a smarter child by immersing that child in a stimulating environment, giving the child a drug, or directly altering the child's brain or genes?

One example of a drug that alters brain chemistry is Prozac, which is a serotonin reuptake inhibitor. Early in life it acts as a nerve growth factor, but it may also alter the brain early in life to make it more prone to stress and anxiety later in life by altering receptor development (Holden 2004). People with a polymorphism that reduced their serotonin activity were more likely than others to become depressed in response to stressful experiences (Holden 2003). Drugs like Prozac and maternal deprivation may have the same biological effects.

If the outcome is the same, why treat biological manipulation differently from environmental manipulation? Not only may a favourable environment improve a child's biology and increase a child's opportunities, so too may direct biological interventions. Couples should maximize the genetic opportunity of their children to lead a good life and a productive, cooperative social existence. There is no relevant moral difference between environmental and genetic intervention.

Third Argument: No Difference from Treating Disease

If we accept the treatment and prevention of disease, we should accept enhancement. The goodness of health is what drives a moral obligation to treat or prevent disease. But health is not what ultimately matters—health enables us to live well; disease prevents us from doing what we want and what is good. Health is instrumentally valuable—valuable as a resource that allows us to do what really matters, that is, lead a good life.

What constitutes a good life is a deep philosophical question. According to hedonistic theories, what is good is having pleasant experiences and being happy. According to desire fulfilment theories, and economics, what matters is having our preferences satisfied. According to objective theories, certain activities are good for people: developing deep personal relationships, developing talents, understanding oneself and the world, gaining knowledge, being a part of a family, and so on. We need not decide on which of these theories is correct in order to understand what is bad about ill health. Disease is important because it causes pain, is not what we want, and stops us engaging in those activities that give meaning to life. Sometimes people trade health for well-being: mountain climbers take on risk to achieve, smokers sometimes believe that the pleasures outweigh the risks of smoking, and so on. Life is about managing risk to health and life to promote well-being.

Beneficence—the moral obligation to benefit people—provides a strong reason to enhance people in so far as the biological enhancement increases their chance of having a better life. But can biological enhancements increase people's opportunities for well-being? There are reasons to believe that they might.

Many of our biological and psychological characteristics profoundly affect how well our lives go. In the 1960s Walter Mischel conducted impulse control experiments in which 4-year-old children were left in a room with one marshmallow, after being told that if they did not eat the marshmallow, they could later have two. Some children would eat it as soon as the researcher left; others would use a variety of strategies to help control their behaviour and ignore the temptation of the single marshmallow. A decade later they reinterviewed the children and found that those who were better at delaying gratification had more friends, better academic performance, and more motivation to succeed. Whether the child had grabbed for the marshmallow had a much stronger bearing on their SAT scores than did their IQ (Mischel *et al.* 1988).

Impulse control has also been linked to socio-economic control and avoiding conflict with the law. The problems of a hot and uncontrollable temper can be profound.

Shyness too can greatly restrict a life. I remember one newspaper story about a woman who blushed violet every time she went into a social situation. This led her to a hermitic, miserable existence. She eventually had the autonomic nerves to her face surgically cut. This revolutionized her life and had a greater effect on her well-being than the treatment of many diseases.

Buchanan and colleagues have discussed the value of 'all purpose goods' (Buchanan *et al.* 2000). These are traits that are valuable regardless of the kind of life a person chooses to live. They give us greater all-round capacities to live a vast array of lives. Examples include intelligence, memory, self-discipline, patience, empathy, a sense of humour, optimism, and just having a sunny temperament. All of these characteristics—sometimes described as virtues—may have some biological and psychological basis capable of manipulation using technology.

Technology might even be used to improve our *moral character*. We certainly seek through good instruction and example, discipline, and other methods to make better children. It may be possible to alter biology to make people predisposed to be more moral by promoting empathy, imagination, sympathy, fairness, honesty, etc.

In so far as these characteristics have some genetic basis, genetic manipulation could benefit us. There is reason to believe that complex virtues like fair-mindedness may have a biological basis. In one famous experiment a monkey was trained to perform a task and rewarded with either a grape or a piece of cucumber. He preferred the grape. On one occasion he performed the task successfully and was given a piece of cucumber. He watched as another monkey who had not performed the task was given a grape and he became very angry. This shows that even monkeys have a sense of fairness and desert—or at least self-interest!

At the other end, there are characteristics that we believe do not make for a good and happy life. One Dutch family illustrates the extreme end of the spectrum (Brunner *et al.* 1993*b*; Savulescu *et al.* 2006). For over thirty years this family recognized that there were a disproportionate number of male family members who exhibited aggressive and criminal behaviour (Morell 1993). This was characterized by aggressive outbursts resulting in arson, attempted rape, and exhibitionism (Brunner *et al.* 1993*a*). The behaviour was documented for almost forty years by an unaffected maternal grandfather, who could not understand why some of the men in his family appeared to be prone to this type of behaviour. Male relatives who did not display this aggressive behaviour did not express *any* type of abnormal behaviour. Unaffected males reported difficulty in understanding the behaviour of their brothers and cousins. Sisters of the males who demonstrated these extremely aggressive outbursts reported intense fear of their brothers. The behaviour did not appear to be related to environment and appeared consistently in different parts of the family, regardless of social context and degree of social contact. All affected males were also found to be mildly mentally retarded, with a typical IQ of about 85 (females had normal intelligence) (Brunner 1993*a*).[1] When a family tree was constructed, the pattern of inheritance was clearly X-linked recessive. This means, roughly, that women can carry the gene without being affected; 50 per cent of men at risk of inheriting the gene get the gene and are affected by the disease.

Genetic analysis suggested that the likely defective gene was a part of the X chromosome known as the monoamine oxidase region. This region codes for two enzymes that assist in the breakdown of neurotransmitters. Neurotransmitters are substances that play a key role in the conduction of nerve impulses in our brain. Enzymes like the monoamine oxidases are required to degrade the neurotransmitters after they have performed their desired task. It was suggested that the monoamine oxidase activity might be disturbed in the affected individuals. Urine analysis showed a higher than normal amount of neurotransmitters being excreted in the urine of affected males (Morell 1993). These results were consistent with a reduction in the functioning of one of the enzymes (monoamine oxidase A).

How can such a mutation result in violent and antisocial behaviour? A deficiency of the enzyme results in a build-up of neurotransmitters. These abnormal levels of neurotransmitters result in excessive, and even violent, reactions to stress. This hypothesis was further supported by the finding that genetically modified mice that lack this enzyme are more aggressive.

---

[1] I have discussed this example and another in considering the difference between genetic selection and manipulation in Savulescu *et al.* (2006). I have not considered issues of whether enhancement alters the identity of the individual enhanced. It is only with significant alterations of mental capabilities that questions of identity alteration arise. Enhancement decisions then become like selection decisions. Issues relating to enhancement and identity have been considered by Persson (1997) and more recently by De Grazia (2005).

This family is an extreme example of how genes can influence behaviour: it is the only family in which this mutation has been isolated. Most genetic contributions to behaviour will be weaker predispositions, but there may be some association between genes and behaviour that results in criminal and other antisocial behaviour.

How could information such as this be used? Some criminals have attempted a 'genetic defence' in the United States, stating that their genes caused them to commit the crime, but this has never succeeded. However, it is clear that couples should be allowed to test to select offspring who do not have the mutation that predisposes them to act in this way, and if interventions were available, it might be rational to correct it since children without the mutation have a better chance of a good life.

'Genes, Not Men, May Hold the Key to Female Pleasure' ran the title of one recent newspaper article (*The Age* 2005), which reported the results of a large study of female identical twins in Britain and Australia. It found that 'genes accounted for 31 per cent of the chance of having an orgasm during intercourse and 51 per cent during masturbation'. It concluded that the 'ability to gain sexual satisfaction is largely inherited' and went on to speculate that 'The genes involved could be linked to physical differences in sex organs and hormone levels or factors such as mood and anxiety.'

Our biology profoundly affects how our lives go. If we can increase sexual satisfaction by modifying biology, we should. Indeed, vast numbers of men attempt to do this already through the use of Viagra.

Summary: The Case for Enhancement

What matters is human well-being, not just treatment and prevention of disease. Our biology affects our opportunities to live well. The biological route to improvement is no different from the environmental. Biological manipulation to increase opportunity is ethical. If we have an obligation to treat and prevent disease, we have an obligation to try to manipulate these characteristics to give an individual the best opportunity of the best life.

HOW DO WE DECIDE?

If we are to enhance certain qualities, how should we decide which to choose? Eugenics was the movement early in the last century that aimed to use selective breeding to prevent degeneration of the gene pool by weeding out criminals, those with mental illness, and the poor, on the false belief that these conditions were simple genetic disorders. The eugenics movement had its inglorious peak when the Nazis moved beyond sterilization to extermination of the genetically unfit.

What was objectionable about the eugenics movement, besides its shoddy scientific basis, was that it involved the imposition of a state vision for a healthy population and aimed to achieve this through coercion. The movement was aimed not at what was good for individuals, but rather at what benefited society. Modern eugenics in the form of testing for disorders, such as Down syndrome, occurs very commonly but is acceptable because it is voluntary, gives couples a choice of what kind of child to have, and enables them to have a child with the greatest opportunity for a good life.

There are four possible ways in which our genes and biology will be decided:

1. nature or God;
2. 'experts' (philosophers, bioethicists, psychologists, scientists);
3. 'authorities' (government, doctors);
4. people themselves: liberty and autonomy.

It is a basic principle of liberal states like the United Kingdom that the state be 'neutral' to different conceptions of the good life. This means that we allow individuals to lead the life that they believe is best for themselves, implying respect for their personal autonomy or capacity for self-rule. The sole ground for interference is when that individual choice may harm others. Advice, persuasion, information, dialogue are permissible. But coercion and infringement of liberty are impermissible.

There are limits to what a liberal state should provide:

1. safety: the intervention should be reasonably safe;
2. harm to others: the intervention (like some manipulation that increases uncontrollable aggressiveness) should not result in harm. Such harm should not be direct or indirect, for example, by causing some unfair competitive advantage;
3. distributive justice: the interventions should be distributed according to principles of justice.

The situation is more complex with young children, embryos, and fetuses, who are incompetent. These human beings are not autonomous and cannot make choices themselves about whether a putative enhancement is a benefit or a harm. If a proposed intervention can be delayed until that human reaches maturity and can decide for himself or herself, then the intervention should be delayed. However, many genetic interventions will have to be performed very early in life if they are to have an effect. Decisions about such interventions should be left to parents, according to a principle of procreative liberty and autonomy. This states that parents have the freedom to choose when to have children, how many children to have, and arguably what kind of children to have.

Just as parents have wide scope to decide on the conditions of the upbringing of their children, including schooling and religious education, they should have similar freedom over their children's genes. Procreative autonomy or liberty should be extended to enhancement for two reasons. First, reproduction: bearing and raising children is a very private matter. Parents must bear much of the burden of having children, and they have a legitimate stake in the nature of the child they must invest so much of their lives raising (Savulescu 2002).

But there is a second reason. John Stuart Mill argued that when our actions only affect ourselves, we should be free to construct and act on our own conception of what is the best life for us. Mill was not a libertarian. He did not believe that such freedom is valuable solely for its own sake. He believed that freedom is important in order for people to discover for themselves what kind of life is best for themselves. It is only through 'experiments in living' that people discover what works for them and others come to see the richness and variety of lives that can be good. Mill strongly praised 'originality' and variety in choice as being essential to discovering which lives are best for human beings.

Importantly, Mill believed that some lives are worse than others. Famously, he said that it is better to be Socrates dissatisfied than a fool satisfied. He distinguished between 'higher pleasures' of 'feelings and imagination' and 'lower pleasures' of 'mere sensation' (Mill 1910: 7). He criticized 'ape-like imitation', subjugation of oneself to custom and fashion, indifference to individuality, and lack of originality (1910: 119–20, 123). Nonetheless, he was the champion of people's right to live their lives as they choose.

I have said that it is important to give the freest scope possible to uncustomary things, in order that it may appear in time which of these are fit to be converted into customs. But independence of action, and disregard of custom, are not solely deserving of encouragement for the chance they afford that better modes of action, and customs more worthy of general adoption, may be struck out; nor is it only persons of decided mental superiority who have a just claim to carry on their lives in their own way. There is no reason that all human existence should be constructed on some one or small number of patterns. If a person possesses any tolerable amount of common sense and experience, his own mode of laying out his existence is the best, not because it is the best in itself, but because it is his own mode. (Mill 1910: 125).

I believe that reproduction should be about having children with the best prospects. But to discover what are the best prospects, we must give individual couples the freedom to act on their own value judgement of what constitutes a life with good prospects. 'Experiments in reproduction' are as important as 'experiments in living' (as long as they don't harm the children who are produced). For this reason, procreative freedom is important.

There is one important limit to procreative autonomy that is different from the limits to personal autonomy. The limits to procreative autonomy should be:

1. safety;
2. harm to others;
3. distributive justice;
4. *such that the parent's choices are based on a plausible conception of well-being and a better life for the child*;

5. *consistent with development of autonomy in the child and a reasonable range of future life plans.*

These last two limits are important. It makes for a higher standard of 'proof' that an intervention will be an enhancement because the parents are making choices for their child, not themselves. The critical question to ask in considering whether to alter some gene related to complex behaviour is: Would the change be better for the individual? Is it better for the individual to have a tendency to be lazy or hardworking, monogamous or polygamous? These questions are difficult to answer. While we might let adults choose to be monogamous or polygamous, we would not let parents decide on their child's predispositions unless we were reasonably clear that some trait was better for the child.

There will be cases where some intervention is plausibly in a child's interests: increased empathy with other people, better capacity to understand oneself and the world around, or improved memory. One quality is especially associated with socio-economic success and staying out of prison: impulse control. If it were possible to correct poor impulse control, we should correct it. Whether we should remove impulsiveness altogether is another question.

Joel Feinberg has described a child's right to an open future (Feinberg 1980). An open future is one in which a child has a reasonable range of possible lives to choose from and an opportunity to choose what kind of person to be; that is, to develop autonomy. Some critics of enhancement have argued that genetic interventions are inconsistent with a child's right to an open future (Davis 1997). Far from restricting a child's future, however, some biological interventions may increase the possible futures or at least their quality. It is hard to see how improved memory or empathy would restrict a child's future. Many worthwhile possibilities would be open. But it is true that parental choice should not restrict the development of autonomy or reasonable range of possible futures open to a child. In general, fewer enhancements will be permitted in children than in adults. Some interventions, however, may still be clearly enhancements for our children, and so just like vaccinations or other preventative health care.

OBJECTIONS

Playing God or Against Nature

This objection has various forms. Some people in society believe that children are a gift, of God or of nature, and that we should not interfere in human nature. Most people implicitly reject this view: we screen embryos and fetuses for diseases, even mild correctable diseases. We interfere in nature or God's will when we vaccinate, provide pain relief to women in labour (despite objections of some earlier Christians that these practices thwarted God's will), and treat cancer. No one would object to the treatment of disability in a child if it were possible. Why, then, not treat the embryo with genetic therapy if that intervention is safe? This is no more thwarting God's will than giving antibiotics.

Another variant of this objection is that we are arrogant if we assume we could have sufficient knowledge to meddle with human nature. Some people object that we cannot know the complexity of the human system, which is like an unknowable magnificent symphony. To attempt to enhance one characteristic may have other unknown, unforeseen effects elsewhere in the system. We should not play God since, unlike God, we are not omnipotent or omniscient. We should be humble and recognize the limitations of our knowledge.

A related objection is that genes are pleiotropic—which means they have different effects in different environments. The gene or genes that predispose to manic depression may also be responsible for heightened creativity and productivity.

One response to both of these objections is to limit intervention, until our knowledge grows, to selecting between different embryos, and not intervening to enhance particular embryos or people. Since we would be choosing between complete systems on the basis of their type, we would not be interfering with the internal machinery. In this way, selection is less risky than enhancement (Savulescu *et al.* 2006).

But such a precaution could also be misplaced when considering biological interventions. When benefits are on offer, such objections remind us to refrain from hubris and over-confidence. We must do adequate research before intervening. And because the benefits may be fewer than when we treat or prevent disease, we may require the standards of safety to be higher than for medical interventions. But we must weigh the risks against the benefits. If confidence is justifiably high, and benefits outweigh harms, we should enhance.

Once technology affords us the power to enhance our own and our children's lives, to fail to do so would be to be responsible for the consequences. To fail to treat our children's diseases is to wrong them. To fail to prevent them from getting depression is to wrong them. To fail to improve their physical, musical, psychological, and other capacities is to wrong them, just as it would be to harm them if we gave them a toxic substance that stunted or reduced these capacities.

Another variant of the 'Playing God' objection is that there is a special value in the balance and diversity that natural variation affords, and enhancement will reduce this. But in so far as we are products of evolution, we are merely random chance variations of genetic traits selected for our capacity to survive long enough to reproduce. There is no design to evolution. Evolution selects genes, according to environment, that confer the greatest chance of survival and reproduction. Evolution would select a tribe that was highly fertile but suffered great pain the whole of their lives over another tribe that was less fertile but suffered less pain. Medicine has changed evolution: we can now select individuals who experience less pain and disease. The next stage of human evolution will be rational evolution, according to which we select children who not only have the greatest chance of surviving, reproducing, and being free of disease, but who have the greatest opportunities to have the best lives in their likely environment. Evolution was indifferent to how well our lives went; we are not. We want to retire, play golf, read, and watch our grandchildren have children.

'Enhancement' is a misnomer. It suggests luxury. But enhancement is no luxury. In so far as it promotes well-being, it is the very essence of what is necessary for a good human life. There is no moral reason to preserve some traits—such as uncontrollable aggressiveness, a sociopathic personality, or extreme deviousness. Tell the victim of rape and murder that we must preserve diversity and the natural balance.

Genetic Discrimination

Some people fear the creation of a two-tier society of the enhanced and the unenhanced, where the inferior, unenhanced are discriminated against and disadvantaged all through life.

We must remember that nature allots advantage and disadvantage with no gesture to fairness. Some are born horribly disadvantaged, destined to die after short and miserable lives. Some suffer great genetic disadvantage while others are born gifted, physically, musically, or intellectually. There is no secret that there are 'gifted' children naturally. Allowing choice to change our biology will, if anything, be more egalitarian, allowing the ungifted to approach the gifted. There is nothing fair about the natural lottery: allowing enhancement may be fairer.

But more importantly, how well the lives of those who are disadvantaged go depends not on whether enhancement is permitted, but on the social institutions we have in place to protect the least well off and provide everyone with a fair chance. People have disease and disability: egalitarian social institutions and laws against discrimination are designed to make sure everyone, regardless of natural inequality, has a decent chance of a decent life. This would be no different if enhancement were permitted. There is no necessary connection between enhancement and discrimination, just as there is no necessary connection between curing disability and discrimination against people with disability.

The Perfect Child, Sterility, and Loss of the Mystery of Life

If we engineered perfect children, this objection goes, the world would be a sterile, monotonous place where everyone was the same, and the mystery and surprise of life would be gone.

It is impossible to create perfect children. We can only attempt to create children with better opportunities of a better life. There will necessarily be difference. Even in the case of screening for disability, like Down syndrome, 10 per cent of people choose not to abort a pregnancy known to be affected by Down syndrome. People value different things. There will never be complete convergence. Moreover, there will remain massive challenges for individuals to meet in their personal relationships and in the hurdles our unpredictable environment presents. There will remain much mystery and challenge—we will just be better able to deal with these. We will still have to work to achieve, but our achievements may have greater value.

Against Human Nature

One of the major objections to enhancement is that it is against human nature. Common alternative phrasings are that enhancement is tampering with our nature or an affront to human dignity. I believe that what separates us from other animals is our rationality, our capacity to make normative judgements and act on the basis of reasons (Savulescu 2003). When we make decisions to improve our lives by biological and other manipulations, we express our rationality and express what is fundamentally important about our nature. And if those manipulations improve our capacity to make rational and normative judgements, they further improve what is fundamentally human. Far from being against the human spirit, such improvements express the human spirit. To be human is to be better.

Enhancements Are Self-Defeating

Another familiar objection to enhancement is that enhancements will have self-defeating or other adverse social effects. A typical example is increase in height. If height is socially desired, then everyone will try to enhance the height of their children at great cost to themselves and the environment (as taller people consume more resources), with no advantage in the end since there will be no relative gain.

If a purported manipulation does not improve well-being or opportunity, there is no argument in favour of it. In this case, the manipulation is not an enhancement. In other cases, such as enhancement of intelligence, the enhancement of one individual may increase that individual's opportunities only at the expense of another. So-called positional goods are goods only in a relative sense.

But many enhancements will have both positional and non-positional qualities. Intelligence is good not just because it allows an individual to be more competitive for complex jobs, but because it allows an individual to process information more rapidly in her own life, and to develop greater understanding of herself and others. These non-positional effects should not be ignored. Moreover, even in the case of so-called purely positional goods, such as height, there may be important non-positional values. It is better to be taller if you are a basketball player, but being tall is a disadvantage in balance sports such as gymnastics, skiing, and surfing.

Nonetheless, if there are significant social consequences of enhancement, this is of course a valid objection. But it is not particular to enhancement: there is an old question about how far individuals in society can pursue their own self-interest at a cost to others. It applies to education, health care, and virtually all areas of life.

Not all enhancements will be ethical. The critical issue is that the intervention is expected to bring about more benefits than harms to the individual. It must be safe and there must be a reasonable expectation of improvement. Some of the other features of ethical enhancements are summarized below.

What Is an Ethical Enhancement?

An ethical enhancement:

1. is in the person's interests;
2. is reasonably safe;
3. increases the opportunity to have the best life;
4. promotes or does not unreasonably restrict the range of possible lives open to that person;
5. does not unreasonably harm others directly through excessive costs in making it freely available;
6. does not place that individual at an unfair competitive advantage with respect to others, e.g. mind-reading;
7. is such that the person retains significant control or responsibility for her achievements and self that cannot be wholly or directly attributed to the enhancement;
8. does not unreasonably reinforce or increase unjust inequality and discrimination—economic inequality, racism.

What Is an Ethical Enhancement for a Child or Incompetent Human Being?

Such an ethical enhancement is all the above, but in addition:

1. the intervention cannot be delayed until the child can make its own decision;
2. the intervention is plausibly in the child's interests;
3. the intervention is compatible with the development of autonomy.

CONCLUSION

Enhancement is already occurring. In sport, human erythropoietin boosts red blood cells. Steroids and growth hormone improve muscle strength. Many people seek cognitive enhancement through nicotine, Ritalin, Modavigil, or caffeine. Prozac, recreational drugs, and alcohol all enhance mood. Viagra is used to improve sexual performance.

And of course mobile phones and aeroplanes are examples of external enhancing technologies. In the future, genetic technology, nanotechnology, and artificial intelligence may profoundly affect our capacities.

Will the future be better or just disease-free? We need to shift our frame of reference from health to life enhancement. What matters is how we live. Technology can now improve that. We have two options:

1. Intervention:
   * treating disease;
   * preventing disease;
   * supra-prevention of disease—preventing disease in a radically unprecedented way;
   * protection of well-being;
   * enhancement of well-being.
2. No intervention, and to remain in a state of nature—no treatment or prevention of disease, no technological enhancement.

I believe that to be human is to be better. Or, at least, to strive to be better. We should be here for a *good* time, not just a *long* time. Enhancement, far from being merely permissible, is something we should aspire to achieve.

REFERENCES

AGAR, N. (2003), *Liberal Eugenics* (Oxford: Blackwell).

The Age (2005), 'Genes, Not Men, May Hold the Key to Female Pleasure', 9 June.

ANNAS, G. (2000), 'The Man on the Moon, Immortality and Other Millennial Myths: The Prospects and Perils of Human Genetic Engineering', *Emory Law Journal*, 49/3: 753–82.

BRUNNER, H. G., NELEN, M., *et al.* (1993*a*), 'Abnormal Behaviour Associated with a Point Mutation in the Structural Gene for Monoamine Oxidase A', *Science*, 262/5133: 578–80.

—— *et al.* (1993*b*), 'X-Linked Borderline Mental Retardation with Prominent Behavioural Disturbance: Phenotype, Genetic Localization, and Evidence for Disturbed Monoamine Metabolism', *American Journal of Human Genetics*, 52: 1032–9.

BUCHANAN, A., BROCK, D., DANIELS, N., and WIKLER, D. (2000), *From Chance to Choice* (Cambridge: Cambridge University Press).

CHEITLIN, M. D., HUTTER, A. M., *et al.* (1999), 'ACC/AHA Expert Consensus Document JACC: Use of Sildenafil (Viagra) in Patients with Cardiovascular Disease', *Journal of the American College of Cardiology*, 33/1: 273–82.

DAVIS, D. (1997) 'Genetic Dilemmas and the Child's Right to an Open Future', *Hastings Center Report*, 27/2 (Mar.–Apr.), 7–15.

DE GRAZIA, D. (2005), 'Enhancement Technologies and Human Identity', *Journal of Medicine and Philosophy*, 30: 261–83.

DE MARCHI, N., DANIELE, F., and RAGONE, M. A. (2001), 'Fluoxetine in the Treatment of Huntington's Disease', *Psychopharmacology*, 153/2: 264–6.

DICKENS, W., and FLYNN, J. (2001), 'Heritability Estimates Versus Large Environmental Effects: The IQ Paradox Resolved', *Psychological Review*, 108/2: 346–69.

ELLIOTT, C. (2003), *Better Than Well: American Medicine Meets the American Dream* (New York: W. W. Norton).

FEINBERG, J. (1980), 'The Child's Right to an Open Future', in W. Aiken and H. LaFollette (eds.), *Whose Child? Parental Rights, Parental Authority and State Power* (Totowa, NJ: Rowman and Littlefield), 124–53.

FUKUYAMA, F. (2003), *Our Posthuman Future: Consequences of the Biotechnology Revolution* (London: Profile).

HABERMAS, J. (2003), *The Future of Human Nature* (Cambridge: Polity Press).

HARRIS, J. (2000), 'Intimations of Immortality', *Science*, 288/5463: 59.

—— (2002), 'Intimations of Immortality: The Ethics and Justice of Life Extending Therapies', in M. Freeman (ed.), *Current Legal Problems* (Oxford: Oxford University Press), 65–95.

—— (2004), 'Immortal Ethics', in A. D. N. J. de Grey (ed.), 'Strategies for Engineered Negligible Senescence: Why Genuine Control of Aging May Be Foreseeable', *Annals of the New York Academy of Science*, 1019: 527–34.

HOLDEN, C. (2003), 'Don't Go Off the Prozac', *Science*, 301: 760.

—— (2004), 'Treatment of Newborn Mice Raises Anxiety', *Science*, 306: 792.

HOLLOWAY, M. (1999), 'Flynn's Effect', *Scientific American*, 280/1 (Jan.), 37.

KAMM, F. (2005), 'Is There a Problem with Enhancement?', *American Journal of Bioethics*, 5/3: 5–14.

KASS, L. R. (2002), *Life, Liberty and the Defense of Dignity: The Challenge for Bioethics* (San Francisco: Encounter Books).

LIM, M. (2004), *Nature*, 429: 754–7.

LIU, Z. J., RICHMOND, B. J. A., *et al.* (2004), 'DNA Targeting of Rhinal Cortex D2 Receptor Protein Reversibly Blocks Learning of Cues that Predict Reward', *Proceedings of the National Academy of Sciences*, 101/33: 12336–41.

MILL, J. S. (1910), *On Liberty* (London: J. M. Dent).

MISCHEL, W., SHODA, Y., and PEAKE, P. K. (1988), 'The Nature of Adolescent Competencies Predicted by Preschool Delay of Gratification', *Journal of Personality and Social Psychology*, 54/4: 687–96.

MORELL, V. (1993), 'Evidence Found for a Possible "Aggression Gene"', *Science*, 260: 1722–3.

PALMA, V., LIM, D., *et al.* (2005), 'Sonic Hedgehog Controls Stem Cell Behaviour in the Postnatal and Adult Brain', *Development*, 132: 335–44.

PERSSON, I. (1997), 'Genetic Therapy, Person-Regarding Reasons and the Determination of Identity: A Reply to Robert Elliot', *Bioethics*, 11/2: 161–9.

PRESIDENT'S COUNCIL ON BIOETHICS (2003), *Beyond Therapy: Biotechnology and the Pursuit of Happiness* (New York: Dana Press).

RIETZE, R., VALCANIS, H., *et al.* (2001), 'Purification of a Pluripotent Neural Stem Cell from the Adult Mouse Brain', *Nature*, 412: 736–9.

SANDEL, M. (2004), 'The Case Against Perfection', *Atlantic Monthly* (Apr. 2004), 51–62.

SAVULESCU, J. (2002), 'Deaf Lesbians, "Designer Disability," and the Future of Medicine', *British Medical Journal*, 325/7367: 771–3.

_____ (2003), 'Human–Animal Transgenesis and Chimeras Might Be an Expression of Our Humanity', *American Journal of Bioethics*, 3/3: 22–5.

_____ HEMSLEY, M., NEWSON, A., and FODDY, B. (2006), 'Behavioural Genetics: Why Eugenic Selection Is Preferable to Enhancement', *Journal of Applied Philosophy*, 23/2: 157–71.

SOCIETY FOR NEUROSCIENCE (2004), 'Early Life Stress Harms Mental Function and Immune System in Later Years According to New Research', 26 Oct., <http://apu.sfn.org/content /AboutSFN1/NewsReleases/am2004_early.html>, accessed Feb. 2006.

SPIRES, T., GROTE, H., *et al.* (2004), 'Environmental Enrichment Rescues Protein Deficits in a Mouse Model of Huntington's Disease, Indicating a Possible Disease Mechanism', *Journal of Neuroscience*, 24/9: 2270–6.

SULLIVAN, F. R., BIRD, E. D., ALPAY, M., and CHA, J. H. (2001), 'Remotivation Therapy and Huntington's Disease', *Journal of Neuroscience Nursing*, 33/3: 136–42.

URNOV, F. D., MILLER, J. C., *et al.* (2005), 'Highly Efficient Endogenous Human Gene Correction Using Designed Zinc-Finger Nucleases', *Nature*, 435: 646–51.

VAN DELLEN, A., BLAKEMORE, C., *et al.* (2000), 'Delaying the Onset of Huntington's in Mice', *Nature*, 404: 721–2.

CHAPTER 23

PHARMACOGENOMICS: ETHICAL AND REGULATORY ISSUES

MATTHEW DECAMP AND ALLEN BUCHANAN

INTRODUCTION

PHARMACOGENOMICS and pharmacogenetics attempt to elucidate the role of genetic variation in human responses to compounds introduced into the body, such as medications.[1] Although the notion of genetic determinants of drug response and toxicity dates to at least the 1950s (Weber 2001), new molecular techniques and the completion of the Human Genome Project promise to reveal genetic variations

---

[1]   The difference between pharmacogenomics and pharmacogenetics is not fixed in the literature. For example, some (Lindpainter 2003) suggest that -*genomics* be limited solely to gene expression analyses, whereas -*genetics* be used primarily to denote any number of inherited differences in DNA sequences (e.g. single nucleotide polymorphisms, or SNPs) that correlate with differential drug response. In this chapter we use 'pharmacogenomics' as a more inclusive term that incorporates pharmacogenetics as well as the genome-wide expression analyses (e.g. DNA microarrays) of pharmacogenomics. Only where necessary will we distinguish the two.

at an unprecedented rate. Already, some institutions use pharmacogenomic tests to avoid adverse drug effects, via dosing changes, that sometimes result from the anti-coagulant warfarin (Higashi *et al.* 2002) and the chemotherapeutic drug 6-MP (Marshall 2003). In late 2003 Roche Diagnostics released information on its AmpliChip™ technology, which would test genetic variations of the cytochrome P450 enzymes crucial to drug metabolism (Roche Diagnostics 2003). On the horizon are pharmacogenomic tests to aid cancer therapy (Marsh and McLeod 2004), asthma treatment (Dewar and Hall 2003), and prediction of response to anti-hypertensive agents (Kreutz 2004), among others. The end of 'one size fits all' medicine–and the beginning of 'personalized medicine'—appears to be near, with pharmacogenomics playing a major role (Langheier and Snyderman 2004).

The potential benefits of pharmacogenomic methodologies are multifarious and could dramatically change the health care system. Adverse reactions resulting from medications are a major cause of morbidity and mortality, as well as a cost for health care systems, as a recent report from the US Institute of Medicine Committee on Quality of Health Care in America has shown (Kohn *et al.* 2000). Although many adverse reactions result from human error, others are caused by individual differences in drug absorption, distribution, metabolism, and excretion that are the result of genetic variation. A better understanding of these factors may reduce adverse drug reactions (Phillips *et al.* 2001; O'Kane *et al.* 2003), as recent research with the HIV drug abacavir suggests (Hughes *et al.* 2004). In addition, advocates of pharmacogenomics anticipate a streamlined drug development process, both by focusing on specific drug targets (for example, particular receptors) and through the use of smaller clinical trials restricted to individuals whose genotypes make them more likely to respond and less likely to suffer a serious adverse event. Finally, pharmacogenomics might rescue drugs abandoned in the past owing to serious toxic side effects if researchers can show that only a genetic subpopulation suffered the toxic response. These are but a few of the highly publicized benefits of pharmacogenomics.

Not everyone is taken by this excitement, however. Some criticize the pharmacogenomic methodology itself. For example, from a scientific standpoint, van Aken *et al.* (2003) recognize the impact of pharmacogenomics, specifically on the use of 6-MP, but also note that a larger percentage of adverse reactions could be unrelated to genetic polymorphisms. Why devote so many resources to a small, though important, part of adverse drug reactions if more adverse reactions result from preventable human error? Moreover, one should not ignore the role of multiple mutations (e.g. if a test reveals an individual to be a slow metabolizer of 6-MP, but another, unused test could reveal him or her to also be a fast excretor, thereby compensating for the original variant), polygenic traits, overlapping metabolic pathways, other environmental influences, or concomitant disease status, such as kidney and liver disease (Nebert *et al.* 2003).

Holtzman (2003) further substantiates this healthy skepticism with an analysis that shows the predictive value of most current pharmacogenomic tests to be relatively low. Unfortunately, some findings are nevertheless being prematurely applied via direct-to-consumer Internet marketing of pharmacogenomics, causing some to question the regulation of these tests, or the lack thereof.[2]

To take these scientific concerns seriously is to acknowledge the speculative nature of some of what follows but does not make the discussion fruitless. Instead, discussion and deliberation may help shape the technological development of pharmacogenomics in a beneficial way (Hedgecoe and Martin 2003). Moreover, it may be more prudent to explore a range of possible issues, some of which may not arise, than to be overtaken by events owing to the failure to think ahead.

It is fruitful to distinguish between concerns about pharmacogenomics as a methodology and concerns arising from the embodiment of the methodology in particular technologies. Some issues may be invariant to the choice of technologies; others may be specific to them.

While acknowledging the potential benefits of pharmacogenomics as a methodology, a number of comprehensive reports in the past several years examine a multitude of ethical, legal, and social factors that may limit the extent to which these benefits are realized—and realized in ethically acceptable ways (Buchanan *et al.* 2002; Consortium on Pharmacogenetics 2002; Freund and Wilfond 2002; Robertson *et al.* 2002; Melzer *et al.* 2003; Nuffield Council on Bioethics 2003; Rothstein 2003). Our purpose in this chapter is to identify and explore the most basic ethical and regulatory issues that are likely to arise if pharmacogenomics becomes widely enough used to have a significant impact on research and clinical practice. First, however, we address the question of whether pharmacogenomic tests are unique when compared to other genetic tests and thus deserving of more or less stringent ethical and regulatory requirements.

Is Pharmacogenomics Unique?

In a now frequently cited article, Roses (2000) makes the claim that pharmacogenomic tests are distinct from other genetic tests, specifically those genetic tests that are related to disease genes.[3] Roses argues that because pharmacogenomic tests are employed to determine likely medicine response, they do not carry the problematic ethical, legal, and social implications of genetic tests for diseases or predispositions

---

[2] For one example, see <http://www.bankdna.com/index.html>, accessed 5 July 2006.

[3] It is interesting to note that this view, which might be called 'pharmacogenomic exceptionalism', runs counter to 'genetic exceptionalism' more broadly construed. On the latter view, all genetic information is somehow unique and deserves *more* stringent protections, whereas the pharmacogenomic version seeks to carve pharmacogenomic information out of this circle and place it back with other, 'less threatening', medical information. In fact, neither form of exceptionalism is tenable, and for similar reasons. For one argument against genetic exceptionalism, see Green and Botkin (2003).

to diseases. Freund and Wilfond (2002) add that the uniqueness of pharmacogenomic technologies may be their distinct function: to help identify an appropriate and available intervention. One might conclude from these characterizations that pharmacogenomic tests require less stringent regulatory protections, for example, regarding the confidentiality of pharmacogenomic data, because these data are less likely to result in harm when compared to genetic tests for disease or the risk of genetic disease in one's offspring. Less stringent regulatory requirements could be advantageous because they might enable research to proceed without being hindered by the many ethical debates that have occurred in other areas of genetics (e.g. the US ethical, legal, and social implications program for the Human Genome Project).

A closer analysis, however, reveals that the supposed bright line distinction between pharmacogenomic tests and other genetic tests is in fact rather blurry (Lindpaintner 2003). Immediately after Freund and Wilfond (2002) make their proposal, they note that regulatory decisions might need to be made on a case-by-case basis, not on the basis of 'pharmacogenomic' versus 'other' genetic tests. The attempt to draw such a sharp distinction breaks down on several fronts.

First, pharmacogenomic tests will not solely be used to select one intervention from among several equivalent alternatives. Some tests might reveal that no safe intervention is available, whereas others might reveal that a therapeutic intervention is available but at an extremely high price. Both scenarios could raise concerns about discrimination regarding insurance coverage or cost. For example, suppose a pharmacogenomic profile of tissue from an individual with breast cancer reveals that standard therapy will be ineffective at preventing metastasis. This yields information about the type of treatment that will be needed and perhaps about future disease prognosis, both of which might interest an insurance company.

Second, in some cases, pharmacogenomic tests will be associated with 'disease' information. For example, the same genetic marker used in a pharmacogenomic test may also indicate a predisposition to a particular disease. Similarly, because the same genes are often involved in drug metabolism and environmental substance detoxification (drugs, after all, are merely a controlled environmental exposure), information from pharmacogenomic tests might also reveal the potential for environmentally mediated disease (Schulte et al. 1999). Were this not the case, one would not expect the US National Institute of Environmental Health Sciences to devote a substantial portion of its initial Environmental Genome Project budget to pharmacogenomics. So it is a mistake to assume either that pharmacogenomic information only conveys likelihood of drug response or that information about the likelihood of drug response is devoid of psychosocial significance.

Lindpainter (2003) goes a step further by noting that pharmacogenomics may in fact be *more* likely to evoke ethical issues. First, he surmises that because genetic information about drug response will be available to more people in the health care process, from physician to nurse to pharmacist to administrator, the risks of disclosure are greater. Second, he notes that in certain cases an individual might be found not only to be at high risk of a particular disease via a 'disease' genetic test, but also at high risk not to respond to conventional therapy via a pharmacogenomic test. Under these conditions, the pharmacogenomic test results become even more important from a strictly financial insurance standpoint.

On balance, then, there seems to be no reason to require less or more stringent protections for pharmacogenomic tests as a group. It is more reasonable to remain open-minded as one explores the alternative technologies in which the methodology may come to be employed and the social, legal, and economic context in which these technologies are likely to be utilized.

ETHICAL ISSUES IN TECHNOLOGICAL DEVELOPMENT

Who Will Develop Pharmacogenomics, and For Whom?

Although it may be unconventional to raise economic incentives as the first 'ethical' issue arising in pharmacogenomics, we do so because who receives the eventual benefits of pharmacogenomic advances (and who bears its costs) will be partly determined by economic considerations. Because the economic incentive structure will help determine who benefits and how these benefits are distributed, it is subject to evaluation from the standpoint of justice. Often, ethical analyses *conclude* with discussions of justice; unfortunately this encourages the false assumption that issues of justice regarding access to and distribution of benefits and costs can be adequately addressed independently of evaluating the production process. To make this assumption is to ignore the possibility that a particular production process, once in place, may seriously limit the possibilities for how its products may be distributed. A widely cited statistic is that 90 per cent of the world's disease burden receives 10 per cent of the funding for relief of this burden. If this is true, either the 'distribute later' approach would need to be of Herculean proportions, or an alternative means is necessary in order to achieve a more just global distribution (Advisory Committee on Health Research 2002). Changing the nature of the production process by modifying the incentives of those who decide which products to try to develop may be a necessary element in any realistic strategy to secure a more equitable distribution of benefits from medical research. As we shall see shortly, one factor that may shape incentives is the nature of the intellectual property rules under which research and development occurs.

One major economic concern of pharmacogenomics is the effect of market segmentation. Market segmentation would occur if drugs that would otherwise be available to everyone with a particular condition became available only to a subset people with a particular genotype. The question is whether such a situation would prevent the development of particular drugs (because the target market is not large enough to support them) or prevent access (because the costs of drug development would be spread over a smaller number of individuals). This could result in the identification of 'orphan genotypes' that do not have markets large enough to attract pharmaceutical investment (Rothstein and Epps 2001). As Reeder and Dickson (2003) point out, however, the situation is complex; as noted below, pharmacogenomics might at the same time reduce the costs of drug development with better and more efficient drug targets as well as smaller, more efficient clinical trials. Furthermore, smaller pharmaceutical companies might fill the leftover niche and develop these small market pharmacogenomic drugs.

One example of a prospective effort to promote a more just distribution of therapeutics is the 1983 US Orphan Drug Act.[4] This law requires the US Food and Drug Administration (FDA) to assist companies that are developing a drug for a disease afflicting fewer than 200,000 individuals or a drug that has no reasonable expectation of recouping expenditures via US sales. The Act creates economic incentives for pharmaceutical companies to develop drugs they might otherwise find unprofitable. These incentives are provided by tax breaks and small grants for clinical trials, but also by what amounts to a minor modification of the existing intellectual property rules: if a company develops an 'orphan drug', then the FDA will approve no competing drugs for the same condition for seven years after the original marketing approval.

The tacit assumption behind the Orphan Drug Act is that the most effective way to redress an inequity in the distribution of health care is to modify the process by which health care benefits are produced. Although not designed with orphan genotypes in mind, the Act could presumably be reinterpreted or amended to cover them.

Before such a strategy is seriously considered, two questions need to be answered. First, is the use of pharmacogenomics in drug development likely to lead to new 'orphan' problems? At this point, it is probably too early to tell. Second, how well has the US Orphan Drug Act (and its analogues in Japan and the European Union) worked in addressing the inequities it was designed to ameliorate? Many consider it to be already a success in the United States, noting that over 230 orphan products were developed in the nine years after the Act passed, compared to ten in the preceding decade, many of which were by large pharmaceutical companies (Haffner *et al.* 2002). Rai (2002*b*) argues that if the Act is extended to pharmacogenomic 'orphan genotype' groups, gains in equity could be made in a cost-effective manner.

However, the plausibility of relying on orphan drug acts should not preclude other forms of forward thinking about better means of attaining distributive justice regarding the availability of valuable medicines. Many orphan diseases have yet to pique the interests of pharmaceutical companies. If the number of persons for whom

---

[4] For more information, see <http://www.fda.gov/orphan/oda.htm>, accessed 5 July 2006.

effective therapies are not developed increases as a result of so-called 'orphan genotypes'—identified by the use of pharmacogenomic tests—what some consider to be an already underfunded system (only $US13.5 million in grants are awarded each year, an amount that has been relatively stable) will be inadequate (Stevens 2003).

In addition, some argue the drugs covered by the Orphan Drug Act are of marginal clinical utility; for example, a particular drug to treat amyotrophic lateral sclerosis has been shown to increase life expectancy by three months (Miller 2003). In other words, the Act may not adequately distinguish between relatively good and relatively poor efficacy drugs. And even if one solution might be to modify the Orphan Drug Act, as Rohde (2000) suggests, this leaves open the solution to distributive justice at the global level (Trouiller and Olliaro 1999; Pang 2003). Clearly, if the wider use of pharmacogenomics in drug development contributes to the problem of lack of availability of medicines for certain groups of patients, more work is needed to determine whether an Orphan Drug Act approach will be effective.

Will Intellectual Property Stifle or Stimulate Pharmacogenomic Technologies?

A related economic factor may serve to limit the usefulness of pharmacogenomics. DNA microarrays consisting of sequences from multiple if not hundreds of genes are a staple of contemporary pharmacogenomics and genomics in general. Many have expressed concern that the viability of microarray technology may be endangered by genomic patent rights awarded over the past several years (Rouse and Hardiman 2003). For example, suppose a DNA microarray to assess the pharmacogenomic profile of an individual's breast cancer utilizes ten genes which together yield a test with high predictive value. Take any single gene sequence out, and the predictive value is substantially reduced. Now suppose several companies own patents on these genes. For optimal predictive value, all of the genes are needed, but if even one company enforces its intellectual property rights with cost prohibitive licensing (or the denial of licensing), society may be forced to accept a lower quality test. Furthermore, as the number of genes increases, so do the transaction costs necessary to obtain licensing, and the costs can add up quickly.

This predicament has been labeled the 'anti-commons' problem (Heller and Eisenberg 1998) because strong intellectual property rights paradoxically deter the use of resources to develop new products (in this case, pharmacogenomic microarray tests). Similar concerns led Rai (2002a) to question whether research platforms (not just genomic ones) should be patented, even if the downstream products they produce are patentable.

On the other hand, one should not confuse strong intellectual property rights with how those rights are exercised. Interview data suggest that many research stakeholders find ways around strong intellectual property rights via permissive 'licensing, inventing around patents, going offshore, the development and use of public databases and research tools, court challenges, and simply using the technology without a license' (Walsh *et al.* 2003). Nevertheless, many remain concerned about how intellectual property rights will affect the basic science research necessary prior to product development. From an ethical standpoint, the topic of this section echoes the previous one: the rules and frameworks that create incentives and disincentives to various types of product development are subject to ethical evaluation because they affect not only who will have access to what gets produced, but also what gets produced in the first place.

Here it is crucial to understand that the evaluation of alternative intellectual property rights regimes is not a strictly technical question, and certainly not reducible to the question of selecting the optimal means for achieving a single, uncontroversial goal. The current debate over strong (i.e. broadly awarding patent rights to DNA sequences and their potential uses) and weak (i.e. narrowly awarding such rights) intellectual property rights mistakenly proceeds as if the maximization of innovation were the only good involved; it does not often consider the distribution of these innovations, whether the innovations themselves are good (or good on balance given their negative features or effects), or from whose standpoint they are regarded as good. Quite simply, there are some innovations, such as nuclear weapons, that we might arguably be better without. Similarly, some contend that some possible genomic innovations (such as genetic interventions to 'enhance' human embryos or treatments involving human embryos as sources for stem cells) are morally unacceptable in themselves or likely to contribute to significant social harms. To the extent that the regulation of research and development in pharmacogenomics is affected by policy choices concerning intellectual property rules, it raises these same perplexing, though largely neglected, ethical issues.

Streamlining Clinical Trials—At What Cost?

As noted in the Introduction, pharmacogenomics may come to enhance the efficiency of clinical trials at almost every stage in drug development: from identifying drug targets to preclinical studies to all phases of clinical trials, including postmarketing surveillance (Manasco and Arledge 2003). The basic notion is simple: one could rationally design clinical trials to exclude those likely to experience toxic side effects and include those more likely to respond to a given experimental drug. These strategies could thereby identify more drug targets and then test them faster and more efficiently than under the previous scheme. However, such a streamlining strategy raises two critical questions: First, how does the use of pharmacogenomic testing in clinical trials affect the ethics of clinical research (Issa 2002)? And second, are there costs associated with this increased efficiency?

Issa (2002) cites the ethical principles proposed by Emanuel *et al.* (2000) and analyzes their applicability to pharmacogenomic clinical trials. At least three of their seven proposed criteria are particularly applicable in this context: value to society, fair subject selection, and minimization of risks. If pharmacogenomics delivers on its promise to identify genetic variations that affect drug response, the value of pharmacogenomically driven research will be clear. Furthermore, fair subject selection and the minimization of risks may not simply *allow* pharmacogenomic clinical trials—it may *require* them, for example, if a drug reaction to be avoided is particularly severe or likely, and it is also adequately predicted based on a pharmacogenomic test.

However, this increased efficiency comes at a cost. First, the eventual clinical trial results, because they are based on a select population, will only be generally applicable to that population. This could be important if the individuals excluded from the trial have no other therapeutic options. Should they take the approved drug? To draw an analogy with a non-genetic drug, consider a recent debate about whether tamoxifen—a therapeutic agent thought to be effective only in breast tumors that have estrogen receptors—should be given to women with a known genetic risk of breast cancer to prevent recurrence of the disease. Some small studies suggest that even if these women have tumors that lack estrogen receptors, tamoxifen might be effective in certain circumstances (Foulkes *et al.* 2002). Whether or not this particular finding is validated, the general message is that researchers might, as a result of 'rational' design processes, mistakenly exclude individuals from a treatment that could otherwise benefit them. In some cases, no substitute exists but to perform the trial.

A second cost of smaller, faster clinical trials is that the detection of rare, unanticipated adverse drug responses might be even further decreased than at present. To compensate, society might need a more extensive postmarketing surveillance system, thereby offsetting some of the potential cost savings of streamlined clinical trials. It is important to recognize, then, that the increased efficiency of clinical trials will come at a price. Further reflection on these costs may be needed before pharmacogenomically directed trials proceed on a broad scale.

Pharmacogenomics: Reifying Race and Ethnicity, or Transcending It?

Clinical trials, whether in pharmacogenomic or other research areas, sometimes raise politically charged questions about the use of race in medicine and in biomedical publication (Risch *et al.* 2002; Bamshad *et al.* 2003; Holden 2003; Kaplan and Bennett 2003). For example, the HIV study noted in the Introduction (Hughes *et al.* 2004) differentiates between Whites, Blacks, and Hispanics, and also draws conclusions from these groupings. Another recent controversy surrounds a heart failure drug (BiDil) that may be marketed specifically to African Americans (Kahn 2003). In addition, a major international project to create a haplotype map (the International HapMap) includes samples characterized by origins in Africa, Asia, and Europe.[5] The literature on this topic has grown quickly, reaching the popular scientific press (Bamshad and Olson 2003). The primary concern is that pharmacogenomic findings might reinforce preexisting ethnic or racial stereotypes or create new ones, for example, if a particular group is associated with a higher frequency of 'difficult to treat' diseases. This is the pharmacogenomic analogue of worries on the part of Ashkenazi Jews that they would be stigmatized as having bad 'Jewish genes' as a result of the finding that a genetic predisposition to breast cancer occurred at a slightly higher frequency in their population.

At the same time, others might believe that preexisting social categories might be used in order to help remove health disparities; for example, Howard University has created the Genomic Research in the African Diaspora Biobank to help address health issues specific to those of African descent.[6]

In order to conceptualize the literature on the role of race in research, Weijer and Miller (2004) divide arguments into three separate categories. One view takes race to be biologically irrelevant; it is entirely a social construct, so its use in pharmacogenomics would be generally unjustified (Schwartz 2001). A second considers race at least partly biological, but often inappropriately applied; on this view the challenge is to distinguish between legitimate and illegitimate uses (Burchard et al. 2003). Finally, a third suggests that the imprecision of socially defined race and ethnicity should be replaced by scientifically (i.e. genetically) defined groups (Foster et al. 2001). Weijer and Miller (2004) do not try to determine which approach is best, but note that each has obvious policy implications.

What can be said regarding these options? One should distinguish between stating that race and ethnicity are genetically based versus stating that race and ethnicity correlate, no matter how weakly or strongly, with genetic differences between groups. Regarding the former assertion, it is perhaps clear that race and ethnicity are not genetically based or somehow wholly caused by genetics; racial and ethnic categories can change over time, often depend on self-reporting, and may lead to genetically heterogeneous populations being grouped together. For example, in one study, genetic frequencies differed between black individuals from Nigeria versus black individuals in the United States (Cooper et al. 2000), yet both might be called 'African American' in a research study. This reveals a weakness of scientific reliance on social labels to approximate genetic homogeneity.

On the other hand, it also seems uncontroversial to assert, from a population genetics standpoint, that phenomena such as the 'founder effect' and differing selection pressures might lead to different gene frequencies among different populations.

---

[5] For updated information, see <http://www.hapmap.org>, accessed 5 July 2006.
[6] For more information, see <http://www.genomecenter.howard.edu>, accessed 5 July 2006.

If no differences existed between different populations, no matter how they are defined, there would be nothing to report. The statement that all humans are 99.9 per cent identical, though often used as support for the thesis that race and ethnicity are entirely separate from genetics, is misleading. What matters is whether the remaining 0.1 per cent of the 3 billion base pairs is significantly variable, not simply its absolute number. Therefore, part of the race and genomics quandary remains a scientific problem, and until we have a better idea of how well social categories do (or do not) approximate genetic homogeneity or heterogeneity, the question is partly unanswered. The second thesis—that race and ethnicity may have *some* relation to genetic diversity—seems most plausible, even if the degree to which a particular social category correlates or does not correlate may fluctuate or disappear over time.

Paradoxically, it may be necessary to rely on racial and ethnic categories for a time in order eventually to transcend them. Imagine a day, for example, when everyone has his or her genome on a CD-ROM. Rather than prescribing BiDil because someone is self-identified as African American, a physician might prescribe on the basis of a pharmacogenomic profile from the CD-ROM that better correlates with positive drug response. But, at present, it may make sense—in some well-validated contexts—to proceed on the assumption that some drugs should be prescribed for particular racial or ethnic groups. An important part of this decision process will involve the harm that might occur if the identification does not correlate with the biological characteristic in question.

This line of argument has two important caveats. First, others might argue that research using racial categories as preliminary markers for genetic differences will only reify the social categories in question, making them more difficult to eliminate later, perhaps because the individuals in question end up identifying strongly with the purely social characterization for reasons other than scientific ones. Second, a more recent article by Foster (2003) notes that even if present social categories of race and ethnicity are one day replaced, other social identities (such as the 'orphan genotypes' alluded to above) will no doubt emerge.

How one answers these difficult questions depends in part on whether the social aspects are seen as separate from the scientific ones, or whether the two may actually interact in a process of coproduction (Reardon 2001). Whereas the past saw science operating to help vindicate already established social categories, it may be that the future sees social categories responding more to science. One should therefore resist the temptation to think that science will make these and other important social issues disappear. In the meantime, although race or ethnicity labels might reasonably be used when no other more direct measures of variation exist, researchers should pay close attention to how these labels are defined in both the design and eventual reporting of research results. Above all, the inference from pharmacogenomic variation among members of two different social categories to the statement that all members of this group share a common trait should be avoided.

Pharmacogenomic Research: Finding the 'Community' in Community Review

The issue of race and ethnicity in genetics leads into another issue researchers continue to struggle with: community review. Whether or not social categories correspond with genetic diversity, so long as they are used in the recruitment or analysis of research findings, the question of community review is sure to arise. The premise behind community review is quite simple. Certain harms, like the ones alluded to above regarding the Ashkenazi Jewish population, do not accrue only to those individuals who participate in a study, but also to anyone who is a member of the group being studied. An individual need not participate in the study to suffer this type of 'group-based' harm. Group-based harms are not specific to pharmacogenomics, or even genetic research more generally (any research finding, genetic or not, associated with a group has the potential for this harm). The US National Bioethics Advisory Commission (1999) recognized the need to anticipate and prevent these harms, but, unfortunately, neither is simple to do. Requiring individuals to anticipate these risks and address them with individual informed consent may not be enough; informed consent was not intended for this purpose. Furthermore, the relatively homogeneous composition of ethics review committees might make the identification of culturally specific risks (e.g. threats to identity as a result of genomic research) exceedingly difficult.

A way of dealing with the risk of group-based harms in genomics developed out of the experience with the Human Genome Diversity Project (HGDP).[7] 'Group consent' emerged as a way to mitigate these group-based harms (Greely 1997). However, in the time since its proposal, many have either criticized group (or 'community') consent (Juengst 2000) or modified it from its original conception. Most agree that giving groups or communities 'consent' over individuals' personal decisions would be morally problematic, if not illegal, and therefore group or community consent are not often used. Thus, 'community review' and 'community consultation' have become preferred terms. Instead of group or community *consent*, some recommend a spectrum of increasing community involvement and control, beginning with community dialogue and proceeding through consultation, approval, and long-term partnership (Sharp and Foster 2000). The goals of all are roughly the same: to show respect for the community under study and encourage the cooperation of members in a research partnership.

In a recent article Weijer and Miller (2004) argue that the time is right to consider community consultation of two types: consultation and consent, or community consultation alone (another option, of course, is no added protections beyond

---

[7] In 1991 the HGDP sought to collect DNA from approximately 500 indigenous or isolated populations for anthropologic purposes. The HGDP is recognized for what it has *not* accomplished, partly because of concern over groups. After more than ten years of ethical and scientific wrangling, it only recently began collecting samples. See Greely (2001).

existing requirements of individual consent). They first note the risks of pharmaco-genomics to communities, such as the perception of being 'hard to treat' or a 'drain on the system', or the disruption of community identity (if pharmacogenomics were to reveal different genetic evidence regarding a community's anthropologic history, for example). Next, they elaborate the morally relevant features of communities: a legitimate political authority, a representative group, and a communication net-work. Different communities will share these features to different degrees, which will lead to one of the three policy options (consent, consultation alone, or no added protections). Only those communities with legitimate political authorities are eli-gible for community consent and consultation. Racial and ethnic groups—lacking some of the relevant features, such as legitimate political authorities—might fall into the second category requiring consultation alone, whereas 'bald men', though socially identifiable, are not the sort of group for which community consent or consultation are appropriate.

Although this approach appears plausible, it raises more questions than it answers. One problem throughout the literature on community review occurs because the model for community consent and consultation involves communities, such as Native Americans in the United States, that exist as legitimate political entities within defined geographic regions of a larger political state. These populations already require something akin to community consent or approval. Of course, one should not confuse mere approval with community consultation or partnership: simply approving a study does not mean that the community has been consulted in any meaningful way, and we are not suggesting that the present system of ethics committee approval by these communities is in all cases sufficient.

The problem of translating these success stories to other communities and defining the scope and feasibility of community consultation alone, however, is a difficult one (Sharp and Foster 2002). Who represents the African American community or the Ashkenazi Jewish community? How much control should the community have over the publication of results that may be damaging to their community identity? What types of benefit from research should be shared with the community? Although consensus is emerging that community review adds valuable insight to research protocols (National Institutes of Health n.d.), and that benefits should be shared with these communities (HUGO Ethics Committee 2000), such recommendations lack the force of regulatory requirements—as well as the necessary funding to execute them.

One actual example of required community consultations is worth mentioning and frequently goes unnoticed in the present context. In 1996 the FDA and the Department of Health and Human Services codified the permissibility of emergency and resuscitation research without consent (Biros 2003). One proviso, among others (see Figure 1), requires consultation with the community of potential subjects and the community where the research will be performed. The guidelines unfortunately give little definition of what adequate community consultation

The investigator must reveal:

- Nature and purpose of the study
- Meaning of informed consent
- Risks and benefits of the research

The investigator must answer community questions about the research and listen to their concerns.

The investigator must ask the community:

- How can those who do not wish to be enrolled be prospectively identified?
- How does this study interact with local cultural beliefs?

Suggestions for fulfilling the regulations:

- Identify and use existing community networks to actively engage the community
- Ask community gatekeeping groups for assistance
- Standard civic meetings
- School, club, and church meetings
- Set up special open community meetings around the topic of the research
- Include a public health message
- Discuss prevalence/prognosis of disease(s) under study
- Incorporate local health related information
- Identify and consult with representatives or leaders of the community
- Invite members of the community to serve as ethics committee members
- Develop a representative advisory panel to provide continuing consultation

Fig. 1 Key elements of community consultation in emergency and resuscitation research. From Biros (2003)

requires, probably because each situation is highly context dependent, even though the information requirements are explained. Unfortunately, the experience with community consultation appears mixed at best; researchers and ethics committees often have a difficult time engaging the community in a process that can add much time and expense to a research study (Kremers *et al.* 1999).

In these authors' experience on ethics committees, it is not uncommon for the community to show little interest in attending dialogues and meetings to discuss the protocols. This could reflect lack of community interest or inadequate engagement by the researchers and ethics committees, but the burden of proof should be on those who believe the former. Of course, these protocols deal with geographically defined communities that may exhibit less social or community identity when compared to racial or ethnic groups (it is unclear if Weijer and Miller's analysis would consider these protocols as deserving consultation). Nonetheless, those interested in community consultation in pharmacogenomics should not ignore the lessons of consultation in emergency research.

Might Technological Innovation Transform Debates About Informed Consent?

No matter how thorough community review is, the interests of the group toward research participation do not trump the free choice of individuals about whether to participate. However, defining the scope of individual informed consent has been a challenge in genomic, and therefore in pharmacogenomic, research. From its beginnings in the Nuremberg Code to its elaboration in the Belmont Report, US Code of Federal Regulation, and other international regulations, the principle of informed consent is essential for the ethical conduct of research. Traditionally, this involves allowing an individual to give informed consent to a specific research project for a defined period of time, a principle that is suitable for most purposes.

The resource requirements of some genetic research, however, may lead one to question how well this principle works in some contexts. For example, large population databases involve a tremendous investment of time and resources—investments that make replication infeasible or inefficient: the UK Biobank plans to collect 500,000 DNA samples from adults at a cost of approximately $73 million (*Nature Genetics* 2003). Recognizing this, the National Institutes of Health recently emphasized the need for data sharing, or an explanation of why sharing is not possible, for grants in excess of $500,000 (National Institutes of Health 2003). These situations highlight the need for appropriate data sharing practices, but should researchers be able to share data for new, 'secondary' research uses without the informed consent of the individuals who donated their DNA or tissue?

The issue is not unique to samples *collected* for the purpose of genetic research; it has been previously considered in the context of genetic research on *stored* tissue samples (Clayton *et al.* 1995). As (Winickoff 2003) points out, three ethical positions emerged on informed consent for secondary data uses.[8] On one end of the spectrum, the National Bioethics Advisory Commission (1999) in the United States concluded (though not unanimously) that it is permissible for research subjects to give 'broad' or 'blanket' consent to any future uses of their research

---

[8] Although one might suggest complete anonymization of samples, so that they could no longer be linked to individual research subjects (save perhaps by DNA fingerprinting itself), anonymous samples have a notable cost: they prevent the correlation of useful medical or phenotypic data with genotype. In addition, they make recontacting subjects impossible, should the research result in valid information of suitable clinical importance with appropriate medical advice and treatment available (National Bioethics Advisory Commission 1999). Our discussion here focuses on identifiable samples, as opposed to anonymous ones, though the latter certainly do not fall outside the regulation of research.

data. This proposal undercuts a chief purpose of informed consent: giving the subject the opportunity to decide whether or not to participate on the basis of information relevant to assessing the costs and benefits to him or her of participating (Consortium on Pharmacogenetics 2002). At the other extreme, Annas (1993) argues for requiring 'narrow' authorization for each and every use of data or tissue, a proposal that could be cost prohibitive for researchers to recontact and reconsent every subject. Somewhere between these two, Greely (1999) suggested that subjects might reasonably give consent to future research, so long as it is relatively limited in scope and well defined. For example, on this moderate view, a subject entering a study to identify genetic variations that influence response to a particular antihypertensive might also consent to future uses of his or her data for other hypertension medications or cardiovascular studies for a defined period of time with a recontact agreement. However, he or she would not thereby consent to future uses of the data for unrelated research, such as on the genetics of Alzheimer's disease or addiction. Because the moderate view seems to balance respect for autonomy with recognition of the costs and desire for scientific progress, it seems most plausible. Nevertheless, it is still necessary to set principled limits on what counts as 'related' research areas.

Advances in information technology may render the debate over the proper scope of informed consent considerably more tractable. For example, First Genetic Trust—an information technology company that provides services to large-scale genetic research sponsors—has developed a proprietary Dynamic Informed Consent Process (Penelope Manasco, personal communication).

When information about a subject enters the databank, he or she is given a personal account from which to give informed consent and control uses of his or her genetic data and other personal medical information. The account is accessible via either the Internet or the telephone, to help ensure availability for those without regular Internet access. Broad or blanket consent, as described above, is not permitted; after initial enrollment, subjects can elect to consent and opt in to future studies that desire their data (i.e. it is not an opt-out system, so if a subject never returns to his or her account no future uses will be permitted). Subjects are recontacted at time intervals of their choosing, but at least once every four years. Finally, subjects may withdraw their samples from the bank at any point, though data already collected remain in the system. This could present a problem, depending on the amount of genetic data already collected, because the notion of 'withdrawal' becomes less meaningful.

This centralized access system via a trusted intermediary has several advantages, including the ability to maintain contact with research subjects over time and to enroll geographically dispersed research populations. Given that adverse drug reactions are often quite rare, this second advantage can be quite important. Furthermore, the information technology can reduce the burden, and presumably part of the financial cost, on researchers to recontact study participants for consent.

Nevertheless, the Dynamic Consent Process technology remains in its infancy, and many questions remain. Do subjects utilize the options this system provides, or do they find doing so too burdensome? At present the system more closely approximates the narrower more than the broader model of informed consent. What if subjects simply do not behave as if they desire tight control over their data? Should an option for broad consent be introduced? This technology does not remove the debate over the scope of consent, but it at least has the capacity to incorporate both the narrow and a broader scope for informed consent. Eventually, it may offer individuals a choice of a range of alternatives.

There is another important question to ask about technologies like Dynamic Informed Consent: how does the informed consent process in this computerized system compare to the traditional, face-to-face process? As research proceeds (the company has agreements with Howard University's Genomic Research in the African Diaspora Biobank and Pfizer, Inc., among others), evidence will develop for answering these empirical questions. It is worth emphasizing that First Genetic Trust's system, though to the authors' knowledge the first of its kind, may not and need not be the sole provider of such a dynamic informed consent process. Moreover, this sort of process need not be restricted to for-profit 'trusted intermediaries'. One important pharmacogenomics policy question is whether a profit system, a public system, or, more likely, a combination of both types would be optimal to balance the protections of subjects with the progress of science.

Privacy and Confidentiality: Does Who Owns the Biobank Matter?

Informed consent, though a crucial and important safeguard, is not sufficient for the ethical conduct of research with human subjects (Emanuel *et al.* 2000). Besides informed consent, an oft-discussed ethical issue in genomics is the protection of privacy and confidentiality. Why is this important? The literature on the economic, psychological, and social risks of genetic information is vast. Suffice it to say that pharmacogenomic information, if disclosed, has the potential to cause all three, most notably as a result of discrimination for insurance purposes or stigmatization of 'difficult to treat' genotypes. Furthermore, risks can be magnified if collateral information from a pharmacogenomic test is linked to other disease predispositions or results (e.g. non-paternity) for which the test was not intended.

Appropriate safeguards for privacy and confidentiality can mitigate this risk, either by limiting access to the information or by limiting its use. Here, as in most cases, risks can never be eliminated entirely, at least not at a reasonable cost. The challenge, then, is not to reduce risk to zero, but to achieve adequate risk reduction without undue costs. And it is important to understand that one cost of elaborate risk reduction mechanisms is that they may raise the cost of pharmacogenomic testing to the detriment of access.

A recent example illustrating 'limited use' is the US Genetic Information Nondiscrimination Act, a bill introduced several times over the past few years that routinely passes in the Senate but stalls in the House of Representatives. At the time of this writing, the 2005 version of the bill has unanimously passed in the Senate and awaits a vote by the House of Representatives. Another is the current moratorium on the use of DNA test results for most insurance premiums in the United Kingdom. However, in this section we explore the prior option—control over access—by focusing on a recent debate over the use of trusted intermediaries as repositories of genetic and medical information for research.

Trusted intermediaries, sometimes called biobanks, serve to regulate research activities by forcing researchers to access clinical data, tissue samples, and genetic information through them, rather than the research subject. Biobanks need not be linked to the informed consent process, though they often are. Many biobanks already exist, the most notable being ventures in Iceland and the United Kingdom (Kaiser 2002).

The controversy over biobanks primarily concerns ownership. Often it is assumed that 'public, non-profit' biobanks are superior to 'private, for-profit' ones from an ethical standpoint and that something as important as the privacy and confidentiality of biosamples and related medical records should not be trusted to private entities. However, not all private biotech companies are for-profit and in some cases public and private ventures are linked or even merged (e.g. the SNP Consortium). The fact that few biobanks or databases fit these clear categories should cause ethicists to pause when making blanket statements about 'public' versus 'private' or 'for-profit' versus 'non-profit' entities. Nor should one assume that for-profit or private entities are more trustworthy than non-profit or public ones. What matters is the behavior of the entity or collaboration in question, not simply its legal status or official goals.

Nonetheless, recent arguments seem to support the idea that some commercial biobanks, though giving adequate attention to many of the important ethical issues already described (Otten et al. 2004), may differ in important ways from those that operate as part of non-profit endeavors. Take, for example, the deCODE Genetics combination of an Icelandic Health Sector Database (HSD; contains computerized medical records that deCODE itself will develop and implement) and the Genealogy Genotype Phenotype Resource (contains genealogy and DNA sequence information) deCODE has exclusive licensing to the linking of the two databases for future commercial purposes, and has given attention to some of the ethical issues arising as a result of this project (Gulcher and Stefansson 2000).

However, a recent analysis suggests the deCODE project may differ in ethically significant ways from more public, non-profit biobanks (Merz et al. 2004). Merz et al. worry that the content of the HSD as well as its design may inappropriately serve the research purposes of the company rather than the interests of the Icelandic people and government. They note that the situation is more complicated than it seems; deCODE is not simply the funder of an otherwise governmental health databank, because a publicly funded venture would make samples and related data more widely available to the Icelandic research community instead of granting exclusive access to the funder. In addition, there is the possibility that this arrangement will undermine the trust of patients in their medical system.

For now, these accusations are conjectures, but if they prove true, this may lead to amending the deCODE agreement or encourage a move toward a 'charitable trust' model that has been recently proposed (Winickoff and Winickoff 2003, 2004). On this model, the general public, not shareholders, serve as the primary beneficiary toward whom the biobank or trust has a fiduciary duty. The charitable trust model does not exclude private funding but separates the funding and control functions. Whether this model will eventually supplant or coexist with others is an open question. To help answer it, a priori evaluations of alternative models are inadequate; only informed, comparative analysis of performance will determine which model or combination of models is best.

Bringing Research Findings
to the Clinic

Most of this chapter has dealt with the more important ethical issues arising in pharmacogenomic research. The last part focuses on two critical questions concerning the transition of pharmacogenomic technologies to the clinic: how they should be regulated and how physicians should use them.

Who Should Regulate Pharmacogenomics, and How?

Although we place regulatory questions in this section, it should be pointed out that a section on regulation could just as easily have been the first issue considered; one question is whether research will drive regulation, or whether regulation will drive research. The correct answer is probably both, but because many regulatory issues arise only after pharmacogenomic products are available, we consider three of them here rather than in the earlier discussions of research issues: the regulation of tests prior to marketing, appropriate labeling practices, and direct marketing to consumers.

A recent report by Melzer *et al.* (2003) highlights some of the regulatory difficulties posed by pharmacogenomics and emphasizes a meaningful distinction: some pharmacogenomic tests may be marketed with a drug by the same pharmaceutical company that markets the drug (or via a contractual agreement with another company), whereas other pharmacogenomic tests may be offered as independent laboratory services. In certain respects, the latter could be more controversial. Why might this be?

An example of 'co-development' between a drug and its test is trastuzumab for the treatment of certain breast cancer subtypes (i.e. those with Her-2/neu gene amplification). Success of the drug depended on the development of an adequate diagnostic test. Presumably, cases such as these do not require specific regulations because it is in the interest of all stakeholders to develop an appropriate diagnostic test to bring the drug to market; otherwise, the drug might fail in clinical trials unless a particular genotypic subpopulation is tested. Unfortunately, these situations may be relatively uncommon; success in the absence of regulation does not itself conclusively argue against regulation. One way such regulation might occur is if a pharmaceutical company develops or uses a pharmacogenomic test in conjunction with a new drug application; regulatory agencies, such as the US FDA, may then review the analytic and clinical data associated with it. An alternative is the evaluation of diagnostic kits prior to their sale. There may be other options as well.

The regulation of certain independently offered diagnostic tests or services, including pharmacogenomic ones, has come under increasing scrutiny both in Europe and in the United States. There is concern that regulations currently allow for their premature use, prior to adequate clinical validation. For example, the US FDA has subcategories of medical devices and 'analyte specific reagents', or ASRs, which require no demonstration of clinical safety or effectiveness prior to marketing. Tests informally known as 'home brews', unlike diagnostic kits offered for sale, are assembled by the user and can be exempt from oversight. Even if the laboratory performing the test achieves certification according to regulatory standards, such as those of the US Clinical Laboratory Improvement Act, this guarantees only analytic validity (how well the test measures what it says it does), not clinical validity or utility (broadly, how useful the test is in helping achieve positive clinical outcomes).

Do pharmacogenomic tests and microarrays fall into this category? Some might. This issue came to a head when the FDA denied ASR status to Roche's AmpliChip™ in October 2003, recommending instead that Roche submit premarket review data (Kling 2003). In the United States recognition of the need for greater regulation by the FDA and the unprincipled nature of 'home brew' exemptions has led to the formulation of draft guidelines for the submission of pharmacogenomic data by industry (Hackett and Lesko 2003; US Department of Health and Human Services 2003). The draft guidelines encourage data collection by the FDA with voluntary compliance by industry. Importantly, they are not a move toward greater regulation or the full regulation of 'home brew' tests, but they do signify an interest on the part of the FDA to collect and examine pharmacogenomic data. If additional oversight is initiated, it is not clear whether it will be accomplished through a new regulatory category, or through other measures.

The second regulatory issue is the labeling of pharmacogenomic tests. Current US regulations require drug labels to describe the evidence and tests available should a particular drug affect certain defined subpopulations in terms of safety or efficacy (US 21 CFR 201.57). For example, the labeling of atomoxetine notes that laboratory tests are available to identify poor metabolizers of the drug who experienced statistically significant differences in the frequency of adverse events, sometimes twice as often (Lesko 2003). The important point is that current labels and package inserts describe the evidence and tests but make no recommendation about when testing may be required. Are these label warnings enough? Currently, the onus is on health care providers to decide whether testing is required (see below). One important question for pharmacogenomic policy is whether this decision should be left to the discretion of individual physicians or whether regulations or 'consensus conference' guidelines from appropriate health care professional organizations should be developed.

A final regulatory issue deserves mention. A recent report from the HGC (Human Genetics Commission 2003) focuses on the direct marketing of genetic tests to consumers. Genetic tests for paternity, disease risk, nutraceuticals, and likely drug response to a cluster of prescription and nonprescription drugs whose metabolism is affected by genetic variations in the cytochrome P450 enzymes are already widely available. Many of these escape regulation because of 'home brew' status and disclaimers about educational—not diagnostic—purposes. The HGC report notes two harms that might result from the unregulated availability of self-administered, direct marketed genetic tests: the possibility of obtaining information about others, including children, without their consent, and the risk of inaccurate predictive information. Other risks include possible breaches of confidentiality or privacy once a test provider has collected test data. The possibility of overseas and Internet marketing, both of which are difficult to control, magnifies the risk of these harms. One way of dealing with these issues would be to prohibit direct marketing of self-administered tests altogether; another would be to do nothing pending more information about whether these possible harms are actually occurring.

Perhaps surprisingly, the HGC did not recommend a blanket prohibition; instead, they recommended a prohibition on some, but not all, tests. At least initially, and until the science of pharmacogenomics becomes better developed, the HGC believes that most tests should not be marketed directly to consumers. Drawing on an analogy between genetic test regulation and the regulation of pharmaceuticals, they note that not all genetic tests will necessarily involve complicated, risky, or socially complex information. If this is true, some might reasonably be marketed as 'over-the-counter' tests, even if the number of tests fitting these criteria is quite small.

Any proposals for restricting direct-to-consumer genetic tests should take into account their benefits as well as the risks. Direct availability may improve access, particularly if individuals prefer to be tested without going through traditional providers and creating a record of the test information; they might see this as less risky from the standpoint of insurance discrimination. In addition, tests might be less expensive if marketed directly to consumers rather than through intermediaries.

The HGC's recommendations also include measures to ensure access to needed tests (e.g. via a national genetics service in the United Kingdom) and to improve consumer education. An example of the latter is GeneWatch UK,[9] a non-profit group that monitors biotechnologies for the public interest. GeneWatch recently claimed partial responsibility for the withdrawal of a particular company's direct-to-consumer genetic tests, some of which were pharmacogenomic, from retail stores.

Whether a defensible distinction can be made between those tests that require strict controls and those that do not is a difficult question. In the United States the Secretary's Advisory Committee on Genetic Testing attempted to develop a linear scheme but could not come to consensus on how to flesh it out (Secretary's Advisory Committee on Genetic Testing 2001). They considered various features, such as whether a test was diagnostic or predictive, whether it involved a rare or common disease, and whether it would be used for population screening. However, it appears that (at the very least) adequate oversight for genetic tests generally, including pharmacogenomic tests, would require a company to submit its data to the FDA or its analogue in other countries, prior to marketing its test, either directly to the public or via health care providers. To determine what special oversight provisions, if any, would be appropriate for direct-marketed, self-administered genetic tests, it would first be necessary to determine the size of the market for such tests, the practices of those companies that offer them, and the likelihood that additional tests will become available and widely used.

How Will Pharmacogenomics Affect Standards of Care and Professional Obligations?

In the Introduction of this chapter, we noted that basic knowledge of pharmacogenomics has existed for many years. In addition, tests for the various cytochrome P450 enzymes crucial to drug metabolism are not new. Some expect drugs with a narrow therapeutic index (i.e. a small difference between a therapeutic dose and a toxic one) to be the initial targets for widespread and effective use of pharmacogenomic tests (Oscarson 2003). But if some of this knowledge is not new, and if pharmacogenomics will revolutionize medicine, why are we only now discussing it? Are there other reasons clinicians have not used pharmacogenomics testing?

---

[9] <http://www.genewatch.org>, accessed 5 July 2006.

The simple answer is that the science remains in its infancy. However, a more nuanced answer—and one that points toward what is necessary for further development of the methodology—requires an examination of the ways in which standards of care evolve and are implemented by clinicians.

Legal mechanisms, such as malpractice liability, are one way to implement standards of care. In this case, a clinician might be found negligent if he or she does not reasonably follow accepted standards of how others would treat a patient in similar circumstances. In other words, if a pharmacogenetic test is available and considered standard by his or her peers, the clinician may be liable if he or she does not use it prior to prescribing a particular drug. Moral and professional obligations to 'do no harm' might also shed some light on whether a clinician utilizes a specific test before prescribing. Finally, cost-driven criteria imposed on physicians by private insurers or a national health system could determine whether a clinician is required or permitted to use a pharmacogenomic test. In this last case, as we saw earlier, the possible use of pharmacogenomic testing as a 'gatekeeper' for access to drugs in the context of a 'rational drug policy' implicates the familiar tension between what is best from a population health perspective and what may be best for an individual patient (Consortium on Pharmacogenetics 2002; Moldrup 2002). In an era when rationing is becoming more explicit and systematic in the context of population-based health services (whether private, as in managed care, or public, as in national health services), the standard of care cannot literally be what is best for the individual patient. Taking this point seriously calls into question the truthfulness of concepts like 'personalized medicine' if they are used in an absolute sense.

Under these conditions, greater reliance is being placed on cost-effectiveness as a determinate of the standard of care. In some cases, recourse to pharmacogenomic tests will be cost-effective, in others it will not. For example, pharmacogenomic tests may be one way to determine dosing of the blood thinning drug warfarin, but routine blood tests might be more cost-effective. Alternatively, a clinician operating under cost-containment incentives or simply trying to economize on her own time might elect not to prescribe a drug that requires a pharmacogenomic test before it is to be prescribed if another drug exists that does not require a pharmacogenomic test, even if the former is somewhat more effective.

Although all these factors may influence the patterns of physician behavior that eventually crystallize into a standard of care, the dissemination of 'user-friendly' knowledge to physicians is of critical importance. It seems likely that pharmacogenomic methodologies will become integrated at the point of care when general practitioners recognize that they need to know information about a particular patient's likely response to a particular drug, prior to prescribing. The prior question the clinician faces, of course, is, When should she seek 'personalized' knowledge about a patient's likely drug response, instead of simply relying on highly general information about rare adverse reactions?

The first question is: From where will this information come, and what sorts of sources are likely to be most accessible and up to date? Analyses suggest that online resources for general practitioners are lacking in both the United States and the United Kingdom (Pagon *et al.* 2001; Stewart *et al.* 2001). A major pharmacogenomics knowledge base, PharmGKB, is available[10] and promotes the sharing of pharmacogenomic data between scientists and clinicians alike. However, its present format is not likely to be useful as a clinical decision tool.

Physicians are not the only actors in the health care process whose obligations and knowledge needs will change under the impact of pharmacogenomics. Another critical piece of input into clinical practice will necessarily come from pharmacists, who are already adept at developing drug management practices, helping ensure drug safety, and educating others (Brushwood 2003). Pharmacists occupy a unique role in the health care process, one that has changed over time from dispenser of drugs to patient protector and educator. Pharmacogenomics may again change pharmacists' professional obligations while also requiring their invaluable contribution for pharmacogenomics to be successfully implemented.

A second question pertains to the role of health care providers with specialized genetic knowledge. If pharmacogenomics becomes integrated with general medical practice, will it require the sophisticated, extensive genetic counseling many advocate in other genetic testing scenarios? The answer to this question will depend on whether the information is especially confusing for patients to understand or is associated with psychosocial risks of the same magnitude as those attendant on some other genetic tests. The risk of psychosocial harm could be mitigated, but probably not eliminated, by test result reports that indicate only the information relevant to the clinical decision at hand.

Furthermore, it is important to emphasize that the requirement of patient understanding not be interpreted too robustly. After all, present clinical practice does not require counseling when interpreting or informing patients of even relatively simple diagnostic tests, such as electrocardiograms.

A related issue surrounds the necessity of obtaining informed consent in this setting. Should detailed informed consent be required for these tests? Consent should be obtained, of course, no matter what the test, but in the clinical setting informed consent may be more or less extensive. For example, HIV tests often involve written consent whereas many other blood tests do not. Thus, much will depend on the specific nature of the test in question. If the test cannot be performed without revealing complicated, sensitive information about an individual or perhaps his or her family, it may be necessary to obtain written informed consent from the patient. It could also be necessary to aid patient understanding or mitigate physician liability. For example, in the unfortunate situation where a patient's test reveals a high likelihood of an adverse event from the only available treatment, the

[10] <http://www.pharmgkb.org>, accessed 5 July 2006.

consent form might protect the physician by providing evidence that the risk was communicated.

The situation in which a diagnostic test reveals the availability of a single, potentially toxic treatment is not unique to pharmacogenomics, and to require more than minimal informed consent in all cases seems unreasonable and costly. It is unreasonable because a simple pharmacogenomic test that directs a clinician to one drug or another and does not reveal any other potentially damaging information does not seem to require any more formal informed consent than other diagnostic tests. If pharmacogenomics comes to play an important role in general clinical practice, requiring written informed consent of a complex nature could divert time and resources that could be better directed toward patient care.

A third and especially critical issue is how regulations might deal with the commonplace off-label usage of many medical therapeutics. Will pharmacogenomic tests have labels that simply suggest using the test, as noted above, or will they require it? If they do require it, will off-label uses of the drug—that is, uses in the absence of a prior pharmacogenomic test—be permitted? For example, suppose a patient cannot afford the pharmacogenomic test but nevertheless desires a particular drug that usually requires such a test. Currently, the United States is liberal in regard to off-label uses of medication, but will pharmacogenomics force rethinking of this issue? Should the patient be allowed to assume the risk if this drug is the only available treatment? A case can certainly be made that this off-label use would be morally justified (Robertson et al. 2002).

Finally, although many of the aforementioned reports note that a general knowledge problem regarding genetics exists, and that current resources for remedying this deficiency appear insufficient, they do not take the next step and make concrete recommendations regarding the needed information technology and the means of putting it into play. Given limitations of space, we can only hint at what such tools will look like, drawing on the expanding literature on clinical decision support systems, or CDSSs.

The basic premises behind CDSSs are simple. Medical information increases at a seemingly exponential rate and changes frequently. It becomes difficult for practicing clinicians to remain current and memorize treatment guidelines as they become available. Moreover, guidelines often require the integration of an enormous amount of data. Therefore, why not present the relevant guidelines at the critical time when they are needed? One should not infer the incompetence of clinicians from their need to rely on such systems; instead, these systems might support more humanistic and caring clinicians who can spend more time comforting their patients than trying to recall memorized prescription or clinical care guidelines. Lest one be concerned that clinicians become mere robots following recipes on computer screens, one should recall the warning of Holtzman (2003) that pharmacogenomic tests will not tell the whole story of a patient's response to a particular drug. The goal is not to replace the physician's judgment, but to aid it.

> 1. Speed is everything.
> 2. Anticipate needs and deliver in real time.
> 3. Fit into the user's workflow.
> 4. Little things (i.e. being user-friendly) can make a big difference.
> 5. Recognize that physicians will strongly resist stopping.
> 6. Changing direction is easier than stopping.
> 7. Simple interventions work best.
> 8. Ask for additional information only when you really need it.
> 9. Monitor impact, get feedback, and respond.
> 10. Manage and maintain your knowledge-based systems.

Fig. 2 The 'Ten Commandments' of Clinical Decision Support. From Bates *et al.* (2003)

Although CDSSs are still under development, requiring both further evaluation and standardization, preliminary results at improving patient safety are promising (Kaushal *et al.* 2003; Potts *et al.* 2004). At present none of these systems are widely used. In consequence, much empirical research examines the features of CDSSs that predict their utilization, several of which are worth mentioning. Immediate, non-optional feedback is one important predictor (Kawamoto and Lobach 2003). Others (see Figure 2) have noted the importance of speed as one of the 'Ten Commandments' of CDSSs (Bates *et al.* 2003).

Not surprisingly, CDSSs raise ethical and legal issues of their own, both for the clinicians who use them and the companies who design them (Berner 2002). If they come to play a key role in clinical practice, these systems may themselves one day require regulatory oversight.

A final critical issue about CDSSs concerns the locus of primary ethical responsibility for developing them. Should society rely on market forces to provide them, or should public funding be used for at least their initial development? Should they be privately or publicly owned? Would a private–public partnership work best? The answers to these questions will almost certainly depend upon the nature of the health care system in which these information technologies are to function.

CONCLUSION

This chapter began with questions about the production of pharmacogenomic technologies (i.e. the instantiation of a particular scientific methodology) and ended with questions about the production of the knowledge tools needed to integrate these technologies into clinical practice. This is not surprising. If the ethical issues raised by a particular scientific methodology depend on how it is instantiated, attention should be given to how such technologies develop, by whom they are likely to be developed, and under what incentives.

In between these two framing questions, we noted several areas where more specific questions of technological instantiation are already being explored. For example, the methodology of pharmacogenomics, when used in clinical trials, can achieve smaller, faster clinical trials, but at the cost of more generalizable knowledge about adverse reactions. Although this point has been grasped in the growing literature on pharmacogenomics, there is no consensus on how the trade-off should be made or who should decide how it should be made.

We also noted that emotionally and politically charged concerns about the use of racial and ethnic labels intersect pharmacogenomics in both research and clinical practice. The concerns here are that unscientific social labels may become even more entrenched and that in some cases such labels may be poor surrogates for genetic variations that affect medicine response. However, under certain circumstances, these labels might be appropriate. By not requiring the genotyping of all individuals, but instead relying in some cases on 'race' as a surrogate, efficiency in health care delivery may increase, and individuals concerned about control over their genetic data might welcome not needing to have a genetic test prior to receiving a particular drug.

As technologies for pharmacogenomics continue to develop in the research setting, care should be taken to ensure that appropriate standards are met for informed consent, privacy, and confidentiality. The challenge here is to meet these fundamental ethical standards while at the same time allowing exchanges and integration of information that will both facilitate fruitful research and directly benefit particular individuals.

In the coming years critical public policy choices will have to be made if this challenge is to be met. For example, if 'trusted intermediary' entities are to play an important role, should they be public agencies on the 'charitable trust' model or for-profit enterprises, or is a mix of public and private approaches optimal? More generally, what role can and should market forces play in developing the new information technologies required for the ethical use of pharmacogenomics?

We have also emphasized that the implementation of pharmacogenomics is likely to require new types of regulatory oversight and changes to professional obligations for physicians and others involved with health care delivery, such as pharmacists. The development of 'user-friendly' knowledge tools will be critical, not only to enable physicians to satisfy emerging standards of care, but to reduce the costs of their utilizing the technology to the point that they are willing to make it an important part of the practice of medicine.

Finally, pharmacogenomics, like other potentially beneficial methodologies, raises familiar issues of distributive justice. The most obvious is whether the technologies through which the methodology is deployed will be broadly affordable. In the United States the two critical questions are whether important pharmacogenomic tests will come to be included in the standard benefit packages of those who are fortunate enough to have health insurance and whether the number of those who lack health insurance is likely to be reduced. In other developed countries, where health care coverage is much more nearly universal, the increasing costs of aging populations are already leading to significant and increasingly explicit and systematic rationing of beneficial services. In these countries it is unclear whether a significant range of pharmacogenomic tests will be regarded as sufficiently valuable as to be included in a standard benefit package. Given the relatively short time-horizon of electoral politics, there is the risk that policy makers may regard the costs of introducing a new technology to be politically unacceptable, even in cases where the eventual benefits of the technology would far exceed the start-up costs. In less developed countries the potential benefits of pharmacogenomics may be considerable, but the infrastructure and training needed for effective deployment of pharmacogenomic technologies, as well as the cost of the technologies themselves, make it unlikely that these benefits will be realized.

Another, less evident, ethical issue concerns the role of pharmacogenomic 'gatekeeping' as a factor in determining who among those who have health care coverage will have access to particular medications. The tension between the good of society and the good of the individual may become more apparent when a pharmacogenomic test reveals that the most effective drug is also the most expensive or when a drug that is a particular patient's only hope is denied to her on the grounds that her genotype increases the risk of adverse reaction.

More generally, if cost-effective technologies are developed and physicians and insurers have sufficient incentives to accept the transition costs of introducing them into practice, pharmacogenomics may come to play a 'gatekeeping' role in 'rational drug policies' for organizations—whether public or private—that must serve the health care needs of populations of patients within the constraints of limited budgets. There is no reason to think that the ethics of rationing issues raised by the use of pharmacogenomic testing as a factor in determining access to medications will be novel. But if pharmacogenomics becomes a prominent tool of rationing in the context of more systematic and widespread reliance upon 'rational drug policies', these issues may become more salient and more politically charged.

Few (if any) of the ethical and regulatory issues we have explored in this chapter are unique to pharmacogenomics. However, the particular forms these issues take will be influenced by the character of the specific technologies in which the methodology of pharmacogenomics is deployed and by the social, economic, and cultural context in which the technologies are developed. As these technologies continue to evolve, become more widely implemented, and change in response to problems that cannot be fully foreseen prior to implementation, new issues may emerge.

REFERENCES

ADVISORY COMMITTEE ON HEALTH RESEARCH (2002), *Genomics and World Health: Report of the Advisory Committee on Health Research* (Geneva: World Health Organization).

ANNAS, G. J. (1993), 'Privacy Rules for DNA Databanks: Protecting Coded "Future Diaries" ', *JAMA* 270/19: 2346–50.

BAMSHAD, M. J., and OLSON, S. E. (2003), 'Does Race Exist?', *Scientific American*, 289/6: 78–85.

—— *et al.* (2003), 'Human Population Genetic Structure and Inference of Group Membership', *American Journal of Human Genetics*, 72/3: 578–89.

BATES, D. W., *et al.* (2003), 'Ten Commandments for Effective Clinical Decision Support: Making the Practice of Evidence-Based Medicine a Reality', *Journal of the American Medical Informatics Association*, 10/6: 523–30.

BERNER, E. S. (2002), 'Ethical and Legal Issues in the Use of Clinical Decision Support Systems', *Journal of Healthcare Information Management*, 16/4: 34–7.

BIROS, M. H. (2003), 'Research Without Consent: Current Status, 2003', *Annals of Emergency Medicine*, 42/4: 550–64.

BRUSHWOOD, D. B. (2003), 'The Challenges of Pharmacogenomics for Pharmacy Education, Practice, and Regulation', in Rothstein (2003: 207–25).

BUCHANAN, A., *et al.* (2002), 'Pharmacogenetics: Ethical Issues and Policy Options', *Kennedy Institute of Ethics Journal*, 12/1: 1–15.

BURCHARD, E. G., *et al.* (2003), 'The Importance of Race and Ethnic Background in Biomedical Research and Clinical Practice', *New England Journal of Medicine*, 348/12: 1170–5.

CLAYTON, E. W., *et al.* (1995), 'Informed Consent for Genetic Research on Stored Tissue Samples', *JAMA* 274/22: 1786–92.

CONSORTIUM ON PHARMACOGENETICS (2002), *Pharmacogenetics: Ethical and Regulatory Issues in Research and Clinical Practice*, <http://www.bioethics.umn.edu/news/pharm_report.pdf>, accessed 5 July 2006.

COOPER, R. S., *et al.* (2000), 'Heritability of Angiotensin-Converting Enzyme and Angiotensinogen: A Comparison of US Blacks and Nigerians', *Hypertension*, 35: 1141–7.

DEWAR, J. C., and HALL, I. P. (2003), 'Personalised Prescribing for Asthma: Is Pharmacogenetics the Answer?', *Journal of Pharmacy and Pharmacology*, 55/3: 279–89.

EMANUEL, E. J., WENDLER, D., and GRADY, C. (2000), 'What Makes Clinical Research Ethical?', *JAMA* 283/20: 2701–11.

FOSTER, M. W. (2003), 'Pharmacogenomics and the Social Construction of Identity', in Rothstein (2003: 251–65).

—— SHARP, R. R., and MULVIHILL, J. J. (2001), 'Pharmacogenetics, Race, and Ethnicity: Social Identities and Individualized Medical Care', *Therapeutic Drug Monitoring*, 23/3: 232–8.

FOULKES, W. D., *et al.* (2002), 'Tamoxifen May Be an Effective Adjuvant Treatment for BRCA1-Related Breast Cancer Irrespective of Estrogen Receptor Status', *Journal of the National Cancer Institute*, 94/19: 1504–6.

FREUND, C. L., and WILFOND, B. S. (2002), 'Emerging Ethical Issues in Pharmacogenomics: From Research to Clinical Practice', *American Journal of Pharmacogenomics*, 2/4: 273–81.

GREELY, H. T. (1997), 'The Control of Genetic Research: Involving the "Groups Between"', *Houston Law Review*, 33/5: 1397–1430.

—— (1999), 'Breaking the Stalemate: A Prospective Regulatory Framework for Unforeseen Research Uses of Human Tissue Samples and Health Information', *Wake Forest Law Review*, 34: 737–66.

—— (2001), 'Human Genome Diversity: What About the Other Human Genome Project?', *Nature Reviews Genetics*, 2: 222–7.

GREEN, M. J., and BOTKIN, J. R. (2003), '"Genetic Exceptionalism" in Medicine: Clarifying the Differences Between Genetic and Nongenetic Tests', *Annals of Internal Medicine*, 138/7: 571–5.

GULCHER, J. R., and STEFANSSON, K. (2000), 'The Icelandic Healthcare Database and Informed Consent', *New England Journal of Medicine*, 342/24: 1827–30.

HACKETT, J. L., and LESKO, L. J. (2003), 'Microarray Data: The US FDA, Industry and Academia', *Nature Biotechnology*, 21/7: 742–3.

HAFFNER, M. E., WHITLEY, J., and MOSES, M. (2002), 'Two Decades of Orphan Product Development', *Nature Reviews Drug Discovery*, 1/10: 821–5.

HEDGECOE, A., and MARTIN, P. (2003), 'The Drugs Don't Work: Expectations and the Shaping of Pharmacogenetics', *Social Studies of Science*, 33/3: 327–64.

HELLER, M. A., and EISENBERG, R. S. (1998), 'Can Patents Deter Innovation? The Anticommons in Biomedical Research', *Science*, 280/5364: 698–701.

HIGASHI, M. K., *et al.* (2002), 'Association Between CYP2C9 Genetic Variants and Anticoagulation-Related Outcomes During Warfarin Therapy', *JAMA* 287/13: 1690–8.

HOLDEN, C. (2003), 'Race and Medicine', *Science*, 302/5645: 594–6.

HOLTZMAN, N. A. (2003), 'Clinical Utility of Pharmacogenetics and Pharmacogenomics', in Rothstein (2003: 163–85).

HUGHES, A. R., *et al.* (2004), 'Association of Genetic Variations in HLA-B Region with Hypersensitivity to Abacavir in Some, But Not All, Populations', *Pharmacogenomics*, 5/2: 203–11.

HUGO ETHICS COMMITTEE (2000), 'Hugo Ethics Committee Statement on Benefit Sharing', *Clinical Genetics*, 58: 364–66.

HUMAN GENETICS COMMISSION (2003), *Genes Direct: Ensuring the Effective Oversight of Genetic Tests Supplied Directly to the Public* (London: Department of Health); <http://www.hgc.gov.uk/UploadDocs/DocPub/Document/genesdirect_full.pdf>, accessed 5 July 2006.

ISSA, A. M. (2002), 'Ethical Perspectives on Pharmacogenomic Profiling in the Drug Development Process', *Nature Reviews Drug Discovery*, 1/4: 300–8.

JUENGST, E. T. (2000), 'Commentary: What "Community Review" Can and Cannot Do', *Journal of Law, Medicine and Ethics*, 28/1: 52–4.

KAHN, J. (2003), 'Getting the Numbers Right: Statistical Mischief and Racial Profiling in Heart Failure Research', *Perspectives in Biology and Medicine*, 46/4: 473–83.

KAISER, J. (2002), 'Population Databases Boom, from Iceland to the U.S.', *Science*, 298: 1158–61.

KAPLAN, J. B., and BENNETT, T. (2003), 'Use of Race and Ethnicity in Biomedical Publication', *JAMA* 289: 2709–16.

KAUSHAL, R., SHOJANIA, K. G., and BATES, D. W. (2003), 'Effects of Computerized Physician Order Entry and Clinical Decision Support Systems on Medication Safety: A Systematic Review', *Archives of Internal Medicine*, 163/12: 1409–16.

KAWAMOTO, K., and LOBACH, D. F. (2003), 'Clinical Decision Support Provided Within Physician Order Entry Systems: A Systematic Review of Features Effective for Changing Clinician Behavior', *American Medical Informatics Association Annual Symposium Proceedings*, 361–5.

KLING, J. (2003), 'Roche's Microarray Tests US FDA's Diagnostic Policy', *Nature Biotechnology*, 21/9: 959–60.

KOHN, L. T., CORRIGAN, J., and DONALDSON, M. S. (eds.) (2000), *To Err Is Human: Building a Safer Health System* (Washington, DC: National Academy Press).

KREMERS, M. S., WHISNANT, D. R., LOWDER, L. S., and GREGG, L. (1999), 'Initial Experience Using the Food and Drug Administration Guidelines for Emergency Research Without Consent', *Annals of Emergency Medicine*, 33/2: 224–9.

KREUTZ, R. (2004), 'Pharmacogenetics of Antihypertensive Drug Response', *Current Hypertension Reports*, 6/1: 15–20.

LANGHEIER, J. M., and SNYDERMAN, R. (2004), 'Prospective Medicine: The Role for Genomics in Personalized Health Planning', *Pharmacogenomics*, 5/1: 1–8.

LESKO, L. J. (2003), *Impact of Pharmacogenomics on FDA's Drug Review Process*, <http://www4.od.nih.gov/oba/SACGHS/meetings/October2003/Lesko.pdf>, accessed 5 July 2006.

LINDPAINTNER, K. (2003), 'Pharmacogenetics and the Future of Medical Practice', *Journal of Molecular Medicine*, 81/3: 141–53.

MANASCO, P. K., and ARLEDGE, T. E. (2003), 'Drug Development Strategies', in Rothstein (2003: 83–97).

MARSH, S., and MCLEOD, H. L. (2004), 'Cancer Pharmacogenetics', *British Journal of Cancer*, 90/1: 8–11.

MARSHALL, E. (2003), 'Preventing Toxicity with a Gene Test', *Science*, 302/5645: 588–90.

MELZER, D., *et al.* (2003), *My Very Own Medicine: What Must I Know? Information Policy for Pharmacogenomics* (Cambridge: Department of Public Health and Primary Care, University of Cambridge).

MERZ, J. F., MCGEE, G. E., and SANKAR, P. (2004), '"Iceland Inc."? On the Ethics of Commercial Population Genomics', *Social Science and Medicine*, 58: 1201–9.

MILLER, R. (2003), 'Riluzole for ALS: What Is the Evidence?', *Amyotrophic Lateral Sclerosis and Other Motor Neuron Disorders*, 4/3: 135.

MOLDRUP, C. (2002), 'Ethical, Social and Legal Implications of Pharmacogenomics: A Critical Review', *Community Genetics*, 4/4: 204–14.

NATIONAL BIOETHICS ADVISORY COMMISSION (1999), *The Use of Human Biological Materials in Research* (Bethesda, Md.: National Bioethics Advisory Commission).

NATIONAL INSTITUTES OF HEALTH (n.d.), *Bioethics Resources on the Web*, <http://bioethics.od.nih.gov/named_populations.html >, accessed 5 July 2006.

—— (2003), 'Final NIH Statement on Sharing Research Data', <http://grants1.nih.gov/grants/guide/notice-files/NOT-OD-03–032.html>, accessed 5 July 2006.

Nature Genetics (2003), 'Bankable Assets?', Editorial, 33: 325–36.

NEBERT, D. W., JORGE-NEBERT, L., and VESELL, E. S. (2003), 'Pharmacogenomics and "Individualized Drug Therapy": High Expectations and Disappointing Achievements', *American Journal of Pharmacogenomics*, 3/6: 361–70.

NUFFIELD COUNCIL ON BIOETHICS (2003), *Pharmacogenetics: Ethical Issues* (London: Nuffield Council on Bioethics).

O'KANE, D. J., WEINSHILBOUM, R. M., and MOYER, T. P. (2003), 'Pharmacogenomics and Reducing the Frequency of Adverse Drug Events', *Pharmacogenomics*, 4/1: 1–4.

OSCARSON, M. (2003), 'Pharmacogenetics of Drug Metabolising Enzymes: Importance for Personalised Medicine', *Clinical Chemistry and Laboratory Medicine*, 41/4: 573–80.

OTTEN, J., WYLE, H. R., and PHELPS, G. D. (2004), 'The Charitable Trust as a Model for Genomic Biobanks', *New England Journal of Medicine*, 350/1: 85–6.

PAGON, R. A., PINSKY, L., and BEAHLER, C. C. (2001), 'Online Medical Genetics Resources: A US Perspective', *British Medical Journal*, 322/7293: 1035–7.

PANG, T. (2003), 'Impact of Pharmacogenomics on Neglected Diseases of the Developing World', *American Journal of Pharmacogenomics*, 3/6: 393–8.

PHILLIPS, K. A., *et al.* (2001), 'Potential Role of Pharmacogenomics in Reducing Adverse Drug Reactions: A Systematic Review', *JAMA* 286/18: 2270–9.

POTTS, A. L., *et al.* (2004), 'Computerized Physician Order Entry and Medication Errors in a Pediatric Critical Care Unit', *Pediatrics*, 113/1, pt. 1: 59–63.

RAI, A. K. (2002*a*), 'Genome Patents: A Case Study in Patenting Research Tools', *Academic Medicine*, 77/12, pt. 2: 1368–72.

—— (2002*b*), 'Pharmacogenetic Interventions, Orphan Drugs, and Distributive Justice: The Role of Cost–Benefit Analysis', *Social Philosophy and Policy*, 19/2: 246–70.

REARDON, J. (2001), 'The Human Genome Diversity Project: A Case Study in Coproduction', *Social Studies of Science*, 31/3: 357–88.

REEDER, C. E., and DICKSON, W. M. (2003), 'Economic Implications of Pharmacogenomics', in Rothstein (2003: 229–50).

RISCH, N., BURCHARD, E., ZIV, E., and TANG, H. (2002), 'Categorization of Humans in Biomedical Research: Genes, Race and Disease', *Genome Biology*, 3/7, comment 2007.

ROBERTSON, J. A., *et al.* (2002), 'Pharmacogenetic Challenges for the Health Care System', *Health Affairs*, 21/4: 155–67.

ROCHE DIAGNOSTICS (2003), 'Microarray ("DNA Chip") and Roche Amplichip™ CYP450 Backgrounder', press release, <http://www.roche-diagnostics.com/media/pdf/press_release/2003/background_amplichip_450.pdf>, accessed 5 Jul. 2006.

ROHDE, D. D. (2000), 'The Orphan Drug Act: An Engine of Innovation? At What Cost?', *Food and Drug Law Journal*, 55/1: 125–43.

ROSES, A. D. (2000), 'Pharmacogenetics and the Practice of Medicine', *Nature*, 405/6788: 857–65.

ROTHSTEIN, M. A. (ed.) (2003), *Pharmacogenomics: Social, Ethical, and Clinical Dimensions* (Hoboken, NJ: John Wiley).

—— and EPPS, P. G. (2001), 'Ethical and Legal Implications of Pharmacogenomics', *Nature Reviews Genetics*, 2/3: 228–31.

ROUSE, R., and HARDIMAN, G. (2003), 'Microarray Technology: An Intellectual Property Retrospective', *Pharmacogenomics*, 4/5: 623–32.

SCHULTE, P. A., LOMAX, G. P., WARD, E. M., and COLLIGAN, M. J. (1999), 'Ethical Issues in the Use of Genetic Markers in Occupational Epidemiologic Research', *Journal of Occupational and Environmental Medicine*, 41/8: 639–46.

SCHWARTZ, R. S. (2001), 'Racial Profiling in Medical Research', *New England Journal of Medicine*, 344/18: 1392–3.

SECRETARY'S ADVISORY COMMITTEE ON GENETIC TESTING (2001), *Development of a Classification Methodology for Genetic Tests: Conclusions and Recommendations of the Secretary's Advisory Committee on Genetic Testing* (Bethesda, Md.: National Institutes of Health), <http://www4.od.nih.gov/oba/sacgt/reports/Addendum_final.pdf>, accessed 5 Jul. 2006.

SHARP, R. R., and FOSTER, M. W. (2000), 'Involving Study Populations in the Review of Genetic Research', *Journal of Law, Medicine and Ethics*, 28/1: 41–51.

——— (2002), 'Community Involvement in the Ethical Review of Genetic Research: Lessons from American Indian and Alaska Native Populations', *Environmental Health Perspectives*, 110, suppl. 2: 145–8.

STEVENS, L. (2003), 'Orphan Drug Act at 20: Big Gains, Some Strains', *American Medical News*, 46/29: 36.

STEWART, A., HAITES, N., and ROSE, P. (2001), 'Online Medical Genetics Resources: A UK Perspective', *British Medical Journal*, 322/7293: 1037–9.

TROUILLER, P., and OLLIARO, P. L. (1999), 'Drug Development Output: What Proportion for Tropical Diseases?', *The Lancet*, 354/9173: 164.

US DEPARTMENT OF HEALTH AND HUMAN SERVICES (2003), *Guidance for Industry: Pharmacogenomic Data Submissions*, <http://www.fda.gov/cder/guidance/5900dft.pdf>, accessed 25 Mar. 2004.

VAN AKEN, J., SCHMEDDERS, M., FEUERSTEIN, G., and KOLLEK, R. (2003), 'Prospects and Limits of Pharmacogenetics: The Thiopurine Methyl Transferase (TPMT) Experience', *American Journal of Pharmacogenomics*, 3/3: 149–55.

WALSH, J. P., COHEN, W. M., and ARORA, A. (2003), 'Science and the Law: Working Through the Patent Problem', *Science*, 299/5609: 1021.

WEBER, W. W. (2001), 'The Legacy of Pharmacogenetics and Potential Applications', *Mutation Research*, 479/1–2: 1–18.

WEIJER, C., and MILLER, P. B. (2004), 'Protecting Communities in Pharmacogenetic and Pharmacogenomic Research', *Pharmacogenomics Journal*, 4/1: 9–16.

WINICKOFF, D. E. (2003), 'Governing Population Genomics: Law, Bioethics, and Biopolitics in Three Case Studies', *Jurimetrics Journal*, 43: 187–228.

——— and WINICKOFF, R. N. (2003), 'The Charitable Trust as a Model for Genomic Biobanks', *New England Journal of Medicine*, 349/12: 1180–4.

——— (2004), 'The Charitable Trust as a Model for Genomic Biobanks', *New England Journal of Medicine*, 350/1: 85–6.

PART VII

RESEARCH ETHICS

CHAPTER 24

CLINICAL EQUIPOISE: FOUNDATIONAL REQUIREMENT OR FUNDAMENTAL ERROR?

ALEX JOHN LONDON

A PROFOUND moral tension lies at the heart of research ethics (Jonas 1969; London 2003). On the one hand, medical research is an important and socially valuable activity whose goals are to advance our limited understanding of health-related issues by utilizing scientific and statistical methods to investigate clinically relevant questions. By pushing forward the boundaries of knowledge, medical research ultimately aims to improve the standard of medical care available to future patients. On the other hand, medical research requires the participation of individuals, each of whom has his or her own interests and needs. As high-profile scandals in research ethics powerfully illustrate, the pursuit of sound science and statistical validity may require research activities that diverge from—or which are simply antithetical to—the best interests of present participants. One of the fundamental challenges of research ethics, therefore, has been to articulate a framework for advancing scientifically meritorious research without also sacrificing the interests of research participants to the greater good of scientific progress.

One of the most promising frameworks holds that as a necessary condition for ethically acceptable human-subjects research, clinical trials must begin in and be designed to disturb a state of equipoise. The concept of 'equipoise' was first articulated by the philosopher Charles Fried in the mid-1970s. Fried claimed that physicians owe a 'duty of personal care' to their individual patients, a duty that may be in tension with important features of the gold standard for medical research, the randomized clinical trial (RCT). According to Fried, it would be consistent with the duty of personal care to enroll a particular patient in a clinical trial only as long as the physician was uncertain about the relative therapeutic merits of the interventions to which the patient could be randomly assigned in the trial (Fried 1974). He referred to this state of uncertainty—being equally poised between the available options—as 'equipoise'.

Perhaps the clearest and most ambitious use of the concept of equipoise appeared roughly a decade later in the work of Benjamin Freedman (Freedman 1987, 1990). Freedman argued that equipoise is a necessary—though not always a sufficient—condition for ethical human-subjects research, but he rejected Fried's formulation of equipoise. Since that time, the equipoise requirement has played an important role in research ethics and subsequent thinkers have gone on to offer a variety of interpretations or refinements of the concept. From its inception, however, the equipoise requirement has also been the subject of searching criticism and vociferous debate. The turn of the new millennium has brought what may be the most concerted and far-reaching criticisms of this approach. As a result, research ethics may now be at a critical juncture as the field struggles to clarify issues that touch on its very foundations (Kaebnick 2003).

The most prominent and critically significant criticisms of the equipoise requirement can be grouped under three general headings. Objections from *indeterminacy* point to proliferating conceptions of equipoise and question the extent to which the concept has a determinate meaning. In the first section below I clarify important features of competing conceptions of equipoise to reveal a *set* of well-formed conceptions of equipoise. In order to assess the merits of these various formulations, I turn to objections from *utility*. These objections hold that the equipoise requirement does not resolve the inherent tension between advancing science and safeguarding the interests of individual participants. I argue that these criticisms are either misplaced, or apply only to a limited subset of possible formulations of the concept. Among those formulations to which they do not apply, I claim, is what Freedman calls clinical equipoise.

Any view of equipoise, however, faces perhaps the most radical and far-reaching objections from *moral foundations*. These objections hold that the equipoise requirement conflates the ethics of medical research and the ethics of clinical medicine. Once this conflation is recognized, this position holds, research can be given a new foundation on the imperative to avoid exploiting research participants. I argue that what is novel in this critique is not as successful as its proponents claim and that the ultimate success of this approach actually hinges on a version of the objection from utility. Nevertheless, this criticism highlights the limited scope of applicability of the equipoise requirement. I conclude, therefore, by describing the outlines of what I call an 'integrative approach' to clinical trials. This approach represents one way in which the normative requirements of equipoise and the non-exploitation approach might be unified under a single, broad framework.

Objections from Indeterminacy: Whose Uncertainty? Which Equipoise?

One very basic charge leveled against the equipoise requirement is that it is something of a misnomer to speak of 'the' equipoise requirement. Rather, the growing literature on this topic is littered with alternative conceptions of equipoise and numerous interpretations of the corresponding equipoise requirement. Confronted with such variety, even those who are sympathetic to the ambitions of the equipoise requirement may be frustrated at the lack of clarity and uniformity that surrounds the subject (Ashcroft 1999; Miller and Weijer 2003). A less sanguine appraisal, however, holds that until proponents of this approach provide a determinate account of the concept of equipoise and its associated moral requirements it is not possible to evaluate the merits of this approach or to implement it consistently in practice (Sackett 2000).

To illustrate something of the diversity that motivates this charge, consider the following extended example. When Freedman opens his seminal paper 'Equipoise and the Ethics of Clinical Research', he writes:

In the simplest model, testing a new treatment B on a defined population P for which the current accepted treatment is A, it is necessary that the clinical investigator be in a state of genuine uncertainty regarding the comparative merits of treatments A and B for population P. If a physician knows that these treatments are not equivalent, ethics requires that the superior treatment be recommended.   (Freedman 1987: 141)

In this general introductory statement, Freedman follows Fried's formulation in which the uncertainty that is required to justify the trial is situated in the mind of the individual clinical investigator. Freedman does not himself endorse this view, however. He associates this position with what he calls 'theoretical equipoise', which he rejects. He refers to the view which he endorses as 'clinical equipoise', according to which the requisite uncertainty is located in the larger expert medical community. Equipoise obtains, on the latter view, when 'there is no consensus within the expert

clinical community about the comparative merits of the alternatives to be tested'
(Freedman 1987: 144).

Confusion about this feature of clinical equipoise persists in the literature,
however. For example, Ashcroft (1999: 320), describes clinical equipoise as:

equipoise in the mind of the intending physician regarding treatment options. In many
ways, this remains the best formulation. For clinical equipoise is a necessary condition on
entering a patient into a trial, and if any clinician is not in clinical equipoise regarding a
patient or a trial, then this (or any other of his patients) should not be entered by him or
her into the trial. The ethical duty of the physician here is clear enough.

What Ashcroft refers to as 'clinical equipoise', however, is not what Freedman
articulated. Freedman explicitly states that clinical equipoise can exist when there
is 'a split in the clinical community, with some clinicians favoring A and others
favoring B', and that clinical equipoise is 'consistent with a decided treatment
preference on the part of the investigators. They simply recognize that their less
favored treatment is preferred by colleagues whom they consider to be responsible
and competent' (Freedman 1987: 144).

What Ashcroft identifies as 'clinical equipoise', therefore, is actually what Freedman identified as 'theoretical equipoise' and what Fried had referred to simply as
'equipoise'. Adding to the complexity, within literature from the United Kingdom
this position is also commonly referred to under the name of 'the uncertainty principle' (Hill 1963; Peto et al. 1976; Peto and Baigent 1998; Sackett 2000). In contrast,
what Freedman actually describes as 'clinical equipoise', Ashcroft calls 'collective or
professional equipoise', terms that are also more common among writers from the
United Kingdom (e.g. Chard and Lilford 1998).

As this example illustrates, the proliferation of different nomenclatures and ter-
minologies has exacerbated the difficulty of isolating and evaluating the underlying
positions to which those terms are intended to refer. Putting such confusions aside,
however, it is possible to construct as many conceptions of equipoise as there are
combinations of alternative positions on four central issues.

The first issue, illustrated above, concerns *who ought to be in equipoise* or,
in other words, *where the relevant uncertainty ought to be located*. In addition
to the possibilities mentioned already, a view sometimes referred to as 'narrow
patient equipoise' (Ashcroft 1999: 321) requires that the individual patient have
no preference between treatment alternatives (Johnson et al. 1991; Veatch 2002),
whereas 'wide patient equipoise or *community equipoise*' requires not only that
patients and care givers be in equipoise, but that family members and the broader
'community' be in equipoise as well (Gifford 1995; Karlawish and Lantos 1997).
Although these different accounts of where equipoise ought to be located are
often treated as mutually exclusive, several writers have argued for the necessity
of equipoise at more than one of these levels (Chard and Lilford 1998; Miller and
Weijer 2003; Mann et al. 2005).

Such differences over where to locate the relevant uncertainty are only the first of four possible dimensions along which alternative conceptions of equipoise can be distinguished. In addition to deciding whose uncertainty is relevant for establishing equipoise we must also explain *what the epistemic threshold is for the state of uncertainty*. For example, Freedman was eager to reject the view that he attributed to Fried and which he referred to as 'theoretical equipoise', because he associated this position with a particularly fragile epistemic threshold. A fragile epistemic threshold is disturbed as soon as there is any reason to think that the odds that one treatment will be more successful than another are tipped past 50:50 (Freedman 1987: 143). On this model, equipoise requires an 'exact balance' between the prospects for benefit between each alternative, where such a balance can be tipped by something as flimsy as a hunch or a gut feeling.

In contrast, Freedman claimed that 'clinical equipoise' embodies a more robust epistemic threshold. According to this view, equipoise persists until evidence for the superiority of one intervention emerges that would be sufficient to forge a consensus in the relevant expert clinical community. This more robust epistemic threshold requires that the evidence supporting a claim to superiority be sufficiently compelling that it will influence the practice behavior, not just of one physician, but of the community of physicians. Clinical equipoise thus rests on an epistemic threshold that is set by the presence or absence of consensus in the relevant expert medical community. A third set of alternatives rely on decision theoretic tools to deal with this issue. For example, the Kadane–Sedransk–Seidenfeld design (KSS Model) creates computer models of the clinical judgments of expert clinicians and then applies methods from Bayesian decision theory to update those models as new data are generated from the trial. In such a decision theoretic approach, the epistemic threshold is operationalized as the point at which the data is sufficient to change the treatment allocations recommended by the decision models (Kadane 1996).

Conceptions of equipoise can be also be distinguished according to a third dimension: *the evaluative focus of the decision maker's concern*. A one-dimensional conception of equipoise focuses critical attention on a single attribute of the set of interventions in question, usually their relative efficacy. Efficacy here refers to an intervention's brute impact on a single, dominant clinical endpoint, such as tumor reduction or infection control. In contrast, a multidimensional conception of equipoise focuses critical attention on an all-things-considered evaluation of the various factors that determine the attractiveness of the interventions in question (Chard and Lilford 1998; Gifford 2000; London 2001). Freedman (1987: 143) refers to this as an intervention's 'net therapeutic index', in which its efficacy is evaluated along with factors such as its side-effect profile, ease of administration and use, and so on.

Finally, different interpretations of the equipoise requirement can be distinguished in terms of *the way they ground the moral obligation* to ensure that equipoise obtains in clinical trials. Nearly all extent defenses of the equipoise requirement appeal to role-related obligations of physicians. For example, Fried was motivated by a concern for the 'duty of personal care' that clinicians owe to their patients (Fried 1974), and Marquis refers to a similar concern under the heading of the 'therapeutic obligation' which he explicates as follows: 'A physician should not recommend for a patient therapy such that, given present medical knowledge, the hypothesis that the particular therapy is inferior to some other therapy is more probable than the opposite hypothesis' (Marquis 1983: 42).

In both cases, the equipoise requirement is a constraint that is grounded in an obligation that physicians owe to their patients. Because Marquis's view of the therapeutic obligation builds in controversial features from some of the dimensions of equipoise mentioned here, others have chosen to ground the requirement simply in the clinician's fiduciary relationship to the patient (Miller and Weijer 2003). The latter approach views the duty of personal care in a way that is consistent with a more robust epistemic threshold, but it retains the traditional emphasis on role-related obligations that stem from the doctor–patient relationship.

In the integrative approach that I develop below, the equipoise requirement is grounded in a set of general values whose moral force does not depend on or emerge within the doctor–patient relationship. As I argue below, grounding the integrative approach in a broader set of social values gives it a significantly broader scope than traditional versions of the equipoise requirement. It also enables the integrative approach to avoid a tension that I argue undermines Freedman's attempt to embrace both the therapeutic obligation as the normative foundation of the equipoise requirement and a conception of equipoise that locates the relevant uncertainty, not in the mind of the individual clinician, but in the broader expert medical community (London 2006a, b).

This very brief discussion at least provides a sense of *the matrix of possible formulations of the equipoise requirement that emerge from different combinations of views on each of the above dimensions.* This matrix of possibilities is mapped out for a sample of representative views in Figure 1. It should be emphasized, though, that Figure 1 presents a fairly crude matrix. It is sufficient to show, for example, that what Freedman termed 'theoretical equipoise' and what is often referred to as 'the uncertainty principle' are the same view. However, some categories, such as decision theoretic approaches to the epistemic threshold, are too crude to reveal genuine differences that may exist between models that use different decision theoretic methods. These details can be put aside for the present discussion, however.

Although this brief analysis establishes that there are a variety of determinate formulations of equipoise, it provides little guidance for narrowing these options to a more attractive subset. To determine which of these alternatives is most philosophically and practically attractive, we must turn to objections from utility.

	Whose uncertainty				Epistemic threshold			Evaluative focus		Normative grounds	
	Patient	Clinician	Medical community	Larger community	50:50 fragile	Community consensus	Decision theoretic	One-dimensional	Multidimensional	Role related	Broader moral values
Freedman's clinical equipoise (1987)		X				X			X	X	
Theoretical equipoise (Fried as understood by Freedman)	X				X			X		X	
Uncertainty principle		X			X			X		X	
Fried as understood by Miller and Weijer (2003)		X				X			X	X	
Miller and Weijer (2003)		X	X			X			X	X	
Chard and Lilford (1998)	X	X	X	X			X		X	X	
Integrative approach	X		X				X		X		X

Fig. 1 Matrix of dimensions along which versions of the equipoise requirement may be constructed.

OBJECTIONS FROM UTILITY

The most significant challenge to the utility of equipoise is the charge that it fails to reconcile (*a*) the duty to safeguard the interests of present participants with (*b*) the statistical and scientific requirements necessary to generate reliable, generalizable data. This perceived failure is what underwrites widespread claims that the equipoise requirement is too restrictive because it sacrifices scientific progress to a misplaced desire to protect certain perceived interests of participants. As I will indicate later on, this perceived failure also underwrites claims that some formulations, such as clinical equipoise, are too permissive because they permit participant interests to be sacrificed to the perceived interests of scientific progress.

Claims that the equipoise requirement cannot resolve the tension between these competing ends hinge centrally on two independent issues. The first concerns the nature and extent of the duty to safeguard the interests of present participants. Call this the *responsiveness to participant interests condition*. The second concerns the proper epistemic threshold and evaluative focus of the equipoise requirement. Call this the *content of equipoise condition*. Claims that the equipoise requirement is overly restrictive usually presuppose a symmetric account of these conditions in which both the duty to safeguard the participant's interests and the content of equipoise embody a fragile epistemic threshold located in the mind of the individual clinician. Marquis's formulation of the therapeutic obligation is probably the clearest example: 'A physician should not recommend for a patient therapy such that, given present medical knowledge, the hypothesis that the particular therapy is inferior to some other therapy is more probable than the opposite hypothesis' (Marquis 1983: 42).

As Marquis and others argue (Gifford 1986; Hellman 2002), only in relatively rare circumstances will a physician believe that it is equally probable that two or more therapeutic options offer a particular patient the same degree of benefit. Without such a fragile state of equipoise, however, a clinical trial between therapeutic alternatives could not ethically be initiated. Alternatively, if it were the case that such a fragile state of equipoise obtained, critics argue, then it would not persist long enough to bring a clinical trial to its desired conclusion. As soon as the trial generates its first data points the physician is obligated to look for trends. If one option appears to fare better than another, the hypothesis that one option is inferior to the other would be more probable than its opposite. Once this fragile state of uncertainty is disturbed, the trial can no longer be justified on the grounds that equipoise obtains.

The equipoise requirement therefore appears to be overly restrictive because it would effectively prohibit the vast majority, if not the entirety, of clinical research. As a result, many reason that, since clinical research is such an important and socially valuable activity, what the above argument actually shows is that we must reject the equipoise requirement altogether. If we cannot reconcile the therapeutic obligation with the demands of sound science, then the necessity of scientific progress can legitimize the abrogation of the therapeutic obligation. In other words, if the interests of present participants must be weighed against the value of scientific knowledge and benefits to future patients, then it must be permissible to subordinate the former to the latter (Marquis 1983; Gifford 1986; Hellman 2002; Miller and Brody 2003).

In his defense of clinical equipoise, Freedman claimed to be able to avoid this particular objection from utility. The nature of Freedman's argument, however, remains poorly understood and is frequently misrepresented. In particular, critics often fail to realize that Freedman too offers a symmetric account of the responsiveness to participant interests condition and the content of equipoise condition. However, Freedman's account is symmetric because both conditions embody a robust epistemic threshold located in the state of consensus in the clinical community. In other words, while it is widely appreciated that Freedman rejects a view of equipoise that embodies a fragile epistemic threshold, critics often overlook the fact that he also offers a distinctive account of the nature and extent of the duty to safeguard the interests of participants which rejects this fragile epistemic threshold. For Freedman, the obligation to safeguard participant interests is determined by the requirements of sound medical practice but, like Fried before him, he thinks that the requirements of sound medical practice are determined by the consensus of the expert medical community (Freedman 1987: 144; Miller and Weijer 2003). Let me explain.

It is best to begin with Freedman's view of the content of the equipoise requirement. Consider the following pair of situations. In one case, the members of the expert medical community are uncertain about the relative therapeutic merits of two interventions, A and B. Such a state of affairs might obtain, for example, if A is the current treatment for a medical condition, say A is an antibiotic treatment for a particular bacterial infection, and treatment B is a new antibiotic that has shown promise in treating this infection. In the laboratory and in Phase I and II clinical trials B has been shown to be safe and promising in humans. Assume further that A is often not well tolerated by patients because of its side-effects and that one of the hopes for treatment B is that it will have similar efficacy with less burdensome side-effects. At the current time, however, there is not enough experience with B to predict reliably whether it is sufficiently efficacious and well tolerated in patients as to be equally attractive or more attractive than A. We can refer to this sort of uncertainty in the clinical community as *clinical agnosticism* to reflect the idea that the members of the expert medical community have not yet made determinate judgments about the relative therapeutic merits of A and B.

The second scenario presents a case of what we might call uncertainty as *clinical conflict*. Imagine that things are largely as they were in the previous scenario with the following exception. In this new case, more is known about the therapeutic merits of B, and members of the expert medical community have formed definite opinions about the relative therapeutic merits of A and B. Now imagine, however, that the community of expert clinicians is divided in their preferences, with some preferring A over B and some preferring B to A. The division need not be 50:50, since what is at stake is not an issue of popularity (London 2000). Rather, the community may be in conflict as long as a 'reasonable minority' of informed and reflective expert clinicians would offer advice to patients that conflicts with the advice of the majority (Freedman 1987; Kadane 1996; Miller and Weijer 2003).

Unfortunately, Freedman lumps both clinical agnosticism and clinical conflict together as cases of uncertainty in the expert medical community. As I argue below, clearly distinguishing these scenarios helps to avoid confusion and adds an additional level of sophistication to the defense of the equipoise requirement. Nevertheless, Freedman seems to hold, correctly, that in each of these scenarios it is permissible to carry out a randomized clinical trial in which patients with the particular bacterial infection are assigned at random to either treatment A or treatment B (Freedman 1987: 144). That is, in each case clinical equipoise obtains because there is no consensus in the relevant expert medical community about which treatment is best for patients with the relevant medical condition. This lack of consensus also provides the proper target for clinical research in that there is great social and clinical value in trials that are designed to disturb or to eliminate such a state of agnosticism or conflict. As a result, in addition to playing an important ethical role in clinical research, Freedman took the concept of equipoise to play an important epistemic or scientific role by identifying the proper focus of clinical research initiatives.

Freedman should be understood, therefore, as defending clinical equipoise on the ground that it not only allows clinical trials to be initiated, but permits their being carried out until such a time as they generate data that is sufficient to eliminate clinical agnosticism or to resolve the state of conflict in the clinical community. Finally, by targeting clinical research at questions about which the expert clinical community is conflicted, clinical equipoise ensures that clinical research targets important questions whose resolution will advance the care of future persons. As such, it ensures that clinical research has both scientific and moral merit.

It is at this point, however, that critics charge clinical equipoise with being overly permissive in allowing the interests of participants to be sacrificed to the perceived interests of scientific progress. Consider that within standard, fixed sized RCTs researchers stipulate in advance a P value or significance level (usually $\leq .05$) for ruling out the possibility of mistakenly accepting the hypothesis that the experimental intervention is superior to the control. As data are acquired over time, trends may emerge. Critics hold that in any trial that ultimately produces statistically significant results, there will be some point prior to reaching the desired level of statistical significance at which the hypothesis that one intervention is inferior to the other is sufficiently probable that allowing another patient to enroll in the trial, or allowing the trial to continue for current participants, violates the therapeutic obligation (Gifford 2000). Such scenarios are most compelling when they occur in a trial that is intended to eliminate clinical agnosticism. Surely, the critic claims, there is some point before the trial reaches the desired level of statistical significance at which it is sufficiently clear that one intervention is inferior to another that continuing with the trial violates the therapeutic obligation.

Three responses, however, are open to the proponent of clinical equipoise. First, if the interim data from the trial are sufficiently persuasive that they resolve the agnosticism of the clinical community in favor of one intervention over another, then the trial should be stopped because equipoise has been disturbed. Second, if, in contrast, only some clinicians are persuaded by the interim data, then we have only moved from a state of clinical agnosticism to a state of clinical conflict. In this case, however, equipoise still obtains and it is *permissible* to carry out the trial until consensus emerges and the conflict is resolved.

Third, and more fundamentally, however, this criticism of the equipoise requirement retains a view of the therapeutic obligation that Freedman rejects. That is, the objection presupposes an asymmetric relationship between the conditions above according to which the responsiveness to participant interests condition embodies a fragile epistemic threshold in the mind of the individual clinician and the content of the equipoise condition embodies a more robust epistemic threshold situated in the clinical community. Freedman's account of these conditions, however, is symmetric in that both conditions embody a robust epistemic threshold located in the state of consensus in the clinical community. This is a point worth emphasizing.

Freedman claims that the content of the obligation to safeguard the interests of trial participants is determined by the norms of sound medical practice. When there is conflict in the clinical community, however, he claims that ' "good medicine" finds the choice between A and B indifferent' (Freedman 1987: 144). The use of the term 'indifferent' in this context is somewhat misleading because it treats cases of clinical conflict as though they were cases of clinical agnosticism. It is more accurate, therefore, to say that in cases of clinical conflict good medicine is conflicted. Moreover, when good medicine is conflicted, 'it is likely to be a matter of chance that the patient is being seen by a clinician with a preference for B over A, rather than by an equally competent clinician with the opposite preference' (Freedman 1987: 144). In this respect, enrolling in a clinical trial in which one is randomized to either A or B is not significantly different from chance determining that one sees a clinician with one treatment preference rather than an equally competent clinician with the opposite treatment recommendation. In both cases, the individual receives a therapeutic option that is favored by some clinicians, but not by others (see also Kadane 1996).

There is another respect, however, in which these situations do differ dramatically. Conducting the clinical trial has the advantage of generating the data that is necessary to resolve the conflict in the medical community by clarifying the relative net therapeutic advantages of A and B. As a result, the option of conducting the clinical trial dominates the option of not doing so because, in both cases, patients and participants receive a treatment that is recommended for them by at least a reasonable minority of the expert medical community over a contrary recommendation from others in the expert medical community, but when this happens within the context of a clinical trial there is the added advantage of generating the data that will resolve the conflict to the benefit of future patients.

This response on behalf of clinical equipoise helps to motivate additional refinements to the theory that avoid further unnecessary confusion. For example, Freedman and others often speak as though equipoise concerns the relative therapeutic advantage of a set of treatment options relative to a *population of patients*. This has led some critics to claim that equipoise requires individual clinicians to abandon their commitment to the interests of individual patients (Hellman 2002). The reason is that it is possible for a clinician to be uncertain about the relative therapeutic merits of two interventions for a large population of people, but not to be uncertain in this regard when presented with a particular individual with particular symptoms and needs. If equipoise is applied at the level of treatment populations, so the objection goes, it would permit clinicians to enroll an individual in a clinical trial even though, in their considered medical opinion, one of the options in the trial is dominated by another for that particular person.

While this objection rests on some serious and important issues, it does not apply to the interpretation of equipoise that I have outlined here. As my treatment of equipoise in this section illustrates, equipoise should be understood as focusing on individual potential trial participants and whether, in each case, the expert medical community is agnostic or in conflict over the relative therapeutic merits for treating this particular individual. Clearly, good clinical medicine will always provide recommendations to individuals only in so far as they instantiate a more general clinical profile. And there is nothing wrong with speaking of 'well-defined patient populations' if what we mean is sets of individuals described at the finest level at which sound medicine can discriminate. As a purely interpretive matter, I think this is probably what Freedman has in mind when he uses similar terminology. It is important to be clear about this point, however, because we want to avoid a focus on populations that would give rise to well-known statistical problems of the relevant reference class in which a treatment could be beneficial for the aggregate population but harmful to all but one sub-population of the aggregate (Kadane 1996; London 2001, 2006a).

This, however, is a point about the conditions on which participating in a clinical trial can be justified as an admissible option for potential individual participants. It should not be confused with a very different claim, namely, that individual physicians must somehow disavow their own conscience and hide their treatment preferences from their patients. Quite the opposite, in fact. Even Freedman claims that if the individual physician has a particular treatment preference, this should be disclosed to the patient and the physician should be free to advise the patient as their conscience dictates (Freedman 1987: 144). However, this liberty of conscience does not eliminate the obligation to disclose to the patient that there exists sufficient disagreement in the expert medical community that different experts might provide treatment recommendations that conflict with this physician's advice (Chard and Lilford 1998).

There is a more radical argument, however, that can be made against objections to clinical equipoise that rely on a view of the therapeutic obligation that incorporates a fragile epistemic threshold in the mind of the individual clinician. In particular, such views embody an unjustified vestige of medical paternalism in research ethics. They are paternalistic because they limit the set of admissible options from which a patient may choose to those that happen to be recommended by a particular physician, regardless of what other equally competent experts would recommend to the same patient. Simplifying for this example an approach used in the KSS model (Kadane 1996), we can define a therapeutic option as 'admissible' if it would be recommended for a particular patient by at least a reasonable minority of clinicians in the expert medical community. In the case of clinical conflict, if both A and B are admissible interventions, so would be the option of participating in a clinical trial in which one would be randomized to either A or B. To prevent individuals from using their own values to choose from among the options of A, B, and the trial of A & B is to place an arbitrary restriction on individual choice. This restriction is arbitrary because it treats the opinions of a single expert as sovereign in the face of dissenting views from equally competent experts.

It is worth noting, however, that the above example reveals a fundamental tension within Freedman's account of clinical equipoise. In particular, it provides strong grounds for questioning whether the moral basis of the equipoise requirement ought to be located in the role-related obligations of the individual clinician. This is because such role-related obligations are traditionally understood as binding individual clinicians; each clinician is obligated to minister to the best interests of his or her patients. As a result, such role-related obligations require a conception of equipoise that locates the relevant uncertainty in the mind of the individual clinician. Freedman's position, therefore, appears to be untenable; one must either locate the relevant uncertainty in the expert medical community and find a different normative basis for the equipoise requirement, or one must accept the physician's duty of personal care as the moral basis of equipoise and locate the relevant uncertainty in the mind of the individual clinician (London 2006a).

To drive home the above point, consider the above situation from the standpoint of the patient. Each patient seeks advice that reflects the background beliefs and expert understanding of the physician, combined with an analysis of the available data regarding the therapeutic alternatives, to yield treatment advice that is tailored to the specific situation of the particular patient. The reflective patient may also realize, however, that different physicians may have different background beliefs, different interpretations of the available data about the therapeutic alternatives, and possibly different beliefs about the patient's specific clinical situation. Less idealistically, 'ordinary' patients may encounter these conflicting recommendations in person if they are able to seek several opinions about their case, or within the medical literature if they are able to research into the state of expert medical opinion. If the patient cannot determine with confidence which body of expert opinion is most likely to be correct, why would it be less reasonable to allow one's treatment to be allocated at random than to randomly decide to believe one expert rather than another? It should be noted, for example, that Marquis now appears to endorse this approach as a response to the conflict between the demands of clinical research and the therapeutic obligation (Marquis 1999).

To be clear, there may be reasons that might lead a potential trial participant to prefer one treatment over another even though expert opinion is conflicted. For example, a Christian Scientist might prefer treatment B to A if A involves an invasive surgical procedure while treatment B is medical in nature. In such a case, the patient's all-things-considered judgment about the available treatment options may not be conflicted once all of the patient's personal values are brought to bear on the decision. When this is the case, participating in a clinical trial may not be a permissible option for that particular patient. However, participation would still be permissible for patients whose values are not sufficiently clear or not of sufficient personal priority to generate a determinate treatment preference in the face of conflicting medical advice. In these cases, both the patient and the clinician could endorse participation in a properly designed clinical trial as a means of resolving clinical conflict in the larger medical community. This example of clinical conflict provides additional reason to endorse a claim that others have made to the effect that equipoise ought to exist at a variety of levels (Chard and Lilford 1998). It also provides a clear focus for the goals of the informed consent process: to ensure that only those individuals participate in research who see the clinical trial as a reasonable option in light of the conflict or uncertainty that exists in expert medical opinion.

It is difficult to overstate the significance of this view of clinical trials as a legitimate response to conflicted opinion at the level of the expert clinical community and in the mind of the individual trial participant. In particular, this insight plays a foundational role in what I refer to below as an integrative approach to clinical trials. In order to motivate this transition, however, it is necessary to consider objections from moral foundations that have recently been raised against clinical equipoise.

OBJECTIONS FROM MORAL FOUNDATIONS

Perhaps the most radical critique of clinical equipoise holds that this entire approach is built upon the mistaken foundational presupposition that the ethics of clinical research must be derived from and constrained by the ethics of clinical medicine (Miller and Brody 2002, 2003). According to this view, the dilemma to which the equipoise requirement was meant to respond is actually a false dilemma. It appears compelling only under the false assumption that clinical research and clinical medicine are contiguous activities. These critics claim, however, that the goals of clinical medicine and the goals of clinical research are 'logically incompatible' (Brody and Miller 2003: 332). Unlike clinical medicine, the purpose of clinical research is not to administer treatment; it is to investigate scientific hypotheses and gather generalizable data. Once we jettison this misconception, we are told, we jettison half of the dilemma with it. We are thus left with the permissibility of pursuing clinical research as a socially valuable activity, but clinical researchers are no longer saddled with the therapeutic obligation. In fact, investigators explicitly do not have 'a fiduciary relationship with research subjects' (Brody and Miller 2003: 336). Instead, they have an obligation to conduct sound science on society's behalf and to prevent and avoid the exploitation of research participants in the process.

To be clear, the proponents of equipoise and the proponents of the non-exploitation approach agree that a variety of conditions must be met in order for a clinical trial to be morally permissible. For instance, Emanuel, Wendler, and Grady point to seven necessary conditions: scientific or social value, scientific validity, fair subject selection, favorable risk-benefit ratio, independent review, informed consent, and respect for research participants (Emanuel *et al.* 2000). They endorse clinical equipoise as a means of ensuring that research is scientifically valid and as a necessary condition for medical research to be carried out when informed consent cannot be obtained. Implicit in the latter claim is that the existence of equipoise helps to ensure a favorable risk–benefit ratio. Proponents of the 'non-exploitation' approach agree with these seven conditions, but they reject any role for clinical equipoise in determining their content (Miller and Brody 2003: 26). In particular, they hold that the limits of morally permissible medical research do not have to remain within the restrictive boundaries of good clinical medicine—as in the equipoise requirement—but only within the more permissible boundary of the social obligation not to exploit research participants.

For the non-exploitation view, the content of the concept of exploitation is defined entirely in terms of the relationship between the risks to the interests of participants and the potential gains in scientific progress. When the risks to participants are justified by, proportionate to, or outweighed by the potential gains to science then research is not exploitative. When the risks are disproportionate to, not compensated by, or outweighed by the gains in science, then research is exploitative.

How successful is this critique of the moral foundations of equipoise? At best, this objection shows only that the equipoise requirement cannot govern the entire domain of clinical research if (*a*) as a constraint on permissible medical research equipoise is grounded in an obligation to provide a level of care for the needs of participants that falls within the boundaries of good clinical medicine and (*b*) some areas or aspects of clinical research do not directly involve treating, or testing a potential treatment for, participant needs. However, this limitation has been recognized and embraced by proponents of the equipoise requirement. Most notably, Weijer argues that the equipoise requirement applies only to those elements of a clinical trial that are being evaluated to clarify their potential value as therapeutic options. Elements of a clinical trial that are not candidates for therapeutic use, but which are instead necessary elements of a sound scientific and statistical design, must be evaluated in terms of the risks they post to participants. In particular, it must be determined whether the risks are necessary, whether they have been minimized, and whether they are justifiable in light of the potential benefits of the research to scientific progress (Weijer 1999, 2000, 2002; Emanuel *et al.* 2000: 2705–6).

Of course, proponents of the non-exploitation approach want to make a more radical claim, namely, that the entire enterprise of medical research falls under the scope of (*b*) above since the point and purpose of research *as such* is not to minister to patient needs but to generate reliable scientific information. This is the point of their claim that the ends of clinical medicine and the ends of clinical research are 'logically incompatible'. Unfortunately, this argument for their more radical claim suffers from several serious flaws.

First, the notion of 'logical incompatibility' is ambiguous. Certainly it is true that *at a purely conceptual level* the guiding purpose of clinical medicine and the guiding purpose of clinical research are distinct. But it does not follow that these conceptually distinct ends either are, or should be, mutually exclusive *in practice*. That is, it does not follow that these ends cannot both be integrated in practice by a single activity or that it is always desirable to keep them separate. For example, driving to work and showing concern for the interests of others are conceptually distinct activities. But that doesn't mean that they cannot be pursued simultaneously in practice or that it would always be advantageous to separate them! Similarly, when a patient receives conflicting advice about how to treat her medical condition, participating in a clinical trial that randomly assigns her to one of those competing options represents a means of pursuing the end of clinical research in a way that is consistent with her receiving a level of care that is consistent with what at least one group of competent clinicians would recommend. There is nothing inconsistent about claiming that these conceptually distinct goals are each being pursued in a single activity. It is necessary, however, to recognize that these distinct conceptual ends create tensions within the single practical activity, and these tensions must be addressed openly and explicitly in order to avoid confusion.

Such a straightforward position is very different from pretending either that this activity is only pursuing the goal of providing treatment or that it is only conducting clinical research. The former error is morally problematic because it prevents participants from recognizing the potential divergence between the needs of research and their own best interests. The latter error is also morally problematic, however, if it is taken to provide a justification for researchers to be insensitive to the basic interests of research participants. This point is especially important in those cases when research and treatment could not be neatly separated in practice, as when research focuses on precisely those needs that would be the subject of treatment in a clinical context. To say that these ends are 'logically distinct', therefore, is not to say anything about how those conceptually distinct ends ought to be treated when they cannot both be pursued separately in actual practice.

Second, by focusing on the fact that these activities are conceptually distinct, the non-exploitation approach risks begging the central moral issue. In particular, the non-exploitation view presupposes that the ethical constraints that are appropriate for an activity are properly determined by the *conceptual goals* or *guiding purpose* of the activity. The proper moral norms of clinical medicine, this view holds, are internal to or derived from the purpose of that activity and, similarly, the proper moral norms of research are internal to or derived from the purpose of that activity. Since these purposes are different, the ethical requirements are different (Brody and Miller 1998; 2003: 332). This position can therefore be represented as contrasting two forms of consequentialism. Clinicians are required to act according to a *patient-centered consequentialism* according to which the goal is to maximize the welfare of the individual patient. Researchers on the other hand are required to act according to a *general consequentialism* that seeks to 'promote the medical good of future patients' (Miller and Brody 2003: 21).

Even if we grant (1) that the ends of clinical medicine and clinical research are conceptually distinct and (2) that the ethical constraints that are appropriate for an activity are determined by its conceptual goals, it does not follow (3) that in order to advance science it is permissible in practice for researchers to provide a level of care for participant interests that falls below the level of care that would be recommended by sound medical practice. The reason that (3) does not follow from (1) and (2) is that (1) and (2) entail only (3*) that clinical research requires that the interests of present participants be weighed against the interests of science and benefits to future patients. *This proposition, however, does not say anything about the specific weights that it is permissible to assign to these competing interests.* In other words, from (1) and (2) we can derive the need to weigh or compare competing interests of different individuals but there are many possible ways of doing this and (1) and (2) alone are not so specific as to mandate that these trades be made in a particular way.

In order to go beyond (3*) to (3) without simply begging the question, therefore, we need a substantive argument to justify setting the relevant weights in a way that allows the interests of present participants to be directly outweighed by gains to the interests of future patients. Proponents of the non-exploitation view often speak of research ethics as a utilitarian enterprise. In this spirit, one way to derive (3) from (3*) would be to hold that the interests of each individual should count for one, and no more than one, and that the interests of each future person should be summed together with the interests of each present person. Research initiatives that produce the highest utility score for the resulting aggregate would be morally justified. While such a utilitarian calculus would yield (3*) it would also permit researchers to exact significant sacrifices from research participants since for any new drug in development there will be a relatively small group of research participants whose interests would be greatly outweighed by the thousands or millions of future patients who would benefit from access to the medication. So, not only does (3) not follow directly from (1) and (2) but at least some of the most common means of deriving (3*) from (3) yield pernicious consequences that are antithetical to much of contemporary research ethics.

It is worth pointing out, therefore, that it would also be consistent with (3*) to adopt a different kind of *consequentialist calculus* according to which it is permissible to consider the interests of future patients in designing a clinical trial only if it is possible to ensure first that present participants receive a level of care that is consistent with what would be recommended in their case by at least a minority of expert clinicians. If a great many people would stand to benefit from a particular research initiative, these numbers might provide a reason to give priority to that research relative to other endeavors. But ever greater numbers would not license exacting ever greater sacrifices from research participants. I will return to such a view in the final section below.

This analysis points out two sources of deficiency in the current debate. First, linking the normative force of the equipoise requirement to duties that are specific to the role of the physician makes it appear that proponents of the equipoise requirement must be committed to claim (2) above. However, as I will illustrate in a moment, the equipoise requirement can be grounded in values that are not derived from role-related duties. Second, the perception that both proponents and critics of equipoise endorse (2) above makes it easier to confuse conclusion (3*) with (3). It thereby exacerbates the difficulty in seeing that *the equipoise requirement can itself be understood as consequentialist calculus that provides the content to (3*) by detailing when tradeoffs in individual welfare for benefits to future patients become exploitative.*

Proponents of the non-exploitation approach do have an additional argument that they hope will make (3) above appear more attractive than a position that relies on equipoise to provide content to the tradeoffs required by (3*) above. However, this is simply a version of the argument from utility in which equipoise is associated with a duty to safeguard patient interests that embodies a fragile epistemic threshold in the mind of the individual clinician. Proponents of the non-exploitation approach have been able to leverage this argument more fruitfully than their predecessors, however, because they have focused on an area where proponents of the equipoise requirement have not always offered advice that is consistent with the specifics of their own theory, namely, the use of placebo controls in clinical trials (Emanuel and Miller 2001; Miller and Brody 2002).

Briefly put, proponents of the non-exploitation approach criticize proponents of equipoise for holding that it is only permissible to employ a placebo control in a clinical trial when no alternative treatment for the condition in question exists. Critics then point out that this would prohibit the use of placebo controls for studies in which subjects are not subject to more than the most mild risks, such as forgoing a current treatment for baldness or an analgesic for minor headaches. They charge in response that 'This argument conflates clinical research with clinical care. Clinicians frequently do not treat such ailments and patients often forgo treatment, indicating that there can be no ethical necessity to provide it' (Emanuel and Miller 2001: 916).

It is not that this argument conflates clinical research and clinical care, since, as the critics themselves point out, there are many instances where effective medical care exists *but non-treatment remains an admissible treatment option.* The problem lies, rather, in a misunderstanding of the responsiveness to participant interests condition discussed above. That is, as the above comment nicely illustrates, the problem here lies with a view of the duty of personal care or the therapeutic obligation that embodies a fragile epistemic threshold and that requires treatment for absolutely any problem. As a result, proponents of equipoise should simply accept this point and argue that placebo controls are permissible if no effective therapeutic option exists or if such options do exist but non-treatment remains an admissible therapeutic option. Recent treatments of equipoise make just this move (Weijer and Glass 2002; Weijer and Miller 2004). In the following section I provide a more careful analysis of the latter condition. For the moment I simply want to claim that conceptions of equipoise that adopt a multidimensional evaluative focus and a robust epistemic threshold are not committed to the simplistic attitude toward placebo controls that critics often saddle them with.

Finally, one must also ask how successful the non-exploitation approach is in offering an alternative to the equipoise requirement. In particular, if one rejects the equipoise requirement as a method for determining when research participants are being exploited, then what is the substantive criterion according to which exploitative and non-exploitative research can be discriminated? If medical research is concerned with promoting the good of future patients, then is it permissible, for example, to withhold effective medical care for a severe (what about debilitating or life threatening) medical condition if the trial in question will generate an intervention that could potentially help thousands (what about tens of thousands or millions) of future patients?

Unfortunately, this aspect of the non-exploitation approach has not been fully worked out. Although the partisans of this view are clear that it is permissible to trade the welfare of participants for gains in science, we are only told that the limit of permissible tradeoffs is imprecise or fuzzy and a matter of judgment. In other words, the talk of 'weighing' or 'trading off' is purely metaphorical since the underlying judgments cannot be explicitly quantified. This is particularly disappointing for an approach that views medical research as an inherently utilitarian enterprise. It is also a significant limitation for a theory that will be needed most in precisely those cases where well-intentioned people are likely to disagree (London and Kadane 2003; London 2006a).

To be clear, it would be a mistake to think, as proponents of the non-exploitation approach sometimes seem to imply, that these are tradeoffs that cannot be quantified. The problem, I submit, is exactly the opposite—there are uncountably many different tradeoff schedules that could be specified. It is not that no such calculus exists, therefore, so much as that there are too many possible calculi from which to choose and what we need are non-arbitrary reasons for narrowing the class down to an admissible set or, if possible, a preferred schedule. It is also worth stressing that while this problem is more pressing for the non-exploitation view—since it relies on such judgments as the sole means of determining when the risks posed to subjects are morally appropriate—it must also be faced by proponents of the equipoise requirement in those areas of research to which equipoise does not apply.

At best, therefore, proponents of the non-exploitation view can be seen as underscoring the claim that clinical equipoise cannot alone govern the entire domain of human-subjects research. While they are clear in their assertions that a more comprehensive framework will be consequentialist in nature, their view remains sufficiently undefined as to be consistent with uncountably many different accounts of how to make the requisite tradeoffs. Clearly, however, not just any consequentialism can function as a defensible foundation for research ethics. For example, assigning the same weight to the interests of each future patient and each present research participant would effectively license exposing present participants to an unbounded degree of risk since the number of future beneficiaries of any successful research initiative is potentially unlimited. Fortunately, however, the space of viable options is populated by more reasonable approaches than this relatively anemic framework of moral accounting.

THE INTEGRATIVE APPROACH TO CLINICAL TRIALS

In the previous section I suggested that the degree of fragmentation at the foundations of research ethics is greatly exaggerated. In this final section I amplify this claim by sketching the outlines of a view of research ethics that has been more fully developed and articulated elsewhere (London 2006a, b). This outline should be sufficient to illustrate how the equipoise requirement itself can be seen as a means of specifying the content of the requirement not to exploit research participants and, therefore, as illustrating how what are currently perceived to be mutually exclusive ethical ideals can be united under a single heading.

Like the non-exploitation approach, the integrative approach holds that the social justification for the institutions of clinical research lies in their capacity to advance the common good of community members by investigating socially significant questions using sound scientific methods. It also holds that it is sometimes permissible to subordinate the individual good of particular persons to the common good. The integrative approach, however, rejects the idea that the individual good and the common good refer to the complete set of interests of two different entities, one of which is an individual and the other an aggregate of individuals united into a corporate body. Rather, these terms distinguish *two sets of interests, each of which can be attributed to every individual person* (London 2003).

In liberal democratic communities, individuals often differ radically in their *personal interests*. These are defined as interests that individuals have in virtue of the particular projects and life plans embraced by that individual. The integrative approach identifies the personal or *individual good* of agents with the pursuit of the goals and ends that constitute their personal interests. This diversity in personal interests can frustrate social decision making because it is often the source of disagreements about how to value risks, activities, goals, and ends.

Amidst this diversity in personal goods, however, individuals in liberal democratic communities share a higher order interest in being able to cultivate and to exercise the basic human capacities they need in order to pursue their personal interests. This shared higher order interest provides a social perspective from which the members of such communities can identify a set of *basic interests*. These are interests that each individual has in being able to cultivate and to exercise their capacities for reflective thought and practical decision making, to develop and exercise their affective or emotional capacities, and in having the external necessities to exercise those capacities in pursuit of particular projects and meaningful social relationships. The integrative approach identifies the *common good* with this set of basic interests and the basic social interest of every community member in ensuring that their basic interests are secured and advanced by the social structures of their community. It then uses this set of basic interests to define the space of social equality, the domain with respect to which each community member has a just claim to equal treatment.

Because the basic interests of individuals can be profoundly restricted or defeated by sickness and disease, each can recognize a reason to support medical research as a social institution in so far as it strives to advance the state of medical science and, with this, the standard of care that is available to future patients. The institutions of clinical research represent one element within a larger social division of labor that must be justifiable to the members of the community whose basic interests those institutions are supposed to serve (London 2005). As such, the integrative approach holds that clinical research must pursue this goal of advancing the interests of future patients in a way that is consistent with an equal regard for the basic interests of the present persons whose participation makes those results possible.

In light of this requirement, the integrative approach adopts the following definition of reasonable risk:

Definition of reasonable risk: Risks to individual research participants are reasonable just in case they (1) require the least amount of intrusion into the interests of participants that is necessary in order to facilitate sound scientific inquiry and (2) are consistent with an equal regard for the basic interests of study participants and the members of the larger community whose interests that research is intended to serve. (London 2006*a*)

This requirement of equal regard is intended to reflect the claim that although there is a moral imperative to carry out research that will advance the basic interests of community members in the future, this imperative is not sufficient to legitimize sacrificing or forfeiting the basic interests of other community members in the process. To say that it may be morally permissible, when necessary, to subordinate the individual good of particular persons to the common good is not to set up a calculus in which all of an individual's interests are weighed in a balance against the interests of the other individuals in the community or against the interests of future individuals. It is, instead, to say that it is permissible to ask individuals to modify or even to sacrifice some of the particular goals and ends that are a part of their individual good in order to provide others with the conditions necessary to cultivate and engage those basic capacities for agency and sociability that constitute their share of the common good. The integrative approach, therefore, seeks to create the social conditions in which community members can take on, as a personal project, the goal of assisting future patients, while being assured that their basic interests are treated with the same moral concern as that which provides the moral motivation for the research enterprise itself.

Operational criteria for this conception of reasonable risk are generated by considering how the basic interests of community members are safeguarded and advanced in other areas of the social division of labor. When the basic interests of individuals are threatened or restricted by sickness, injury, or disease, this job falls in large part to the health care system. The integrative approach therefore adopts the following as the first of two operational criteria:

First operational criterion: Equal regard for the basic interests of research participants and non-participants requires that when the basic interests of an individual participant are threatened or compromised by sickness, injury, or disease, the basic interests of that individual must be protected and advanced in a way that does not fall below the threshold of competent medical care. (London 2006a)

This operational criterion invokes the threshold of competent medical care, not as a source of the normativity of this framework, but as a standard for determining what is required in order to show equal regard for the basic interests of individuals whose basic interests are threatened or restricted by sickness, injury, or disease. Similarly, its scope is limited to the basic interests of individuals because this criterion delineates the level of risk that it is permissible to *offer* to prospective research participants. Participants are then free to decide for themselves whether the risks that remain are acceptable in light of their various goals and commitments.

This focus on basic interests also reflects the normative claim that it is permissible to ask individual research participants to alter, risk, or even to sacrifice some of their personal interests in an effort to advance the basic interests of others. This means that it is permissible to ask individuals to undergo intrusive, painful, and otherwise uncomfortable experiences in order to advance scientifically meritorious research. The constraint is simply that the risks that such research poses to the basic interests of participants must be consistent with the requirement of equal regard expressed in the above operational criterion.

The following practical test can then be used to determine whether or not a particular clinical trial satisfies this operational criterion.

Practical test for first criterion: A specific intervention s is admissible for an individual i just in case there is either uncertainty among, or conflict between, expert clinicians about whether s is dominated by any other intervention or set of interventions that are recognized as options for treating individual i. For each individual in a clinical trial, the care and protection afforded to that individual's basic interests falls within the threshold of competent medical care just in case each intervention to which that individual might be allocated within the clinical trial is admissible for that individual. (Adapted from London 2006a)

This practical test is similar to Freedman's clinical equipoise, but there are important differences. First, the scope of this requirement is limited to the basic interests of participants and its moral force is grounded, not in the role-related obligations of physicians, but in broader claims about the need for basic social structures to provide equal regard for the basic interests of all community members. Second, this practical test explicitly distinguishes uncertainty in the mind of expert clinicians from the state of clinical conflict between such clinicians. Third, where the equipoise requirement is often applied to entire trial populations, the above practical test is applied to each individual trial participant.

The integrative approach therefore permits the use of a placebo control as an admissible arm of a clinical trial:

1. if no effective therapeutic option exists, or
2. if an effective therapeutic option exists but the condition in question is such that non-treatment remains an admissible therapeutic option because either
    (a) the condition being treated does not threaten the individual's ability to function in a way that would adversely affect their basic interests, or
    (b) the condition is more severe but an all-things-considered evaluation of the benefits and burdens of the existing interventions reveals that they do not necessarily offer a clear net therapeutic advantage over non-treatment.

When these conditions cannot be met, a placebo control will not be an admissible option. Alternative means of generating scientific information will have to be pursued that provide an admissible treatment option to research participants. If this makes science in the service of the common good more costly in terms of time and other resources, then such inefficiencies must be tolerated as an unfortunate byproduct of a fundamental commitment to safeguarding and protecting for each individual the very basic interests that justify initiating the research enterprise itself.

When research involves individuals whose basic interests are not compromised or threatened by sickness and disease, the equipoise requirement does not apply. However, the more general requirements of the integrative approach remain in force. The integrative approach uses the following, second, operational criterion to make operational in this context the goal of advancing science in a way that is consistent with an equal regard for the basic interests of all community members.

Second operational criterion: In all cases, the cumulative incremental risks to the basic interests of individuals that derive from purely research-related activities that are not offset by the prospect of direct benefit to the individual must not be greater than the risks to the basic interests of individuals that are permitted in the context of other socially sanctioned activities that are similar in structure to the research enterprise. (London 2006a)

Respect for the moral equality of individuals cannot require that individuals be prohibited from voluntarily assuming some risk to their basic interests, since such a standard simply cannot be achieved. This proposal therefore seeks to identify social activities that are structurally similar to the research enterprise and to ensure that the incremental risks to the basic interests of participants associated with purely research-related activities do not exceed the incremental risks to the basic interests of individuals associated with those structurally similar social activities.

I have proposed elsewhere criteria that might be used to construct practical tests for this second operational criterion (London 2006a). For my present purposes I merely want to indicate how a single overarching approach to research ethics might provide a foundation for research ethics within which the equipoise requirement itself might be seen as a means of specifying the content to the ideal of not exploiting research participants. Clearly, key concepts within this approach have to be explicated more carefully and then wedded to a particular decision theory in order to provide more precise guidance to practical decision making. Nevertheless, even these broad outlines are sufficiently suggestive as to provide a motivation to take up such a project in earnest. At the very least, they should provide a clear indication that the foundations of research ethics may appear to be more fragmented than they actually are and that, with effort, we may yet find a philosophical theory that brings unity to this apparent diversity.

References

ASHCROFT, R. (1999), 'Equipoise, Knowledge and Ethics in Clinical Research and Practice', *Bioethics*, 13/3–4: 314–26.

BRODY, H., and MILLER, F. G. (1998), 'The Internal Morality of Medicine: Explication and Application to Managed Care', *Journal of Medicine and Philosophy*, 23: 384–410.

―― ―― (2003), 'The Clinician–Investigator: Unavoidable but Manageable Tension', *Kennedy Institute of Ethics Journal*, 13/4: 329–46.

CHALMERS, T. C. (1978), 'The Ethics of Randomization as a Decision-Making Technique and the Problem of Informed Consent', in T. L. Beauchamp and L. Walters (eds.), *Contemporary Issues in Bioethics* (Encino, Calif.: Dickenson), 426–9.

CHARD, J. A., and LILFORD, R. J. (1998), 'The Use of Equipoise in Clinical Trials', *Social Science and Medicine*, 47/7: 981–98.

EMANUEL, E. J., and MILLER, F. G. (2001), 'The Ethics of Placebo Controlled Trials—A Middle Ground', *New England Journal of Medicine*, 345/12: 915–19.

―― WENDLER, D., and GRADY, C. (2000), 'What Makes Clinical Research Ethical?', *JAMA* 283/20: 2701–11.

FREEDMAN, B. (1987), 'Equipoise and the Ethics of Clinical Research', *New England Journal of Medicine*, 317: 141–5.

____ (1990), 'Placebo Controlled Trials and the Logic of Clinical Purpose', *IRB: A Review of Human Subjects Research*, 12/6: 1–6.

FRIED, C. (1974), *Medical Experimentation: Personal Integrity and Social Policy* (Amsterdam: North-Holland).

GIFFORD, F. (1986), 'The Conflict Between Randomized Clinical Trials and the Therapeutic Obligation', *Journal of Medicine and Philosophy*, 11/4: 347–66.

____ (1995), 'Community-Equipoise and the Ethics of Randomized Clinical Trials', *Bioethics*, 9: 127–84.

____ (2000), 'Freedman's "Clinical Equipoise" and "Sliding-Scale All-Dimensions-Considered Equipoise" ', *Journal of Medicine and Philosophy*, 25/4: 399–426.

HELLMAN, D. (2002), 'Evidence, Belief, and Action: The Failure of Equipoise to Resolve the Ethical Tension in the Randomized Clinical Trial', *Journal of Law, Medicine, and Ethics*, 30: 375–80.

HILL, A. B. (1963), 'Medical Ethics and Controlled Trials', *British Medical Journal*, 1: 1043–9.

JOHNSON, N., LILFORD, R. J., and BRAZIER, W. (1991), 'At What Level of Collective Equipoise Does a Clinical Trial Become Ethical?', *Journal of Medical Ethics*, 17: 30–4.

JONAS, H. (1969), 'Philosophical Reflections on Experimenting with Human Subjects', *Daedalus*, 98/2: 219–47.

KADANE, J. B. (ed.) (1996), *Bayesian Methods and Ethics in a Clinical Trial Design* (New York: John Wiley).

KAEBNICK, G. E. (2003), 'From the Editor: No Wonder Research Ethics Is So Confusing', *Hastings Center Report*, 33/3: 2.

KARLAWISH, J. H. T., and LANTOS, J. (1997), 'Community Equipoise and the Architecture of Clinical Research', *Cambridge Quarterly of Healthcare Ethics*, 6: 385–96.

LEMMENS, T., and MILLER, P. B. (2002), 'Avoiding a Jekyll-and-Hyde Approach to the Ethics of Clinical Research and Practice', *American Journal of Bioethics*, 2/2: 14–17.

LILFORD, R. J. (2003), 'Ethics of Clinical Trials from a Bayesian and Decision Analytic Perspective: Whose Equipoise Is It Anyway?', *British Medical Journal*, 326: 980–1.

LONDON, A. J. (2000), 'The Ambiguity and the Exigency: Clarifying "Standard of Care" Arguments in International Research', *Journal of Medicine and Philosophy*, 25/4: 379–97.

____ (2001), 'Equipoise and International Human-Subjects Research', *Bioethics*, 15/4: 312–32.

____ (2003), 'Threats to the Common Good: Biochemical Weapons and Human Subjects Research', *Hastings Center Report*, 33/5: 17–25.

____ (2005), 'Justice and the Human Development Approach to International Research', *Hastings Center Report*, 35/1: 24–37.

____ (2006a), 'Reasonable Risks in Clinical Research: A Critique and A Proposal for the Integrative Approach', *Statistics in Medicine*, 25/17: 2869–2885.

____ (2006b), 'Sham Surgery and Reasonable Risks', in D. Benatar (ed.), *Cutting to the Core: Exploring the Ethics of Contested Surgeries* (New York: Rowman & Littlefield), 211–28.

____ and KADANE, J. B. (2002), 'Placebos that Harm: Sham Surgery Controls in Clinical Trials', *Statistical Methods in Medical Research*, 11: 413–27.

____ ____ (2003), 'Sham Surgery and Genuine Standards of Care: Can the Two Be Reconciled?', *American Journal of Bioethics*, 3/4: 61–4.

MANN, H., LONDON, A. J., and MANN, J. (2005), 'Equipoise in the Enhanced Suppression of the Platelet IIb/IIIa Receptor with Integrilin Trial (ESPRIT): A Critical Appraisal', *Clinical Trials*, 2: 233–43.

MARQUIS, D. (1983), 'Leaving Therapy to Chance', *Hastings Center Report*, 13/4: 40–7.

_____ (1999), 'How to Resolve an Ethical Dilemma Concerning Randomized Clinical Trials', *New England Journal of Medicine*, 341/9: 691–3.

MILLER, F. G. (2003), 'Sham Surgery: An Ethical Analysis', *American Journal of Bioethics*, 3/4: 41–8.

_____ and BRODY, H. (2002), 'What Makes Placebo-Controlled Trials Unethical?', *American Journal of Bioethics,* 2/2: 3–9.

_____ _____ (2003), 'A Critique of Clinical Equipoise: Therapeutic Misconception in the Ethics of Clinical Trials', *Hastings Center Report*, 33/3: 19–28.

_____ and WEIJER, C. (2003), 'Rehabilitating Equipoise', *Kennedy Institute of Ethics Journal*, 13/2: 93–118.

PETO, R., and BAIGENT, C. (1998), 'Trials: The Next 50 Years', *British Medical Journal*, 317: 1170–1.

_____ *et al.* (1976), 'Design and Analysis of Randomized Clinical Trials Requiring Prolonged Observation of Each Patient: I. Introduction and Design', *British Journal of Cancer*, 34: 585–612.

SACKETT, D. L. (2000), 'Equipoise, a Term Whose Time (If It Ever Came) Has Surely Gone', *Canadian Medical Association Journal*, 163/7: 835–6.

SCHWARTZ, D., FLAMANT, R., and LELLOUCH, J. (1980), *Clinical Trials*, trans. M. J. R. Healy (London: Academic Press).

VEATCH, R. M. (2002), 'Indifference of Subjects: An Alternative to Equipoise in Randomized Clinical Trials', *Social Philosophy and Policy*, 19: 295–323.

WEIJER, C. (1999), 'Thinking Clearly About Research Risk: Implications of the Work of Benjamin Freedman', *IRB: A Review of Human Subjects Research*, 21/6: 1–5.

_____ (2000), 'The Ethical Analysis of Risk', *Journal of Law, Medicine and Ethics*, 28: 344–61.

_____ (2002), 'When Argument Fails', *American Journal of Bioethics*, 2/2: 10–11.

_____ and GLASS, K. C. (2002), 'The Ethics of Placebo Controlled Trials', *New England Journal of Medicine*, 346: 382–3.

_____ and MILLER, P. B. (2004), 'When Are Research Risks Reasonable in Relation to Anticipated Benefits?', *Nature Medicine*, 10/6: 570–3.

CHAPTER 25

RESEARCH ON COGNITIVELY IMPAIRED ADULTS

JASON KARLAWISH

INTRODUCTION

THE ethical conduct of human subjects research relies on a matrix of protections: institutional review board (IRB) review, fair subject selection, and informed consent. These protections are derived from the principles of research ethics: beneficence, justice, and respect for persons (National Commission for the Protection of Human Subjects of Biomedical and Behavioral Research 1979). Among these protections, investigators and IRBs (or research ethics boards, REBs) devote substantial attention to one of them: the requirement for informed consent from the subject (Bell *et al.* 1998: 86).[1] In the United States, for example, research regulations detail procedures investigators and IRBs must follow to assure compliance with the elements of informed consent including requirements for an investigator to disclose up to

---

[1] Bell and colleagues' (1998) survey of 255 investigators' interactions with IRBs found that 99 per cent of the investigators reported IRB modifications to the consent forms and procedures, and 6 per cent reported IRB modifications to the scientific design. These sharply divergent proportions suggest that IRBs rely on informed consent rather than modifying the design of research to achieve human subjects' protection.

sixteen distinct categories of information to a potential subject (Department of Health and Human Services 1991, sect. 46.116).

The preeminence of informed consent in human subjects protections reflects Western democratic societies' ethical and political commitments to secure each citizen against both coercive and paternalistic influences of other people. Society permits adults extensive personal discretion in choices such as where to live, what to eat, how to dress, and whether to be in research. In short, individuals are afforded extensive discretion in choosing what to do and what is in their own best interests.

Informed consent to enroll in research is especially important because research necessarily involves procedures such as randomization and blinding that are done to assure that the project will produce generalizable knowledge (Freedman 1987a; Weijer 2000). Hence, subjects who are exposed to these procedures are exposed to the risks, costs, hassles, or discomforts of interventions that are not justified by benefits to their health and well-being, as is the case in treatment, but instead by the value of the knowledge the research is expected to produce. For example, research studies of surgical interventions that use a sham surgical procedure as a control group (Macklin 1999) assign some subjects to a control group who receive some but not all of the surgical procedure: anesthesia, an incision, and sutures. The justification for exposing subjects to these risks is the importance of the knowledge that would be gained. However, society requires an important constraint on this kind of experimentation: an insistence on the subjects' informed consent. A critical component of informed consent is understanding the risks of participation. A trial that compared arthroscopic knee surgery to a sham procedure for the treatment of degenerative joint disease required subjects to give written statements that they understood they could be assigned to the sham arm (Moseley *et al.* 2002). The investigators argued that this assurance that the subjects understood key research procedures and risks justified exposing them to the harms of sham surgery in order to develop generalizable knowledge. Other examples of this ethical tension are clinical trials that use a placebo-only control arm in the study of a promising intervention for a disease that has effective treatments, thereby requiring some subjects to forgo taking accepted therapies.

Democratic nations do recognize circumstances when it is appropriate to forgo the individual's informed consent and thereby sacrifice liberty for the collective good, such as epidemics and war, when mandatory vaccination and conscription are acceptable.[2] But as valuable as research may be to advance the health and well-being of a nation, no one is obligated to enroll in research to advance the diagnosis and treatment of diseases. Even in the setting of 'declaring war' against common, costly, and devastating diseases such as cancer, we no longer conscript

---

[2] Research that involves soldiers is outside the focus of this chapter but it offers a useful study of the conflict between issues of national security and the common good versus the personal choice of the potential subject in research that involves subjects who are under the command of superiors, e.g. soldiers. See e.g. Advisory Committee of Human Radiation Experiments (1996).

participants into research (Beecher 1966). Altruism is a personal choice. Hence, the voluntary choice of a competent adult to enroll in research is an essential practice to assure the ethical conduct of human subjects research and was a core subject protection in one of the first codes of research ethics, the Nuremberg Code (1949).

Unfortunately, in certain kinds of research, informed consent may not be feasible, in particular, in research that enrolls persons who are 'cognitively vulnerable'. The term describes having impairments in the abilities to understand, appreciate, reason, or make a choice that are severe enough that a reasonable person would judge them as lacking capacity and therefore not competent to make the decision. The spectrum of causes of impairments in decision making capacity is diverse. They can be developmental such as in children,[3] or acquired. The acquired causes can be further classified based on their chronicity and potential reversibility. Common chronic and progressive conditions include dementia from diseases such as Alzheimer's disease, whereas acute and potentially reversible conditions including emergent illness from trauma, acute psychosis, and critical illness. While the spectrum of causes that can impair decision making capacity is diverse, their common and ethically relevant feature is that the subjects may be unable to provide an informed consent because they lack the capacity to make the decision.

Research that involves persons who are cognitively vulnerable presents a dilemma: after removing the protection of informed consent from the subject of the research, are the remaining human subjects protections adequate? Or, does the absence of this protection render all research that would enroll them unethical? These questions frame a dilemma between the value of research to improve the health and welfare of persons with conditions that cause cognitive impairment versus the value of protecting such persons from exposure to research risks and discomforts. The sides of this dilemma are clear, contentious, and have been repeatedly recast along arguments that began in the early 1970s.

In the United States two national commissions (Department of Health Education and Welfare 1978; National Bioethics Advisory Commission 1998) and multiple advisory panels and expert groups have proposed guidelines for research that involves adults with cognitive impairment (Fletcher *et al.* 1985; Melnick *et al.* 1985; American College of Physicians 1989; National Institutes of Health, Office of Extramural Research 2001). With the exception of the focused issue of 'emergency research' (Department of Health and Human Services, Food and Drug Administration 1996), none of these guidelines have become regulations. They simply have not received sufficient support from researchers, subjects, and ethicists to serve as

---

[3] By law, children, that is persons under 18, are not competent. However, at a certain developmental stage they may be capable of making a decision to enroll in research. Hence, a child who has attained sufficient cognitive development and literacy may be as competent as an adult, but by law is still deemed not competent. The investigator must obtain informed consent from the child's parents and assent from the child (Department of Health and Human Services 1991, subpart D).

the basis for guidance on research on cognitively impaired persons.[4] Four questions frame the content of these guidelines and the controversies that have thwarted consensus:

How much research risk is permissible to expose a noncompetent adult?
What is an appropriate process for assessing research risks and benefits?
How should we decide an adult cannot provide an informed consent?
When is proxy informed consent appropriate?

The answers to these questions require both ethical and historical analyses. Historical analysis shows that it has been difficult to achieve consensus in answering these questions because even though the ethical principles used to work through the issues have been generally accepted, key participants' understanding of the issues is changing and the principles give no direction on how to resolve trade-offs when they are in conflict.

BACKGROUND: HISTORICAL OVERVIEW

The focus of this history is events in the United States that began in the 1970s with the work of the National Commission for the Protection of Human Subjects of Biomedical and Behavioral Research (hereafter referred to as the National Commission). The advantage of focusing on the United States is that its research infrastructure brings together many of the relevant political, social, and scientific actors. Its political order is grounded in a constitution that articulates the rights of the citizen, as opposed to the obligations of the subject to the state. Both public and private funding of increasingly allied academic and industrial research infrastructures make the United States the largest producer of scientific research. In the 1970s, in part as a result of scandals in the design and conduct of research (Beecher 1966),[5] Congress authorized a National Commission to develop a code of research

---

[4] The degree of controversy over these issues has been sharp even within the Commissions. Both the National Commission's Department of Health Education and Welfare (1978) and the National Bioethics Advisory Commission's (1998) proposed regulations included Commission members' dissents from specific proposals.

[5] Beecher's summary of multiple cases of unethical research was among the pivotal catalysts in the recognition that human subjects researchers could not alone regulate themselves. Notably, in the introduction to Beecher (1966) he suggested that financial and academic pressures are at least in part to blame for this. He chronicled the increase in research funding at both his own institution (Massachusetts General Hospital) and the National Institutes of Health and suggested that this pressure of funding, coupled with the requirement for success in research as a measure of academic success, spurred even more research, and, by inference, that without reform there would be more unethical research of the kinds he meticulously described.

ethics to guide all research conducted with federal funds or under Food and Drug Administration (FDA) regulations.[6]

But these regulations are incomplete. Although the United States has regulations for selected vulnerable populations—children, pregnant women and fetuses, and prisoners—the world's largest producer and consumer of human subject research still does not have specific guidance for research that involves the general class of cognitively vulnerable subjects. The only regulations to govern the conduct of research that involves adults with cognitive impairment are regulations for a narrowly defined group: adults with an acute, serious, and life threatening condition from whom informed consent from either the subject or the subject's proxy cannot be 'practicably obtained', commonly referred to as the 'emergency research regulations' (Department of Health and Human Services, Food and Drug Administration 1996).

The origins of this gap and the conditions that sustain it make the United States an excellent case study in the social, political, scientific, and ethical factors that determine what conditions, if any, must be fulfilled before enrolling an adult in research without that person's informed consent. The purpose of this section is to examine these factors with attention to demonstrating how this regulatory gap reflects continued changes in the framing of who is the focus of ethical concern. Specifically, we will examine changes in the political orientation of the mental illness community towards research, and in concepts of what it means to be competent to consent. In short, consensus on guidelines has been elusive because we are still working out what we are talking about.

Thirty years ago the focus of this chapter would not have been research that involves 'cognitively impaired adults'. Instead, it would be research that involves persons with 'mental illness'. This transformation reflects changes in concepts of mental illness from a concept distinct from other conditions that can impair cognition, to being within the category of one of many conditions that can cause cognitive impairment.

The National Commission's 1978 proposed regulations were focused on research involving persons who were 'institutionalized as mentally infirm' (Department of Health Education and Welfare 1978). This title, assigned in the 1974 National Research Act, reflected the ascendancy of the mental health rights movement, whose concerns were dramatized in films such as *Titicut Follies* and *One Flew Over the Cuckoo's Nest* (a gripping documentary and drama respectively of the oppressive life in mental institutions) and galvanized with scandals such as the Jewish Chronic Disease Hospital, in which investigators sought to examine the immune response

---

[6] Although the requirement that the common rule and its subparts for children, prisoners, and pregnant women covers all research conducted using federal funds from agencies who have signed on to the common rule and privately sponsored research, e.g. the pharmaceutical industry, conducted under FDA authority, the regulations are not the 'law of the land'. Congressional efforts to make the regulations a statute that governs all human subjects research have consistently failed.

of elderly residents of a long term care facility to injected cancer cells (Katz 1972). During this time several states adopted laws that limited the kinds of research that could enroll persons who were residents of institutions or under legally appointed guardianship.

But conditions for the treatment of the mentally ill were changing. The National Commission noted in its report that 'stereotyped notions' about the causes and treatment of psychiatric illnesses no longer applied. The changes included a transformation in concepts of mental illness from psychodynamic to biological pathogenesis. Biological psychiatry saw the proposed guidelines as a barrier to valuable research. In addition, public policy for the care of the mentally ill was changing. States were adopting an approach of 'deinstitutionalization' of the mentally ill. In short, the National Commission wrote recommendations for an era that was coming to a close.

The second reason for the change in focus was that organized advocates for the mentally ill began to divide in their view of research. The general attitude was no longer that persons with mental illness should be protected from research. Instead, groups such as the National Alliance for the Mentally Ill (NAMI) advocated that more research was needed to improve the care of the mentally ill. NAMI advocated clinical trials in the United States to obtain FDA approval of the anti-psychotic clozapine for the treatment of acute psychosis (Fried 1998). Unlike clozapine, available anti-psychotic medications had the risk of a disabling movement disorder, but clozapine had the risk of a sudden decline in infection-fighting white blood cells. It is a testament to the power of a patient advocacy group aligned with a pharmaceutical company and investigators that the research necessary to obtain FDA approval occurred in spite of these risks and the absence of regulations to guide research that involves persons with acute psychosis, a condition that can cause cognitive impairment.

Related to this political transformation was a change in the understanding of how mental illness impacts on a person's ability to make a decision. Prior to the 1980s much of the writing on informed consent focused on legal perspectives. For example, the National Commission invoked the concept of a 'legally valid informed consent', which referred to the competency of the person who granted it. But the law recognized at least three legal concepts of competency: a rational reasons standard, capacity to reach a reasonable result, and capacity to make a decision. It is notable that the third—the capacity to make a decision—was the view of only a minority of courts and would later become the most widely recognized standard.

Instead, the most widely recognized standards for competency assessment were the first two: a person is competent if his or her answer was what a reasonable person would choose or the person's reasons were 'rational'. While such a standard may have limited legitimacy in clinical care decisions when the balance of benefits clearly outweighs harms and risks, it is entirely inadequate for decisions where reasonable people disagree, such as the merits of enrolling in research.

Medicine and medical researchers had little if any interest in the issue of what it means to be competent to consent. For example, the Commission's review of the informed consent practices for mental health research does not discuss if the investigators made an effort to assess the subject's capacity to consent. In all likelihood, they did not. This reflected medicine's and medical research's attitude about informed consent that ranged from indifference to open hostility (Demy 1971; Ingelfinger 1972). Although psychiatrists were recognized as experts in judging competency, it was not until the 1980s that the field began to articulate a conceptual framework of competency and then develop a social science to validate it empirically.[7]

Medicine and medical research have transformed how they decide whether a person is competent to consent from judgments of competency that were based largely on the diagnostic label and whether the person makes a 'reasonable' or 'rational' choice—i.e. a person with acute schizophrenia is competent if he agrees to be hospitalized—to an assessment of the functional consequences of cognitive impairment: diminished decision making capacity. A key finding from decision making capacity research is that labels do not match how a person performs on a measure of capacity. Being labeled 'mentally ill' did not substantially equate with being not competent. For example, most persons hospitalized with schizophrenia perform as well on measures of their decision making abilities as age and education matched non-schizophrenic persons (Carpenter et al. 2000).

The recognition that the ability to make a decision, the foundation of being competent, could be assessed and measured has slowly influenced the practice of informed consent in clinical research. It was not until the latter part of the 1990s that researchers began to assess explicitly the ability of a potential subject to provide informed consent,[8] and some medical journals required investigators to state how they obtained informed consent from the subjects (Charney et al. 1999).

In the years that followed the National Commission's never-adopted guidelines, both public and private organizations repeatedly noted the lack of federal regulations to provide specific guidance for the conduct of research that involves adults with disorders that could impair their competency to provide an informed consent (Fletcher et al. 1985; Melnick et al. 1985; American College of Physicians 1989; National Institutes of Health, Office of Extramural Research 2001). As these organizations attempted to fill this gap, they struggled to settle on a coherent language to

[7] The mental health network supported by the MacArthur Foundation were leaders in developing this conceptual framework (Appelbaum and Grisso 1988; Grisso and Appelbaum 1998b) and empirically testing it with instruments to assess the capacity to make research (Appelbaum and Grisso 1995) and treatment (Grisso and Appelbaum 1995) decisions.

[8] At the Alzheimer's Disease Center, where I conduct research, all persons with Alzheimer's disease who enroll in clinical trials or greater than minimal risk research are required to complete a quiz that assesses their understanding of the key elements of the research project. This quiz is used to assist in the judgment of subject competency, and the informed consent form includes a section to document whether the subject is competent to consent, and, if not, is assenting to participation.

describe what class of subjects they were trying to protect and the problem that pre-cipitated the whole issue in the first place—the concept of competence to consent. For example, proposed guidelines issued by the American College of Physicians in 1989 addressed 'cognitively impaired subjects' (American College of Physicians 1989) and the last national effort to write guidelines, by the National Bioethics Advisory Commission (NBAC) in 1998, was titled 'Research Involving Persons with Mental Disorders that May Affect Their Decisionmaking Capacity' (National Bioethics Advisory Commission 1998). NBAC's title reflects a tension between two views. On the one hand, there was the argument that the focus on 'mental illness' was necessary because of the stigma and history of abuse and exploitation such persons face. In contrast, persons schooled in the science of competency assessment argued that the focus simply perpetuated a historical stigma of mental illness while at the same time neglected the category of disorders that are not mental illnesses but can still impair decision making capacity, such as critical illness that requires sedation and ventilation.

Recent events suggest there is consensus on the focus of ethical concern: disorders that cause cognitive impairment (one of which is mental illness) that may impair the ability to make a decision. In 2002 the National Human Research Protections Advisory Committee, a multi-disciplinary advisory panel to the Federal office that oversees the regulation of human subjects research, the Office of Human Research Protections, issued recommendations modeled after the NBAC guidelines but changed the focus to research that involves all adults who lack decisional capacity for any reasons (National Human Research Protections Advisory Committee 2002). Similarly, a Department of Health and Human Services working group on the NBAC Report endorsed the position that the scope of the NBAC recommendations applies to all persons with decisional impairment, irrespective of the cause of the decisional impairment (National Institutes of Health, Office of Extramural Research 2001).

THE ETHICAL FRAMEWORK

Competent adults are allowed extensive discretion in their choice of whether enrolling in research is in their best interests. These interests can include hopes for personal benefit or the fulfillment of altruistic values (Daugherty et al. 1995). The general ethical framework for research that involves cognitively impaired adults who are not capable of making this choice themselves does not grant their proxies or IRBs this same degree of discretion over another person's life. Instead, proxy consent or even no informed consent is appropriate within a framework of subject protections that rely on further specification of the principles of research ethics.

The architecture of this framework is that the research is relevant to the subject's condition, its risks and benefits fit within certain categories, and efforts are taken to assess the subject's competency and to protect the autonomy of the noncompetent subject. Each aspect of this framework is discussed below.

How Much Research Risk Is Permissible to Expose a Noncompetent Adult?

During the 1970s the National Commission addressed whether it is possible to conduct research ethically without the subject's informed consent. The Commission addressed the ethics of research that involves selected subject populations from whom informed consent was not possible: children (Department of Health and Human Services 1991, subpart D) and persons with mental illness severe enough to warrant institutionalization (Department of Health Education and Welfare 1978). The Commission also addressed categories of research in which written informed consent from the subject was either not feasible (Department of Health and Human Services 1991, sect. 46.116), such as deception research, or seemed an excessive subject protection, such as a study that used existing samples taken for clinical purposes (Department of Health and Human Services 1991, sects. 46.117(c)(2), 101(b)(4)).

The conceptual framework the Commission developed to address these situations was a substantial step away from the strict requirement for informed consent. By relaxing informed consent as an absolute requirement for all human subjects research the Commission established a standard that recognized that the social worth of research could outweigh a strict adherence to informed consent. In sum, vulnerable subject populations should have access to research and its potential benefits, and many kinds of valuable research not otherwise practicable without a waiver or modification of informed consent were viewed as being permissible.

The conceptual framework relied on more nuanced applications of the principles of beneficence and justice (Weijer 2000). Waivers and modifications of written informed consent from the subject are permissible if the research risks and potential benefits fulfilled specific criteria: the necessity requirement and specific categories of research risks and benefits. The 'necessity requirement' describes the finding that the research is relevant to the vulnerable subject population and could not be otherwise done with a nonvulnerable population who themselves can consent to be in the research. 'Relevant' means the research addresses a problem that is encountered in the daily lives of the vulnerable population. This requirement is an absolute requirement. In other words, no amount of other reasons or subject protections can justify research that does not fulfill the necessity requirement.

The second criterion addressed by the Commission described categories of research risk and benefit that circumscribe when it is appropriate to enroll a subject who cannot consent. The Commission proposed a framework based on three concepts: minimal risk, potential benefit, and the importance, or value, of the knowledge to be gained from the research. Proxy consent is appropriate if the research risks meet a criterion of minimal risk. In the case of greater than minimal risk research, further subclasses were created. The increment could be just a minor increment above minimal risk, or the research might have a reasonable prospect of potential benefit to the subject. If neither of these criteria could be met, then the research had to be reviewed and approved by a national panel. With the exception of emergency research, subsequent proposals for research that involves cognitively impaired adults (as well as children) have all used this basic framework.

The conceptual model for this framework justifies research risks based on balancing risks against two things: the potential benefits to the subjects and the importance of the knowledge that could reasonably be expected to result from the research. This model was consistent with two of the Commission's recommendations in the general guidelines for human subjects research. The guidelines for IRB review of research required that the IRB judge risks reasonable to the potential benefits to subjects and to the importance of the knowledge that could reasonably result from the research (Department of Health and Human Services 1991, sect. 46.111(A)(2)) and that the risks of research are minimized wherever possible by linking research procedures to existing procedures done for clinical purposes (Department of Health and Human Services 1991, sect. 46.111(A)(1)). This model creates two risk assessments: a risk to potential benefit assessment and a risk to knowledge assessment.

But the Commission never addressed two shortcomings in its conceptual model. The failure to do so is the source of substantial disagreements in the ethics of research that involves noncompetent adults (Karlawish and Hall 1996; Weijer 2000; McRae and Weijer 2002). First, the Commission never clarified what risks should be balanced against the potential benefits to subjects and what risks should be balanced against the importance of the knowledge to be gained from the research. Consider the case of a clinical trial of a promising new intervention for sepsis that plans to enroll persons who are critically ill and therefore typically unable to communicate and thus to provide an informed consent. A common perspective on the risks and benefits of this study is that it is potentially beneficial and also presents risks that are greater than minimal but the subjects are so sick that those risks may not be too great. This 'whole protocol' approach to research risk assessment balances all the research risks against the potential benefits to the subjects. While such an approach makes sense in clinical care, it does not fit with the nature of research. Research studies inherently involve procedures designed not to benefit subject but to benefit science by producing generalizable knowledge. It is thus potentially exploitative to justify risks of interventions done solely to gather knowledge with the potential benefits of the intervention.

The second shortcoming in the Commission's model was that it did not clearly articulate how to interpret the minimal risk definition: 'The probability and magnitude of harm or discomfort anticipated in the research are not greater in and of themselves than those ordinarily encountered in daily life or the performance of routine physical or psychological examinations or tests' (Department of Health and Human Services 1991, sect. 46.102(i)). A clear limitation in this definition is the absence of a comparison group, that is an anchor upon which an IRB could answer the question to whose daily life should the IRB compare the risks of the research? Should the IRB compare the risks of the research to the risks encountered in the daily lives of the potential subjects of the research or in the daily lives of healthy persons? The draft regulations stated healthy persons but this was dropped to yield the definition that makes reference to no comparison group (Department of Health Education and Welfare, Office of the Secretary 1979). The commentary to the final rule stated that the definition referred to the risks faced by the subjects of the research (Department of Health Education and Welfare, Office of the Secretary 1979). The authors of the regulations explained that this revision was intended to permit a waiver of informed consent for research that involved persons with head injury (McCarthy 1995). Unfortunately, this was a quick fix without the necessary public discussion of a substantial modification in the nature and intent of the rules for waiver and modification of informed consent in research that involves vulnerable subjects. It was politically ambitious and ethically simplistic to think that a single word modification in the definition of minimal risk with an explanation in the commentary section would settle the issue of when it is appropriate to waive informed consent.

Recent scholarship has attempted to reconcile the shortcomings in the conceptual model. The proposal developed by Charles Weijer and adopted by the National Bioethics Advisory Commission is called 'component analysis' (Weijer 2000). Component analysis begins with the recognition that research involves at least one of two kinds of distinct components: therapeutic and nontherapeutic. Therapeutic components describe interventions that may help subjects, such as a promising drug for which there is legitimate but uncertain evidence it is safe and effective. The risks and benefits of these interventions are justified by the epistemic condition of equipoise: the honest professional disagreement that a new intervention is at least as good as the current standard of care (Freedman 1987b). Research also includes interventions that are solely done to gather generalizable knowledge. These components, such as additional blood draws and randomization, are part of the nontherapeutic components of research. The risks of these interventions are justified by the value of the research results, that is, the importance of the knowledge to be gained from the research.

Component analysis provides a useful tool to answer the critical question in the ethics of research that involves the cognitively impaired: how much risk is appropriate to expose a noncompetent subject? The answer to this question is in the degree of nontherapeutic risk that is deemed acceptable. Persons who oppose exposing noncompetent subjects to any risk not justified by potential benefits to the subjects would answer 'none'. Hence, noncompetent subjects, including children, could not be in any kind of research as all research involves some procedures that are done solely to generate generalizable knowledge, however trivial those procedures may be. The general consensus is that this position is extreme. Instead, assuming the research has passed the necessity requirement, it is acceptable to expose noncompetent subjects to risks that are no greater than minimal risk.

The remaining controversy is how to assess whether research risk is minimal risk. The definition lacks a comparison group, that is, an anchor upon which an IRB could answer the question to whose daily life should the IRB compare the risks of the nontherapeutic components of the research. A reasonable answer is based on what is the point of research: to create valuable knowledge that can benefit society. In accord with the principle of justice, the increment of risk noncompetent subjects face to contribute to society's well being should be minimal and the assessment of this degree of risk should not be based on the severity of the subject's illness. To base the assessment of minimal risk on the severity of the subject's illness effectively means sicker subjects could be exposed to greater research risks because they are sick. Such an approach exploits subjects on the basis of their vulnerability. Instead, to determine whether the nontherapeutic components present minimal risk (or some accepted increment above it), the IRB should compare the risks of the nontherapeutic components to the risks faced in the routine medical and psychological tests encountered in the lives of an average person.

The failure to reconcile what risks apply to the minimal risk criteria and how to interpret the definition of minimal risk has led to incoherent standards for acceptable research risks. Perhaps the most egregious example is the emergency research regulations. The regulations created a category of permissible research risk and benefit called a 'potential . . . to provide a direct benefit to the individual subjects' (Department of Health and Human Services, Food and Drug Administration 1996). The IRB is instructed to judge whether a study met this standard based on a tripartite risk benefit assessment: 'risks associated with the investigation are reasonable in relation to (1) what is known about the medical condition of the potential class of subjects, (2) the risks and benefits of standard therapy, if any, and (3) what is known about the risks and benefits of the proposed intervention or activity' (Department of Health and Human Services, Food and Drug Administration 1996).

The standard suggests three risk assessments. Research risks should be compared to the severity of medical condition, the risks and benefits of standard therapy, and the risks and benefits of the proposed intervention. There are a number of shortcomings to this tripartite standard (McRae and Weijer 2002). First, it suggests that the potential benefits of a promising intervention can justify the risks of interventions that are designed to answer the research questions, such as additional monitoring, that is, the potential benefits of therapeutic components can justify the risks of nontherapeutic components. Second, the assessment of risk against the severity of medical condition suggests that the sicker the subject population is, the more appropriate are increasing research risks. While this is accepted in clinical care, it is not at all appropriate that increasing vulnerability justifies exposing people to increasing risks of nontherapeutic components. Third, the balancing of 'risks associated with the investigation' to 'risks and benefit for the proposed intervention' is at least vague and even incoherent. What risks of the investigation are distinct from the risks of the proposed intervention? Fourth, the balance between risk and the importance of the knowledge that may reasonably result is entirely absent. In short, while the idea that some kinds of research can be potentially beneficial and present minimal risks to subjects is intuitively sensible and a justification for enrolling persons who themselves cannot consent, the emergency research risk and benefit standard shows how considerable conceptual ambiguity exists in how to make this assessment.

Component analysis clears up the kinds of conceptual ambiguity found in the emergency research regulations. Consider the case of a clinical trial of a promising new intervention for sepsis that plans to enroll persons who are critically ill and therefore typically unable to communicate and thus to provide an informed consent. A common perspective on the risks and benefits of this study is that it is potentially beneficial and also presents risks that are greater than minimal but the subjects are so sick those risks may not be too great.

Component analysis reaches a different and conceptually more coherent assessment. The therapeutic elements of the research—in this case the promising new intervention—may present substantial risks, such as a serious allergic reaction. But these risks are not part of the minimal risk assessment. They are justified by the potential benefits of the intervention and the equipoise condition. In contrast, the nontherapeutic interventions such as the additional tests done on the subjects to assure that the results are gathered in a manner that is scientifically rigorous are justified by the importance of the scientific question—a better treatment for sepsis. These risks should not be greater than minimal or perhaps some increment above minimal, depending on the comparison group used to interpret the minimal risk definition. This study would be considered potentially beneficial and *minimal risk*. Depending on the nature and extent of other subject protections, the waiver of informed consent or the use of proxy consent would be permissible.

The addition of risky research procedures to answer scientific questions demonstrates how component analysis provides a more coherent risk assessment than one that does not distinguish between therapeutic and nontherapeutic components and links the judgment that risks are acceptable to the severity of the subjects' condition. Suppose the study included the placement of a right heart catheter to monitor how sepsis affected pulmonary pressures. This intervention is not part of the efficacy or safety assessments. It is done solely to gather knowledge about sepsis. Hence, it is part of the nontherapeutic components of the study and needs to pass the minimal risk standard. Such a procedure presents risks that are greater than those ordinarily encountered in the lives of reasonable persons. This potentially beneficial study is also greater than minimal risk. The waiver of informed consent or the use of proxy consent would be highly controversial or even prohibited.

In summary, the ethical framework of research risk and benefit assessment that articulates conditions when it is acceptable to obtain informed consent from someone other than the subject or even a waiver of informed consent relies on two features. First, there is the 'necessity requirement'. The recruitment of the subject population must be necessary and not simply convenient. This avoids scandals such as the Jewish Chronic Disease Hospital case (Katz 1972). Second, the research risks and benefits should pass component analysis. Components that are part of therapeutic elements of research, such as the intervention and its control group, are justified if there is legitimate disagreement within the community over which intervention is beneficial. Components that are part of nontherapeutic elements of the research, such as the techniques to assure that the knowledge gained from the research is generalizable, should fulfill a standard of being no more than minimal risk or some acceptable increment above that threshold.

What Is an Appropriate Process for Assessing Research Risks and Benefits?

The standards outlined above describe the categories of research risks and benefits that are acceptable to allow investigators either to obtain informed consent from a proxy or to waive informed consent from the subject and proxy. The judgment that the research fits within the categories of potential benefit and minimal risk is informed not only by knowledge of the science of the intervention, but also by the experience of the daily lives of the subjects.

The need for the perspective of the daily lives of the subjects suggests that the research review process needs to include the perspective of the subject community and, for subjects who are vulnerable, the people who care for them. IRB membership must include a representative of the community and the IRB is empowered to bring in additional members as necessary to assist in reviewing a study (Department of Health and Human Services 1991, sect. 46.106) and is in particular encouraged (but not required) to call on a member of or advocate for any vulnerable study populations, but the process of research design and review may not adequately foster this kind of input. There are a number of reasons why.

Typically, studies are designed by the expert medical community and then reviewed by each study site's IRB. This expert medical community often includes persons who have substantial interests in the commercialization of the results of the research. Hence, their judgments about whether legitimate uncertainty exists and the design of the trial that will settle this uncertainty are influenced not only by the considerations of medical science but also by corporate concerns of profit and patent protection (Krimsky 2003). The IRB does not routinely seek the input of the potential subjects of the research. The results of IRB review are not routinely shared with other IRBs reviewing the same protocol. Although the point of research is to produce generalizable knowledge, public disclosure of results is not required, and, in the case of some research, it may not occur.

In the case of research that involves cognitively impaired adults, the principles of beneficence and justice warrant greater attention to involving the subjects in the research risk and benefit assessment. Perhaps the best example of the requirement for involving the subject community is the emergency research regulations (Department of Health and Human Services, Food and Drug Administration 1996). They require the study sponsor and investigator to consult with representatives of the communities from which the subjects will be drawn, and, prior to starting the research, public disclosure to these communities of the plans for the research and its risks and expected benefits. In the event that an IRB does not approve of a study, the regulations require the IRB to document why it cannot approve it, and the sponsor is required to disseminate this report to other investigators and IRBs who are involved in the research. During the course of the research, a data safety and monitoring board should review the conduct of the study. Finally, at the close of the research, the sponsor must disclose the results to the community where the research was conducted. The general theme of this process is an open and public discussion at both the start and the end of the social worth of the research.

Among these requirements, the most innovative are the requirements for community consultation and public disclosure and a sharing of other IRBs' determinations. This model of democratic deliberation is novel to the social structure for research review, approval, and monitoring. The requirement that the sponsor and the investigator consult with representatives of the community from which subjects will be drawn includes suggestions for public meetings to discuss the protocol, creating a panel of community members from which the subjects will be drawn and consultants to the IRB, and adding community members who are not affiliated with the institution to the IRB. The goal of these efforts is to promote the public's comprehension of the study and the proposed waiver of informed consent and elicit community opinions and input. While there are not formal requirements for the community to approve the research or alter its design, the acts of consultation and disclosure provide the community the opportunity to weigh in on what are permissible risks in the pursuit of research to develop new therapies.

Community consultation makes conceptual sense. The histories of AIDS and schizophrenia research suggest that there is a need to involve the community of potential subjects proactively into the process of research review (Epstein 1996; Karlawish and Lantos 1997). In AIDS research, patients with the disease sharply and vocally disagreed with the standard approach that investigators proposed to determine whether a drug was a safe and effective AIDS treatment. The ensuing debate resulted in changes in the design and conduct of AIDS clinical trials. The NAMI was instrumental in convincing Sandoz Pharmaceuticals of the social worth of pursuing studies of clozapine for schizophrenia (Fried 1998).

Community consultation has a clear role to assure that the research risks are reasonable with respect to both potential benefits to subjects as well as the social worth of the research. But as appealing as community input into the research risk and benefit assessment is, the social structure of research is not set up to assure that subjects' rights and interests are adequately represented. Research training does not include how to interact with the subject community. And disease advocacy groups, such as the Alzheimer's Association and the NAMI, do not have a prespecified role in setting research policy. Moreover, their membership policies, leadership structure, and how they interact with researchers and the for-profit research industry are not uniform or deliberately structured to address the assessment of research risks and benefits. Hence, the legitimacy of any one group's 'representation' may be questioned.

How Should We Decide that an Adult Cannot Provide an Informed Consent?

The review of research to assure that it fits within certain categories of risk and benefit and the conduct of that review to include input from the subject community are designed to assure that the principles of beneficence and justice are adequately fulfilled. This balances the relaxation or even waiver of respect for the subject's autonomy by means of an informed consent. But all adults are presumed competent until proven otherwise. How do we arrive at the judgment that a person is not competent in a manner that does not rely on labels (such as mental illness) or judgments based on what the investigator thinks is a 'reasonable choice'?

Substantial progress has occurred in the last thirty years on developing a conceptual model for competency to consent to research and treatment. The judgment that a person is not competent to consent relies on an assessment of the person's decision-making capacity. This capacity is determined by their performance on four decision-making abilities: understanding, appreciation, choice, and reasoning (Grisso and Appelbaum 1998a). Understanding, the ability that is most widely recognized as essential for competence to consent, means knowing the meaning of the information disclosed. Appreciation describes recognizing how facts can apply to one's personal situation. Reasoning describes inferring consequences of a choice to one's life. Choice describes the ability to state a preference consistently.

An investigator can assess a potential subject's performance on each of these abilities by asking the individual questions tailored to the specifics of the decision at hand. For example, to assess understanding, an investigator can ask a subject to 'say back in their own words' certain facts, such as how it is decided what subjects receive in the clinical trial. In the case of enrollment in a randomized clinical trial, the question 'How is it decided what subjects receive in this study?' assesses the ability to understand randomization. A subject who answers 'You do it by chance, a flip of the coin' would demonstrate adequate understanding of randomization.

Studies of persons with conditions that can cause cognitive impairment show that their performance on measures of decision making ability vary largely on the severity of their cognitive impairments. Much of this variance in performance is explained by the degree of impairment in executive function, a term that describes a person's ability to organize, plan, and categorize information (Marson and Harrell 1999).

The constructs of capacity and decision-making abilities and the methods to assess them have had a tremendous impact on the judgment of competency. They provide structure and a conceptual framework for what can otherwise be a highly idiosyncratic judgment based on a variety of characteristics that have nothing to do with the decision at hand, such as whether the person is mentally ill or makes a choice other people consider 'reasonable'. But there are two challenges to applying the conceptual model.

What Is the Best Way to Assess Capacity?

One of the most widely studied methods to assess a person's decision making abilities, the MacArthur Competency Assessment Tool for Clinical Research (MacCAT-CR), uses a semi-structured interview (Appelbaum and Grisso 2000). For each ability, the subject's answers to a set of questions are scored. The sum of scores constitutes a score for that ability. For example, the MacCAT-CR measure of understanding asks thirteen questions to assess understanding, each of which is scored 0, 1, or 2, generating an understanding score that ranges from 0 to 26. Should this twenty minute long interview be the standard for all kinds of research that involves cognitively impaired subjects? Alternative methods include a quiz that asks true–false or multiple choice questions or simply an informal interview modeled after MacCAT-CR style questions but that is not scored.

The general issue is how much rigor should an assessment of decision making abilities involve. A balancing principle is needed to assure that the capacity assessment does not take longer than participation in the actual research project. A reasonable guideline is that the rigor of an assessment should be commensurate with the degree of research risks to the subjects, especially risks of the nontherapeutic components. Hence, a study that involves developing a brief memory test arguably would require a minimal assessment of capacity, such as understanding that the project is research and that it involves a memory test. In contrast, a study that involves substantial research risks, such as a test of the pharmacology of a drug that involves an inpatient stay, would require a more rigorous assessment of decision making capacity.

What Kinds of Deficits in Decision-Making Ability Are Severe Enough that the Person Is Not Competent?

Related to the issue of the method of assessing capacity is how to arrive at a judgment that the person is not competent. That is, what degree of impairment in decision making ability describes a person who is not competent? For example, the range of scores on a MacCAT-CR assessment of understanding is 0 to 26. Short of a 26, there is no single score that defines 'adequate understanding'. This lack of a clear cut-off score that defines acceptable understanding reflects the absence of a 'gold standard' that defines a person as not competent. A judgment of competency is a moral judgment. It is not a diagnosis.

A reasonable position recognizes that competency to make a decision is presumed until shown otherwise and that it is specific to that task. Hence, reasonable people can agree upon core things a person has to understand to be competent, just as reasonable people can agree on what a person needs to know to be competent to drive a car or pass out of the ninth grade math class and into the tenth grade class. For example, to be competent to consent to a study to test the pharmacology of a drug that involves an inpatient stay a person may need to understand that the project involves certain procedures, that it is research, and its purpose. Such up front conditions can be written into a protocol to define what it means to be competent to consent to a particular study.

When Is Proxy Informed Consent Appropriate?

An assessment of patient capacity to provide an informed consent to enroll in a research study may result in the judgment that the cognitively impaired subject cannot provide an informed consent. This chapter has discussed two conditions designed to assure that enrolling the noncompetent subject is ethical: the judgment that the research risks fit within the categories of minimal risk or some acceptable increment above minimal risk, and that an appropriately representative IRB made this risk assessment. This section addresses a third set of conditions: respect for subject assent and dissent, and limits on who can serve in the proxy role and how they should make their decision.

Respecting Subject Assent and Dissent

Competency is a categorical judgment. A person is either competent or not competent. But this judgment is derived from an assessment of a person's performance along a continuum of four abilities (understanding, appreciation, reasoning, and choice). Persons who are judged not competent may still coherently express aspects of these abilities. For example, while a substantial number of persons with mild to moderate Alzheimer's disease may not be capable of an informed consent to enroll in a trial, many of them are capable of a choice and can embellish this choice with plausible reasons that draw on limited degrees of understanding, appreciation, and reasoning, and are involved in decision making with their family members (Karlawish *et al.* 2002*a*, *b*). The ethical consequences of this are substantial and the issue was a cause of dissenting views among members of both the National Commission and the National Bioethics Advisory Commission. What responsibility does an investigator have to listen to a potential subject's assent, dissent, or attempt to withdraw, once enrolled?

The answer to this question engages an important but largely unsettled effort to respect the autonomy of persons who are not competent. Guidelines for research that involve the cognitively impaired differ on an investigator's responsibility vis-à-vis each of these. The National Commission argued that investigators had to obtain subject assent and respect dissent (Department of Health Education and Welfare 1978). In contrast, the National Bioethics Advisory Commission focused only on the investigator's obligation to respect a subject's dissent (National Bioethics Advisory Commission 1998). Each of these requirements—soliciting assent or respecting dissent—has intuitive appeal. It is good that people are in agreement with what is happening to them, even if they do not fully grasp the plan, and the indignity of forcing someone who says 'no' to undergo research procedures is prima facie unacceptable.

But assent and dissent are undifferentiated constructs. As such, investigators and IRBs do not have clear guidelines for how to operationalize them. Absent such guidance, as appealing as the sentiment of respecting an assent or dissent is, investigators cannot coherently apply it.

What constitutes an assent? The higher standard of competency to consent requires evidence of some degree of adequate understanding, appreciation, reasoning, and choice. How much less of these abilities does a person have who while not capable of consent, is still capable of assent? The National Commission described assent as authorization by a person 'whose capacity to understand and judge is somewhat impaired by illness or institutionalization, but who remains functional' (Department of Health Education and Welfare 1978, 11332). The Commission defined assent as the subject 'know[s] what procedures will be performed in the research, choose[s] freely to undergo those procedures, communicate[s] this choice unambiguously, and [is] aware that subjects may withdraw from participation' (Department of Health Education and Welfare 1978, 11332). Thus, according to the Commission, assent is not simply saying 'yes'. It means having the ability to understand procedures and voluntariness, and the ability to choose.

But why require only the ability to choose and to understand research procedures and voluntariness? Why not require more evidence of abilities in order to assent? For example, why not require that, in addition to the Commission's standard, a subject also needs to reason about how enrolling in the research could affect his or her everyday life? The point of these questions is that the construct of assent is contingent upon what we decide it is. The only boundaries to its requirements are that they not be the same as consent and, at the other extreme, that there must be at least some evidence of a choice.

A more reasonable construct of assent ties it to the purpose of eliciting it in the first place. Assent is a means to assure subject protection from research risk. The general principle is that, as the risks of the research increase, there is a greater need to protect subjects and, hence, for a stricter standard that assures that the subject understands the risks of the research. Thus in a study involving only minimal risks, assent may simply be the choice to enroll and an understanding that the project is research. In the case of a greater than minimal risk project, assent will need additional requirements such as understanding the risks of the procedures that are an increment above minimal risk.

Dissent has not been operationalized with the same detail as assent. The NBAC proposal argued that 'any potential or actual subject's objection to enrollment or continued participation in a research protocol must be heeded in all circumstances' (National Bioethics Advisory Commission 1998, recommendation 7). Hence, an investigator should respect as a valid dissent any utterance that suggests 'no'. NBAC did not define a dissent in the detail that the National Commission defined assent. It defended this broad and undefined standard as a means to maximize subject protection from research risks and also effectively to eliminate the dignitary harm of enrolling someone in research who simply does not want to be in it.

NBAC's standard effectively eliminates the unappealing image of restraining a subject who repeats 'no' and makes physical efforts to leave the research setting. But a blanket policy of respect for dissent of any kind and at any time in the course of a research project may be counterproductive to one of the justifications for the requirement. Specifically, blanket respect for dissent may not maximize subject protection from research risks if withdrawing from the research would place the subject at some risk as a result of withdrawing.

Consider the case of a subject who is enrolled in a study that involves the permanent placement of stem cell tissue in the brain of persons with Alzheimer's disease. After seven months of being in the study, the subject is attending a clinical assessment and during the cognitive testing says 'No—I don't want to do this'. Is the research assistant who is doing the testing obligated there and then to cease the testing and notify the investigator that the subject has withdrawn from the research? Or is this 'no' only applicable to the testing session? It is reasonable that the assistant find out the reason for the objection and attempt to address it. It may be that the subject needs to take a break or simply does not want to do the cognitive testing but will engage in the remainder of the study visit (such as the physical exam). Suppose the subject's 'no' was about overall participation in the research. In such a case, it is reasonable that the investigator and the subject's proxy discuss the subject's dissent with the subject in order to make sure that dropping out is in the subject's best interests.

The claim that enrolling in research can be in a subject's best interests is controversial because research is not treatment. But once a person is in research, withdrawing may present risks. In this case example, the implanted cells are permanent. There is a need for continued monitoring for the purposes of safety assessment. Hence, an investigator should respect the decision of subject who consistently says 'no' and understands the risks of no longer being assessed. In the case of a subject who says 'no' but does not understand the risks of dropping out, there is a strong warrant to make sure the subject's proxy and caregiver are aware of the dissent, to agree that the subject does not understand the consequence of dropping out, and to have a plan to make sure the subject continues to receive assessments necessary for safety. Additionally, the investigator has a responsibility to determine whether this 'no' is part of other behavioral problems. For example, it may be that the subject is not only resisting study procedures; the caregiver may report that the person is also resisting dressing and bathing. In such a case, the person may benefit from treatment for agitation. Options include environmental manipulations—including stopping the research, caregiver education, and even pharmacotherapy.

Guidelines on Who Can Serve in the Proxy Role and How the Proxy Should Make a Research Enrollment Decision

There are two instances in research that involves persons who are cognitively impaired and not competent that are especially ethically challenging: (1) research that proposes to enroll subjects who are not capable of an assent, and (2) research that presents risks that are greater than some acceptable threshold of risk, such as minimal risk. The combination of these two instances within a single research project, that is, enrolling subjects incapable of assent into greater than minimal risk research, creates an even greater ethical challenge.

The following case illustrates these ethical challenges. Mr Smith, a previously well man, becomes critically ill from a pneumonia. His treatments require mechanical ventilation and sedation. Throughout his stay in the intensive care unit, his physicians talk with his wife to make decisions for a variety of therapeutic interventions such as the placement of an arterial line in order to monitor closely Mr Smith's labile blood pressure.

In general, society is comfortable with Mrs Smith serving in this role of making clinical care decisions on behalf of her husband. She does not need legal authorization. Instead, this role follows naturally from her close relationship with her husband. But what if an investigator wishes to recruit Mr Smith into a clinical trial to test a new critical care technique? Mr Smith is so cognitively impaired that he cannot grant an assent or express dissent. Is an informed consent from his wife an appropriate extension of her role as a proxy for clinical care decisions? This question raises two issues: whether she can serve in this role, and, even if she can, how she should make the decision.

Thirty years ago guidelines for research that involves persons who are cognitively impaired required Mrs Smith to have legal authorization to serve as a research proxy. Since then, there has been a general loosening of this requirement. Instead, guidelines argue that the model for clinical care decision making should apply to research decision making. Close family who serve as a proxy for clinical decisions can also serve as a proxy for research decisions (National Bioethics Advisory Commission 1998; National Human Research Protections Advisory Committee 2002).

But while requirements for who can serve in the role of a research proxy resemble the practice used in clinical care decision making, requirements for how that person should make a decision differ from clinical care guidelines. In clinical care, a proxy should exercise a substituted judgment. To refer to the case described above, this means that Mrs Smith should choose what Mr Smith would choose if he were capable of making that choice. If Mr Smith had previously written a document called a 'living will' that specifically sets out future preferences for care, Mrs Smith should follow that document. But what if Mrs Smith does not have sufficient information about her husband's preferences to make a substituted judgment? Absent such knowledge, she is then expected to decide what is in her husband's best interests.

This conceptual framework for clinical care decision making seems incompatible with research decision making. Absent a substituted judgment that the noncompetent person would have wanted to be in research, there is no best interests justification for enrolling a person in research. Research is not an activity designed solely for a subject's best interests. It follows then that a proxy can only grant an informed consent to enroll a noncompetent person in research on the basis of a substituted judgment. This requirement for a substituted judgment as an absolute condition for research enrollment has led to the recommendation that a proxy can only enroll a noncompetent person in greater than minimal risk research that does not offer the prospect of benefit to the subjects if the person had previously executed an advance directive that expressed a willingness to be in such research (National Bioethics Advisory Commission 1998). In contrast, most guidelines accept that a substituted judgment is not necessary for proxy informed consent for minimal risk research. The defense of this position is based on a utilitarian argument that the value of the knowledge to society exceeds the risks to subjects and the dignitary harm of putting someone in research that they may not have wanted to participate in. Thus, the degree of research risk is the central determinant of whether we take a stance of either strictly protecting autonomy or advancing the common good.

These requirements presume that they in fact do reflect how people would want their proxy to make research enrollment decisions. Studies of people's willingness to grant their family members authority to serve as proxy decision makers suggest that this may not reflect their ethic. Most people are comfortable with granting trusted family members' discretion in making choices that may even violate a research advance directive. Instead, people want their proxy to balance substituted judgment with what is in their best interests. A survey of family members of persons with Alzheimer's disease found the vast majority willing to execute a research advance directive, but when offered the opportunity to execute one, few did it (Wendler *et al.* 2002). The majority preferred to have their research advance planning instructions followed over a family member's choice, but the majority also permitted a family member to overrule these instructions in the case of potentially beneficial research.

Although the investigators did not examine the contentious issue of the discretion people would give to a proxy over enrollment in research that is judged nonpotentially beneficial or whose risks of nontherapeutic procedures are greater than minimal, these results suggest that the requirements that a proxy can only enroll a noncompetent person in more than minimal risk research on the basis of a substituted judgment or that a proxy can enroll persons in minimal risk research in the absence of a substituted judgment may not reflect how people conceptualize respect for their autonomy when they are themselves no longer capable of asserting their autonomy. 'Best interests' is an unusual standard in research settings where there is no plausible individual benefit or where there are real chances of risk to the research participant. In these situations, 'best interests' might be understandable only as an appreciation for the altruistic intents of either the subject or the proxy and the willingness of the subject to grant their proxy discretion in exercising this altruism regardless of the degree of research risk.

Conclusion

Human subjects research presents an ethical dilemma between advancing the interests of society while protecting individuals from harms encountered in an effort to accomplish the research. Democratic society's standard approach to resolving this dilemma is a procedural solution: informed consent. But in the case of research that involves subjects who have cognitive impairments this solution has unacceptable consequences, including an absolute prohibition on research on entire segments of the population. To avoid these consequences, society must find a standard that allows for vital research while at the same time providing adequate protection for vulnerable individuals.

Thirty years of scholarship have proposed a set of subject protections that attempt to justify research with either proxy consent or even a waiver of any consent. The failure of these proposed protections to achieve a consensus reflects continued ambiguity in how to justify research risks, the meaning of an assent and dissent, and the ambiguity on whether substituted judgments are essential when a proxy makes a research decision.

CHAPTER 26

RESEARCH IN DEVELOPING COUNTRIES

FLORENCIA LUNA

RESEARCH ethics already has a history of its own. Just as bioethics focused initially on autonomy and individual rights, and recently on questions about public health, justice, and social rights, research ethics has also turned from problems of autonomy and informed consent to more general ones that embrace obligations to research subjects and the community, such as nonexploitation. The situation of societies with vulnerable and marginal populations is now being analyzed thoroughly. For these populations, informed consent is merely the first step in a far more complex and problematic process. This shift in the focus of interest is related to the problems that developing countries have brought to the international debate.

In this chapter I examine the problems that research ethics confronts in developing countries and the impact that research in developing countries has had on research ethics. In order to show this I shall analyze the first paradigmatic cases that gave rise to the 'classic' analysis of research ethics. Hence, in this first part, many of the ethical concerns apply wherever research is conducted and are not particular to developing countries. Secondly, I shall describe the complex process of research by analyzing different research actors and their interests in the current research process. Thirdly, I shall sketch some of the recent cases that have prompted fierce ethical debate surrounding research in developing countries. I shall indicate a new battlefield: the ethical guidelines for research, in particular the Declaration of Helsinki (1996). The standard of care for control groups, the use of placebos, and post-trial benefits were and still are intensely debated. These involve issues about responsibilities, obligations during and after research, justice, and exploitation.

I

CLASSIC CASES

The first cases to reveal the importance of establishing guidelines in research ethics were the abuses during the Second World War. Nazi physicians forced people to drink seawater to find out how long a man could survive without fresh water. In Dachau, Russian prisoners were immersed in icy waters to see how long a pilot might live when shot down over the English Channel and to find out what kinds of protective gear or warming techniques were most effective. At Fort Ney, near Strasbourg, fifty-two prisoners were exposed to phosgene gas, a biological-warfare agent, in 1943 and 1944 to test possible antidotes. Again in Dachau, Ernst Grawitz infected prisoners with a broad range of pathogens to test homeopathic preparations. Nazi military authorities were worried about exotic diseases that German troops might contract in Africa or eastern Europe, and physicians in the camps reasoned that the 'human materials' at their disposal could be used to develop remedies. Hundreds of people died in these experiments, and many of those who survived were forced to live with painful physical or psychological scars (Annas and Grodin 1992).

These experiments were perpetrated during wartime and by Nazis. Germany at that time was scientifically highly advanced, and these experiments were conducted by German physician–researchers. In contrast to what was asserted in post-war apologies, physicians were never forced to conduct these experiments (Annas and Grodin 1992). However, these experiments represent aberrations in the field of nontherapeutic research; research subjects were prisoners of war in a situation of total subordination without any question of consent.

Variations on these kinds of abuse in times of peace and prosperity are the cases that were conducted during the so-called 'gilded age of research' in the United States. These cases were revealed by the anesthesiologist Henry Beecher in 1966 (Rothman 1991). For example, researchers explored different physiological responses, in one case inserting a special needle through a bronchus into the left atrium of the heart. This was done in an unspecified number of subjects, some with cardiac disease, some with normal hearts. The technique was a new approach whose hazards at the beginning were quite unknown. The subjects with healthy hearts were used, not for their personal benefit, but for that of patients in general. In other cases researchers experimented to determine the period of infectivity of infectious hepatitis. Artificial induction of hepatitis was carried out in an institution for mentally defective children in which a mild form of hepatitis was endemic. As part of a study of cancer immunity live cancer cells were injected into twenty-two human subjects. According to a recent review, the subjects (hospitalized patients) were 'merely told they would be receiving "some cells"... the word cancer was entirely omitted' (Rothman 1991). All of these cases risked the lives and health of the individuals without their consent or approval. Beecher reported that only two of the original fifty protocols mentioned obtained consent; thus, his cases do not represent simply a few rare examples, but describe how mainstream investigators in the period between 1945 and 1965 exercised their broad discretion.

Baruch Brody illustrates this same point and adds data from other sources and countries. For example, he cites M. H. Pappworth, who published *Human Guinea Pigs* (Pappworth 1967), in which he alleged similar problems in British research. In Canada much attention was focused in the 1960s on the Halushka case, in which a subject in a study who had not received adequate information about what was involved suffered serious injury after the use of a new drug and invasive monitoring. In New Zealand investigations in the 1980s focused on research in the 1960s and 1970s in which women with cervical cancer were left untreated in order to study the natural history of the disease. As was expected, many developed invasive carcinoma, from which some died (Rothman 1991).

This is not merely a matter for nontherapeutic research. It concerns therapeutic research, isolated populations, and subjects with a deficient education who were being misled. All of these cases occurred in so-called 'industrialized countries' and express a characteristic problem of early bioethics: that of inadequate respect for the autonomy of the research subjects, where a solution would have been to enforce informed consent as a means of avoiding these mistakes. It is interesting that AIDS, in its early period, takes this model of research ethics to an extreme. AIDS patients—research subjects proposed that informed consent should be the only element to restrict research ethics (Merrigan 1990). However, the model does not hold: research ethics cannot be reduced to informed consent; even if it is a necessary condition for all research, it is not sufficient (see Luna 2001a).

During these early cases some safeguards were brought in, constituting the basis of early research ethics. The most relevant were: informed consent, the risk–benefit ratio, ethics committees, and confidentiality.

CLASSIC PROBLEMS

Research ethics initially focused on informed consent. The celebrated Nuremberg Code (1947), a consequence of the trials following the atrocities of the Nazi physicians, broke new ground. The document, produced by lawyers, focused on nontherapeutic research. Its obligation of informed consent was quite demanding and required that the subject be legally capable.

However, informed consent in itself has lost its privileged place: it was the first article of the Nuremberg Code but in the Declaration of Helsinki it is to be found in Article I.9 (WMA 1996). Informed consent is unquestionably one of the fundamental factors in research ethics. Based on the principle of respect for persons as outlined in the Belmont Report (National Commission for the Protection of Human Subjects of Biomedical and Behavioral Research 1979), it implies the recognition of the autonomy of research subjects and the need for their authorization to participate in a clinical trial. It is worth stressing the emphasis on informed consent that is given in the analyses of research ethics stemming from the above cases (Brody 1998). But note that, despite the long tradition in implementing informed consent, it still poses problems. For example, we have to consider the amount and kind of information that must be presented—some consents appear to overwhelm the research subjects rather than inform them. Even if there is consent; respect for voluntariness appears to evade the rules in the case of research subjects who are so needy that the trial is their only access to treatment; or in the case of rural or very isolated communities where certain members have no decision-making power, for example, women.

However, as was mentioned earlier, consent alone cannot serve as the sole condition for acceptable research ethics. Other fundamental elements have begun to play important roles. One is the risk–benefit ratio (based on the principle of beneficence described in the Belmont Report). This implies two assessments: the first, to minimize possible risks; the second, to ensure that the possible benefits outweigh the possible risks to subjects (Brody 1998). It is a difficult assessment that deals with various factors, for example, the seriousness of the disease, the available alternative treatments, or the adverse effects of such treatments. Thus, the risk–benefit ratio of a treatment for AIDS at the onset of the epidemic when no treatment existed and the only alternative was death was different than it is today with drugs that improve patients' quality of life.

Another factor that has begun to play an interesting role is the need for independent review, for example, through research ethics committees. These committees must assess the research protocols and check whether the ethical requirements have been thoroughly fulfilled. This practice began in the United States with the so-called institutional review boards (IRBs) and is currently accepted worldwide, although variations exist (Brody 1998).

Finally, among the crucial factors, confidentiality is key, for example, in the case of some diseases that can stigmatize patients such as psychiatric illness or the sexually transmitted diseases such as AIDS.

It is interesting to note how during this first period these analyses were shared internationally. After examining the Nuremberg Code, the Declaration of Helsinki, the International Ethical Guidelines for Biomedical Research Involving Human Subjects, also known as the CIOMS Guidelines (CIOMS–WHO 1993), as well as some European and international documents, Baruch Brody says:

A clear-cut consensus has emerged in all of these official policies about the basic conditions for the permissibility of research on human subjects. Procedurally, such research needs to be approved in advance by a committee that is independent of the researchers. Substantially, informed voluntary consent of the subjects must be obtained, the research must minimize risks and involve a favorable risk–benefit ratio, there should be an equitable non-exploitative selection of subjects and the privacy and the confidentiality of the data must be protected. (Brody 1998)

II

Socio-Economic Changes and Actors in Research

Nowadays, this broad consensus on protections and obligations to research subjects has disappeared (Schüklenk 2004). To understand the dynamics and complexity of research today, the current debate, and the impact research has on developing countries, let us briefly examine the interests, concerns, and influence of the various actors in international research. They share the objective that clinical trials should be conducted correctly, although their agendas, interests, and main concerns may differ.

The Research Subject

One of the main actors in clinical trials is the person who constitutes the 'research subject'. Obligations toward research subjects will depend on our conceptualization of them. Judith P. Swazey and Leonard Glantz examine society's conception of its ethical obligation to research subjects and argue that the social concept of moral obligation may vary depending on whether we consider them altruistic heroes, gift-givers, willing contractors, or victims (Swazey and Glantz 1982). They propose these models on the specific issue of compensation for injured subjects. However, their analysis can be examined in a broader context, that is, in relation to our conception of a research subject in general. The altruistic hero or gift-giver is not a useful image to determine obligations. Heroes volunteer and assume risks for someone else's sake. Since heroes are not supposed to seek reward, society has no obligation to compensate heroic research subjects. Likewise, with gift-givers, although such donors may not be morally entitled to compensation, society may desire to return the favor by compensating their injuries. In the following I shall only consider the cases of the contractor and the victim, which may be more relevant to the conception of a research subject than the above.

Willing contractors follow the model of the businessman striking a bargain: so long as the negotiation process is just, the contractors have a right to no more than what they bargained for. Victims are those who are treated unjustly or harmed without their consent. They can be especially vulnerable or the target of exploitative behavior and can do little to avoid these harms.

Is the willing contractor model acceptable? It appears to be so in the case of English or Swedish research subjects who can access a universal healthcare system. However, issues to consider are problems like 'therapeutic misconception' (that is, believing that research procedures have therapeutic aims) (Appelbaum *et al.* 1987), as well as the emotional stress caused by the extent of available therapeutic alternatives. Patients with access to current therapies are better off than those without; they can test the best current therapy or participate in a trial, weigh the risks and benefits, and decide. This may be an accurate description if we do not consider the severity of some diseases and the stress that the patient may be undergoing. However, aside from the accuracy of the situation of the Swedish research subject, this is not the case for someone who lives in absolute poverty and/or in a poor country. We have to be very careful when assessing the suitability and limits of informed consent in these situations. There might be variables (for example, extreme needs or distress) that can pose serious challenges to informed consent. How can patients negotiate when their only access to treatment is a clinical trial? Note that these are not perfect contracts. They occur in the real world and depend on the negotiating power of the actors. Onora O'Neill indicates the importance of the possibility of refusal or renegotiation in order to ascertain that consent is not a mere formality (O'Neill 1996). In cases such as this the possibility of refusal is fundamental in order to avoid a merely formal and vacuous consent. Even if it is not always a question of an unjust offer that someone cannot refuse (Wertheimer 1996), such proposals are closely related to potential exploitation. In regard to this possibility Thomas Pogge points out the limits of informed consent, especially in situations of extreme distress. The otherwise impermissible harming of another is not rendered permissible by this person's prior rational consent when such consent is exacted as a condition of saving her from a horrible predicament or as a condition of giving her some chance of being so saved (Pogge 2003).

Should we endorse, then, the image of the victim? Swazey and Glantz assume a total lack of consent (for example, victims of the Nazis or from Tuskegee). The latter are clearly unethical models. On this view, victims appear to be entitled to assistance, having a strong moral claim to compensation, especially where society has facilitated the research or benefited by it (Swazey and Glantz 1982). However, Swazey and Glantz's proposal, focusing solely on the formality of informed consent, appears to take a narrow view of the concept of victim: other, subtle factors seem to weigh, for example, vulnerability.

The CIOMS–WHO Guidelines refer to vulnerable groups as 'people receiving welfare benefits or social assistance and other poor people and the unemployed . . . some ethnic and racial minority groups . . . members of communities unfamiliar with modern medical concepts' (CIOMS–WHO 2002). According to this definition, many research subjects in countries with scarce resources may be deemed vulnerable. The Guidelines specify that to the extent that these and other classes of people have attributes resembling those of classes identified as vulnerable, the need for special protection of their rights and welfare should be reviewed, and applied where relevant.

Having been born destitute also conveys the situation of victim: people are not responsible for the social situation into which they have been born. The 'social lottery' can generate victims (though several analyses of justice try to avoid these 'circumstances' and 'social lottery' factors; Dworkin 1971; Rawls 1971; Sen 1980; Cohen 1993). The situation prior to informed consent may be unjust, and considerations about injustice and exploitation should be taken into account. Even if we cannot modify the initial conditions of the social lottery, we should not profit from its imbalance.

However, choosing one particular image of the research subject may prove simplistic. Neither the image of the willing contractor nor that of the victim is completely applicable to real-world research subjects, and something of each should be reflected in the concept. On the one hand, the individual is a willing contractor (hence the importance of informed consent), but in many cases, the person may also share the features of a victim (hence the importance of proper protection). Thus, in each research situation the model should be reevaluated for whether the individual is a willing contractor or a victim. This will help to establish the correct safeguards.

Who, then, are the actors in clinical research who can provide such an evaluation and protection if applicable?

Researchers

Researchers are principal actors in this process. They can design or influence the design of clinical trials. They also conduct the trials and are responsible for their implementation. Thus, it is in their interest that trials are conducted properly.

They may have diverse personal interests. Academic researchers may be particularly interested in publication, in making brilliant discoveries, or in raising their prestige. If they have been hired by the drugs industry, they may also be interested in matters of salary or in economic incentives.

Another issue that merits examination is the role of the researcher on the 'periphery' of a trial. Given the structure of multicentric trials, researchers in developing countries play a different role from those involved in the 'original' design, which is done at the site that originated the research—generally in a industrialized country. As the same study must be replicated in different populations, there is little flexibility for researchers at other sites—generally in developing countries—to modify the design; thus, their role is quite marginal. This may also apply to researchers in industrialized countries who were not initially involved in the design.

In addition, we should not forget that scientific research has undergone a powerful transformation in recent decades. The paradigm of altruistic research in the name of the 'progress of humankind' has given rise to a kind of highly profitable research governed by market rules. Eloquent article titles illustrate this: 'Academia and Industry: Increasingly Uneasy Bedfellows', 'Uneasy Alliance: Clinical Investigators and the Pharmaceutical Industry' (Weatherall 2000; Bodenheimer 2000).

As Marcia Angell says:

The ties between clinical researchers and industry include not only grant support, but also a host of other financial arrangements. Researchers serve as consultants to companies whose products they are studying, join advisory boards and speakers' bureaus, enter into patent and royalty arrangements, agree to be the listed authors of articles ghostwritten by interested companies, promote drugs and devices at company-sponsored symposiums, and allow themselves to be plied with expensive gifts and trips to luxurious settings. Many also have equity interest in the companies. (Angell 2000)

In fact, prestigious journals have referred to this troubling relationship between science and academia. For example, 27 per cent of discoveries could take over six months to be published; unforeseen or problematic findings may never be published. One problem is under-reporting (Pitch *et al.* 2003; Antes and Chalmers 2003). Researchers must sign strict confidentiality agreements with the drug companies (Angell 2000). In an attempt to solve these conflicts some of the more prestigious medical journals have begun to hold researchers responsible for the content of their articles, and they request that conflicts of interest be duly explained (Angell 2000).

Sponsors

Another category of actor in the research process comprises the pharmaceutical industry and private companies. These sponsors prioritize successfully developed research in order to obtain approval from the new drugs or procedures by regulatory agencies. However, the context and the rules are determined by the market. A day's delay costs the pharmaceutical industry approximately $US1.3 million, so speedy approval is of key importance. Patents expire quickly, although they have recently been extended from fifteen to twenty years. The industry applies for a patent during the preclinical trial phase, before the trial has been concluded. It can take from eight to twelve years to develop all of the studies, and costs can run from approximately $400 million to $600 million.

The faster the drug company can obtain the necessary information for the drug's approval, the greater the financial gains. Certain steps in the research process, like the first phases of the research (Phase I and early Phase II) cannot be condensed, but the final phases in clinical trials (late Phase II and Phase III) can be accelerated (Luna and Salles 1998). One way to achieve this is by recruiting patients in the least possible time. This explains why research is currently conducted in different parts of the world simultaneously. In many cases, a large number of research subjects are included for a brief period with the aim of gathering the necessary information, obtaining the patent, and launching the drug on the market as fast as possible.

'Me-too' drugs are another way in which drug companies seek to maximize profits, at the expense of consumers. 'It's expensive to produce an innovative drug. On average, the bill runs to more than $400 million. So drug companies often take a less costly route to create a new product. They chemically rejigger an oldie but goodie, craft a new name, mount a massive advertising campaign and sell the retread as the latest innovative breakthrough' (Spector 2005). This imposes unnecessary costs on consumers, who are paying considerably more for what is essentially the same drug. A prime example is Nexium, a drug manufactured by AstraZenica for the treatment of stomach acid. When the patent for the original drug expired, other companies were able to create much cheaper generic drugs. So AstraZenica created Nexium, which is not chemically different from their older drug, but simply a different color (the new pill is purple). Although 'the little purple pill' is medically indistinguishable from generic drugs, it has been widely advertised on American television as if it were a major breakthrough in the treatment of acid reflux disease.

Other kinds of sponsor are the research agencies. Although they may not fully share market logic, they are not impervious to it. For example, agencies are fast becoming the owners of patents. Here again there is a difference between the 'leading' agencies of the industrialized world, such as the National Institutes of Health in the United States and its counterpart in European countries, whose budgets are quite high, and those of resource-poor countries, in, for example, much of Latin America, such as CONICET in Argentina. These agencies with very limited budgets may find it very difficult to comply with some of the requirements drawn up for the industry.

The Regulatory Agency

Other actors, until recently overlooked in scientific and ethics literature, are the regulatory agencies, who are responsible for the approval of new drugs. These need reliable information to consider adverse effects since they are responsible for preventing potentially harmful drugs from being launched on the market. The congruence and validity of the information and the design of the research are essential to matters of precision and safety.

One factor that regulatory agencies must consider is their responsibility to the population who will be using the new drug. The main concern of these agencies is to safeguard public health, and incorrect evaluation can affect the life and health of many people. This applies particularly to agencies in industrialized countries since they are responsible for approving the great majority of drugs that are launched worldwide. Regulatory agencies in developing countries have a low rate of approval for new drugs. Drugs generally approved have already been accepted in industrialized countries with high standards of pharmacovigilance. Thus, they do not face the same pressure in analyzing the data.

When approving a new drug, one of the main goals of the regulatory agencies is public health. At the same time, agencies draw up regulations and conduct inspections to protect research subjects. (An example of this is the concern of the US Food and Drug Administration (FDA) for the 'self-satisfied' choice of committees—'IRB shopping'; Dotzel 2002.) These conflicting demands—for the population in general as against the research subjects—create a degree of tension, if not possible conflicts in responsibilities. However, this issue is still to be thoroughly considered.

Research Ethics Committees

We have seen that many of the actors in clinical research—in addition to their particular interests and concerns—share the aim of ensuring that the research process develops appropriately, but can these safeguards guarantee that research subjects are protected?

If we accept the above conception of a research subject, we need an agent that can evaluate the individual's need for protection and provide safeguards. In one way or another the above-mentioned actors are concerned with the well-being of research subjects, but there is one more category of actor whose main objective is to protect research subjects; this is the research ethics committee.

The glossary of the 'Good Clinical Practices Consolidated Guideline' specifies that it is the responsibility of research ethics committees

to ensure the protection of the rights, safety, and well-being of human subjects involved in a trial and to provide public assurance of that protection, by, among other things, reviewing and approving/providing favorable opinion on the trial protocol, the suitability of the investigator(s), facilities, and the methods and material to be used in obtaining and documenting informed consent of the trial subject. (International Conference on Harmonization 1996)

This is accomplished by analyzing and assessing the ethical elements in the research protocol with the help of guidelines and international ethics documents—hence the importance of ethical documents such as the Declaration of Helsinki and the CIOMS Guidelines.

The most recent revision of the Declaration of Helsinki (2000) introduces, in addition, the option for committees to monitor the research process itself. Thus, the responsibility of ethics committees is substantial, though they do not have the power that other actors have, such as regulatory agencies and drug companies. This is an issue that should not be overlooked.

In general, research ethics committees face many obstacles. A frequent concern refers to the gap between what laws or regulations stipulate and what actually occurs (Luna 2002). Another problem focuses on the inadequate constitution of these committees, which are made up mostly of researchers and physicians (Luna 2002). Unlike the model in northern Europe, which has a high percentage of lay members of the community, many Latin American committees, for example, experience serious difficulties in incorporating representatives of the community. This may be because of their highly authoritarian culture and the prevalence of the medical model discourse that filters through this, making members of the community, nongovernmental organizations, and groups of patients difficult to include. In addition, a common problem in many developing countries is the poor training of some of the members, as well as the lack of resources for infrastructure (for example, subscriptions to journals, photocopies, and books) and administrative backup, which undermines the efficacy of the committee. Part of the problem lies in the lack of qualified committees and the lack of a system that can assess the performance of the ethics committees and the accuracy of their work. In contrast to the strong responsibility and demands implied in approving a research protocol, there is a lack of institutional support (for example, committee members may not be given time off work to sit on the committees; physicians or hospital staff may have to attend patients at the same time; or there may be a lack of secretarial support). This is closely related to the status of these committees, but it also has to do with the scarce resources and revenue to finance some of their tasks.

A further complication regarding the adequate functioning and protection of committees is the dissimilarity of policies among ethics committees themselves, even in the same country, region, or city. A South African committee illustrates this point clearly: 'Our committee, established in 1966, is the oldest and most experienced in South Africa and is known to be conservative. Protocols not accepted by us, we know, have been readily approved in the private sector or at other institutions' (Committee for Research on Human Subjects (Medical) 1997). This leads to another flaw in the opportunity for good protection: ethics committee shopping. Research ethics committees' main goal is to protect research subjects.

However, this is an exacting responsibility for an actor who is not as powerful or as well constituted as others.

In the next section we will consider another problem that research ethics committees face regarding the difficulties in having clear guidelines to direct them.

When we examine the situation of research actors in developing countries, we see that the system of safeguards may be weaker here than in industrialized countries. In this respect the following comment by Emanuel *et al.* (2004) may be quite accurate. On the risk of exploitation, they say: 'Furthermore, the regulatory infrastructures and independent oversight processes that might minimize the risk of exploitation may be less well established, less supported financially, and less effective in developing countries.'

III

RECENT CASES

New problematic cases related to research in developing countries have emerged recently. In late 1997 and 1998 a fierce international polemic followed the controversial use of placebos in pregnant women with AIDS (Lurie and Wolfe 1997; Angell 1997; Varmus and Satcher 1997; Mbidde 1998). The studies were conducted in sub-Saharan Africa, Thailand, and the Dominican Republic. The purpose was to find a more economic and effective treatment to prevent vertical transmission of AIDS. The study proposed giving pregnant women short AZT treatments against placebo, that is, the administration of a drug with no therapeutic effects for the control group. The problem arose because an effective treatment had already been available since 1994: the AIDS Clinical Trial Group Protocol 076, which consists of AZT treatment from the sixteenth week of pregnancy, intravenously during delivery, and during the newborn's first six weeks of life. The original controversy focused on the use of placebos in the control group and further questioned the ethics of withholding proven treatment in clinical trials. I shall not discuss the details and development of the debate here (see Luna 2001a).

In February 2001 the FDA seriously considered approving the design of a test for Surfaxin to be conducted in Ecuador, Bolivia, Peru, and Mexico. It proposed a control group of 325 premature newborn children with respiratory distress syndrome. This potentially fatal condition was to be treated with placebos while other surfactants existed. These surfactants had FDA approval and might have saved their lives (Lurie and Wolfe 2001). Approval of the trial would have meant condemning seventeen children to preventable deaths. The drug known to reduce mortality by 34 per cent (Lurie and Wolfe 2001). More questionable yet was the fact that the same laboratory was seeking approval for the drug with a European trial in which the children would receive not the placebo but an FDA-approved surfactant.

Another kind of controversial research was conducted in 1991 with a hepatitis A vaccine in northern Thailand. Forty-thousand children between the ages of 1 and 16 participated. The vaccine only provided protection for one year and was costly. Sponsors knew that the vaccine would not be accessible to or viable for the population that participated in the trial. The studies helped SmithKline Beecham to patent the vaccine, basically for tourists who would be traveling to countries with this kind of pathology (Lie 2000).

CURRENT PROBLEMS

With the increase of research in developing countries, new issues have become the focus of international debate: analyses about obligations during the trials and once they have been concluded, about the vulnerability of some populations, or about access to the benefits of the research.

It is difficult to answer these questions without falling back on slogans. A number of factors are at play in research and a degree of subtlety is essential. The research endeavor combines manifold interests and actors that impact not only on the health and well-being of many people, but also on the economy and the healthcare infrastructure of countries. The problem lies in filtering out abusive research and in promoting good-quality research, which should protect the research subjects while helping to close the gap between prevailing inequalities. It is a matter of considering the peculiarities of each case and of neither imposing unnecessary curbs nor simply consenting to any kind of research.

Because of cases like the AZT trials in sub-Saharan Africa, where the control group received placebos when an effective proven treatment was available, some bioethicists (e.g. Levine 1999) advocated the revision of the main research ethics documents, such as the Declaration of Helsinki and the CIOMS Guidelines. Developing countries caught the attention of the industrialized world, and other documents addressing some of their problems came to light, such as the Nuffield Report (Nuffield Council on Bioethics 2002) and the National Bioethics Advisory Commission Report (National Bioethics Advisory Commission 2001). However, the battlefield was and still is the Declaration of Helsinki.

Why is this attack on ethical codes so important? If it results in new guidance and new ethical documents with conflicting rules, it will impact on the design of research, and especially on the work of research ethics committees, which rely on the ethical guidelines, as do well-intentioned researchers. These attacks erode the moral authority of these documents and create confusion.

In the following sections I shall present the main arguments regarding these new problems, as well as the response given in the Declaration of Helsinki.

Levels of Treatment To Be Offered

The first point in the discussion was the standard of care for research subjects and participants during the research, that is, the obligations researchers have toward research subjects during the research. There are at least two aspects to this question:

1. the type of treatment that must be offered during the clinical trial (best proven treatment, highest attainable treatment, best current treatment, standard of care, etc.);
2. the single-standard versus the double-standard discussion.

This debate took place during the revision of the Declaration of Helsinki. Previous versions of the Declaration stipulated that the 'best proven treatment' be offered to all participants in a trial. Because of the AZT trials in Africa, among other clinical trials, this standard was considered to be too high. Hence, the first draft version of the current document, later rejected, suggested offering the comparator of the 'highest attainable therapy' in the host country (WMA 1999). To accept this would have implied the unacceptable situation of providing no treatment whatsoever. For some countries 'nothing' is the standard. What parameters should we use: the rural or urban population? Who will decide? etc. There are huge gaps between different regions or even within the same country. In Argentina there is good healthcare in some public clinics in the capital city, while 20 miles to the north or south may differ substantially. The situation in some of the poorer provinces of the country is even worse; here, treatment may be highly inadequate. It is even more problematic if we add the 'sustainability condition' as suggested by Robert Levine:

The 'highest attainable' therapy is the best therapy that one could reasonably provide under the conditions of the trial. The 'highest sustainable' therapy refers to the level of therapy that one could reasonably expect to be continued in the host country after the trial had been completed. That is, there should be a reasonable expectation that *the provision of the therapy could be sustained with the resources that would be available after the external support provided by the trial sponsors had been discontinued.* (Levine 1999)

We know that poor countries cannot sustain minimum healthcare conditions. Some countries, for example, allocate less than $10 per person per year (Mbidde 1998 comments that Uganda allocates $6 per person per year). Hence, the 'sustainability' condition would further lower the conditions of care and treatment. There really does not seem to be much difference between the 'highest attainable' and 'standard' care, even if that means no care at all. The notion of 'highest attainable' originates in the World Health Organization's Constitution and in the United Nations Covenant of Social and Economic Rights, in which a person has a 'right' to the 'highest attainable' health. The original meaning is the ideal goal that any country should strive for—nearly the opposite of what it is intended to mean in this context.

A similar proposal is the one that offers 'the standard treatment'. This ambiguous term may imply the standard of everyday practice, that is, the existing treatment. Or it may mean the standard that someone must meet (for example, to be accepted by a university), the objective or ideal that must be attained to be accepted (Macklin 2001). Many advocates of the standard therapy hold the first interpretation. It is not a question of making a minimal effort to improve the base situation. And it is particularly abusive when 'nothing' is the standard. The problem is: Is it acceptable to withhold proven and effective treatment? Is it tolerable to deny treatment that may save those people's lives or avoid a fatal illness? This leads to the next problem: What should the rationale be for the use of placebos?

However, before considering placebos, one point to examine is the introduction of a double standard into research—a standard for industrialized countries that can provide the best existing therapies and another for poor countries with limited funding and a deficient healthcare system.

Why do we speak of a double standard? Proposals such as Levine's (1999) suggest this path. What is the most common rationale in favor of a double standard? It indicates the benefits of research *for developing countries*: successful research will bring benefits and progress to that society, and obstacles to it may do harm in the medium and long term. This kind of reasoning emphasizes the positive consequences of endorsing a double standard: more research and faster results will be available and will benefit these poor societies. However, when we evaluate this argument, the numbers do not add up if the drug or therapies are not available. The argument depends on two factors: good clinical results obtained through research, and effective access to drugs or therapies (Luna 2001*b*). However, this depends not only on scientific endeavor but also on economic and political variables that are quite difficult to meet (Del Rio 1998; Tomas 1998; Schüklenk 2004). If one or any of these factors fails, there will be serious obstacles to achieving the expected benefits, and research subjects may be harmed in the meantime. Hence, the consequentialist rationale for a double standard may function only in an ideal world where economic and political variables are effectively met.

However, we do not live in an ideal world. Inequalities have been growing over past decades. Consider the broader picture: Why should we think that lowering the standards of research will benefit developing countries? There is a deep imbalance in global research funding, with less than 10 per cent of the $50–60 billion spent on health research per year devoted to diseases that account for 90 per cent of the global disease burden (Ahmad 2000), not to mention the wider gaps between the rich and the poor and the known lack of redistribution of wealth. Why should this global tendency make a change for the better? If the research is of no special benefit to these countries, but will benefit richer countries that can access the new drugs and therapies, why are we burdening these already suffering populations with a lower standard of treatment? Would it not be the right thing to do to provide the same treatment for all?

This logic of a double standard is interpreted in different ways. For example, Alex John London argues that a global or local standard of care is less important than the fundamental question of whether the standard ought to be de facto or de jure. London points out that whereas de facto standards are set by the level of care that is actually available in the relevant population, the de jure standard is set by what the expert medical community knows to be effective for treating the relevant illness in the relevant population. He argues that the de jure standard is the most ethically and scientifically defensible standard because of its relation with the disturbance of equipoise (London 2005). Crouch and Arras (1998) provide another interesting interpretation of the standard of care debate. They try to avoid double standards by defending the tailoring of research to the needs and circumstances of the host community. This may result in a research design that would not be proposed in more industrialized countries. They do not claim to endorse the double standard but say that people in the developing world have different needs that must be met in very different circumstances. Trials will have to take these specific circumstances into consideration if they are to prove valuable.

The above may be the case in some exceptional situations. In fact, in Luna (2001*b*) I consider a similar objection that indicates that providing the best therapy would imply distorting the conditions of the study to the extent that its results would not be relevant to the conditions of the host country. I accept that this criticism may sometimes be correct regarding certain sociocultural and socioeconomic conditions. However, we should consider carefully the scope of such an objection. This may be the situation for some specific trials, for example, in last-phase clinical trials with the immediate goal of introducing a new treatment or a drug into a community or country. But not all clinical trials have such goals. Accepting a lower or different treatment must not be the rule but the exception. If we want to address these particular cases, we should do it in a very specific way, including effective safeguards and sophisticated designs with rescue treatments in order to protect the research subjects. In these special cases, effective safeguards plus availability by clear prior agreements should be required (Luna 2001*b*).

In October 2000, following heated debate, the World Medical Association (WMA) approved a new version. It reintroduced the universal sense, avoiding the notorious double standard, and established in paragraph 29 that research subjects be given the best current treatment. Unfortunately, in the Spanish translation the word 'current' appears as 'available' (*disponible* or as *existente*), which has a different connotation.

Correct Use of Placebos

The second point that generated fierce controversy surrounded placebos. It was explicitly included for the first time in the last version of the Declaration of Helsinki and is still being discussed at the time of writing this chapter.

One actor that had not taken part in the previous debates began to participate. In 2001 the regulatory agencies took an aggressive stance. The first to act was the FDA, publishing the *Guidance for Industry: Acceptance of Foreign Clinical Studies*. The document advocated the previous version of the Declaration of Helsinki (1989) and the laws of countries. It said: 'In October 2000, the World Medical Association revised the Declaration. FDA has not taken action to incorporate those revisions into its regulations. FDA is making available this guidance document to clarify that the action of the World Medical Association did not change FDA regulations' (FDA 2001).The document went on to clarify that the FDA had incorporated five previous amendments to the Declaration of Helsinki after carefully examining their impact. It concluded that the FDA was revising its regulations to determine whether new standards or requirements should be incorporated.

In June 2001 the Scientific Committee of the European Medicines Agency (EMEA) also produced a document questioning paragraph 29 of the Declaration of Helsinki. In this case, the European Agency referred directly to the controversial paragraph. It said:

However, trials that seek to prove that a new agent and an active control have similar efficacy are inherently less reliable than trials that seek to prove the superiority of the new agent to a comparator, whether inactive or active. Increasing the size of trials does not alleviate this problem. In some areas of medicine, this lack of reliability means that it is only possible to obtain convincing scientific evidence of the efficacy of a new medicinal product by means of superiority trials. (EMEA–CPMP 2001)

Additionally, it established specific conditions. 'First and foremost, the period during which a placebo is administered *must not entail any additional risk of irreversible harm to the patient*' (my italics). It also referred to the process of informed written consent and the right to withdraw from the trial at any time. The last condition is highly relevant:

Similar ethical standards should be applied in trials performed in the European Union as well as in foreign countries. These aspects fall within the responsibilities of *Ethics Committees* reviewing protocols of clinical trials. (my italics)

Note the responsibility it places on the research ethics committees, a responsibility that is very difficult to fulfill given their lack of power and the problems they face.

Why is there such strong advocacy for the use of placebos? In some cases placebos provide scientific reliability (one of the interests of the regulatory agencies) and help to save time and money. Trials using placebos are shorter and require fewer research subjects (one of the main concerns of the drug companies). Hence, these two powerful actors concur on this point.

After these strong criticisms of the regulatory agencies and the pharmaceutical industry, the WMA published a Note of Clarification in October 2001 (WMA 2000). It supposedly 'endorsed' paragraph 29, but added:

However, a placebo-controlled trial may be ethically acceptable, even if proven therapy is available, under the following circumstances:

- Where for compelling and scientifically sound methodological reasons its use is necessary to determine the efficacy or safety of a prophylactic, diagnostic or therapeutic method; or
- Where a prophylactic, diagnostic or therapeutic method is being investigated for a minor condition and the patients who receive placebo will not be subject to any additional risk of serious or irreversible harm.

Contrary to its goals, this Note of Clarification obscured facts. Of the two clauses in the Note of Clarification, the second is the truly relevant one. The first clause, concerning 'compelling and scientifically sound methodological reasons', is a presupposition of all good research. The second clause establishes the use of placebos in the case of a 'minor condition' and when 'the patients who receive placebo will not be subject to any additional risk of serious or irreversible harm'. It allows placebos in trials with some analgesics, hypnotics, antihistamines, and antiemetics where the disease is minor, and implies no additional risks or irreversible harm, as in the case of, for example, a temporary illness. However, placebos are unacceptable in chemotherapy treatment with antiemetic drugs. The assessment is correctly rooted in the severity of the disease and not in the type of drug (Greco 2002). This flexibility makes placebos admissible in cases that are often considered important, such as moderate hypertension. It also allows for the use of 'add-on' treatments because they do not revoke the treatment of research subjects.

If this second clause is fundamental, the two clauses cannot be coordinated by the disjunction 'or' but by the conjunction 'and'. The two clauses in the Note of Clarification should be taken together, as simultaneous requirements. Recall that the Note of Clarification goes far beyond the EMEA's Guide. As the EMEA points out, the period during which a placebo is administered 'must not entail any additional risk of irreversible harm to the patient' and, even more, it seems to advocate a single standard.

Hence, if the use of placebos is to be expanded to include cases in which current therapies exist, and the limit is a matter of research subjects not being exposed to additional risks or serious and irreversible harms during the trial, it is fundamental to establish clear and sensible limits. The Note of Clarification does not require this. It could end up consenting to unacceptable trials like the Surfaxin trial in Ecuador, Bolivia, Peru, and Mexico.

Post-Trial Obligations

Finally, the last problems are clearly related to the question of justice. What obligations exist once the trial has been concluded? What criteria must be respected to prevent abusive and exploitative research?

The many perspectives and problems to be considered make this quite a complex issue. For example: (1) Which treatments should be provided? In the case of AIDS it could be viral load monitoring, CD cell counts and vaccinations, and antiretroviral therapy. But what about other typical complications during the later stages of AIDS, such as TB or meningitis? (2) A second issue is duration: should this be five years, ten years, a lifetime? (3) To whom should this treatment be provided: the individuals? And what about their families and extended-family members, or the community? (4) Finally, by whom should it be provided? Here we also find alternatives: sponsors or researchers. (This seems to be adequate in the case of the pharmaceutical industry but poses problems for noncommercial, small government research agencies.) What about private donors? (The latter was the choice of the HIV Vaccine Trials Network, which set up a fund using private donations for a trial in Haiti; Fitzgerald *et al.* 2003). Another solution is to allocate responsibility to governments. If access to adequate healthcare is a human right, it should be provided. However, governments sometimes have few resources to spend on healthcare and even fewer on research. Moreover, if this research is to benefit humanity, there should be global help. In this sense, fitting candidates are bilateral and multilateral programs or international funds.

We may find various responses to these questions (Tucker and Slack 2003; Berkley 2003; Fitzgerald *et al.* 2003). Even conscientious researchers may differ when answering how long a treatment should be provided, what kind of treatment is suitable, or how to provide it. Many issues are relevant: for example, the kind of illness, the spread of the illness in the region, and the available infrastructure.

An initial answer to these questions calls on research to be responsive to healthcare needs. However, it is not always easy to establish what this means: Does it consist of studying a disease that is prevalent in the region? Remember the hepatitis A trial that studied a relevant disease but did not satisfy the subjects' needs: the result was a vaccine for tourists. Does this imply, then, that the community must benefit? How? Multiple answers are generated, for example, 'benefiting the community as a whole'. The proposals vary from capacity-building (for example, training suitable researchers or competent physicians) to helping with infrastructure (for example, building hospitals or roads) (Emanuel *et al.* 2000).

Proving that these are complex and pressing questions, Emanuel *et al.* (2004) added an eighth principle to their previous framework for ethical research. They recognize the need to minimize the possibility of exploitation regarding research in developing countries and propose the principle of 'collaborative partnership', elaborating it through benchmarks that specify practical measures.

Another response suggests elaborating prior agreements to access successful findings. For example, the World Health Organization has negotiated some cost-free drugs for specific populations, established ceilings on prices, or withheld licenses or patents, for example, with respect to contraception or diseases like malaria. The International AIDS Vaccine Initiative applied for funding to conduct research and to develop a vaccine for distribution. This proposal regarding the elaboration of prior agreements has already been included in international documents like the CIOMS Guidelines (1993).

Alex London (2005) provides an interesting analysis. He outlines a first model derived mainly from international guidelines that requires researchers to obtain pre-trial assurances that the fruits of successful research programs will be made 'reasonably available' to members of the host population. The second model, known as the 'fair benefits approach', rejects this narrow emphasis on post-trial access, concentrating instead on avoiding exploitation by ensuring that there is a fair exchange of a wider range of benefits. Such benefits could include, but would not necessarily be limited to, bringing economic activity to a community, providing healthcare services that are secondary to the goals of the research initiative, providing educational and employment opportunities, or enhancing the community's infrastructure needs or addressing public health concerns. Host populations should be free to participate in research initiatives that would provide their community with what those community members judge to be a fair level of benefits from among any of these various categories in exchange for participation in research (Participants in the Conference on Ethical Aspects of Research in Developing Countries 2003).

Even if at first sight the model of fair exchange seems promising, there are notorious problems, as London correctly points out. One of the greatest is that, while this framework's reliance on collaborative partnership to negotiate a fair exchange is laudable, this ideal faces a variety of structural impediments in practice that cast into doubt the ability of host populations to access a meaningful range of the possible benefits touted as a strength of this approach. What constitutes a sufficient or fair exchange is then determined by what members of the host population are willing to accept in return for participation. The fair exchange model does not address the structural inequalities in bargaining power or problems regarding political legitimacy concerning who speaks for the host population. There is no serious consideration of real-world problems of inequalities, no correction for structural imbalances. London proposes a model based on human development to function both directly and indirectly to expand the capacity of basic social structures in the host community. It is based on justice grounded in the interest of free and equal persons in having fair equality of opportunity to develop their basic human capacities for agency and community and to be free to pursue a meaningful life plan that is consistent with the liberty of others to do likewise (CIOMS–WHO 1993). On this view, justice is not the outcome of a bargaining procedure in which parties with various differences in power negotiate terms of social cooperation. Rather, the distribution of power and privilege and their effects on the basic interests and liberties of community members are themselves issues that fall under the scope of justice.

In my view the reasonable availability model is a minimum in Phase III trials. It can be complemented by a model such as the human development model. I agree with London that it embodies higher moral aspirations than the fair benefits approach. Its primary strength lies in its focusing on productive pathways for bridging the gap between current conditions and more decent social arrangements. However, the human development approach is too abstract, requiring further clarification and refinement, an issue that London himself recognizes.

This last set of extremely complex issues is concerned with the avoidance of exploitative research. Why is this the case? Classic analysis of research ethics did not center on exploitation. Most research ethics seemed satisfied by attending to informed consent, risk–benefit, independent review, and confidentiality. There were some analyses of categories of research subjects such as children, mentally handicapped individuals, or institutionalized people that were considered vulnerable. And, even if some 'justice' issues were present, they mostly concerned an equitable range of burdens and benefits in the selection of research subjects. These analyses were not central, and the majority of the guidelines bypassed the issue of exploitation.

An exception to this trend was the CIOMS Guidelines (CIOMS–WHO 1993). In its Commentary to Guideline 8 these problems are spelled out very concisely. They ask for the approval of local or national research ethics committees, responsiveness to health needs, reasonable availability of successful drugs, and simultaneity when doing first phases of drug and vaccine trials (Macklin 2004). Contrary to the classic analysis, today exploitation in multicentric research is a key issue and can no longer be ignored. Here Ruth Macklin's examination of the concept of exploitation is quite relevant and useful: 'Exploitation occurs when wealthy or powerful individuals or agencies take advantage of the poverty, powerlessness, or dependency of others by using the latter to serve their own needs (those of the wealthy or powerful) without adequate compensating benefits for the less powerful or disadvantaged individuals or groups' (Macklin 2004).

What Macklin's proposal reveals immediately is that the initial situation is one of asymmetry: on one side are wealthy or powerful individuals or agencies; on the other, the powerless. This is quite a common situation in multicentric research conducted in developing countries, and it is why it is relevant to consider the concept of exploitation in this context. However, this does not mean that all research per se done in developing countries is exploitative. As Macklin correctly points out, other conditions should be present, for example, harms to the vulnerable groups, and herein begins the discussion about the later availability of the benefits of research and the meeting of community needs.

Macklin (2004) proposes some cases as leading candidates in which exploitation can occur:

1. Studies are carried out without the knowledge or voluntary consent of the individual research subjects;
2. Basic research is conducted in an industrialized country on a health problem that exists both in the industrialized and in a developing country; but clinical

trials are done in the developing country because it is simpler or cheaper to do them there. Successful products of the research become available soon afterwards to the industrialized country but become available in the developing country only fifteen to twenty years later, if at all;

3. Clinical trials are conducted in a developing country and could not, for ethical reasons, be conducted in the sponsoring, industrialized country;

4. Randomized clinical trials are conducted in both the industrialized country sponsor and in a developing country, with the control group in both countries receiving the best current treatment for the disease. A successful product resulting from the research becomes available only in the industrialized country because neither the government nor the majority of the population in the developing country can afford the product.

Macklin explains that, in the last case, the research subjects are treated equally in the industrialized country and in developing countries and both groups receive equal benefits during the study. However, the benefits are not provided to the wider population after the study is concluded, for economic reasons. She rightly points out that whether this situation fits the definition of exploitation depends on how the benefits of research are calculated. I agree that this is a difficult case to evaluate. There are reasons to accept this kind of research because it may benefit not only the subjects but also part of the research infrastructure of such a country. Even if some bioethicists would see the latter as exploitative (Glantz *et al.* 1998), I have doubts about this. Part of the problem will be to clarify what is understood by the difficult concept of 'adequate compensating benefits'. Undoubtedly these are very complex and controversial issues, and a case-by-case examination is necessary.

Once again the controversy arose over the Declaration of Helsinki. Following the ethical principle of benefiting from research, paragraph 30 says: 'At the conclusion of the study, every patient entered into the study should be assured of access to the best proven prophylactic, diagnostic and therapeutic methods identified by the study' (WMA 2000). This paragraph again raised strong criticism, which led to an attempt to make another clarification in October 2003. This paragraph puts pressure and implies expenditure, or, at least, responsibility, on the part of the pharmaceutical industry, as well as on the researchers.

The WMA explained that the terminology 'conclusion of the research', 'best methods', and 'identified by the study' was inadequate. They also said that research is not a fitting substitute for an inadequate healthcare system, and that it could inhibit academic research with small budgets. They did recognize that attacking this paragraph implied contradicting paragraph 19, which indicates that 'medical research is only justified if there is a reasonable likelihood that the populations in which the research is carried out stand to benefit from the results' (WMA 2000). In order to counter these criticisms, it is necessary to read this paragraph correctly. It implies the ethical principle of benefiting, but its scope is exaggerated, implying an obligation not on all kinds of research, but on some treatments such as treatment of chronic diseases.

Owing to the strong opposition of some developing countries, the amendment was postponed. Particularly strong throughout these debates was the position of Brazil, which never accepted a double standard and which, for example, provides universal antiretroviral treatment for AIDS. In the case of paragraph 30, Brazil maintained its leading role and the Argentine delegation supported it, even though this did not end the debate. At the time of writing, the WMA Workgroup (2004) *Report on the Revision of Paragraph 30 of the Declaration of Helsinki* was issued. It recommends making no changes and recovering the spirit of the ethical principles that the paragraph establishes, but acceptance of its recommendation is still open to discussion.

Concluding Remarks

Undoubtedly research in developing countries is generating new problems and discussions. We can see how the current analysis brought forward by developing countries goes far beyond informed consent, as well as beyond the first framework of early ethical guidelines. Informed consent is a necessary condition for research, but it is not sufficient. Developing countries' problems show that ethics does not end with the acceptance of a contract; the conditions under which it is accepted are also relevant. Individuals with no other choice may find it difficult to refuse to participate in research. They are not acting as contractors, and they may reflect the characteristics of the victim. The situation of the Swedish research subject who enjoys a public, efficient, and accessible healthcare system is a far cry from the subject in Mozambique or Bolivia who has no access to vital medication. It is not enough just to have a clear initial contract.

If research subjects share some features of a contractor as well as of a victim, adequate informed consent and an effective protection system should be in place. As we have seen, such responsibility seems to be shared by various actors, but this is one interest among many. Research ethics committees seem to have such responsibility; their main goal is the research subject's protection. However, they are not very powerful. They may have many problems in their functioning (such as inadequate membership, education, or expertise for diverse novel protocols). But, most importantly, they rely on ethical documents like the Declaration of Helsinki as a guide for difficult cases. Hence, the attacks on and questionings of the ethical codes are not naive. Not only do they undermine the foundations of research ethics and generate confusion, but they also destroy one of the tools for the evaluation of ethics committees. And even if ethical codes cannot be legally enforced, they do provide moral standards. They can shame researchers and justify criticisms from peers and colleagues. It is essential to maintain this moral and normative power, and it should not be diffused by issuing opposing guidelines or obscure 'clarifications'.

The problems that have been associated with increased research in developing countries have not been solved. They are difficult and complex. In the past there was quite a broad consensus on adequate safeguards, and vulnerability, exploitation, and justice were marginal. At present, these cannot be ignored and imply new challenges. A clear initial contract is merely a first step; other substantial issues should be considered, such as obligations to research subjects during and after research, and the benefit to the populations. Efforts should be made to avoid the moral and legal validation of unfortunate burdens on the vulnerable populations of the world.

REFERENCES

AHMAD, K. (2000), 'Report Reveals Serious Imbalance in Global Research Funding', *The Lancet*, 355: 170.

ANGELL, M. (1997), 'The Ethics of Clinical Research in the Third World', *New England Journal of Medicine*, 337/12: 847–9.

—— (2000), 'Is Academic Medicine for Sale?', *New England Journal of Medicine*, 342/20: 1516–18.

ANNAS, G. J., and GRODIN, M. A. (1992), *The Nazi Doctors and the Nuremberg Code* (Oxford: Oxford University Press).

ANTES, G., and CHALMERS, I. (2003), 'Under-Reporting of Clinical Trials Is Unethical', *The Lancet*, 361: 978–9.

APPELBAUM, P., *et al.* (1987), 'False Hopes and Best Data: Consent to Research and the Therapeutic Misconception', *Hastings Center Report*, 17/2: 20–4.

BERKLEY, S. (2003), 'Thorny Issues in the Ethics of AIDS Vaccine Trials', *The Lancet*, 362: 992.

Bodenheimer, T. (2000), 'Uneasy Alliance: Clinical Investigators and the Pharmaceutical Industry', New England Journal of Medicine, 342/20: 1539–44.

BRODY, B. (1998), *The Ethics of Biomedical Research* (Oxford: Oxford University Press).

CIOMS–WHO (COUNCIL FOR INTERNATIONAL ORGANIZATIONS OF MEDICAL SCIENCES andWORLD HEALTH ORGANIZATION) (1993), *International Ethical Guidelines for Biomedical Research Involving Human Subjects* (Geneva: CIOMS).

—— (2002), *International Ethical Guidelines for Biomedical Research Involving Human Subjects*, Guideline 13 (Geneva: CIOMS–WHO),<http://www.cioms.ch/frame_guidelines _nov2002.htm>.

COHEN, G. A. (1993), 'Equality of What? On Welfare Goods and Capabilities', in M. Nussbaum and A. Sen (eds.), *The Quality of Life* (Oxford: Clarendon Press).

COMMITTEE FOR RESEARCH ON HUMAN SUBJECTS (MEDICAL) (Peter Cleaton-Jones, Chairman) (1997), 'An Ethical Dilemma: Availability of Antiretroviral Therapy After Clinical Trials with HIV Infected Patients Are Ended', *British Medical Journal*, 314: 887–91.

CROUCH, R., and ARRAS, J. (1998), 'AZT Trials and Tribulations', *Hastings Center Report*, 28/6: 26–34.

DEL RIO, C. (1998), 'Is Ethical Research Feasible in Developed and Developing Countries?', *Bioethics*, 12/4: 330.

DOTZEL, M. (2002), *Federal Register*, 67/44: 10115–16.

DWORKIN, R. (1971), 'The Ethical Basis of Liberal Equality', in Dworkin, *Ethics and Economics* (Siena: Universidad de Siena).

EMANUEL, E., WENDLER, D., and GRADY, C. (2000), 'What Makes Clinical Research in Developing Countries Ethical?', *JAMA* 283: 2701–11.

—— KILLEN, J., and GRADY, C. (2004), 'What Makes Clinical Research in Developing Countries Ethical? The Benchmarks of Ethical Research', *Journal of Infectious Diseases*, 189: 930.

EMEA–CPMP (EUROPEAN MEDICINES AGENCY and COMMITTEE FOR PROPRIETARY MEDICINAL PRODUCTS) (2001), *Position Statement on the Use of Placebo in Clinical Trials with Regard to the Revised Declaration of Helsinki*, EMEA/17424/01 (London).

FDA (FOOD AND DRUG ADMINISTRATION) (2001), *Guidance for Industry: Acceptance of Foreign Clinical Studies*, <http://www.fda.gov/cber/gdlns/clinical031301.pdf>.

FITZGERALD, D., *et al.* (2003), 'Provision of Treatment in HIV-1 Vaccine Trials in Developing Countries', *The Lancet*, 362: 993–4.

GLANTZ, L. H., *et al.* (1998), 'Research in Developing Countries: Taking Benefits Seriously?', *Hastings Center Report*, 28: 38–42.

GRECO, D. (2002), 'Comments on the Council for International Organizations of Medical Sciences (CIOMS) on the Revised Draft, January 2002 International Guidelines for Biomedical Research Involving Human Subjects', unpub.

INTERNATIONAL CONFERENCE ON HARMONIZATION (1996), 'Good Clinical Practices Consolidated Guideline', in *Buenas Prácticas de Farmacologì en Investigación Clìnica* (Buenos Aires: CEDIQUIFA).

LEVINE, R. (1999), 'The Need to Revise the Declaration of Helsinki', *New England Journal of Medicine*, 341: 531–4.

LIE, R. (2000), 'Justice and International Research', in R. Levine, S. Gorovitz, and J. Gallagher (eds.), *Biomedical Research Ethics: Updating International Guidelines* (Geneva: CIOMS–WHO), 27 40.

LONDON, A. (2005), 'Justice and the Human Development Approach to International Research', *Hastings Center Report*, 35/1 (Jan.–Feb.), 24–37.

LUNA, F. (2001*a*), *Ensayos de Bioética: Reflexiones desde el Sur* (Mexico: Fontamara Ediciones).

—— (2001*b*), 'Is 'Best Proven' a Useless Criterion?', *Bioethics*, 15/4: 273–88.

—— (2002), 'Research Ethics Committees in Argentina and South America', *Notizie di Politeia*, 13/67: 95–100.

—— SALLES, A. L. F. (1998), *Bioética: Investigación, procreación, muerte y otros temas de ética aplicada* (Buenos Aires: Sudamericana).

LURIE, P., and WOLFE, S. (1997), 'Unethical Trial Interventions to Reduce Perinatal Transmission of the Human Immunodeficiency Virus in Developing Countries', *New England Journal of Medicine*, 337/12: 853–6.

—— (2001), Letter to Secretary Thompson, US Department of Health and Human Services, <http://www.citizen.org/publications/release.cfm?ID=6761>.

MACKLIN, R. (2001), 'After Helsinki: Unresolved Issues in International Research', *Kennedy Institute of Ethics Journal*, 11/1: 17–36.

—— (2004), *Double Standards in Medical Research in Developing Countries* (Cambridge: Cambridge University Press).

MBIDDE, E. (1998), 'Bioethics and Local Circumstances', Editorial, *Science*, 279: 155.

MERRIGAN, T. C. (1990), 'You Can Teach an Old Dog New Tricks: How AIDS Trials Are Pioneering New Strategies', *New England Journal of Medicine*, 323: 1341–3.

NATIONAL BIOETHICS ADVISORY COMMISSION (2001), *Ethical and Policy Issues in International Research: Clinical Trials in Developing Countries* (Bethesda, Md.: NBAC).

NATIONAL COMMISSION FOR THE PROTECTION OF HUMAN SUBJECTS OF BIOMEDICAL AND BEHAVIORAL RESEARCH (1979), *The Belmont Report: Ethical Principles and Guidelines for the Protection of Human Subjects of Research* (Washington, DC: US Government Printing Office).

NUFFIELD COUNCIL ON BIOETHICS (2002), *The Ethics of Research Related to Health Care in Developing Countries*, Ethical and Policy Issues in International Research (Draft Report) (London: NBAC).

O'NEILL, O. (1996), 'Justicia, sexo y fronteras internacionales', in M. Nussbaum and A. Sen (eds.), *La calidad de vida* (Mexico: Fondo de Cultura Económica).

PAPPWORTH, M. H. (1967), *Human Guinea Pigs* (Boston: Beacon).

PARTICIPANTS IN THE CONFERENCE ON ETHICAL ASPECTS OF RESEARCH IN DEVELOPING COUNTRIES (2003), 'Moral Standards for Research in Developing Countries', *Hastings Center Report*, 34/3: 17–27.

PITCH, J., *et al.* (2003), 'Role of a Research Ethics Committee in Follow-Up and Publication of Results', *The Lancet*, 361: 1015–16.

POGGE, T. (2003), 'Probando drogas para paìses ricos en poblaciones pobres de paìses en desarrollo', *Perspectivas Bioéticas*, 15/2: 11–43.

RAWLS, J. (1971), *A Theory of Justice* (Cambridge, Mass.: Harvard University Press).

ROTHMAN, D. (1991), *Strangers at the Bedside* (New York: Basic Books).

SCHÜKLENK, U. (1998), 'Unethical Perinatal HIV Transmission Trials Establish Bad Precedent', *Bioethics*, 12: 312–19.

—— (2004), 'The Standard of Care Debate: Against the Myth of an International Consensus Opinion', *Journal of Medical Ethics*, 30: 194–7.

SEN, A. (1980), 'Equality of What?', in L. McMurrin (ed.), *Tanner Lectures on Human Values* (Cambridge: Cambridge University Press).

SPECTOR, R. (2005), 'Me-Too Drugs: Sometimes They're Just the Same Old, Same Old', <http://mednews.stanford.edu/stanmed/2005summer/drugs-metoo.html>.

SWAZEY, J. P., and GLANTZ, L. (1982), 'A Social Perspective on Compensation for Injured Research Subjects', in Congress of the United States, 'President's Commission for the Study of Ethical Problems in Medicine and Biomedical and Behavioral Research', *Compensating for Research Injuries*, 2: 3–18.

TOMAS, J. (1998), 'Ethical Challenges of HIV Clinical Trials in Developing Countries', *Bioethics*, 12/4: 325–6.

TUCKER, T., and SLACK, C. (2003), 'Not If But How? Caring for HIV-1 Vaccine Trial Participants in South Africa', *The Lancet*, 362: 995.

VARMUS, H., and SATCHER, D. (1997), 'Ethical Complexities of Conducting Research in the Third World', *New England Journal of Medicine*, 337/12: 1003–5.

Weatherall, D. (2000), 'Academia and Industry: Increasingly Uneasy Bedfellows', The Lancet, 355: 1574.

WERTHEIMER, A. (1996), *Exploitation* (Princeton: Princeton University Press).

WMA (WORLD MEDICAL ASSOCIATION) (1996), *Declaration of Helsinki* (Somerset West: WMA).

—— (1999), *Declaration of Helsinki (Draft Version)* (Santiago de Chile: WMA); posted on the WMA website for comments at the time, <http://www.wma.net>.

—— (2000), *Declaration of Helsinki: Note of Clarification on Placebo-Controlled Trials* (Edinburgh: WMA).

WORLD MEDICAL ASSOCIATION WORKGROUP (2004), *Report on the Revision of Paragraph 30 of the Declaration of Helsinki*, <http://www.wma.net/e/ethicsunit/pdf/secretariat_report _rev_paragraph30.pdf>.

CHAPTER 27

ANIMAL EXPERIMENTATION

ALASTAIR NORCROSS

INTRODUCTION

I TAKE the central issue concerning the ethics of animal experimentation to be the moral status of animals.[1] Since most animal experimentation involves treating experimental subjects in ways that would clearly not be morally acceptable if the subjects were human, and since no animal experimentation involves the informed consent of the experimental subject(s), any attempt to justify such experimentation must include a defense of the claim that the moral status of animals differs significantly from that of humans. The influence of animal welfare advocates, in particular Peter Singer, Tom Regan, and their followers, but certainly dating back to Bentham and Mill, seems to have resulted in at least the grudging acceptance by the research community that animals have *some* moral status. That is, that the interests of animals should be taken into account when designing and justifying experiments involving them.

For example, Baruch Brody argues for what he calls 'a reasonable pro-research position on animal research', which is committed to at least the following propositions:

1. Animals have interests (at least the interest in not suffering, and perhaps others as well), which may be adversely affected either by research performed on them or by the conditions under which they live before, during, and after the research.

---

[1] In keeping with common conventions I use the term 'animal' in this chapter to refer to non-human animals.

2. The adverse effect on animals' interests is morally relevant, and must be taken into account when deciding whether or not a particular program of animal research is justified or must be modified or abandoned.
3. The justification for conducting a research program on animals that would adversely affect them is the benefits that human beings would receive from the research in question.
4. In deciding whether or not the research in question is justified, human interests should be given greater significance than animal interests.

(Brody 2003: 262–3)

In clarifying 4, Brody argues that human interests should be given *proportionally* greater significance than animal interests, as opposed to *lexically* greater significance. He does not, therefore, claim that *any benefit whatsoever* for humans can justify the infliction of *any harm, no matter how great* on animals. He doesn't attempt to say precisely how much greater significance should be given to human interests. It seems reasonable to say, though, that if this approach is to justify much (though perhaps not all) of the research that currently involves animals, the difference in significance must be vast. Consider such examples of animal experimentation as the Draize Eye Irritancy Test, in which quantities of cleaning fluids are tested on rabbits' eyes, or the infamous learned helplessness experiments of Martin Seligman, in which dogs were subjected to repeated painful shocks from which they couldn't escape. If these experiments, or many others like them, are to be justified by appeal to the claim that human interests should be given greater significance than animal interests, the difference in significance cannot be small. If human interests are merely *somewhat* more significant than animal interests, it should be acceptable to perform such experiments on humans, so long as the humans suffer *somewhat* less than the animals (or perhaps so long as *somewhat* fewer humans are subjected to the experiments). I know of no defenders of animal experimentation who are also prepared to defend painful experiments on humans just so long as these conditions are met.

Attempts to justify the widespread practice of giving little or no consideration to the vital interests of animals (the most obvious one being the interest in avoiding suffering) have been made from several different ethical perspectives. This chapter will explore three of the most common perspectives—utilitarianism, natural rights theory, and social contract theory—and explain why none of them is likely to justify the claim that the interests of humans are vastly more significant than the like interests of animals. While many people may be somewhat disturbed at learning the details of many medical and psychological experiments involving animals, relatively few seriously challenge the moral permissibility of such practices. The status quo in this regard appears to be that, minor details aside, our treatment of animals raises no serious moral questions. I will discuss the utilitarian approach in the first section, where I will argue that the utilitarian case against the status quo is overwhelming. In the next section I will consider various attempts to defend the status quo from within a natural rights framework, and will argue that all such attempts fail. Finally, I will turn to social contract theory, which appears to hold out the most hope for the defender of the status quo with respect to our treatment of animals. In a recent book, Peter Carruthers has vigorously defended the view that social contract theory can justify the claim that all and only humans have basic moral rights. His approach, he claims, provides the only satisfactory way to justify giving greater weight to the interests of severely retarded humans than to those of animals with equal or greater cognitive capacities. That is, it gives an answer to what is commonly called "the argument from marginal cases". I will argue both that social contract theory fails to give such an answer, and that all the well-known versions of the theory actually beg the question against attributing basic moral standing to animals. The ways in which both a natural rights approach and a social contract approach attempt to answer the argument from marginal cases embody a deeply flawed view of morality.

Utilitarianism

Most forms of utilitarianism consist of both a theory of the good and a theory of the right. The theory of the good tells us what states of affairs are intrinsically valuable or desirable, while the theory of the right tells us what actions are right or wrong, morally obligatory or morally forbidden. The standard utilitarian account of the good is that happiness, or more broadly, well-being, is intrinsically good, and unhappiness is intrinsically bad. The early utilitarians Jeremy Bentham and, to a certain extent, John Stuart Mill equated happiness with pleasure and unhappiness with pain. More recent utilitarians give a broader account of well-being, some including desire-satisfaction as an essential component, but most agree that pain and other forms of suffering are intrinsically bad. *All* suffering is bad, not just my suffering, or that of my family, or nation, or race, or species. The standard utilitarian account of the right is that the right action is that action, of all possible alternatives, that results in the greatest balance of good over bad. If more than one action results in the same balance of good over bad, and no actions result in a greater balance, all such actions are right, although none is obligatory. Any action that is not right is wrong. This approach to the rightness and wrongness of actions can also be applied to moral evaluations of character, rules, social practices and institutions, and so on. So, for example, a system of government will be judged morally acceptable or unacceptable by a utilitarian depending on whether there are any viable alternative systems that would result in a greater net balance of happiness.

So what does utilitarianism say about the moral status of animals? Consider an animal abuser who tortures dogs and cats out of malevolent curiosity. Our common moral sensibilities are appalled by such behavior. Utilitarianism provides a clear explanation of what is wrong with the abuser's behavior. The dogs and cats are made to suffer for no sufficient reason. In this respect, the utilitarian answer accords with ordinary intuitions. But the utilitarian approach also calls into question much commonly accepted animal experimentation (and animal agriculture). Many experimental subjects, such as rats, mice, rabbits, and monkeys, are made to suffer, sometimes severely, in the process of medical, pharmaceutical, and psychological research. Perhaps we could deny the moral significance of this treatment of animals by denying that they feel pain. It is often claimed that this was Descartes's position, though the truth, as I will explain shortly, is more complicated. Whatever Descartes and his contemporaries may have thought, however, it is hard to find anyone today who seriously claims that animals don't feel pain. The evidence that they do, both physiological and behavioristic, is simply overwhelming. It seems, then, that in order to justify the widespread infliction of animal suffering, a utilitarian will have to argue for a pretty hefty outweighing benefit. What are the prospects for such an argument to succeed?

Perhaps a utilitarian defender of the status quo will deny that she needs to argue for a large benefit to outweigh animal suffering. Perhaps she will say that I was mistaken to claim that *all* suffering is intrinsically bad. It is only human suffering that is intrinsically bad, she might say. Or perhaps she will admit that animal suffering is, indeed, bad, but nothing like as bad as human suffering. What reason could she supply for such differential concern for animal suffering? Perhaps she will claim that animal suffering is of lesser (or no) moral significance, because animals themselves are of lesser (or no) moral significance. They have less intrinsic value than humans, or maybe none at all. While this line of reasoning is fairly common in discussions of the moral status of animals, it is not one to which a utilitarian can appeal. Utilitarians hold that certain types of states have intrinsic value and disvalue, not types of creatures. Talk of an individual creature's intrinsic value is best understood in terms of the intrinsic value of the life of the individual, which in turn amounts to the intrinsic value of the states (usually the mental states) that comprise the life. Given the theoretical primacy of judgements about the intrinsic value of mental states of individuals, claims about the intrinsic value of the individuals themselves cannot be used to justify claims about the intrinsic value of the individuals' mental states. It may well be that the typical human life is of greater intrinsic value than the typical canine life, but this will be because the human life is comprised of a greater and richer variety of experiences, emotions, hopes, aspirations, and the like. The sufferings, however, of a dog, considered in and of themselves, are of no lesser (or greater) moral significance than the like sufferings of a human being.

There is one other line of reasoning open to a utilitarian to deny moral significance to animal suffering. Consider the following partial characterization of what Derek Parfit calls *Preference-Hedonism*: 'On the use of "pain" which has rational and moral significance, all pains are when experienced unwanted, and a pain is worse or greater the more it is unwanted' (Parfit 1984: 493). Some might even claim that it is part of the very concept of pain that it is unwanted. Even if we deny this, it seems plausible to say that a pain is only bad to the extent that it is unwanted. If someone really doesn't care about a pain, in and of itself, it is hard to see how the pain could be intrinsically bad. So what does this have to do with animals? Recall Descartes. Although he didn't deny that animals have sensations, such as pain, he did deny that they have what he called "thoughts", which included both beliefs and desires. (His argument for this, which I won't explore here, has to do with animals' lack of linguistic ability.) If animals are incapable of desire, they are a fortiori incapable of desiring that painful sensations cease. This would also provide a desire-satisfaction utilitarian with a reason to deny moral status to animals.

So, what should we say about the denial that animals have desires? At first sight, it seems almost as unbelievable as the denial that they feel pain. Only a philosopher could make such an obviously false claim with a straight face. Recall some of the other outrageous claims made by philosophers over the ages: motion is impossible; all is flux; all is water; there is no such thing as weakness of will; the physical world is just a collection of ideas; the unregulated free market will work to the benefit of all. Of *course* animals want things. Any pet owner can tell you that. However, as someone who has been known to make some seemingly outrageous claims myself, I cannot dismiss this one without at least examining an argument for it.

A philosopher who argues that animals don't have desires is R. G. Frey. Here, briefly, in his own words is his argument:

I may as well say at once that I do not think that animals can have desires. My reasons for thinking this turn largely upon my doubts that animals can have beliefs, and my doubts in this regard turn partially, though in large part, upon the view that having beliefs is not compatible with the absence of language and linguistic ability.   (Frey 1989: 40)

So, why does Frey claim that desires require beliefs? Here is the example he uses to argue for this claim:

Suppose I am a collector of rare books and desire to own a Gutenberg Bible: my desire to own this volume is *to be traced* to my belief that I do not now own such a work and that my rare book collection is deficient in this regard . . . . without this belief, I would not have this desire.   (Frey 1989: 40)

I don't wish to dwell on this part of Frey's argument, since the more interesting claim is that beliefs depend on linguistic ability. However, it is worth pointing out that, even if we accept his example of the desire for a Gutenberg Bible depending on a belief, it may well be that other, perhaps more basic desires, such as the desire for food, don't depend on beliefs. So, what of his claim that beliefs require linguistic ability? Here he is again, still on the example of the Gutenberg Bible:

Now what is it that I believe? I believe that my collection lacks a Gutenberg Bible; that is, I believe that the sentence 'My collection lacks a Gutenberg Bible' is true. In constructions of the form 'I believe that,' what follows upon the 'that' is a declarative sentence; and *what* I believe is that that sentence is true. The difficulty in the case of animals should be apparent: if someone were to say, e.g., 'The cat believes that the door is locked,' then that person is holding, as I see it, that the cat holds the declarative sentence 'The door is locked' to be true; and I can see no reason whatever for crediting the cat or any other creature which lacks language, including human infants, with entertaining declarative sentences and holding certain sentences to be true.   (Frey 1989: 40–1)

The most obvious flaw with this reasoning is that it generates an infinite regress. According to Frey's approach, my belief that my collection lacks a Gutenberg Bible just is my belief that the sentence 'My collection lacks a Gutenberg Bible' is true. But by the same reasoning, my belief that the sentence 'My collection lacks a Gutenberg Bible' is true just is my belief that the sentence 'the sentence "My collection lacks a Gutenberg Bible" is true' is true. And so on. How plausible is it, for example, that my belief that my collection lacks a Gutenberg Bible just is my belief that the sentence 'the sentence "the sentence 'the sentence "the sentence 'My collection lacks a Gutenberg Bible' is true" is true' is true" is true' is true?

Perhaps a less problematic way of tying beliefs and desires to language could be found, but it seems doubtful that it could do the moral work necessary for justifying the infliction of suffering on animals. There may well be a whole range of beliefs and desires that *does* require linguistic ability. However, the ethically significant ones, such as the desire that a pain cease, do not seem to do so. Even if we define desires in such a way that no nonlinguistic creature has them, there is clearly *some* mental state of the suffering dog that is importantly similar to a human's desire that the pain cease.

So much for any utilitarian attempt to dismiss the intrinsic moral significance of animal suffering. Isn't it nonetheless possible that the suffering involved in animal experimentation is outweighed by the benefits thereby produced? Notice that a utilitarian demands of an action or institution not that it result in a greater amount of happiness than unhappiness, but that it result in a greater *balance* of happiness than available alternatives (ignoring the possibility of ties). This detail is important, though sometimes ignored in discussions of the justifiability of animal experimentation. Let me illustrate the difference, with reference to a common criticism of utilitarianism. Some critics charge that utilitarianism is defective on the grounds that it could be used to justify the institution of slavery. Imagine, they say, a society with a small number of slaves and a large number of free citizens. Perhaps the slaves are exceedingly unhappy. Perhaps, indeed, the unhappiness of each slave is many times greater than the happiness of each free citizen. However, if there are *enough* free citizens, their happiness will outweigh the unhappiness of the slaves. But this is still not enough for the system to be justified on utilitarian grounds. Perhaps the free citizens could have been just as happy, or even happier, in a society without slaves. In which case, assuming that the slaves would have been happier not being slaves, there would have been a bigger balance of happiness over unhappiness in the free society. (The point of this example is not to argue that utilitarianism *couldn't* justify some system of slavery, but to point out that the possibility of such a system being justified on utilitarian grounds is even more remote than it might initially appear.)

The relevance of this point to the moral status of animal experimentation should be clear. To justify a particular practice that inflicts significant suffering on animals it is not enough to argue that the benefits of the practice (probably to humans) are greater than the suffering of the animals. What needs to be argued is that nothing like as much benefit could be achieved without significant animal suffering.

What of the benefits of animal experimentation? Aren't there enormous benefits to humans (and maybe other animals) that can only be achieved through the use of animals in research? I won't explore this empirical question in detail here. It doesn't require more than a cursory glance at the literature, though, to conclude that huge numbers of animal experiments provide little or no benefit, and could never have been reasonably expected to do so. Many drugs are tested on animals in order to compete on a market already glutted with drugs that do the same job. Much psychological research merely confirms what common sense tells us, and serves only to advance the career of the researcher. Even many of those experiments that do, arguably, give results that have beneficial applications may not be justified on utilitarian grounds. Perhaps only a lesser benefit could have been achieved without animal suffering. Nonetheless, the difference in benefit may well be smaller than the suffering in question.

It is sometimes objected that we cannot apply a utilitarian approach to the justification of individual experiments, because we simply never know when we might make a significant breakthrough. If we had to justify each experiment in advance, we wouldn't justify any, and would thereby miss out on those that do lead to great benefits. If the utilitarian approach had been used in the past, it is claimed, we would have missed out on many of the beneficial advances in medicine. This line of reasoning, though, either fails in its own terms or begs the question against the utilitarian approach. Either the benefits from the use of animals in research really do outweigh the animal suffering or they don't. If they do, an expected utility calculation will give the result that at least some experiments are justified. If they don't, the fact that we would miss out on the benefits if we abandoned animal research is not sufficient, morally, to justify such research. But perhaps supporters of research will claim that we simply never know which experiments will result in benefit, even though, on balance, the benefits outweigh the harms. So we can never justify an experiment in advance, on utilitarian grounds, even though we have good reasons to believe that the practice of animal experimentation as a whole can be so justified. This response assumes far too pessimistic a view of our powers of prediction. Researchers don't select lines of enquiry at random, simply hoping to get lucky. There is plenty of evidence on which to base decisions. It is surely reasonable that, in order to justify the certain infliction of suffering on animals, there has to be *some* reason to expect a significant benefit. In the absence of such a reason, we cannot simply resort to the claim that the unexpected sometimes happens. Despite these considerations, there may well be some animal experiments that are justified on utilitarian grounds, but it is likely to be a small fraction of the number actually performed.

To summarize the conclusions of the present section, it seems likely that a utilitarian approach to morality will condemn much, and perhaps most, animal experimentation. Whatever benefit, if any, that comes from most experiments is simply not enough to justify the amount of suffering involved.

NATURAL RIGHTS THEORY

In this section I will discuss an approach to the moral status of animals that, for the sake of convenience, I refer to as "natural rights theory". This approach focuses on identifying certain natural features or properties of individuals or species as the basic grounds for the attribution of differing moral status. So, for example, rationality has often been claimed as the grounds for the superior moral status of human beings over animals. For the purposes of this discussion, to claim that humans have a superior moral status to animals is to claim that it is morally right to give the interests of humans greater weight than those of animals in deciding how to behave. Such claims will often be couched in terms of rights, such as the rights to life, liberty, or respect, but nothing turns on this terminological matter. One may claim that it is generally wrong to kill humans, but not animals, because humans are rational, and animals are not. Or one may claim that the suffering of animals counts less than the suffering of humans (if at all), because humans are rational, and animals are not. These claims may proceed through the intermediate claim that the rights of humans are more extensive and stronger than those (if any) of animals. Alternatively, one may directly ground the judgement about the moral status of certain types of behavior in claims about the alleged natural properties of the individuals involved.

What can a proponent of this approach say about the moral status of animals? The traditional view, dating back at least to Aristotle, is that rationality is what separates humans, both morally and metaphysically, from other animals. With a greater understanding of the cognitive powers of some animals, recent philosophers have often refined the claim to stress the kind and level of rationality required for moral reasoning. Let's start with a representative sample of three. Consider first these claims of Bonnie Steinbock:

While we are not compelled to discriminate among people because of different capacities, if we can find a significant difference in capacities between human and non-human animals, this could serve to justify regarding human interests as primary. It is not arbitrary or smug, I think, to maintain that human beings have a different moral status from members of other species because of certain capacities which are characteristic of being human. We may not all be equal in these capacities, but all human beings possess them to some measure, and non-human animals do not. For example, human beings are normally held to be responsible for what they do. . . . Secondly, human beings can be expected to reciprocate in a way that non-human animals cannot . . . Thirdly . . . there is the 'desire for self-respect'.   (Steinbock 1997: 467–8)

Similarly, Mary Anne Warren argues that 'the rights of persons are generally stronger than those of sentient beings which are not persons'. Her main premise to support this conclusion is the following:

there is one difference [between human and non-human nature] which has a clear moral relevance: people are at least sometimes capable of being moved to action or inaction by the force of reasoned argument.   (Warren 1997: 482)

Carl Cohen, one of the most vehement modern defenders of what Peter Singer calls "speciesism", states his position as follows:

Between species of animate life, however—between (for example) humans on the one hand and cats or rats on the other—the morally relevant differences are enormous, and almost universally appreciated. Humans engage in moral reflection; humans are morally autonomous; humans are members of moral communities, recognizing just claims against their own interest. Human beings do have rights, theirs is a moral status very different from that of cats or rats.   (Cohen 1992: 462)

So, the claim is that human interests and/or rights are stronger or more important than those of animals, because humans possess a kind and level of rationality not possessed by animals. How much of our current behavior towards animals this justifies depends on just how much consideration should be given to animal interests, and on what rights, if any, they possess. Both Steinbock and Warren stress that animal interests need to be taken seriously into account. Warren claims that animals have important rights, but not *as* important as human rights. Cohen, on the other hand, argues that we should actually *increase* our use of animals.

One of the most serious challenges to this defense of the status quo involves a consideration of what philosophers refer to as "marginal cases". Whatever kind and level of rationality is selected as justifying the attribution of superior moral status to humans will either be lacking in some humans or present in some animals. To take one of the most commonly suggested features, many humans are incapable of engaging in moral reflection. For some, this incapacity is temporary, as is the case with infants, or the temporarily cognitively disabled. Others who once had the capacity may have permanently lost it, as is the case with the severely senile or the irreversibly comatose. Still others never had and never will have the capacity, as is the case with the severely mentally disabled. If we base our claims for the moral superiority of humans over animals on the attribution of such capacities, won't we have to exclude many humans? Won't we then be forced to the claim that there is at least as much moral reason to use cognitively deficient humans in experiments (and for food) as to use animals? Perhaps we could exclude the only temporarily disabled, on the grounds of potentiality, though that move has its own problems. Nonetheless, the other two categories would be vulnerable to this objection.

I will consider two lines of response to the argument from marginal cases. The first denies that we have to attribute different moral status to marginal humans, but maintains that we are, nonetheless, justified in attributing different moral status to animals who are just as cognitively sophisticated as marginal humans, if not more so. The second admits that, strictly speaking, marginal humans are morally inferior to other humans, but proceeds to claim pragmatic reasons for treating them, at least usually, *as if* they had equal status.

As representatives of the first line of defense, I will consider arguments from three philosophers, Carl Cohen, Alan White, and David Schmidtz. First, Cohen:

[the argument from marginal cases] fails; it mistakenly treats an essential feature of humanity as though it were a screen for sorting humans. The capacity for moral judgement that distinguishes humans from animals is not a test to be administered to human beings one by one. Persons who are unable, because of some disability, to perform the full moral functions natural to human beings are certainly not for that reason ejected from the moral community. The issue is one of kind . . . What humans retain when disabled, animals have never had.   (Cohen 1992: 460–1)

Alan White argues that animals don't have rights, on the grounds that they cannot intelligibly be spoken of in the full language of a right. By this he means that they cannot, for example, claim, demand, assert, insist on, secure, waive, or surrender a right. This is what he has to say in response to the argument from marginal cases:

Nor does this, as some contend, exclude infants, children, the feeble-minded, the comatose, the dead, or generations yet unborn. Any of these may be for various reasons empirically unable to fulfill the full role of right-holder. But . . . they are logically possible subjects of rights to whom the full language of rights can significantly, however falsely, be used. It is a misfortune, not a tautology, that these persons cannot exercise or enjoy, claim, or waive, their rights or do their duty or fulfil their obligations.   (White 1989: 120)

David Schmidtz defends the appeal to typical characteristics of species, such as mice, chimpanzees, and humans, in making decisions on the use of different species in experiments. He also considers the argument from marginal cases:

Of course, some chimpanzees lack the characteristic features in virtue of which chimpanzees command respect as a species, just as some humans lack the characteristic features in virtue of which humans command respect as a species. It is equally obvious that some chimpanzees have cognitive capacities (for example) that are superior to the cognitive capacities of some humans. But whether every human being is superior to every chimpanzee is beside the point. The point is that we can, we do, and we should make decisions on the basis of our recognition that mice, chimpanzees, and humans are relevantly different types. We can have it both ways after all. Or so a speciesist could argue.   (Schmidtz 1998: 61)

There is something deeply troublesome about the line of argument that runs through all three of these responses to the argument from marginal cases. A particular feature, or set of features, is claimed to have so much moral significance that its presence or lack can make the difference to whether a piece of behavior is morally justified or morally outrageous. But then it is claimed that the presence or lack of the feature in any *particular* case is not important. The relevant question is whether the presence or lack of the feature is *normal*. Such an argument would seem perfectly preposterous in most other cases. Suppose, for example, that ten famous people are on trial in the afterlife for crimes against humanity. On the basis of conclusive evidence, five are found guilty and five are found not guilty. Four of the guilty are sentenced to an eternity of torment, and one is granted an eternity of bliss. Four of the innocent are granted an eternity of bliss, and one is sentenced to an eternity of torment. The one innocent who is sentenced to torment asks why he, and not the fifth guilty person, must go to hell. St Peter replies, 'Isn't it obvious, Mr Ghandi? You are male. The other four men—Adolph Hitler, Joseph Stalin, Richard Nixon, and George W. Bush—are all guilty. Therefore the normal condition for a male defendant in this trial is guilt. The fact that you happen to be innocent is irrelevant. Likewise, of the five female defendants in this trial, only one was guilty. Therefore the normal condition for female defendants in this trial is innocence. That is why Margaret Thatcher gets to go to heaven instead of you.'

As I said, such an argument is preposterous. Is the reply to the argument from marginal cases any better? Perhaps it will be claimed that a biological category such as a species is more "natural", whatever that means, than a category like "all the male (or female) defendants in this trial". Even setting aside the not inconsiderable worries about the conventionality of biological categories, it is not at all clear why this distinction should be morally relevant. What if it turned out that there were statistically relevant differences in the mental abilities of men and women? Suppose that men were, on average, more skilled at manipulating numbers than women, and that women were, on average, more empathetic than men. Would such differences in what was "normal" for men and women justify us in preferring an innumerate man to a female math genius for a job as an accountant, or an insensitive woman to an ultra-sympathetic man for a job as a counselor? I take it that the biological distinction between male and female is just as real as that between human and chimpanzee.

A second response to the argument from marginal cases is to concede that cognitively deficient humans really do have an inferior moral status to normal humans. Can we, then, use such humans as we do animals, and experiment on them (and raise them for food)? How can we advocate this second response while blocking such uses of marginal humans? Warren suggests that 'there are powerful practical and emotional reasons for protecting non-rational human beings, reasons which are absent in the case of most non-human animals' (Warren 1997: 483). Here is Steinbock in a similar vein:

I doubt that anyone will be able to come up with a concrete and morally relevant difference that would justify, say, using a chimpanzee in an experiment rather than a human being with less capacity for reasoning, moral responsibility, etc. Should we then experiment on the severely retarded? Utilitarian considerations aside, we feel a special obligation to care for the handicapped members of our own species, who cannot survive in this world without such care.... In addition, when we consider the severely retarded, we think, 'That could be me'. It makes sense to think that one might have been born retarded, but not to think that one might have been born a monkey.... Here we are getting away from such things as 'morally relevant differences' and are talking about something much more difficult to articulate, namely, the role of feeling and sentiment in moral thinking.   (Steinbock 1997: 469–70)

This line of response clearly won't satisfy those who think that marginal humans really do deserve equal moral consideration with other humans. It is also a very shaky basis on which to justify our current practices. What outrages human sensibilities is a very fragile thing. Human history is littered with examples of widespread acceptance of the systematic mistreatment of some groups who didn't generate any sympathetic response from others. That we do feel a kind of sympathy for retarded humans that we don't feel for dogs is, if true, a contingent matter.

Perhaps we could claim that the practice of giving greater weight to the interests of all humans than of animals is justified on evolutionary grounds. Perhaps such differential concern has survival value for the species. Something like this may well be true, but it is hard to see the moral relevance. We can hardly justify the privileging of human interests over animal interests on the grounds that such privileging serves human interests!

Although the argument from marginal cases certainly poses a formidable challenge to any proposed criterion of full moral standing that excludes animals, it doesn't, in my view, constitute the most serious flaw in such attempts to justify the status quo. The proposed criteria are all variations on the Aristotelian criterion of rationality. But what is the moral relevance of rationality? Why should we think that the possession of a certain level or kind of rationality renders the possessor's interests of greater moral significance than those of a merely sentient being? In Bentham's famous words 'The question is not, Can they reason? nor Can they talk? But, Can they suffer?'

What do defenders of the alleged superiority of human interests say in response to Bentham's challenge? Some, such as Carl Cohen, simply reiterate the differences between humans and animals that they claim to carry moral significance. Animals are not members of moral communities, they don't engage in moral reflection, they can't be moved by moral reasons, *therefore* (?) their interests don't count as much as ours. Others, such as Steinbock and Warren, attempt to go further. Here is Warren on the subject: 'Why is rationality morally relevant? It does not make us "better" than other animals or more "perfect".... But it is morally relevant insofar as it provides greater possibilities for cooperation and for the nonviolent resolution of problems' (Warren 1997: 482). Warren is certainly correct in claiming that a certain level and kind of rationality is morally relevant. Where she, and others who give similar arguments, go wrong is in specifying what the moral relevance amounts to. If a being is incapable of moral reasoning, at even the most basic level, if it is incapable of being moved by moral reasons, claims, or arguments, then it cannot be a moral agent. It cannot be subject to moral obligations, to moral praise or blame. Punishing a dog for doing something 'wrong' is no more than an attempt to alter its future behavior. So long as we are undeceived about the dog's cognitive capacities, we are not, except metaphorically, expressing any moral judgement about the dog's behavior. (We may, of course, be expressing a moral judgement about the behavior of the dog's owner, who didn't train it very well.) All this is well and good, but what is the significance for the question of what weight to give to animal interests? That animals can't be moral *agents* doesn't seem to be relevant to their status as moral *patients*. Many, perhaps most, humans are both moral agents and patients. Most, perhaps all, animals are only moral patients. Why would the lack of moral agency give them diminished status as moral patients? Full status as a moral patient is not some kind of reward for moral agency. I have heard students complain in this regard that it is *unfair* that humans bear the burdens of moral responsibility, and don't get enhanced consideration of their interests in return. This is a very strange claim. Humans are subject to moral obligations, because they are the kind of creatures who *can* be. What grounds moral agency is simply different from what grounds moral standing as a patient. It is no more unfair that humans and not animals are moral agents, than it is unfair that real animals and not stuffed toys are moral patients.

One other attempt to justify the selection of rationality as the criterion of full moral standing is worth considering. Recall the suggestion that rationality is important in so far as it facilitates cooperation. If we view the essence of morality as reciprocity, the significance of rationality is obvious. A certain twisted, but all too common, interpretation of the Golden Rule is that we should 'do unto others in order to get them to do unto us'. There's no point, according to this approach, in giving much, if any, consideration to the interests of animals, because they are simply incapable of giving like consideration to our interests. Inasmuch as there is a consistent view being expressed here at all, it concerns self-interest, as opposed to morality. Whether it serves my interests to give the same weight to the interests of animals as to those of humans is an interesting question, but it is not the same question as whether it is *right* to give animals' interests equal weight. The same point, of course, applies to the question of whether to give equal weight to my interests, or those of my family, race, sex, religion, etc., as to those of other people.

Perhaps it will be objected that I am being unfair to the suggestion that the essence of morality is reciprocity. Reciprocity is important, not because it serves *my* interests, but because it serves the interests of all. Reciprocity facilitates cooperation, which in turn produces benefits for all. What we should say about this depends on the scope of 'all'. If it includes all sentient beings, then the significance of animals' inability to reciprocate is in what it tells us about *how* to give their interests equal consideration. It certainly can't tell us that we should give less, or no, consideration to their interests. If, on the other hand, we claim that rationality is important for reciprocity, which is important for cooperation, which is important for benefiting humans, which is the ultimate goal of morality, we have clearly begged the question against giving equal consideration to the interests of animals.

It seems that any attempt to justify the status quo with respect to our treatment of animals by appealing to a morally relevant difference between humans and animals will fail on at least two counts. It will fail to give an adequate answer to the argument from marginal cases, and, more importantly, it will fail to make the case that such a difference is morally relevant to the status of animals as moral patients as opposed to their status as moral agents.

SOCIAL CONTRACT THEORY

For the would-be defender of the status quo, the most promising moral approach is social contract theory, or contractualism. Given its classical expression in Hobbes's *Leviathan*, Rousseau's *The Social Contract*, and Locke's *Second Treatise on Government*, contractualism views morality as in some sense a human construct. If human beings were to live without rules, in what Hobbes and Rousseau refer to as a 'state of nature', life would be, in Hobbes's memorable phrase 'solitary, poor, nasty, brutish, and short'. It would then be in the interests of everyone to agree to abide by certain rules, such as a rule against killing others, on condition that others also agree. The content of the agreement, or contract, provides the rules of morality. It is no part of the theory that there ever *was* such an agreement. The contract itself is an enlightening fiction, useful to discover the requirements of morality. In the same way, a utilitarian can appeal to the fiction of an ideally informed, impartial, and benevolent observer to explain the content of that theory's requirements. James Rachels expresses the basic idea of contractualism as follows: 'Morality consists in the set of rules, governing how people are to treat one another, that rational people will agree to accept, for their mutual benefit, on the condition that others follow those rules as well' (Rachels 1999: 137). In a recent book, Peter Carruthers has argued that a contractualist approach to ethics supports the status quo with respect to animals. He claims that the most plausible versions of contractualism accord full direct moral status to all humans, including the severely cognitively impaired, and deny direct moral status to all animals. He further claims that such an approach can explain the wrongness of many instances of cruelty to animals, without accepting that animal experimentation (or factory farming) is wrong, or that the animals who are the victims of wrongful cruelty have direct moral significance. Carruthers bases his discussion on two influential contemporary versions of contractualism;

the theories of John Rawls and Thomas Scanlon. Here are Carruthers's summaries of the main points of the two theories:

The basic idea, then, is that we are to think of morality as the rules that would be selected by rational agents choosing from behind what Rawls calls *a veil of ignorance*. While these agents may be supposed to have knowledge of all general truths of psychology, sociology, economics, and so on, they are to be ignorant of their own particular qualities (their intelligence, physical strength, qualities of character, projects and desires), as well as the position they will occupy in the society that results from their choice of rules.... The point of the restrictions is to eliminate bias and special pleading in the selection of moral principles.... Hence his proposal is, in fact, that moral rules are those that we should rationally agree to if we were choosing from a position of complete fairness.... Most importantly, the agents behind the veil of ignorance must not be supposed to have, as yet, any moral beliefs. For part of the point of the theory is to explain how moral beliefs can arise.

[Scanlon's] account of morality is roughly this: moral rules are those that no one could reasonably reject as a basis for free, unforced, general agreement amongst people who share the aim of reaching such an agreement... here the agents concerned are supposed to be real ones, with knowledge of their own idiosyncratic desires and interests, and of their position within the current structure of society. The only idealisations are that choices and objections are always rational... and that all concerned will share the aim of reaching free and unforced agreement... the contractors will know that there is no point in rejecting a proposed rule on grounds special to themselves, since others would then have equal reason to reject *any* proposed rule.   (Carruthers 1992: 37–9)

So, how do animals fare on these approaches? It is fairly clear that they won't be assigned more than indirect moral significance. Since the contractors, on both models, are rational agents motivated by self-interest, 'only rational agents will be assigned direct rights'. The reasoning that leads to this conclusion is slightly different on the two approaches, so I will consider Carruthers's treatment of each in turn. First, Rawls's theory:

Since it is rational agents who are to choose the system of rules, and choose self-interestedly, it is only rational agents who will have their position protected under the rules. There seems no reason why rights should be assigned to non-rational agents. Animals will, therefore, have no moral standing under Rawlsian contractualism, in so far as they do not count as rational agents.   (Carruthers 1992: 98–9)

The story on Scanlon's approach is slightly different, since the contractors are there conceived as real people with differing preferences. In particular, some of them may care deeply about animals, and thus may be inclined to reject a proposed rule that gives little or no weight to the interests of animals. Carruthers objects to this suggestion on the grounds that such a rejection would not have a reasonable basis:

It cannot be reasonable, therefore, to reject a rule merely because it conflicts with some interest or concern of mine. For every rule (except the entirely trivial) will conflict with someone's concerns... If I can reasonably reject rules that accord no weight to the interests of animals, then others can equally reasonably reject rules that allow us to dress and make love as we wish, and to worship or not worship as we please.   (Carruthers 1992: 104)

What rules, then, can reasonably be rejected? Carruthers's answer is 'rules that accord no weight to my interests in general, or rules that allow my privacy to be invaded, or my projects to be interfered with, at the whim of other people . . . the basic principle that we should agree upon is one of respect for the autonomy of rational agents' (Carruthers 1992: 104–5). Of course, if one of my projects is to safeguard the interests of animals, a rule that allows others to disregard those interests *does* allow my project to be interfered with. It seems that respect for autonomy will have to incorporate a very strong moral asymmetry between what is done and what is allowed to happen. Lets assume, for the sake of argument, that such an asymmetry is justified. There are two serious objections that arise from within Carruthers's approach.

First, there is the problem of marginal cases again. For the same reasons that animals don't get assigned moral standing in the contractualist framework, non-rational humans don't seem to count either. Carruthers's response is to suggest two arguments that the contractors would use to justify rules that accord full moral standing to marginal humans. First, there is the following slippery slope argument:

There are no sharp boundaries between a baby and an adult, between a not-very-intelligent adult and a severe mental defective, or between a normal old person and someone who is severely senile. The argument is then that the attempt to accord direct moral rights only to rational agents would be inherently dangerous and open to abuse.   (Carruthers 1992: 114)

It is because starting out with a rule that distinguishes morally between rational and non-rational humans might lead to the mistreatment of rational humans that the rule has to include *all* humans. Excluding animals, on the other hand, wouldn't have the same dangerous consequences. Anyone who argued from the accepted denial of moral standing to chimpanzees to the conclusion that some humans shouldn't have moral standing either would not be taken seriously. Carruthers's second argument has a similar reliance on psychological claims. It is simply a fact about human beings, he says, that they care deeply for their offspring, 'irrespective of age and intelligence'. Given this fact, 'a rule withholding moral standing from those who are very young, very old, or mentally defective is thus likely to produce social instability, in that many people would find themselves psychologically incapable of living in compliance with it' (Carruthers 1992: 117).

There are two pertinent questions with respect to these psychological claims. First, are they true? Second, if they are true, do they provide the appropriate grounds for the claim that the interests of marginal humans have the same moral weight as those of other humans? The answer to both questions is no. We already distinguish between marginal humans and others in the allocation of some rights. The severely mentally defective don't get to vote, neither do they go to college. This selective treatment has led neither to the withholding of such benefits from ordinarily rational humans, nor to widespread social instability. It might be objected that these are examples of different *treatment* of marginal humans, not different consideration of their interests. Severely cognitively deficient humans don't vote or go to college, because it is not in their interests to do so. This distinction is morally significant, but it is only relevant to Carruthers's psychological claims to the extent that it figures in the ordinary thinking of most people, which is hardly at all.

Suppose, though, that Carruthers's psychological claims were true. They would provide a very shaky basis on which to attribute moral standing to marginal humans. To see this, imagine that a new kind of birth defect (perhaps associated with beef from cows treated with bovine growth hormone) produces severe mental retardation, green skin, and a complete lack of emotional bond between parents and child. Furthermore, suppose that the mental retardation is of the same kind and severity as that caused by other birth defects that don't have the other two effects. It seems likely that denying moral status to such defective humans would not run the same risks of abuse and destruction of social stability as would the denial of moral status to other, less easily distinguished and more loved defective humans. Would these contingent empirical differences between our reactions to different sources of mental retardation justify us in ascribing different direct moral status to their subjects? The only difference between them is skin color and whether they are loved by others. Any theory that could ascribe moral relevance to differences such as these doesn't deserve to be taken seriously.

Carruthers might reply that my own treatment of my example undermines its force. My argument demonstrates, he might say, why the denial of moral status to the green-skinned humans really would be subject to the slippery slope and social stability arguments. It is because philosophers such as I can show the moral irrelevance of the differences between the green-skinned humans and other marginal humans that we couldn't justify rules that distinguished between them. But this response is unavailable to Carruthers, of all people. For my demonstration of the moral irrelevance of the differences between green-skinned humans and other humans is no different from other demonstrations of the moral irrelevance of the differences between many animals and humans. If we can appeal to the supposed persuasive force of one argument we can appeal to a similar persuasive force for the other. Unfortunately, neither argument has the requisite psychological force.

Contractarianism fails, then, to give a convincing answer to the argument from marginal cases. It also fails to account for what Carruthers calls our common-sense attitudes towards animals. It seems to deny direct moral status to animals at all. The prevailing view may be that animals' interests are not as significant as those of humans, but it is not that they count for nothing. According to this view, the cat torturer may not be doing something as bad as the child torturer, but his behavior is nonetheless morally abominable. Furthermore, it is what is done to the cat itself that is morally objectionable. A contractarian approach might suggest rules against cruelty to animals, on the grounds of protecting the interests of animal owners and lovers. But this doesn't capture the central wrong of torturing a cat. It would still be wrong, even if it were a stray and no one else found out about it. Carruthers's response to this problem is similar to Kant's, who objected to cruelty to animals on the grounds that 'he who is cruel to animals becomes hard also in his dealings with men. We can judge the heart of a man by his treatment of animals.' Similarly, Carruthers claims that cruelty to animals (in venues other than factory farms and laboratories) is a sign of a defective character. Anyone who treats animals with wanton cruelty will also probably treat rational agents with disregard for their legitimate interests. Rational contractors, therefore, would have a good reason to agree to rules that discouraged the development of such characters.

This argument is subject to the same two objections as Carruthers's response to the argument from marginal cases. Even though there is fairly strong evidence of a correlation between cruelty to animals and antisocial behavior towards people, it is by no means obvious that *everyone* who is wantonly cruel to animals is a danger to people. But even such evidence as exists doesn't apply to factory farms or most laboratory experiments. Are we supposed to say that the interests of such animals don't count at all, because they are tortured in ways that don't warp their torturers' characters? Besides, the ordinary view that the cat torturer's behavior is morally abominable is in no way contingent on the belief that the torturer is also likely to mistreat people. If you were to discover that Mother Theresa routinely tortured cats for fun, you wouldn't think 'Well, what do you know! I guess torturing cats for fun isn't always wrong.' Neither would you think, 'Well, what do you know! I guess Mother Theresa was actually a danger to people. What luck that she died before she got around to torturing any.' You would probably be dismayed to learn that someone who had so much compassion for people could be so callous towards animals. The reason for your dismay, though, would be your belief that such callousness towards animals is wrong in itself.

The problem with the contractarian approach, at least as presented by Carruthers, is that the specification of the rules as those chosen by rational self-interested individuals begs the question against ascribing moral status to the non-rational. So long as the contractors are motivated by self-interest and are aware of their own rationality, the result is bound to favor rational beings over the merely sentient. Of course, we could modify the approach, at least Rawls's version, to eliminate this feature. If we simply specified that the veil of ignorance prevented the contractors from knowing whether they would, in the society whose rules they are choosing, be rational, the result wouldn't give a privileged status to rational beings. Carruthers considers this move, as suggested by Tom Regan. His reasons for rejecting it expose the fundamental defect in the whole contractarian approach:

The real line of reply to Regan is that his suggestion would destroy the theoretical coherence of Rawlsian contractualism. As Rawls has it, morality is, in fact, a human construction. Morality is viewed as constructed *by* human beings, in order to facilitate interactions *between* human beings, and to make possible a life of co-operative community. This is, indeed, an essential part of the governing conception of contractualism . . . [In my own contractualist account of the source of moral motivation] the basic contractualist concept . . . is held to be innate, selected for in evolution because of its value in promoting the survival of our species. (Carruthers 1992: 102–3)

For all I know, Carruthers's claim that the basic contractualist concept is selected for is true. If true, it might tell us something, though it's not clear how much, about the conditions of human flourishing. The *most* that such a claim could generate, though, would be a hypothetical imperative of the form 'in order to promote human flourishing, treat animals and humans in the following ways'. Even if the content of such an imperative included injunctions against making animals suffer, such injunctions would not have the status of basic moral rules. When we ponder the cat torturer's behavior, we may well be moved, and rightly so, by the inconsistency of such behavior with realizing the goal of human flourishing. We are right to regard such considerations as morally relevant. However, if we believe that such considerations exhaust the realm of moral relevance, if, in particular, we believe that the cat's suffering is of no *direct* moral relevance, we have a sadly impoverished view of morality. That the contractualist approach, and some versions of the natural rights approach, relegate the significance of animal suffering to the merely instrumental renders them unacceptable as *moral* theories, as opposed to theories of human flourishing.

In conclusion, to the extent that we view morality as not simply a human creation, a device whose sole purpose is to ensure cooperation among humans, and thereby promote human flourishing, we have powerful reasons to reject the view that the interests of animals are less significant than the like interests of humans. Such a rejection will render much animal experimentation morally unacceptable. This is not a conclusion that will be eagerly embraced by the scientific community. It is, however, the conclusion best supported by a careful examination of the relevant moral reasons.

References

Brody, B. (2003), 'Defending Animal Research: An International Perspective', in E. F. Paul and J. Paul (eds.), *Why Animal Experimentation Matters: The Use of Animals in Medical Research* (New Brunswick, NJ: Transaction Publishers and the Social Philosophy and Policy Foundation, 2001), 131–47; repr. in S. J. Armstrong and R. Botzler (eds.), *The Animal Ethics Reader* (London: Routledge), 262–71.

Carruthers, P. (1992), *The Animals Issue: Moral Theory in Practice* (Cambridge: Cambridge University Press).

Cohen, C. (1992), 'The Case for the Use of Animals in Biomedical Research', *New England Journal of Medicine*, 315 (1987), 865–70; repr. in T. A. Mappes and J. S. Zembaty (eds.), *Social Ethics*, 4th edn. (New York: McGraw-Hill), 458–67.

FREY, R. G. (1989), 'Rights, Interests, Desires, and Beliefs', *American Philosophical Quarterly*, 16 (1979), 233–9; repr. as 'Why Animals Lack Beliefs and Desires', in T. Regan and P. Singer (eds.), *Animal Rights and Human Obligations*, 2nd edn. (Englewood Cliffs, NJ: Prentice Hall), 39–42.

PARFIT, D. (1984), *Reasons and Persons* (Oxford: Oxford University Press).

RACHELS, J. (1999), *The Elements of Moral Philosophy*, 3rd edn. (New York: McGraw-Hill).

SCHMIDTZ, D. (1998), 'Are All Species Equal?', *Journal of Applied Philosophy*, 15/1: 57–67.

STEINBOCK, B. (1997), 'Speciesism and the Idea of Equality', *Philosophy*, 53/204 (1979), 247–56; repr. in J. E. White (ed.), *Contemporary Moral Problems*, 5th edn. (St Paul, Minn.: West), 464–70.

WARREN, M. A. (1997), 'Difficulties with the Strong Animal Rights Position', *Between the Species*, 2/4 (1987), 433–41; repr. in J. E. White (ed.), *Contemporary Moral Problems*, 5th edn. (St Paul, Minn.: West), 479–85.

WHITE, A. (1989), *Rights* (New York: Oxford University Press, 1986); repr. in T. Regan and P. Singer (eds.), *Animal Rights and Human Obligations*, 2nd edn. (Englewood Cliffs, NJ: Prentice Hall), 119–21.

PART VIII

PUBLIC AND GLOBAL HEALTH

CHAPTER 28

THE IMPLICATIONS OF PUBLIC HEALTH FOR BIOETHICS

JEFFREY KAHN AND
ANNA MASTROIANNI

THE seminal 1988 Institute of Medicine report *The Future of Public Health* defines public health as 'what we as a society do collectively to assure the conditions in which people can be healthy' (IOM 1988, 2002). The emphasis of public health is thus on societal action, rather than individual action, and public health interventions are usually implemented by governments instead of the private sector (Kass 2001). The scope of public health is vast, as commonly accepted definitions of health broadly encompass '[a] state of complete physical, mental and social well-being and not merely the absence of disease or infirmity' (WHO 1948). It can include anything from childhood immunization, ensuring safe water, epidemiologic research, disaster preparedness and relief, smoking restrictions, required use of seatbelts and motorcycle helmets, and reporting of individuals testing positive for sexually transmitted diseases. Since its origins as a discipline more than a century ago, public health's primary objective has been ensuring the advancement of health of populations and communities in contrast to emphasizing health of individuals (Kass 2001). It is this distinctive population perspective that has implications for how bioethics approaches issues in the public health context.

Public health practitioners and policymakers have always encountered and had to resolve ethical issues. The very nature of public health, with its focus on populations and communities, forces recurring and inherent tensions that must be balanced, between actions dominated by social justice and/or utilitarian considerations and the potential infringement of individual liberties. Within the vast enterprise of public health, decisions about issues involving ethics have been and continue to be made on a daily basis without explicit reference to ethical principles and concepts from the formal discipline of bioethics. Indeed, the relatively recent community-based participatory research movement, with its principles for active inclusion of communities in all or many phases of the research process (Israel *et al.* 1998; O'Fallon and Dearry 2002; Community Campus Partnerships for Public Health 2006), appears to have evolved from within the public health research community without reference to standard approaches to bioethics or its literature.

At the same time, bioethics has always taken on issues related to public health, mostly in identifying and trying to address the ethical issues raised by particular public health topics. Until relatively recently, however, a focus on what makes public health unique from an ethics perspective has received less attention in the scholarly literature. Recently Kass (2001) and others (Childress *et al.* 2002) have convincingly argued that public health ethics deserves its own place within bioethics: that public health is distinct in its history and application in comparison to the dominant individual rights orientation reflected in the more established bioethics approaches based in medicine and research. Indeed, the legal literature is ripe with cases involving public health and safety justifications for overriding individual rights, and the post-9/11 world has focused attention on the extent to which the state can and should invoke its police powers in the protection of public health. (See e.g. Gostin *et al.* 2002.) Because of the unique legal force behind public health, it is argued that a distinct ethics framework for addressing public health issues is needed even more to ensure that individual rights are not reflexively overridden (Kass 2001). Public health ethics as a formal disciplinary endeavor within bioethics is thus a relatively recent phenomenon, especially in comparison to the long history of public health. In the first section below, we examine the diverse efforts within bioethics to create formal frameworks for appropriate consideration of public health issues.

As indicated above, at its core, public health introduces tensions between individuals' autonomy and the need to account for perspectives and needs of communities and populations. It further raises social justice issues, including fair allocation of limited resources. In the sections that follow, we examine and elaborate on these tensions and their resolutions using specific public health examples. Experiences in the 1980s and 1990s with HIV/AIDS provide a particularly rich collection of issues that brought ethical issues in public health to the public's attention, and in so doing challenged previously held assumptions about the appropriate consideration of individual rights in the context of population health objectives.

Similarly, public debates in the 1990s and in early 2000 over resource allocation at the macro level of health care decision making forced public consideration of ethical issues, whether as an afterthought or as a formal component of the deliberative process. Lastly, we examine some of the ethical challenges arising in public health applications of recent science and technology advances, specifically the emerging area of public health genomics and the large scale collection and analysis of health information.

FRAMEWORKS FOR ETHICS AND PUBLIC HEALTH

Bioethics scholars are increasing their focus on the frameworks or approaches that might be applied specifically to ethical issues that arise in public health as compared to those in medicine or biomedical research. What they all have in common is the focus on community- and society-level values rather than the individual values found in much of the bioethics literature. Thinking about values for groups such as communities or even the entire society often may lead to different emphases in ethical analysis and to different conclusions about ethically appropriate actions.

As bioethics developed as a discipline in the 1970s, scholars tended to focus on what became known as biomedical ethics—the ethics of medical care and biomedical research. Within this discipline, less attention was paid to understanding ethical issues and their impact at the societal level—issues that are the domain of public health. With few exceptions (Bayer and Moreno 1986; D. E. Beauchamp 1975, 1976a, b, 1980, 1983, 1985, 1986) ethical examinations of particular health policy proposals or the delivery of public health services were not addressed as well-defined topics of study. This is because bioethics, with its origins in the clinical setting, has focused more heavily on ethical issues pertaining to the individual. In public health, of course, the primary ethical issues concern the tension that exists between the rights and interests of individuals and the good of the community or society—such as in policies and programs for mandatory disease testing or reporting.

The mid-1970s saw the explosion of the field of bioethics as a scholarly discipline, born mostly of ethical issues in medicine that required resolution: end of life issues prompted by landmark legal cases such as that of Karen Ann Quinlan, whose parents were granted the right to discontinue respirator support for their daughter who was ventilator-dependent and comatose; new definitions of death prompted by the developing techniques of organ transplantation; and issues in the protection of research subjects prompted by exposés of exploitive research studies. These issues and others like them created an environment in which much of the analysis of ethical issues was occurring in reaction to unethical behavior, e.g. the so-called Tuskegee

Syphilis Study (DHEW 1973). In addition, the general political climate was one of recent empowerment of individuals based on claims of individual rights—civil rights, consumer rights, and patients' rights (Bayer and Fairchild 2004). Therefore, much of the focus of bioethics during this period was on protecting the rights of individuals; whether it was to protect the individual from being taken advantage of (such as in research ethics), or to protect the individual from overzealous and technologically driven medical care (such as in the beginnings of the 'right to die' movement).

The result of this focus was the identification of what has come to be known as the 'principle-based' approach to bioethics; an analysis that relies on mid-level principles as directive in helping resolve ethical issues in medicine and medical research (Beauchamp and Childress 1979, 2001; National Commission for the Protection of Human Subjects of Biomedical and Behavioral Research 1979). The principle-based approach grew to be the reference for helping to think through issues in bioethics. Its four principles—respect for autonomy, beneficence (doing good for others), nonmaleficence (not doing harm to others), and justice—arguably operate best when the perspective of decision making is the individual patient or research subject (Beauchamp and Childress 1979 and later editions). While the architects of this approach might argue that it can do the work required in the context of ethical issues in public health, it was crafted to address issues in medicine and biomedical research and therefore did not fit as seamlessly as an approach crafted for public health. For example, much of the decision making in public health policy is driven by utilitarian considerations. Simply put, what policies will yield the greatest good for the greatest number of people? One strong criticism of such utilitarian approaches is that they fail to account sufficiently for harms to individuals and fairness in the distribution of the burdens and benefits of a policy decision. As this brief explanation demonstrates, there is a fundamental tension between utilitarian approaches that embody the collective values of public health and a principle-based approach that gives strong support for protecting individuals. This is not to suggest that there were not other approaches that tried to expand the reach of ethical frameworks beyond the individual, including communitarian approaches to ethics and policy issues, and work arguing for the importance of relationships to ethics, sometimes categorized 'ethics of care'. These approaches are discussed elsewhere in this volume.

Dan Beauchamp made this point early on in discussions of bioethics, suggesting that traditional frameworks that developed in bioethics would be inadequate for addressing issues in public health (Beauchamp 1975, 1976a, b, 1980, 1983, 1985, 1986, 1995). Beauchamp's work applied concepts from political philosophy to moral issues in public health. His framework considers public health as part of the scope of the government's efforts at 'prevention of disease and premature death through organized community effort' (Beauchamp 1995: 2161). The government's, and therefore the community's, role in public health involves the collection of health information about the population (using biostatistics and epidemiology) and acting upon that information to protect and improve the public health. So far as public health efforts enhance the good of individuals, traditional approaches to bioethics work well in helping address ethical issues. But, as Beauchamp pointed out, the philosophy of public health must address issues outside of the narrow individual interests in health, while acknowledging the claims of individual autonomy and providing justification for state limitation of individual liberty. Public health must approach these issues in ways that respect the community perspective and the common good, as it is understood in terms of the common well-being (Beauchamp 1995). Beauchamp believes that this approach translates into changing 'a social ethic that unfairly protects the most numerous or the most powerful from the burdens of prevention' (Beauchamp 1976a: 3)—primarily an issue of justice. Which models of justice to apply depends on the collective goals of society, or the common good.

Ronald Bayer sounded a similar chord in his work, dating back to the 1980s. The emphasis in his work is society's need to balance the rights of individuals against the need to violate those rights as part of the state's legitimate interests in protecting the public's health. He has written most forcefully about this tension in the health policy decisions that were and continue to be considered in public health's battle against AIDS (Bayer 1989, 1995). One important question that arises in Bayer's work both alone and with others is the extent to which the value of the community's health as a moral end in itself can justify public health policy (Moreno and Bayer 1985).

An alternative approach was taken by John Bryant, and further refined by Daniel Callahan. They emphasized the importance of focusing on equity of health status, or at least on the equitable distribution of the successes of medicine and, by association, public health (Bryant et al. 1997; Callahan 1997). Callahan criticized the emphasis and priorities of modern medicine as working against equity, pointing out that if equity is a value worth pursuing, it 'requires a moral commitment on the part of citizens and their political leaders, and it may require some sacrifice' (Callahan 1997: 125; 1985, 1994).

Through the 1990s, a number of authors began to craft an approach that relied on the language and concept of human rights rather than relying on the language of ethics, especially medical ethics (Gostin and Lazzarini 1997; Gostin and Mann 1994; Mann 1997; Mann et al. 1994; Annas 1988). Mann's effort was cut short by his untimely death, but nonetheless a framework was introduced for broadening ethical considerations in public health to encompass concerns over societal and global determinants of health rather than more limited and medicalized considerations of prevention of death and disability.

Weijer and Emanuel, along with Goldsand, have proposed that communities deserve attention separate from and in addition to individuals participating in biomedical research such that a new principle ought to be recognized: the principle of respect for communities (Weijer et al. 1999; Weijer and Emanuel 2000; Emanuel and Weijer 2005). While their proposal has met with limited acceptance, it was an attempt to move discussion of protectionist research policies to be more explicit in its consideration of group harms and benefits rather than relying on implicit consideration of community issues within the principle of justice.

Not surprisingly, more than twenty years after Dan Beauchamp wrote about the challenges to social justice that ought to be the purview of the ethics of public health, others came to similar conclusions though by quite different routes. Building on these examples of early work in ethics and public health are two recent examples of authors or groups of authors focusing on frameworks for addressing the ethics of public health. Kass (2001) proposes a specific framework for the ethical analysis of public health programs through six analytic questions: (1) what are the public health goals of the program? (2) how effective is the program in achieving its goals? (3) what are its burdens? (4) are there alternatives? (5) is the program implemented fairly? and (6) can burdens and benefits be fairly balanced? Childress *et al.* (2002) identify what they call general moral considerations in the ethics of public health efforts, echoing Kass's emphasis on justice considerations but further highlighting the tension between respect for individual rights and the collective good. This analytic framework includes

producing benefits; avoiding, preventing, and removing harms; producing the maximal balance of benefits over harms and other costs; distributing benefits and burdens fairly and ensuring public participation ... respecting autonomous choices and actions ... protecting privacy and confidentiality; keeping promises ... disclosing information as well as speaking honestly and truthfully; and building and maintaining trust. (Childress *et al.* 2002: 171–2)

When conflicts occur among these considerations, as they inevitably will, the authors proposed resolving conflicts based on which choice would meet the most of five 'justificatory conditions'—in language parallel to Kass: effectiveness of the approach, proportion of benefits over burdens, necessity, least infringement, and public justification.

What are the common threads running through all these approaches? While there are a few, first among them is an emphasis on fairness and equity evident in the principle of justice–from Dan Beauchamp's call for attention to social justice, to Bayer's call for fairness in HIV/AIDS policies, Callahan and Bryant's calls for justice as equity, Mann and Gostin's focus on global justice, Weijer and Emanuel's notion of respect for communities as group justice, and the recent approaches of Kass and Childress *et al.* that have justice as fairness as their centerpieces. The tensions between justice and utilitarian analyses is a thread that is seen in discussions of many of the ethical issues in public health, as we will see below. The various approaches to ethics and public health that have existed and are emerging are attempts to address in a formal way the central and delicate balancing of the rights and interests of the individual with that of community and society. It is not surprising that attempts to articulate frameworks for ethical analysis are increasing. One reason may be that the development of bioethics as a field of study has intersected with increasing attention paid to public health issues in the 1990s; and with such attention has come increasing appreciation for approaches that can accommodate a more nuanced ethical analysis of public health issues. We would go so far as to say that bioethics is in the process of evolving to engage public health questions. This is evident in a number of issues that have recently been debated in the intersection of clinical and public health realms, notably the AIDS epidemic, and more recent concerns over a possible flu pandemic, and preparation for bioterror attacks.

In many cases the foregoing approaches to ethical issues in public health seem to have arisen in isolation, as their introduction, with limited exceptions, frequently offers little explicit reference to other frameworks. There are a number of possible reasons for this that we can offer. First, examining ethical issues in public health is one type of applied ethics—ethics applied to public health issues, just as ethics can be applied to biomedicine and biomedical research, business, the environmental issues, and so on. This creates a diversity of approaches, which is also evident within the scholarship of bioethics. Second, since bioethics is multidisciplinary in origin, drawing on law, medicine, philosophy, and other disciplines, it is not surprising that different approaches have emerged even in addressing common issues. In addition, at the core of these different approaches, however, are sometimes different definitions and understandings of public health—a disagreement that is not unique to bioethics scholars' attempts to address issues in public health.

TOPICS IN ETHICS AND PUBLIC HEALTH

While there are numerous topics in public health that could be discussed for the ethical issues they raise, we have selected only a few as examples. While far from an exhaustive list, these examples may be considered to be representative for the kinds of ethical issues that arise in public health and they work well for explicating how the framework approaches might apply to them.

HIV and AIDS

The HIV/AIDS epidemic served to focus public health professionals, policy makers as well as academics, on the issues of ethics and public health. In many respects, the epidemic and the many issues that it spawned serve as a microcosm of the ethical issues faced in public health, and so it is not surprising that some of the thoughts about frameworks emerged out of thinking about responses to the AIDS crisis (Gostin and Lazzarini 1997; Kass and Gielen 1998).

The HIV/AIDS epidemic is among the defining public health issues of the twentieth century, was unprecedented for its combination of ethics and public health issues, and focused bioethics on public health concerns in ways that had not been experienced during the short history of the field of bioethics. Ethical issues in HIV and AIDS continue to confront public health decision makers, as they have since the beginning of the AIDS crisis. At the same time, advances in HIV and AIDS treatment and research have raised new challenges and ethical issues. As we discuss below, as the illness has changed from acute to chronic, focus has shifted from reporting of HIV status and contact tracing, to issues in international research on HIV, and equitable access to pharmaceuticals—all of which raise inherent tensions among individual rights, justice, and utilitarian considerations.

Reporting and Contact Tracing

Certain types of public health information have long been perceived as posing threats of discrimination and stigmatization to individuals and groups—most notably HIV status and some kinds of genetic information. Remarkable improvements in therapy for HIV infection over a relatively few years sparked efforts to encourage infected individuals to seek treatment as early as possible. From early on in the AIDS epidemic, diagnosis with the disease was reportable to all state health departments. Such AIDS case reporting was based on information needed by public health officials to better understand the course of the epidemic, but at the cost of privacy of individuals and their ability to control highly stigmatizing information about themselves (Bayer 1995).

Justifying mandatory reporting of infection relies on an assessment that protecting the public's health from a communicable disease is important enough to require disclosure to the government of private and very personal information about individuals. In the context of the frameworks' principles, policies requiring disclosure must achieve their goals of protecting the public's health and serving infected individuals in the least intrusive ways, while fairly balancing the benefits and burdens of such approaches. Very important to any successful policy requiring disclosure of sensitive information to the government is the ability to protect the privacy of individuals. Early in the experience with mandatory reporting, in order to protect privacy anonymous HIV testing programs were set up in many states and localities to encourage testing and the knowledge it can provide, without fear of the information being disclosed. But this approach meant little could be learned about the characteristics of those who were infected if identifying information was not collected, and no medical follow-up could be provided to individuals or the contacts of those who tested positive. So in these cases, the value of protecting privacy trumped other public health values such as follow-up with infected and exposed individuals, and good information about the epidemiology of the disease.

The justification was that the public health is better served by programs that encourage greater numbers of individuals to seek testing since their privacy is absolutely protected, even at the dual costs of less information about the epidemic and the inability to track the health or behavior of infected individuals (Bayer 1995).

The presumption toward anonymous testing has changed, with most states requiring reporting not only AIDS cases but also positive HIV tests. The motivation for the change in attitudes was largely the availability of better therapies for HIV infection. Bayer further elucidated three arguments for the move toward HIV reporting: (1) the 'foundation for distinguishing between HIV and AIDS early in the epidemic no longer exist[s]', with early clinical intervention prior to disease symptoms focusing attention from AIDS to HIV disease; (2) 'claims that public health officials need to know who has HIV infection in order to assure adequate clinical follow-up'; and (3) 'only with HIV reporting would it be possible to develop aggressive partner notification programs designed to reach individuals exposed to those with HIV infection' (Bayer 1995: 108–13). The balance tipped toward mandatory reporting when there were better reasons to encourage treatment for those who test positive, as one part of population treatment strategies.

Issues in International Research

Much recent effort to address treatment of HIV infection has focused on the developing world, since much of the successful research in the developed world has led to first-line therapies that require long, expensive, and complex drug therapies that work best in a health care system that offers comprehensive care and has fewer resource constraints. This combination of factors makes these approaches unworkable in many parts of the world, and so research has focused on shorter and less costly approaches (Glantz et al. 1998).

The protocols used in the developing world have not compared new therapies to the accepted treatment regimen, but rather to placebo controls, which has engendered ethical debate among researchers, governments, and the public. The debate revolves around a number of issues, including whether it is ethical to perform such research in the developing world if it would not be permissible in the United States in light of the accepted standard of treatment; whether the resulting benefits of the research would be available to women in developing countries or would only be used to change treatment approaches in the United States; and whether adequate informed consent of subjects could be obtained in settings where little if any health care would otherwise be available (Crouch and Arras 1998; Kahn and Mastroianni 1999; de The et al. 2003; Participants in the 2001 Conference on Ethical Aspects of Research in Developing Countries 2004; Arras 2004; Wendler et al. 2004; Pace and Emanuel 2005; Yearby 2004).

A widely discussed example that prompted attention to this issue are trials of short course AZT therapy for prevention of vertical transmission of HIV from mother to fetus during pregnancy, and which involved US researchers. Some of these trials, performed in Africa, Asia, and Latin America, involved testing the short course regimen against a placebo control arm. This study design was approved even though it had been shown that a regimen involving AZT during pregnancy and labor, and administered to newborns—known as the 076 regimen—reduced the incidence of HIV infection of infants by two-thirds (Sperling *et al.* 1996). One of the reasons the short course trials were approved by US institutions to go forward was that in the countries in which the research was carried out pregnant women infected with HIV would have been unlikely to receive even basic prenatal care, let alone treatment to prevent vertical transmission of HIV. Thus it was argued that use of placebo control was ethically acceptable since assignment to the placebo group would 'not carry a risk beyond that associated with standard practice' (Varmus and Satcher 1997), along with utilitarian arguments about providing important information for a large group of infected women and their future children. The tension arose over claims that research must provide existing 'standard of care' as the control arm of the studies, but whose standard of care? In the United States, standard of care is very different than in many other parts of the world, where no treatment (i.e. placebo) is the norm. It was known before the initiation of the overseas trials that the 076 regimen was effective, and it became standard of care in the United States and other developed countries. But the 076 regimen was so expensive as to be out of reach for use on a widespread basis for nearly every developing country, as well as for some people in the United States. And while placebo controls in a vertical transmission trial could not be justified in the United States, the realities of health care resources are different in the United States than they are in Kenya or Thailand. Numerous authors have argued that to examine a new clinical approach compared to 076 for application in the developing world is to ask the wrong research question (Msamanga and Fawzi 1997; Varmus and Satcher 1997). They contend that it may be better to compare the available treatment (which may sometimes be much more limited or even no treatment at all) against a new and potentially affordable treatment, and that research designs ought to be developed in concert with health ministries of the countries in which they are planned to be carried out (as was the case in the 076 trials) (Abdool 1998; Varmus and Satcher 1997).

Peter Lurie and Sidney Wolfe (1997), along with Marcia Angell (2000) objected to this perspective, and argued that to claim that acceptable standards of care are shaped only by local conditions is to confuse optimal medical care with the quality of the local health care infrastructure. To employ the standard of care in local settings creates incentives to find research subjects with the least access to health care, instead of encouraging research that will best serve those in need.

Different study designs may achieve some middle ground between these positions. Rather than relying on the 'gold standard' of placebo controlled trials, studies in Thailand used active agent controls so that all participants had the chance to receive some therapeutic benefits while in the research, and the research still yielded some information about whether the novel approach was efficacious.

Independent of research design issues, there remain important questions about the dissemination of the benefits of the research, since even less expensive treatment regimens than the standard of care in the West will still be out of reach for the populations of many developing countries (Crouch and Arras 1998; Kahn and Mastroianni 1999; de The *et al.* 2003; Participants in the 2001 Conference on Ethical Aspects of Research in Developing Countries 2004; Arras 2004; Wendler *et al.* 2004; Pace and Emanuel 2005; Yearby 2004). This further fuels the debate over social justice, utilitarian justifications, and the potential for exploitation of subjects in foreign countries, since the results of the research may well be used to implement cheaper therapies for patients in wealthier countries.

This controversy is an example of how ethical issues are now being raised in a world where research is carried out on a global level, but where socioeconomic and political disparities persist. One chapter of this debate ended with the results of a vertical transmission study in Africa (HIVNET012) showing that administration of Nevirapine to an HIV-infected woman in labor, followed by a dose to her infant, reduces the risk of HIV transmission by nearly 50 per cent (Guay *et al.* 1999). The most important aspect of this result is that the newer regimen cost only a few cents, which made it far more likely to be made available throughout the world.

Access to Pharmaceuticals

The many breakthroughs in research on prevention and treatment of HIV infection have brought with them significant issues of justice and access. The issue of access is especially important and acute since the majority of HIV-infected individuals live in the developing world, where drug regimens costing thousands of dollars a year are beyond the means of the local health care system. In addition to cheaper approaches, some organizations and governments in the developed world has sought more equitable access to first-line therapies by negotiating reduced rates for drugs or the right to produce generic versions at much lower cost. One prominent example is former President Bill Clinton's Clinton HIV/AIDS Initiative, which negotiates pricing agreements for both diagnostic tests and drugs to provide increased access to those at risk of HIV infection living in the developing world (Clinton Foundation 2006). These negotiated arrangements with pharmaceutical companies to reduce prices are intended to improve access to lifesaving therapies to a much larger proportion of the population of infected individuals. The arguments have been largely about the ethics of access—based on concepts of social justice as well as the clearly utilitarian argument that access to drugs is more important than profits for pharmaceutical companies (Razum and Okoye 2001; Gostin 2003). For some, these arguments even justify ignoring recognized intellectual property claims such as patents (Shalev 2004; Yamey 2001; Gostin 2003).

Resource Allocation, Access, and Justice Considerations: Health Care Reform in the 1990s

Resource allocation is an ethical issue whenever there are insufficient resources to meet demand, whether for reasons of natural scarcity (such as in the case of solid organs) or created constraints (cost containment in closed systems). There are resource allocation issues throughout the delivery of health care, of course, at the level of paying for patient care, managing the health of populations, and for health care at the macro level. In addition, there are issues surrounding how to allocate specific kinds of resources, such as organs for transplant. This discussion will focus on health care reform and cost containment throughout the 1990s as a historical example of how public health issues have influenced bioethics.

When Faden and Kass (1991) surveyed the landscape of bioethics literature in the 1980s on resource allocation, they found an emphasis in two areas: (1) justice issues, framed as access to health care, including whether and to what extent moral rights or entitlements to health care services existed, and (2) utilitarian considerations, framed as rationing through cost containment. The health care reform efforts in the 1990s and related ethical debates are exemplified by the failure of President Clinton's health care reform proposal.

Debates about the advantages of a single payer system and managed care dominated discussions about health care in the United States during the early part of the 1990s. President Clinton put forth a proposal for comprehensive reform of the US health care system in September 1993 whose centerpiece was referred to as managed competition. The primary objectives of Clinton's Health Security Act were twofold: the provision of health services to all Americans and control of health care costs. There were at least four key initiatives designed to meet these objectives. First, a guarantee of a comprehensive package of benefits to all. Second, a requirement that all employers provide health insurance for their employees (employer mandate) with the opportunity for some premium cost sharing between the employer and employee. Third, government intervention and oversight through the creation of a National Health Board and regional health alliances. These bodies would, among other things, develop the uniform benefits package, contract with health plans, set premiums targets, payment schedules, and budgets (global budgeting), and provide information to consumers about their health insurance options. And fourth, coverage of costs through new taxes and on savings from reform (Cordone 1996–7).

The failure of Clinton's health care reform initiative is well documented (Dougherty 1996; Johnson and Broder 1996; Morone and Belkin 1994; Skocpol 1997). Each of the components was controversial on many levels and supported or opposed by the numerous players involved in the health care system. In addition, the proposal lost public support as people began to feel threatened that their own health care was at risk, prompted in part by a series of advertisements produced by an advocacy group representing health insurers, the Health Insurance Association of America.

The White House Task Force on Health Care included a thirty-one-member ethics working group, known as Working Group 17. Nonetheless, an articulation of ethics concerns was not a central aspect of the Clinton proposal. Indeed, the ethics working group was appointed after all other working groups had already begun their work, and began meeting in March 1993, just six months before the Clinton administration issued their reform proposal.

Among the products delivered to the Task Force was a statement of proposed ethical values and principles of the new health care system. The ethics working group identified fourteen principles, divided into three main sections: (1) *caring for all*, which included universal sharing of risk, financing based on ability to pay, and generations standing together; (2) *making the system work*, which included allocating wisely, treating effectively, ensuring quality, and managing efficiently; and (3) *choice and responsibility*, which included individual choice, personal responsibility, professional integrity, and fair procedures (Secundy 1994).

Daniels (1994) questioned the working group's failure to connect their principles to broader notions or concepts of justice, equality, and community. Instead, the group chose to focus on shared principles that did not require consensus at the level of theory, given their own diversity of opinion and an acknowledgement that similar diversity exists among the American public. In the end, they took their task to be an effort to articulate a working basis for thinking about fairness in the context of health care reform (Daniels 1994).

Both during the time of the Task Force's efforts and now in retrospect, some have speculated as to how much the inclusion of an ethics working group was for the purpose of substantive ethics consideration, and how much was to lend credibility to the process with the 'seal of approval' offered by ethics professionals (Englehardt 1994). While it would be wrong to suggest that their thinking was not reflected in the final product, it is unclear what sort of impact, if any, the working group's conclusions had on the Task Force deliberations, its subsequent report, and the President's ultimate proposal. Finally, the experience of Working Group 17 is instructive in a number of ways: (1) the recognition that health care policy carries ethical implications; and (2) that the role of bioethics in health care policy making has limits, in that it can help describe the contours of the ethics landscape in health care but not provide quick answers to issues (O'Connell 1994). Resolving difficult health policy issues requires contributions from a range of key constituents and areas of expertise, bioethics among them.

The failure of Clinton's health care reform plan stimulated greater attention to the development of incremental approaches to health care reform. Discussions about the value of a single payer system continue to rumble below the surface (DeGrazia 1996; Woolhandler *et al.* 2003). Whatever changes emerge from ongoing and future incremental reform (Medicare Part D, physician pay-for-performance, consumer-driven health care) will bring a host of new ethical issues as the United States struggles to incorporate financial considerations and population-based thinking into the provision of individual health care in the quest for high quality, universal health care coverage coupled with cost containment.

Public Health Genomics

A revolution in new genetic technologies and an explosion of knowledge about genetics emerged in the 1990s and early 2000s. This included the massive under-taking and completion of the Human Genome Project (HGP) to chart the entire genome (NIH–NHGRI 2003; Pennisi 2003) and the initiation by an international consortium of the International HapMap Project designed to map genetic variation within the human genome (NIH–NHGRI 2002; Couzin 2002, 2005). With these advances and technological innovations that speed genomic analysis has come a corresponding interest in understanding how genomics can contribute to improving the public's health through disease prevention and health promotion (Austin *et al.* 2000; Holtzman 1997; Holtzman and Andrews 1997; Khoury 1996, 1997, 2003; Omenn 1996; Schull and Hanis 1990; IOM 2005).

Public health genomics has been described as an 'emerging field [that] assesses the impact of genes and their interaction with behavior, diet, and the environment on the population's health' (IOM 2005: 63). The field covers all the public health sciences, and the scope of activities encompassed within it is vast; e.g. population initiatives in genetic screening and testing, all aspects of research and derivative applications involving genetic epidemiology, pharmacogenetics, ecogenetics, banking and use of tissue samples, and many others. Each of these areas has to contend with traditional ethical tensions that arise in public health policy and practice discussed earlier. In addition, an ongoing debate has emerged in practice and policy as to whether the inherent nature of genetic information requires that it be treated differently and with a heightened level of scrutiny and protection in comparison to other health-related information (Rothstein 2005; Ross 2001; Lemmons and Austin 2001; Murray 1997; Annas *et al.* 1995).

Population-based genomic applications, like research and more individual-ized therapeutic applications, raise ethical issues of privacy and confidentiality, psychosocial risks, discrimination, and stigma (see e.g. Wolf 1995; Stone and Stewart 1996; Annas and Elias 1992; Macklin 1985; Kodish 1997; Holtzman and Watson 1998; Holtzman and Andrews 1997; Gostin 1995; Chadwick 1998; Caulfield 1995; Murphy and Lappe 1994; Campbell and Boyd 1996; APHA 1988; Annas 1995). The potentially high cost of new technologies has also raised classic public health issues of appropriate resource allocation, access by poor and underserved populations to scientific and clinical advancements, and related issues of social justice (see e.g. Buchanan *et al.* 2000; King 1992; Caplan 1994).

Much has been written about the importance of addressing genetic privacy concerns and their attendant psychosocial risks to individuals and families (see e.g. Annas 1995; Gostin 1995; Holtzman 1997; Macklin 1985, 1992; Rothstein 1997; Billings 2005; Beskow *et al.* 2004). Genetic information by its nature may reveal the most basic and private information about inherited disease and susceptibilities about individuals and their families. In the public health context, the collection and use of genetic information in epidemiological efforts to assess disease incidence and prevalence, for example, is critical to our understanding of disease. At the same time, it raises the possibility that such personal information may be linked not only to individuals and families, but to groups or distinct populations, in ways that might embarrass or stigmatize them or even lead to potential employment or insurance discrimination.

Questions are being raised about how best to balance the potential health benefits of genetic information with the attendant privacy risks. For example, removing identifiers from data adds to the protection of individual privacy and confidentiality, but at the cost of losing useful public health information such as the ability to provide health services and follow cases. An alternative is to seek the informed consent of individuals for the collection and use of information about them, an approach that has run into unique challenges such as the unforeseen use of previously collected data and DNA samples (ASHG 1996; Clayton *et al.* 1995; McEwen and Reilly 1994; Sankar 1997).

The transition from individual applications of genetic testing to population-based prevention programs involving genetic screening has raised additional ethical and practical considerations. Early challenges and experiences with government sponsored genetic screening programs date back to the 1960s and included problems with test accuracy, false positives, and misinterpretations and misuses of test results (see e.g. Markel 1997). Despite these problems, ultimately the public health benefits of early interventions offered by newborn screening programs in the United States were determined to outweigh some of the more traditional autonomy-based concerns arising in informed consent; the vast majority of state programs rely on an opt-out approach to parental consent (GAO 2003). Today tandem mass spectrometry technology allows rapid processing of genetic samples and therefore an ability to include greater numbers of genetic tests in screening panels, such as those used in newborn screening. Rather than rely on the market availability of genetic tests to determine the content of screening panels, many have concluded that decisions to include new tests require cautious consideration and oversight with specific attention to ethical, social, and clinical issues (NIH–DOE 1997; NIH–SACGT 2000; Burris and Gostin 1997; Cunningham 1997). Many of the considerations described in the frameworks developed by Childress *et al.* (2002) and Kass (2001), discussed earlier, are echoed in the discussions and criteria developed for adoption and expansion of genetic screening programs, e.g. the probability of population health enhancement, efficient and just uses of resources, resource availability, and public engagement (Burris and Gostin 1997; Chadwick 1998; Cogswell *et al.* 1999; Coughlin *et al.* 1999; Coughlin and Miller 1999; Cunningham 1997). Current issues in the area of newborn screening panels more specifically include the need for 'evidence-based criteria to determine the disorders included in the newborn screening panel, the informed consent process and parent/provider education and assurance of systems of follow up for medical care after screening' (Khoury 2003: 263).

Many ethical issues posed by genetics were highlighted in conjunction with the development of genetic technologies. In fact, a percentage of funding for the HGP (through the U.S. National Institutes of Health and Department of Energy) was earmarked at its initiation for study of its ethical, legal, and social implications (ELSI). The ELSI program has had a profound effect on the bioethics community's research focus, with substantial resources devoted to research on ethics and genetics issues at both the individual and public health levels. Specifically in public health, the US Centers for Disease Control and Prevention (CDC) established the Office of Genomics and Disease Prevention. The CDC has drawn special attention to some of the ethical, legal, and social implications of public health genomics, such as informed consent issues arising in population-based research (Beskow *et al.* 2001). US regions and states have developed genetic service programs (e.g. state departments of health, the Council of Regional Networks for Genetic Services). In addition, US schools of public health, such as those at the universities of Washington, Michigan, and Pittsburgh, now have curricula designed to train future public health researchers and professionals in genetics, and each program includes attention to ethical considerations (Austin *et al.* 2000). This increased interest and attention has provided opportunities for collaboration, discussion, and understanding of the intersection of public health and genomics and its relevant ethical, legal, and social considerations.

Despite the potential benefits accruing from the emerging discipline of public health genomics, public health has had to overcome a history of distrust in this area. Some are wary of public health involvement in genetics, as the eugenics programs of the early twentieth century were motivated and justified by public health goals and principles (Pernick 1997; Proctor 1992; Paul 1994). Other contributing factors leading to the potential for suspicion of public health genetics include the negative and stigmatizing experiences of African Americans with public health screening for sickle cell disease, concerns about our understanding of the public health goal of 'prevention' in the age of prenatal screening and abortion, and stories of genetic engineering (Dula 1991, 1994; Gamble 1993; King 1992). This potential for distrust underscores the need to ensure that genetic information is used by public health authorities in a way that is ethically appropriate. Certainly, a challenge to public health in the future will be how to achieve the public health goals of identification and prevention of genetic diseases in populations while preventing the ethically unacceptable aspects of eugenics, the misuse of genetic information, and the unjust distribution of genetic resources.

Privacy and the Collection of Health Information

While collection of genetic information about populations is a growing concern for the future, collection of other health information about populations is ongoing and increasingly efficient as both states and health care payers use information about groups to guide a variety of health policies. Powerful epidemiological and statistical methods and their applications have been developed to yield important population data of increasingly better quality. The information has tremendous application in service of the public's health, but its collection and use also raise ethical concerns and responsibilities. Access to information about populations is basic to epidemiological research, and larger and more detailed databases promise more and better information about the public's health.

The collection of health-related information about individuals for public health purposes isn't new—many states have registries for vaccinations, birth defects, and cancer cases, and all states collect and test blood samples from live births on Guthrie cards—and this information is often accessible to researchers with a legitimate interest in it (APHA 1996; Coughlin and Beauchamp 1996; McEwen and Reilly 1994). The public health community has rightly argued that the protection of personal information is not absolute, and should be balanced with the societal benefits to be gained by research access to personal data (APHA 1996; Bankowski *et al.* 1991; Chapman 1997; Coughlin and Beauchamp 1996; Gostin 1991; Gostin *et al.* 1996; Schindler 1994; Soskolne 1995).

But the classic tension between public benefit and individual privacy is growing in light of improved access to health information through technological innovations and computerization. The public's fear about potential disclosure of health information reflects concerns about control of personal information and the potential for embarrassment, discrimination, and stigma (Gostin *et al.* 2001). Public concern over the protection of individual privacy has led to heated debate over health data collection efforts and to the restriction of the use of existing medical data (APHA 1996; Bankowski *et al.* 1991; Chapman 1997; Gold 1996; Gostin 1991; Gostin *et al.* 1996; National Research Council 1997; Soskolne 1995; Varmus and Satcher 1997). The reorganization of health care into a system where the majority of people are in some kind of managed care has created the ability to track outcomes for large populations. This creates the opportunity for beneficial epidemiological and outcomes research that may be unprecedented, but at the same time raises ethical concerns. State health departments and health care systems are working together to share information and create even larger and more powerful data sets, but adequate privacy protections may not exist in either setting (Chapman 1997; Coughlin and Beauchamp 1996; Gostin *et al.* 1996; Schindler 1994; Harman 2006).

As privacy concerns and increasing access to better information lead to conflict in population-based research, the tension underscores an important point. The public health and bioethics communities have an opportunity to participate in the debate over privacy and access to health information, and to inform the debate about how to balance the importance and value of data collection and research on groups (important community and utilitarian values) with the important value of individual privacy. Education of the public is crucial and necessary, so as not to undermine the already fragile trust in the government's access to and use of private information about us. Recognition of these issues is leading to new policy initiatives, including restrictions on the use of health information and assurances to individuals of the use, privacy, and security of personal health information (Gostin *et al.* 2001; Harman 2006).

CONCLUSION

We hope to have shown that bioethics and public health is a growing area of scholarship, and an area whose impact will be seen as debate continues about the many public health issues that have ethical dimensions. These efforts will become increasingly relevant as ethics training becomes integrated into the education of public health professionals pursuant to recent Institute of Medicine recommendations identifying ethics as a core component of public health professional education (IOM 2003: 2). Bioethics education, scholarship, and research have all been affected by public health and the growing attention it demands. Bioethics' traditional focus on issues of medicine and biomedical research have understandably led to an emphasis on the importance of respecting individuals and their rights. But this emphasis is challenged by the pressing group interests and population issues faced in public health, with its very real ethical challenges. Bioethics must help address the very real tensions in public health between individual rights and the importance of protecting populations and their interests. Strongly held principles can and do conflict—autonomy versus utility versus justice, and so on. The ethical challenges posed by public health are only likely to increase, as public health programs receive increasing attention in the post-9/11 world. 'Pandemic response programs', 'bioterrorism preparedness', and the like are terms that would have been uttered only as science fiction a few short years ago, but are now with us to stay. Public health issues have assumed a new role in our lives, and bioethics has a role to play in informing how that role takes shape.

REFERENCES

ABDOOL KARIM, S. S. (1998), 'Placebo Controls in HIV Perinatal Transmission Trials: A South African's Viewpoint', *American Journal of Public Health*, 88: 564–6.

ANGELL, M. (2000), 'Investigators' Responsibilities for Human Subjects in Developing Countries', *New England Journal of Medicine*, 342: 967–9.

ANNAS, G. J. (1988), 'Human Rights and Health: The Universal Declaration of Human Rights at 50', *New England Journal of Medicine*, 339: 1777–81.

—— (1995), 'Genetic Prophecy and Genetic Privacy: Can We Prevent the Dream from Becoming a Nightmare?', *American Journal of Public Health*, 85: 1196–7.

—— and ELIAS, S. (1992) (eds.), *Gene Mapping: Using Law and Ethics as Guides* (New York: Oxford University Press).

—— GLANTZ, L., and ROCHE, P. (1995), 'Drafting the Genetic Privacy Act: Science, Policy and Practical Considerations', *Journal of Law, Medicine and Ethics*, 23: 360–5.

APHA (AMERICAN PUBLIC HEALTH ASSOCIATION) (1988), 'Genetics and Public Health', *American Journal of Public Health*, 78: 209–11.

—— (1996), 'Protecting Confidential Data in Disease Registries', *American Journal of Public Health*, 86: 443–4.

ARRAS, J. D. (2004), 'Fair Benefits in International Medical Research', *Hastings Center Report*, 34/3: 3.

ASHG (AMERICAN SOCIETY OF HUMAN GENETICS) (1996), 'ASHG Report: Statement on Informed Consent for Genetic Research', *American Journal of Human Genetics*, 59: 471.

AUSTIN, M. A., PEYSER, P. A., and KHOURY, M. (2000), 'The Interface of Genetics and Public Health: Research and Educational Challenges', *Annual Review of Public Health*, 21: 81–99.

BANKOWSKI, Z., BRYANT, J. H., and LAST, J. M. (1991) (eds.), *Ethics and Epidemiology: International Guidelines* (Geneva: CIOMS).

BAYER, R. (1989), *Private Acts, Social Consequences: AIDS and the Politics of Public Health* (New Brunswick, NJ: Rutgers University Press).

—— (1995), 'AIDS: Public Health Issues', in W. Reich (ed.), *Encyclopedia of Bioethics*, i (New York: Macmillan), 108–13.

—— and FAIRCHILD, A. L. (2004), 'The Genesis of Public Health Ethics', *Bioethics*, 18: 473–92.

—— and MORENO, J. D. (1986), 'Health Promotion: Ethical and Social Dilemmas of Government Policy', *Health Affairs*, 5/2: 72–85.

BEAUCHAMP, D. E. (1975), 'Public Health: Alien Ethic in a Strange Land?', *American Journal of Public Health*, 65: 1338–9.

—— (1976a), 'Public Health as Social Justice', *Inquiry*, 13/1: 3–14.

—— (1976b), 'Exploring New Ethics for Public Health: Developing a Fair Alcohol Policy', *Journal of Health Politics, Policy and Law*, 1: 338–54.

—— (1980), 'Public Health and Individual Liberty', *Annual Review of Public Health*, 1: 121–36.

—— (1983), 'What Is Public About Public Health?', *Health Affairs*, 2/4: 76–87.

—— (1985), 'Community: The Neglected Tradition of Public Health', *Hastings Center Report*, 15/6: 28–36.

—— (1986), 'Morality and the Health of the Body Politic', *Hastings Center Report*, 16/6, suppl., 30–6.

—— (1995), 'Philosophy of Public Health', in W. Reich (ed.), *Encyclopedia of Bioethics*, iv (New York: Macmillan), 2161–6.

BEAUCHAMP, T. L., and CHILDRESS, J. C. (1979), *Principles of Biomedical Ethics*, 1st edn. (New York: Oxford University Press).

BEAUCHAMP, T. L., and CHILDRESS, J. C. (2001), *Principles of Biomedical Ethics*, 5th edn. (New York: Oxford University Press).

BESKOW, L. M., *et al.* (2001), 'Informed Consent for Population-Based Research Involving Genetics', *JAMA* 286: 2315–21.

_____ *et al.* (2004), 'Ethical Issues in Identifying and Recruiting Participants for Familial Genetic Research', *American Journal of Medical Genetics*, 130A: 424–31.

BILLINGS, P. (2005), 'Genetic Nondiscrimination', *Nature Genetics*, 37: 559–60.

BRYANT, J. H., KHAN, K. S., and HYDER, A. A. (1997), 'Ethics, Equity and Renewal of WHO's Health-for-All Strategy', *World Health Forum*, 18: 107–15.

BUCHANAN, A., BROCK, D., DANIELS, N., and WIKLER, D. (2000), *From Chance to Choice: Genetics and Justice* (Cambridge: Cambridge University Press).

BURRIS, S., and GOSTIN, L. O. (1997), 'Genetic Screening from a Public Health Perspective: Some Lessons from the HIV Perspective', in Rothstein (1997: 137–58).

CALLAHAN, D. (1977), 'Health and Society: Some Ethical Imperatives', *Daedalus*, 106/1: 23–33.

_____ (1985), 'Hard Choices: Who Lives, How, and Who Decides? The Ethics of Making National Policy', *Health Matrix*, 3/3: 17–20.

_____ (1994), 'Bioethics: Private Choice and Common Good', *Hastings Center Report*, 24/3: 28–31.

_____ (1997), 'Equity and the Goals of Medicine', *World Health Forum*, 18: 123–5.

CAMPBELL, H., and BOYD, K. (1996), 'Screening and the New Genetics: A Public Health Perspective on the Ethical Debate', *Journal of Public Health Medicine*, 18: 485–6.

CAPLAN, A. L. (1994), 'Handle with Care: Race, Class, and Genetics', in T. F. Murphy and M. A. Lappe (eds.), *Justice and the Human Genome Project* (Berkeley: University of California Press), 30–45.

CAULFIELD, T. A. (1995), 'The Allocation of Genetic Services: Economics, Expectations, Ethics, and the Law', *Health Law Journal*, 3: 213–34.

CHADWICK, R. (1998), 'Genetic Screening', in Chadwick (ed.), *Encyclopedia of Applied Ethics*, ii (San Diego: Academic Press), 445–9.

CHAPMAN, A. R. (1997) (ed.), *Health Care and Information Ethics: Protecting Fundamental Human Rights* (Kansas City, Mo.: Sheed and Ward).

CHILDRESS, J., *et al.* (2002), 'Public Health Ethics: Mapping the Terrain', *Journal of Law, Medicine and Ethics*, 30: 170–8.

CLAYTON, E. W., *et al.* (1995), 'Informed Consent for Genetic Research on Stored Tissue Samples', *JAMA* 274: 1786–7.

CLINTON FOUNDATION (2006),<http://www.clintonfoundation.org/aids-initiative1.htm>.

COGSWELL, M. E., BURKE, W., McDONNELL, S. M., and FRANKS, A. L. (1999), 'Screening for Hemochromatosis: A Public Health Perspective', *American Journal of Preventive Medicine*, 16: 141–5.

COMMUNITY CAMPUS PARTNERSHIPS FOR PUBLIC HEALTH (2006), *Community-Based Participatory Research*,<http://ccph.info>.

CORDONE, J. (1996–7), 'Health Care Reform in the 1990's: From the Clinton Plan to Kassebaum–Kennedy', *Connecticut Insurance Law Journal*, 3/1: 193–219.

COUGHLIN, S. S., and BEAUCHAMP, T. L. (1996), *Ethics and Epidemiology* (New York: Oxford University Press).

_____ and MILLER, D. S. (1999), 'Public Health Perspectives on Testing for Colorectal Cancer Susceptibility Genes', *American Journal of Preventive Medicine*, 16: 111–15.

—— KHOURY, M. J., and STEINBERG, K. K. (1999), 'BRCA1 and BRCA2 Gene Mutations and Risk of Breast Cancer: Public Health Perspectives', *American Journal of Preventive Medicine*, 16: 91–8.

COUZIN, J. (2002), 'HapMap Launched with Pledges of $100 Million', *Science*, 298: 941–2.

—— (2005), 'New Haplotype Map May Overhaul Gene Hunting', *Science*, 310: 601.

CROUCH, R. A., and ARRAS, J. D. (1998), 'AZT Trials and Tribulations', *Hastings Center Report*, 28/6: 26–34.

CUNNINGHAM, G. C. (1997), 'A Public Health Perspective on the Control of Predictive Screening for Breast Cancer', *Health Matrix*, 7/1: 31–48.

DANIELS, N. (1994), 'The Articulation of Values and Principles Involved in Health Care Reform', *Journal of Medicine and Philosophy*, 19: 425–33.

DEGRAZIA, D. (1996), 'Why the United States Should Adopt a Single-Payer System of Health Care Finance', *Kennedy Institute of Ethics Journal*, 6: 145–60.

DE THE, G., *et al.* (2003), 'Ethical Issues in Research on Control of the HIV/AIDS Epidemic: Report from a Workshop of the World Federation of Scientists, Erice, Sicily, Italy, 22–24 August 2003', *Acta Paediatrica*, 93: 1125–8.

DHEW (DEPARTMENT OF HEALTH EDUCATION AND WELFARE) (1973), *Final Report of the Tuskegee Syphilis Study Ad Hoc Advisory Panel* (Washington, DC: US Government Printing Office), <http://biotech.law.lsu.edu/cphl/history/reports/tuskegee/tuskegee.htm>.

DOUGHERTY, C. J. (1996), *Back to Reform: Values, Markets, and the Health Care System* (New York: Oxford University Press).

DULA, A. (1991), 'Toward an African-American Perspective on Bioethics', *Journal of Health Care for the Poor and Underserved*, 2: 259–69.

—— (1994), 'African American Suspicion of the Healthcare System Is Justified: What Do We Do About It?', *Cambridge Quarterly of Healthcare Ethics*, 3: 347–57.

EMANUEL, E. J., and WEIJER, C. (2005), 'Protecting Communities in Research: From a New Principle to Rational Protections', in J. F. Childress, E. H. Meslin, and H. T. Shapiro (eds.), *Belmont Revisited: Ethical Principles for Research with Human Subjects* (Washington, DC: Georgetown University Press), 165–83.

ENGLEHARDT, H. T. (1994), 'Health Care Reform: A Study of Moral Malfeasance', *Journal of Medicine and Philosophy*, 19: 501–16.

FADEN, R. R., and KASS, N. E. (1991), 'Bioethics and Public Health in the 1980s: Resource Allocation and AIDS', *Annual Review of Public Health*, 12: 335–60.

GAMBLE, V. N. (1993), 'A Legacy of Distrust: African Americans and Medical Research', *American Journal of Preventive Medicine*, 9/6, suppl., 35–8.

GAO (UNITED STATES GENERAL ACCOUNTING OFFICE) (2003), *Newborn Screening: Characteristics of State Programs*, GAO-03–449 (Washington, DC: US General Accounting Office), <http://www.gao.gov>.

GLANTZ, L. H., ANNAS, G. J., GRODIN, M. A., and MARINER, W. K. (1998), 'Research in Developing Countries: Taking "Benefit" Seriously', *Hastings Center Report*, 28/6: 38–42.

GOLD, E. B. (1996), 'Confidentiality and Privacy Protection in Epidemiologic Research', in Coughlin and Beauchamp (1996: 128–41).

GOSTIN, L. O. (1991), 'Ethical Principles for the Conduct of Human Subject Research: Population-Based Research and Ethics', *Law, Medicine and Health Care*, 19/3–4: 191–201.

—— (1995), 'Genetic Privacy', *Journal of Law, Medicine and Ethics*, 23: 320–30.

—— (2003), 'The Global Reach of HIV/AIDS: Science, Politics, Economics, and Research', *Emory International Law Review*, 17: 1–54.

GOSTIN, L. O. and LAZZARINI, Z. (1997), *Human Rights and Public Health in the AIDS Pandemic* (New York: Oxford University Press).

_____ and MANN, J. M. (1994), 'Towards the Development of a Human Rights Impact Assessment for the Formulation and Evaluation of Health Policies', *Health and Human Rights*, 1: 58–80.

_____ LAZZARINI, Z., NESLUND, V. S., and OSTERHOLM, M. T. (1996), 'The Public Health Information Infrastructure: A National Review of the Law on Health Information Privacy', *JAMA* 275: 1921–7.

_____ HODGE, J. G., and VALDISERRI, R. O. (2001), 'Informational Privacy and the Public's Health: The Model State Public Health Privacy Act', *American Journal of Public Health*, 91: 1388–92.

_____ *et al.* (2002), 'The Model State Emergency Health Powers Act: Planning for and Response to Bioterrorism and Naturally Occurring Infectious Diseases', *JAMA* 288: 622–8.

GUAY, L. A., *et al.* (1999), 'Intrapartum and Neonatal Single-Dose Nevirapine Compared with Zidovudine for Prevention of Mother-to-Child Transmission of HIV-1 in Kampala, Uganda: HIVNET 012 Randomised Trial', *The Lancet*, 354: 795–802.

HARMAN, L. B. (2006), *Ethical Challenges in the Management of Health Information*, 2nd edn. (Sudbury, Mass.: Jones and Bartlett).

HOLTZMAN, N. A. (1997), 'Genetic Screening and Public Health', *American Journal of Public Health*, 87: 1275–7.

_____ and ANDREWS, L. B. (1997), 'Ethical and Legal Issues in Genetic Epidemiology', *Epidemiological Reviews*, 19: 163–74.

_____ and WATSON, M. S. (1998), *Promoting Safe and Effective Genetic Testing in the United States: Final Report of the Task Force on Genetic Testing. Task Force Created by NIH–DOE Working Group on ELSI of Human Genome Research* (Baltimore: Johns Hopkins University Press).

IOM (INSTITUTE OF MEDICINE) (1988), *The Future of Public Health* (Washington, DC: National Academy Press).

_____ (2002), *The Future of the Public's Health in the 21st Century* (Washington, DC: National Academy Press).

_____ (2003), *Who Will Keep the Public Healthy? Educating Public Health Professionals for the 21st Century* (Washington, DC: National Academy Press).

_____ (2005), *Implications of Genomics for Public Health: Workshop Summary* (Washington, DC: National Academy Press).

ISRAEL, B., SCHULZ, A., PARKER, E., and BECKER, A. (1998), 'Review of Community-Based Research: Assessing Partnership Approaches to Improve Public Health', *Annual Review of Public Health*, 19: 173–202.

JOHNSON, H., and BRODER, D. S. (1996), *The System* (Boston: Little, Brown).

KAHN, J. P., and MASTROIANNI, A. (1999), 'Innocents Abroad? The Ethics of International Research', *Minnesota Medicine*, 82/7: 28–9.

KASS, N. (2001), 'An Ethics Framework for Public Health', *American Journal of Public Health*, 91: 1776–82.

_____ and GIELEN, A. (1998), 'The Ethics of Contact Tracing Programs and Their Implications for Women', *Duke Journal of Gender Law and Policy*, 5: 89–102.

KHOURY, M. (1996), 'From Genes to Public Health: The Applications of Genetic Technology in Disease Prevention', *American Journal of Public Health*, 86: 1717–22.

_____ (1997), 'Relationship Between Medical Genetics and Public Health: Changing the Paradigm of Disease Prevention and the Definition of a Genetic Disease', *American Journal of Medical Genetics*, 71: 289–91.

_____ (2003), 'Genetics and Genomics in Practice: The Continuum from Genetic Disease to Genetic Information in Health and Disease', *Genetics in Medicine*, 5: 261–8.

KING, P. A. (1992), 'The Past as Prologue: Race, Class, and Gene Discrimination', in Annas and Elias (1992: 94–111).

KODISH, E. (1997), 'Commentary: Risks and Benefits, Testing and Screening, Cancer, Genes, and Dollars', *Journal of Law, Medicine and Ethics*, 25: 252–5.

LEMMONS, T., and AUSTIN, L. (2001), 'The Challenges of Regulating the Use of Genetic Information', *ISUMA: Canadian Journal of Policy Research*, 2: 26–35.

LURIE, P., and WOLFE, S. M. (1997), 'Unethical Trials of Interventions to Reduce Perinatal Transmission of the Human Immunodeficiency Virus in Developing Countries', *New England Journal of Medicine*, 337: 853–6.

McEWEN, J. E., and REILLY, P. R. (1994), 'Stored Guthrie Cards as DNA "Banks"', *American Journal of Human Genetics*, 55: 196–200.

MACKLIN, R. (1985), 'Mapping the Human Genome: Problems of Privacy and Free Choice', in A. Milunsky and G. J. Annas (eds.), *Genetics and the Law III* (New York: Plenum Press), 107–14.

_____ (1992), 'Privacy and Control of Genetic Information', in Annas and Elias (1992: 157–72).

MANN, J. M. (1997), 'Medicine and Public Health, Ethics and Human Rights', *Hastings Center Report*, 27/3: 6–13.

_____ et al. (1994), 'Health and Human Rights', *Health and Human Rights*, 1/1: 6–23.

MARKEL, H. (1997), 'Scientific Advances and Social Risks: Historical Perspectives of Genetic Screening Programs for Sickle Cell Disease, Tay-Sachs Disease, Neural Tube Defects and Down Syndrome, 1970–1997, App. 6', in National Human Genome Research Institute, Task Force for Genetic Testing, *Promoting Safe and Effective Genetic Testing in the United States*, <http://www.nhgri.nih.gov/ELSI/TFGT_final/appendix6.html>.

MORENO, J., and BAYER, R. (1985), 'The Limits of the Ledger in Public Health Promotion', *Hastings Center Report*, 15/6: 37 41.

MORONE, J., and BELKIN, G. S. (1994) (eds.), *The Politics of Health Care Reform: Lessons from the Past, Prospects for the Future* (Durham, NC: Duke University Press).

MSAMANGA, G. I., and FAWZI, W. W. (1997), 'The Double Burden of HIV Infection and Tuberculosis in Sub-Saharan Africa', *New England Journal of Medicine*, 337: 849–51.

MURPHY, T. F., and LAPPE, M. A. (1994) (eds.), *Justice and the Human Genome Project* (Berkeley: University of California).

MURRAY, T. (1997), 'Genetic Secrets and Future Diaries: Is Genetic Information Different from Other Medical Information?', in Rothstein (1997: 60–73).

NATIONAL COMMISSION FOR THE PROTECTION OF HUMAN SUBJECTS OF BIOMEDICAL AND BEHAVIORAL RESEARCH (1979), *The Belmont Report: Ethical Principles and Guidelines for the Protection of Human Subjects* (Washington, DC: Government Printing Office).

NATIONAL RESEARCH COUNCIL, COMMITTEE ON MAINTAINING PRIVACY AND SECURITY IN HEALTH CARE APPLICATIONS OF THE NATIONAL INFORMATION INFRASTRUCTURE (1997), *For the Record: Protecting Electronic Health Information* (Washington, DC: National Academy Press).

NIH–DOE (NATIONAL INSTITUTES OF HEALTH and DEPARTMENT OF ENERGY) (1997), *Promoting Safe and Effective Genetic Testing in the United States: Final Report of the Task Force on Genetic Testing Created by the National Institutes of Health—Department of Energy Working Group on Ethical, Legal, and Social Implications of Human Genome Research*,<http://www.genome.gov/10001733>.

NIH–NHGRI (NATIONAL INSTITUTES OF HEALTH and NATIONAL HUMAN GENOME RESEARCH INSTITUTE) (2002), 'News Advisory: International Consortium Launches Genetic Variation Mapping Project',<http://www.genome.gov/10005336>.

_____ (2003), 'News Release: International Consortium Completes Human Genome Project',<http://www.genome.gov/11006929>.

NIH–SACGT (NATIONAL INSTITUTES OF HEALTH SECRETARY'S ADVISORY COMMITTEE ON GENETIC TESTING) (2000), *Enhancing the Oversight of Genetic Tests: Recommendations of the SACGT* (Washington, DC: National Institutes of Health),<http://www4.od.nih.gov/oba/sacgt/reports/oversight_report.pdf>.

O'CONNELL, L. J. (1994), 'Ethicists and Health Care Reform: An Indecent Proposal?', *Journal of Medicine and Philosophy*, 19: 419–24.

O'FALLON, L., and DEARRY, A. (2002), 'Community-Based Participatory Research as a Tool to Advance Environmental Health Sciences', *Environmental Health Perspectives*, 110, suppl. 2, 155–9.

OMENN, G. (1996), 'Comment: Genetics and Public Health', *American Journal of Public Health*, 86: 1701–3.

PACE, C. A., and EMANUEL, E. J. (2005), 'The Ethics of Research in Developing Countries: Assessing Voluntariness', *The Lancet*, 365: 11–12.

PARTICIPANTS IN THE 2001 CONFERENCE ON ETHICAL ASPECTS OF RESEARCH IN DEVELOPING COUNTRIES (2004), 'Moral Standards for Research in Developing Countries: From "Reasonable Availability" to "Fair Benefits"', *Hastings Center Report*, 34/3: 17–27.

PAUL, D. B. (1994), 'Is Human Genetics Disguised Eugenics?', in R. F. Weir, S. C. Lawrence, and E. Fales (eds.), *Genes and Human Self-Knowledge: Historical and Philosophical Reflections on Modern Genetics* (Iowa City: University of Iowa Press), 67–83.

PENNISI, E. (2003), 'Reaching Their Goal Early, Sequencing Labs Celebrate', *Science*, 300: 409.

PERNICK, M. S. (1997), 'Eugenics and Public Health in American History', *American Journal of Public Health*, 87: 1767–72.

PROCTOR, R. N. (1992), 'Genomics and Eugenics: How Fair Is the Comparison?', in Annas and Elias (1992: 57–93).

RAZUM, O., and OKOYE, S. (2001), 'Affordable Antiretroviral Drugs for Developing Countries: Dreams of the Magic Bullet', *Tropical Medicine and International Health*, 6: 421–2.

ROSS, L. F. (2001), 'Genetic Exceptionalism vs. Paradigm Shift: Lessons from HIV', *Journal of Law, Medicine and Ethics*, 29: 141–8.

ROTHSTEIN, M. (1997) (ed.), *Genetic Secrets: Protecting Privacy and Confidentiality in the Genetic Era* (New Haven: Yale University Press).

_____ (2005), 'Genetic Exceptionalism and Legislative Pragmatism', *Hastings Center Report*, 35/4: 27–33.

SANKAR, P. (1997), 'Topics for Our Times: The Proliferation and Risks of Government DNA Databases', *American Journal of Public Health*, 87: 336–79.

SCHINDLER, T. F. (1994), 'Ethics and Information Systems: Making Values Explicit', *Health Progress*, 75/7: 60, 68.

SCHULL, W. J., and HANIS, C. L. (1990), 'Genetics and Public Health in the 1990s', *Annual Review of Public Health*, 11: 105–25.

SECUNDY, M. G. (1994), 'Strategic Compromise: Real World Ethics', *Journal of Medicine and Philosophy*, 19: 407–14.

SHALEV, C. (2004), 'Access to Essential Drugs, Human Rights and Global Justice', *Monash Bioethics Review*, 23: S56–74.

SKOCPOL, T. (1997), *Boomerang: Health Care Reform and the Turn Against Government* (New York: W. W. Norton).

SOSKOLNE, C. L. (2004), 'Public Health, IV. Methods', in S. Post (ed.), *Encyclopedia of Bioethics*, 3rd edn. (New York: Macmillan Reference USA), iv. 2215–21.

SPERLING, R. S., *et al.* (1996), 'Maternal Viral Load, Zidovudine Treatment, and the Risk of Transmission of Human Immunodeficiency Virus Type 1 from Mother to Infant', *New England Journal of Medicine*, 335: 1678–80.

STONE, D. H., and STEWART, S. (1996), 'Screening and the New Genetics: A Public Health Perspective on the Ethical Debate', *Journal of Public Health Medicine*, 18: 3–5.

VARMUS, H., and SATCHER, D. (1997), 'Ethical Complexities of Conducting Research in Developing Countries', *New England Journal of Medicine*, 337: 1003–5.

—— (1997), 'Ethical Complexities of Conducting Research in Developing Countries', *New England Journal Medicine*, 337: 1003–5.

WEIJER, C., and EMANUEL, E. J. (2000), 'Protecting Communities in Biomedical Research', *Science*, 289: 1142–4.

—— GOLDSAND, G., and EMANUEL, E. J. (1999), 'Protecting Communities in Research: Current Guidelines and Limits of Extrapolation', *Nature Genetics*, 23: 275–80.

WENDLER, D., EMANUEL, E. J., and LIE, R. K. (2004), 'The Standard of Care Debate: Can Research in Developing Countries be Both Ethical and Responsive to Those Countries' Health Needs?', *American Journal of Public Health*, 94/6: 923–8.

WHO (WORLD HEALTH ORGANIZATION) (1948), *Preamble to the Constitution of the World Health Organization as Adopted by the International Health Conference, New York, 19–22 June, 1946; Signed on 22 July 1946 by the Representatives of 61 States (Official Records of the World Health Organization, no. 2, p. 100) and Entered into Force on 7 April 1948*, <http://www.who.int/about/definition/en>.

WOLF, S. M. (1995), 'Beyond "Genetic Discrimination": Toward the Broader Harm of Geneticism', *Journal of Law, Medicine and Ethics*, 23: 345–53.

WOOLHANDLER, S., *et al.* (2003), 'Proposal of the Physicians' Working Group for Single-Payer National Health Insurance', *JAMA* 290: 798–805.

YAMEY, G. (2001), 'US Trade Action Threatens Brazilian AIDS Programme', *British Medical Journal*, 322: 383.

YEARBY, R. (2004), 'Good Enough to Use for Research, but Not Good Enough to Benefit from the Results of That Research: Are the Clinical HIV Vaccine Trials in Africa Unjust?', *DePaul Law Review*, 53: 1127–54.

CHAPTER 29

···

GLOBAL HEALTH

···

RUTH MACKLIN

HEALTH is a primary good for individuals. 'Primary goods' are things that every rational person would want because they are needed to carry out a personal life plan (Rawls 1971). Since populations are the sum of individuals in a country, it follows that health is also a primary good for populations. Public health is a public good, and in today's world public health is global health. If governments have any obligations that go beyond their national boundaries, they have obligations to promote global public health. An assumption of this chapter is that governments do have obligations that go beyond their own borders, and, consequently, they have obligations to help prevent the spread of disease, to provide financial or technical assistance to countries too poor to afford medical care and treatment for their own populations, and to adopt policies that preserve and promote health throughout the world.

But what is the source of obligations to protect and promote public health throughout the world? Is it a global obligation of beneficence, to maximize health benefits and minimize harms to health wherever those benefits and harms may exist? Is it an obligation based on a principle of justice that calls for helping the least advantaged populations, those too impoverished or lacking the knowledge or technical capacity to help themselves? Is it simply a matter of enlightened self-interest, an obligation to the population in one's own country to ensure that the developing world is not a reservoir for deadly infectious diseases or instability stemming from the devastating effects of ill health in large numbers of the population? Do obligations flow from human rights as specified in such

This chapter includes excerpts from my book *Double Standards in Medical Research in Developing Countries* (Cambridge: Cambridge University Press, 2004).

documents as the Declaration of Human Rights, the International Covenant on Economic, Cultural, and Social Rights, and customary international law?

In addressing these questions, this chapter deals with four topics in global health: (1) the accelerating rate of spread of communicable diseases throughout the globe; (2) the inequities among industrialized and developing countries in their populations' access to medical treatments; (3) the role of the World Trade Organization (WTO) and industrialized countries in maintaining barriers to poor countries' access to drugs; and (4) the relation between global health and human rights. What ties these topics together is the phenomenon of globalization in the broadest sense of that term.

Intercontinental transportation makes it possible for microbes as well as airline passengers to travel farther and more quickly than at any time in history. Tuberculosis and HIV/AIDS affect populations on every continent, but only a small minority of the world's population has access to effective treatments for these and other diseases. The vast increase in growth and power of transnational companies continues to produce increasingly worrisome environmental consequences, as well as occupational health hazards that affect populations in poor countries. Most such countries have neither the means (or desire) to resist giant industries nor the regulatory structure to protect the health of their own populations. The major multinational pharmaceutical companies, bolstered by the wealthy countries in which they are based, have successfully resisted weakening of patent protections in order that their profits remain as high as possible.

This chapter focuses on access of people in developing countries to medications and medical services that are readily available to inhabitants of industrialized countries. There are, of course, other critical dimensions of public health that require action on a global scale. These include relief for large numbers of people who are starving or living at nearly subsistence levels; provision of a supply of clean, potable water for populations deprived of that essential resource; and the consequences for local agricultural production in countries in which globalization has led to deforestation of vast portions of the land. The focus here on access to health services and needed medications is not intended to minimize the importance of these other areas of global health.

WHAT IS GLOBALIZATION?

Whatever globalization is, it has its strong proponents and opponents. Most people associate globalization with economics, world trade, and especially the establishment by huge international corporations of outposts in developing countries where labor in factories and agriculture is cheap. The fierce opposition to globalization is never more apparent than at the annual meetings of the WTO, where protesters gather to disrupt the travel of delegates as well as the proceedings of the meetings.

According to one definition, 'globalization' means 'openness to trade, to ideas, to investment, to people, and to culture' (Feachem 2001). This definition, with its positive connotation, seems overly broad. If that is all it means, it is hard to see why the phenomenon would give rise to such fierce opposition. Besides, it implies that globalization is nothing new; it has been around for a long time. A somewhat narrower definition takes globalization to be 'the trend of growing economic integration among nations' (Ricupero 2001: 3). Yet even that narrower definition does not describe anything new or, in the view of one commentator, particularly radical: 'Historians have traced its origins as far back as the great sea voyages of Renaissance Europe, and a small academic industry has been built around comparisons of the process of global economic integration today and in the decades before the First World War' (Ricupero 2001: 3).

Still another account, similar but taking the meaning beyond economic integration—'the increasing interconnectedness of people and nations through economic integration, communication and cultural diffusion'—also claims it is nothing new (Labonte 2003: 1). Noting that 'the history of most humankind has been one of pushing against borders, expanding, conquering, and assimilating', this account proceeds to specify a series of health risks that arise as a result of today's version of globalization. These include the harms resulting from resource depletion and pollution, increased transportation-based fossil-fuel emissions, and decreasing amounts of safe water, among others.

A comprehensive definition that is perhaps the most authoritative is provided by Joseph Stiglitz, winner of the 2001 Nobel Prize for Economics: 'Fundamentally, it is the closer integration of the countries and peoples of the world which has been brought about by the enormous reduction of costs of transportation and communication, and the breaking down of artificial barriers to the flow of goods, services, capital, knowledge, and (to a lesser extent) people across borders' (Stiglitz 2002: 9). Stiglitz argues that globalization has had global impacts, and to deal with those, global collective action is required. He cites global environmental issues as an example of such needed action, and the spread of diseases like AIDS, which respect no boundaries, as another. Stiglitz emphasizes the importance of 'global public goods' as values that transcend a country's own national interests. This contrasts starkly with the view expressed by George W. Bush: 'We will not do anything that harms our economy, because first things first are the people who live in America' (Singer 2002: 1–2).

In his book on the ethics of globalization, Peter Singer provides a more nuanced meaning of the term: 'implicit in the term "globalization" rather than the older "internationalization" is the idea that we are moving beyond the era of growing ties between nations and are beginning to contemplate something beyond the existing conception of the nation-state' (Singer 2002: 8). Whatever that 'something' is, it has implications for how nation-states do—and perhaps should—interact with one another. It raises the question whether, in a globalized world, nations have moral obligations that go beyond their own economic self-interest.

Factors other than the growth in power and wealth of transnational companies are at play in globalization. The role of the World Bank and the International Monetary Fund (IMF) in imposing a variety of economic reforms in developing countries has been a significant factor only indirectly related to world trade, if at all. The Bank and the IMF have required various forms of privatization and imposed 'structural adjustment' policies on poor countries as conditions of lessening or forgiving debts those countries are unable to repay. Stiglitz identifies the World Bank, the IMF, and the WTO as the main institutions that govern globalization.

Is globalization good or bad for human health? There are evidence and arguments on both sides of this debate. One view takes the unequivocal position that globalization is good for health:

The evidence that openness to trade and investment is good for economic growth is compelling and goes back several centuries. . . . Because gross national product per capita correlates so strongly with national health status, we can conclude that, in general, openness to trade improves national health status.

And further:

Globalisation, economic growth, and improvements in health go hand in hand. Economic growth is good for the incomes of the poor, and what is good for the incomes of the poor is good for the health of the poor. Globalisation is a key component of economic growth. (Feachem 2001)

The author of these remarks was the Director of Health, Nutrition, and Population at the World Bank from 1995 to April 1999. Given the role of the Bank in fostering globalization, this statement may be viewed as antecedently biased in its favorable assessment of the consequences.

While not denying that globalisation has had some positive influence on the health of poor people in developing countries, another commentator nevertheless provides evidence for the view that globalization can be bad for health. Globalization's negative impacts produce health risks in at least the following areas:

- Poverty and inequality—poverty being the single greatest determinant of disease.
- The environment—the disease perils of over-consumption, pollution and climate change are well known.
- The capacities of national governments—binding trade rules and multi-lateral institutions like the World Trade Organization . . . undercut institutions that support public health and social well-being.

(Labonte 2003: 1)

The promotion by the United States of a market model for delivery of health care has had negative consequences for developing countries that formerly had more robust public health systems. One article notes that 'a policy that promotes "market models" for the delivery of health care in less developed countries is an example of political, administrative globalisation rather than the global reach of for-profit health-care companies' (Pappas *et al.* 2003: 100). The increasing privatization of health in middle-income developing countries, such as Argentina and Brazil, has led to increasing costs for poorer segments of the population, as well as a wider gap in the quality of health care between the public and private sectors. In addition, there is evidence that the global economic policies of the World Bank, the WTO, and the IMF have contributed to chronic and severe malnutrition in many developing countries (Pappas *et al.* 2003).

An intermediate view is that globalization is a mixed blessing from a public health perspective. On the positive side are economic growth and technological advances that have improved the health status of populations in developing countries. On the negative side is the accelerated rate at which a decline in public health and the spread of disease can occur in those same countries. Among the public health consequences of globalization is the role of multinational tobacco companies, which are mostly based in the United States, the United Kingdom, and Japan. The tobacco industry has focused marketing campaigns on developing countries, chiefly in Asia and Africa. The World Health Organization (WHO) estimates that by about 2020 deaths due to tobacco will reach 10 million and 70 per cent of these deaths will be in developing countries (Ram 2001). This is occurring at the same time that anti-smoking campaigns and restrictive anti-smoking laws have resulted in a decline in the number of smokers in the United States and some other industrialized countries. In recognition of the toll tobacco has increasingly taken in developing countries, Gro Harlem Brundtland, the former Director-General of WHO, launched a major anti-tobacco initiative during her tenure at the organization.

WHO is the leading public health organization seeking to improve conditions in developing countries through both disease prevention and treatment programs. Stiglitz (2002) notes that globalization has led to renewed attention to this and other long-established intergovernmental organizations, which have generally been a force for good in the world. In this connection one could also add international nongovernmental agencies that do humanitarian work related to diseases and disasters, such as the International Red Cross and Médecins sans Frontières (MSF).

GLOBAL SPREAD OF COMMUNICABLE DISEASES

Several factors contribute to the current situation in which diseases that emerge in one part of the world spread—slowly or rapidly, but almost inevitably—to all parts of the globe. The best single example of that today is HIV/AIDS, which is believed to have begun in Africa when a simian (chimpanzee) strain of the virus jumped to humans. In a matter of years, a communicable disease that took root in Africa and spread with increasing rapidity in several countries on that continent came to affect millions of people throughout the world. By the end of 2003, an estimated 40 million people were living with HIV/AIDS and more than 3 million died in that year alone.

Early in the epidemic, epidemiologists confirmed the role of international travel as contributing to the speed with which the AIDS virus spread when they tracked down a single individual who became known as 'patient zero'. This individual was a Canadian flight attendant whose occupation called for worldwide travel. Researchers who analyzed a number of early cases of HIV/AIDS found that the Canadian flight attendant was either directly or indirectly involved in sexual contacts that spread the infection to these other persons.

It is not only HIV/AIDS, but also other communicable diseases that can spread rapidly by similar means. According to one report:

Infectious diseases are a global hazard that puts every nation and every person at risk. The recent SARS outbreak is a prime example. Knowing neither geographic nor political borders, often arriving silently and lethally, microbial pathogens constitute a grave threat to the health of humans. Indeed, a majority of countries recently identified the spread of infectious disease as the greatest global problem they confront.   (Institute of Medicine 2003)

However, HIV/AIDS, SARS (Severe Acute Respiratory Syndrome), avian influenza, and other current examples are not the first known instance of worldwide spread of diseases. One third of the population of Europe died in the Black Death epidemic of 1347, which was a direct result of international trade. When European explorers and colonial powers went to the Americas from about 1500 and through the next two centuries, they brought smallpox and other infectious diseases that decimated entire native populations. The influenza pandemic of 1918–19 killed between 40 and 50 million people in a single winter, and this was before the scale of modern transportation in today's world. With the constant movement of immigrants, refugees, military personnel, and travelers for business and tourism, the prospect of rapid global spread of diseases is greatly enhanced.

Among the recent examples is West Nile virus, which experts say is unlikely to be eradicated now it has reached the shores of North America, but at best can only be contained by vigilance and other methods. In the first three years after the virus first appeared in New York City, it spread to thirty-nine states in the United States, infecting thousands of people and killing several hundred (Institute of Medicine 2003). Avian influenza, or bird flu, is at the time of writing still confined to transmission from chickens and birds to humans in several countries in Asia. But public health and infectious disease experts are worried that if people become infected with both bird flu and other forms of influenza that people pass on to other people, the virus could recombine and render bird flu transmissible from human to human. Although the first cases of bird flu in humans were reported in Vietnam and subsequently in Thailand, avian influenza has been fatal in chickens in South Korea and Japan, as well as in the two countries where human disease has appeared.

This phenomenon of global spread of infectious diseases has given rise to multinational public health efforts, often led by WHO and with the cooperation of other governments and their agencies, such as the Centers for Disease Control and Prevention (CDC) in the United States. The experience with SARS is an interesting case study of the way a global health concern prompts a transnational response, raising public health, political, and ethical issues—as well as fears. The quarantine of infected individuals and those who had close contact with them is one example of a relatively rare response to an outbreak of disease in recent times.

SARS first appeared in Guangdong province, China, in November 2002, and quickly spread to other Asian countries and to Canada. The first worldwide outbreak killed 774 people by the end of 2003. By early 2004 new cases were detected in China. A highly infectious disease, SARS spread rapidly in densely populated areas despite the fact that China had a fairly elaborate system of public health law, designed to detect communicable diseases, prevent their spread, and enforce violation of the provisions of the laws. Those include the authority to quarantine and isolate people, close factories, schools, and shops, and even confiscate homes. Some new public health laws in China were put in place as a direct response to the SARS epidemic.

Meanwhile, because SARS had become a global threat, WHO was tracking the epidemic and became aware that China was underreporting SARS cases. WHO publicly rebuked China for failure to provide a full account of the number of cases—an unusual action for the international agency since WHO typically does not criticize its member states. The Chinese government itself also took an unusual political step when it permitted WHO to visit Taiwan to monitor the epidemic there, a move that it had earlier blocked. Coming less than a month after WHO's criticism of its underreporting, this signaled China's willingness to cooperate in what was now seen as a global health threat. According to one report, 'international political and economic realities led the PRC to institute massive isolation and quarantine and other measures to contain the spread of SARS' (Institute for Bioethics, Health Policy and Law 2003).

Whereas public health and governmental officials in China were slow to provide full and accurate reports of the disease, that information was forthcoming from other sources within China as a result of modern telecommunications and the Internet. Only after non-governmental sources provided information to WHO and the media did the official, governmental reports follow. In contrast, the government of Vietnam cooperated fully with WHO from the start. Taiwan also cooperated, although it is not a member nation of WHO.

The steps taken by the United States and other countries to determine whether travelers were infected when they arrived from countries where there was an outbreak of SARS were unusual, to say the least. Symptomatic passengers had their temperatures checked at airports, and passengers arriving by ship, maritime crews, and others crossing international borders faced the same procedures. Singapore, Taiwan, Hong Kong, and other areas where SARS cases were reported took similar measures. Although such surveillance measures are justifiable at the height of an epidemic, how long should they continue when there is no longer a perceived threat? One example cited is thermal sensors used to detect fever in international travelers entering a country. Thermal imaging and other screening measures were implemented without a thorough scientific knowledge of their effectiveness (Institute for Bioethics, Health Policy and Law 2003). Without such knowledge, there is a risk of false positives and false negatives, a risk that may be temporarily acceptable during the crisis. However, once the emergency situation abates, these and other intrusive measures should be suspended and evidence for their effectiveness carefully gathered.

The efforts made to contain the spread of SARS raise the perennial question of how to strike an ethical balance between protecting public health and preserving civil liberties. Isolation and quarantine in the SARS epidemic proved dramatically successful in containing the spread of the epidemic once the disease was recognized and these measures were put in place. Yet they are indisputably extreme measures in restricting individual liberty and intruding on privacy, arguably justified for the protection of public health. Still, critics could contend that the death rate from SARS was sufficiently low to question the use of extreme measures and the resulting worldwide fears that media reports caused. Was Taiwan justified in requiring that all airline passengers from SARS-infected areas wear masks? Was it justifiable to quarantine visitors from infected areas even if they had no disease symptoms, a measure imposed by India and Thailand?

Such questions could be answered fully only by using the gold standard in scientific methodology: controlled experiments in public health. To do that would raise practical, political, and ethical problems. The main practical problems are: Who would mount such experiments? And what would be the unit of analysis? The country? Different airplanes in Taiwanese airlines? Political problems would ensue if, for example, WHO were to conduct such experiments. Permission would have to be granted by the governments of any countries involved, and that would almost certainly give rise to objections by governments that would not consent to have their country randomized in a controlled experiment.

A likely ethical objection to randomized, controlled public health experiments would be the absence of individual informed consent, a standard requirement for research involving human beings. However, individual consent cannot be obtained for the type of experiments in which the unit to be randomized is a hospital or a community, yet those experiments are arguably necessary for answering certain types of questions. The most telling response to the concern about informed consent is that when public policies of all sorts are put in place, there is no informed consent by the public and, most often, no possibility of opting out. The only way of opting out of such policies (or experiments) would be choosing not to travel at all during health emergencies like SARS. All things considered, it would be preferable to seek to conduct such experiments if the practical and political barriers could be overcome.

In sum, the ethical issues that arise from infectious disease epidemics include the classic dilemma in public health: the trade-off between limiting the liberty of individuals suspected of having or carrying transmissible diseases and the public health need to halt or mitigate the spread of those diseases. With globalization, this tension—which formerly occurred within countries and primarily at the level of individuals—has been transformed into one that affects nations and calls for governments to establish policies and procedures, often those recommended by the World Health Organization.

The SARS outbreak resulted in limitations on travel of entire populations and the closing of borders of countries where disease outbreaks occurred. While some public health officials argued that these steps were desirable and necessary, others contended that the measures were unduly restrictive and alarmist. What is clear, however, is that the types of restrictive measures taken to contain the spread of SARS could never be justified in the case of HIV/AIDS. Although some people did promote such measures in the early stages of the AIDS pandemic, and Cuba actually did for a time impose mandatory isolation for people living with AIDS, that response was not only the most restrictive (and unwarranted) alternative, but also, as demonstrated in Cuba, ineffective in preventing the spread of HIV in the population.

GLOBAL DISEASES AND INEQUITABLE ACCESS TO TREATMENT

One of the more striking disparities in the global picture is the inequality in access to medical treatment among different populations in the world. The burden of disease is heaviest in developing countries, whereas access to treatments (not always cures) is greatest in the industrialized world. Many studies have demonstrated that health disparities between socioeconomic classes exists within countries—including wealthy ones—as well as in poorer countries. But the global disparity among rich and poor nations is an even greater inequity because the majority of the population in poor countries lacks access to medical treatment (as well as to clean water and adequate nutrition, in many cases). Until the early 1990s the response to this global inequity on the part of wealthier nations was, at best, some aid in the form of what is best described as charity. The traditional picture began to change with the establishment of international public–private partnerships between and among a variety of organizations. Private, nonprofit foundations, national governments, the WHO, newly created entities such as the Global Fund to Fight AIDS, Malaria, and Tuberculosis, and for-profit companies have formed various alliances aimed at making medical treatments affordable and accessible in countries where the majority of the population lacks access to such treatments.

Numerous factors besides lack of money hinder access to drugs in many developing countries, although poverty is the single most important reason why people in developing countries cannot obtain the drugs they need. These other factors include inefficiency and waste in health care delivery systems, inadequate systems for distribution of drugs within a country, lack of reliable scientific information and appropriate education and training of health care personnel, and local perceptions and beliefs about illness and medicine (Page 2002). The relatively poor health care infrastructure in many developing countries is a leading factor that inhibits access to drugs by large numbers of people. It would not be easy to remove these diverse barriers to adequate access to much-needed drugs, even if cheaper medications are made available and the Global Fund provides financing for drugs to treat AIDS, malaria, and tuberculosis.

These background conditions pose a question about the responsibility of industrialized countries to seek to redress the inequities in health status and access to treatment between the industrialized and developing world. The increasing number of public–private partnerships is evidence of a growing recognition that such a responsibility exists. Two of the latest efforts are described below.

The Global Fund

One of the initially most promising developments was the initiative taken by several United Nations agencies in establishing the Global Fund to Fight AIDS, Tuberculosis and Malaria. The call for the creation of a huge fund to combat diseases that kill or disable millions of people in poor countries came from both Gro Harlem Brundtland, the former Director-General of WHO, and Kofi Annan, the Secretary-General of the United Nations. Both leaders envisaged the need for commitments from government in rich and poor countries alike, as well as from private foundations, nongovernmental agencies, and the private sector to mount this effort. It would require funds not only for the purchase of drugs from manufacturers, but also to mount better educational and prevention programs, build new clinics or enhance existing ones, train health care workers, and strengthen the infrastructure in other ways.

Secretary-General Kofi Annan called for the establishment of a global fund on AIDS and health at the Organization of African Unity summit in Abuja in April 2001. In his 'Call to Action' Annan urged greater coordination among nations and a strong political and financial commitment to support efforts to combat AIDS

(UNAIDS 2001). Soon thereafter, pledges to the fund began coming in, with the United States initially pledging $200,000,000 and the United Kingdom an equal amount. A United Nations General Assembly Special Session on HIV/AIDS took place in New York in June 2001, and the United Nations adopted a declaration of commitment that set out clear goals for a global battle against HIV/AIDS. As of April 2003 pledges to the Global Health Fund totaled more than $US3 billion. The majority of the pledges were from governments, including contributions from rather poor African countries (Uganda and Zimbabwe).

The Global Fund formally adopted the stance of encouraging poor countries to purchase generic drugs instead of the more costly brand-name drugs still under patent protections by the big pharmaceutical companies. This approach was designed to enable manufacturers of generics in countries like Brazil and India, which have that capability, to sell their products to other resource-poor countries. However, the WTO's intellectual property agreement has been a major barrier to full access by poor countries to generic copies of medications that are still under patents held by the huge pharmaceutical companies (see discussion of the WTO in the next section).

Despite the promise inherent in the creation of the Global Fund, many have expressed extreme disappointment at the level of contributions, especially from the United States. In February 2002 the *New York Times* reported that donations to the fund had fallen far short of the amount initially sought by Secretary-General Kofi Annan—at least $7 billion a year—when the fund was established. Advocates for the fund blamed the White House, claiming that the $200 million pledge by the United States sets a poor example for other countries. However, much to the surprise of many people, in January 2003 President George W. Bush proposed his own Emergency Plan for AIDS Relief. Bush asked Congress to commit $15 billion over the subsequent five years, including nearly $10 billion in new money. The money was slated for the most afflicted nations of Africa and the Caribbean (Stolberg and Stevenson 2003). It was not clear at the time the announcement was made how much of those funds would go to the Global Fund.

One year later Bush's AIDS initiative appeared to be faltering, as well as succumbing to ideological and self-serving interests. By February 2004 the US government was about to make a first round of grants—only $350 million of the proposed $15 billion. While this initiative could easily have committed a significant portion of its promised money to the Global Fund, the Bush administration declined to do so. Instead, the individual appointed to run the program (a former chief executive of the huge pharmaceutical company Eli Lilly) decided to give much of the money to American contractors rather than to African groups. In addition, decisions about how to set priorities for use of the funds are delegated to the American ambassador in each country in which the United States provides technical assistance. Moreover, the director of this initiative is a supporter of the form of AIDS education that focuses only on abstinence, ignoring instructions on using and negotiating the use of condoms. Thus, despite the enthusiasm and optimism with which the Global Fund to Fight AIDS, Tuberculosis, and Malaria was launched, it has been in financial trouble almost from its inception and will continue to suffer a significant shortfall without the financial contribution the United States could readily make.

The WHO/UNAIDS 3 × 5 Initiative

One of the latest efforts to provide access to treatment for people in developing countries is the World Health Organization's 3 × 5 Initiative, a program WHO launched in December 2003 aimed at providing antiretroviral (ARV) treatment to 3 million people living with AIDS in developing countries by the year 2005 (WHO 2003). Only time will tell whether the hope and promise of this initiative by WHO and the Joint United Nations Programme on HIV/AIDS (UNAIDS) will be more successful than the Global Fund has been in seeking to fulfill its target. WHO and UNAIDS will not provide a major portion of the funding for this ambitious effort, but are taking a leadership role in partnerships that will include governments of WHO member nations along with industry and other organizations in the private sector.

Initiatives such as 3 × 5 bring with them new ethical challenges: as treatment programs are rolled out, how to select who goes first? Is there a clear and uncontroversial way of determining which groups in a population should be given first priority when all cannot be treated, at least initially? Is this challenge best met by coming up with a fair process for decision making rather than by seeking substantive criteria for equitable access to medical treatments? In its announcement and description of the 3 × 5 Initiative, WHO and UNAIDS included the following among the guiding principles:

- Ethical Standards. The Initiative will identify options for an ethical approach to meeting 3 by 5 targets.
- Equity. The Initiative will make special efforts to ensure access to antiretroviral therapy for people who risk exclusion because of economic, social, geographical or other barriers.

(WHO–UNAIDS 2003: 10)

Ideally, the 3 × 5 Initiative would provide ARV treatment free of charge through public health care institutions. This would ensure not only that the poor will not be excluded from the scaling up of ARV treatment, but also that priority will be given to the large numbers of people in developing countries for whom existing treatments have not been affordable and who would continue to be excluded if they had to pay out-of-pocket for ARV treatment. Moreover, on a practical level evidence from existing programs in which people in developing countries have had to pay for some or all of the cost of ARVs demonstrates an array of negative medical and social consequences, including interruption of therapy, deteriorating health status, poor adherence, and development of drug resistance (Attawell and Mundy 2003).

Although not everyone agrees that the poor should be given preference in scaling up ARV treatment, an argument in favor of giving preference to the poor is supported by a leading ethical principle: concern for the worst off, or the least advantaged—a principle known by the infelicitous term 'prioritarianism'. It means, essentially, that it matters morally that we help those who are least well off. The prioritarian principle calls for giving preference to those who are worst off in some relevant respect. In the context of health care delivery, this is usually understood to refer to those who are worst off in terms of health status, but it could also apply to the poorest members of society; the lowest socioeconomic class; the most vulnerable (for example, children, especially orphans); groups that are marginalized or most discriminated against (in many societies, intravenous drug users, sex workers, and men who have sex with men). Although the principle sets up a presumption in favor of least advantaged and most vulnerable groups, it does not call for giving strict priority to those groups.

Several ethical principles in addition to the prioritarian principle are potentially relevant and can provide justifications for choosing one or another scheme for access to ARV treatment. The *utilitarian* principle, applied specifically to health policy, aims at maximizing *health benefits* for the society as a whole. The best policy would be one that embodies a mix of health care services that produces the greatest overall health effects. An *egalitarian* principle of equity in this context would call for distributing resources equally among persons, or distributing goods, such as health care services, or health, equally among different groups. This could mean either that everyone should receive the same amount of *resources* for health care; or that everyone should receive the same amount of health care *services*; or that as far as possible, *health status* among different groups should be minimized. This principle is the basis for schemes that emphasize health equity over health maximization; there is thus a conflict with the utilitarian approach. The goal is to reduce disparities in health status among different groups or strata in society: the poor, women, people living in rural areas, ethnic or racial minorities, and others.

The three principles described here are likely candidates for a justifiable scheme that might be used by policy makers to set priorities within countries. These principles point to criteria or concerns that must be considered; but the principles can conflict, and it then becomes necessary to balance competing concerns. There is no uniquely correct way of doing this balancing. Moreover, there is no consensus on how the different principles ought to be weighted, or on how the goal of maximizing health should be weighted against other social goods. Different people often have different weightings. For these reasons, leading commentators have urged that emphasis has to be placed on fair processes (Daniels and Sabin 2002). To the extent that decision makers in each country can agree on principled ways to set priorities for equitable access among the various individuals and groups eligible for ARV treatment, the aforementioned principles can be used to justify their decisions. Even given such agreement, the use of fair procedures remains necessary since equity demands adherence to both substantive and procedural aspects of ethics.

In publicizing the 3×5 initiative, WHO described the situation regarding HIV/AIDS in developing countries as a 'public health emergency'. This raises the question of what follows from labeling a situation as an 'emergency'. Does it call for a response different from that in which the health needs of large numbers of people are identified as 'urgent'? In the WTO's agreement known as TRIPS—Trade Related Aspects of International Property—the concept of a national health emergency is a key condition that opens the door to loosening the strict patent protections that have reigned under the influence of the global pharmaceutical industry.

The World Trade Organization and Barriers to Access

In addition to the failure of market forces to ensure access to drugs, another significant factor contributing to the establishment of public–private partnerships has been the restrictions imposed by intellectual property rights. The question is whether the goal of promoting health merits exemption from the rules that govern world trade in all other commercial products. The stated purpose of intellectual property rights—patents, in particular—is to encourage commercial investments in research and development. Industry spokespersons maintain that patent protections are necessary for promoting research, and the resulting products benefit everyone, poor nations included.

The international trade agreements that protect the financial interests of patent holders in world markets have come under increasing scrutiny in the health arena. Critics of globalization claim that the WTO's protection of patents is responsible for the many ills that globalization produces, including poor health of vast numbers of people in developing countries (Singer 2002; Bloch and Jungman 2003). The TRIPS agreement, which became operative in January 1995, requires all member countries to respect the patents held by pharmaceutical and biotechnology companies and to pass laws respecting medical patents. Although the patent system serves the interests of manufacturers, the system is viewed by many to be in the public interest, as well as a benefit to the financial interest of industry. One description of the TRIPS agreement describes it as 'an attempt at the multilateral level to achieve the difficult task of balancing the public health interest in providing incentives for research and development into new drugs with the public health interests of making existing drugs as accessible as possible' (Watal 2001).

There is one provision in this agreement that enables countries to make an exception to the rule that requires respecting the patent rights of pharmaceutical companies. That provision permits countries to manufacture copies of patented drugs in case of a 'national emergency'. The mechanism for this is to obtain a 'compulsory license' to make a generic copy of a drug, and the patent holder is paid a reasonable royalty under this arrangement. Somewhat less certain under this provision has been the ability of a country to import a generic copy of a patented drug. An obvious question is what constitutes a 'national emergency'? Arguably, the AIDS epidemic in countries with a high prevalence rate would qualify. Does the same hold for countries with a high incidence and prevalence of malaria and tuberculosis?

Drug companies and their international umbrella organization, the International Federation of Pharmaceutical Manufacturers Associations, have long resisted efforts to invoke the provision that would allow countries to make or import generic copies of patented drugs under the compulsory licensing clause. Over a four-year period the United States came to soften its initial strong opposition to allowing South Africa (and by implication, other countries) to seek compulsory licensing for AIDS drugs.

Although many observers expected a reversal of the softened US stance with the arrival of the pro-business Bush administration, that did not happen with respect to South Africa. In fact, thirty-nine multinational drug companies that had brought a suit against South Africa began to negotiate to settle the lawsuit, especially after the European Union, WHO, and the National AIDS Council in France publicly supported South Africa's position (Swarns 2001). In April 2001 the companies withdrew their suit, thus allowing South Africa to import cheaper anti-AIDS drugs and other medications.

This move did not end other ongoing battles, however. Since 1998 Brazil has been a major challenger to the international pharmaceutical industry by copying and manufacturing AIDS drugs. State-owned laboratories in that country have produced generic copies of several patented AIDS drugs. Another country in the forefront of this development is India, where private companies have been manufacturing generic drugs. The most prominent of these companies is Cipla.

In May 2001 the Bush administration threatened trade sanctions against Brazil. The head of the Brazilian HIV/AIDS program called the US position 'unacceptable' (Crossette 2001a). In a surprising reversal, in June 2001 the United States withdrew the complaint it had made against Brazil in the WTO, agreeing to settle its dispute out of court. This decision by the United States was announced on the first day of a three-day meeting at the United Nations General Assembly devoted to the global AIDS crisis. The agreement between Brazil and the United States proposed to establish a joint panel that would deal with patent cases (Crossette 2001b).

Advocates of compulsory licensing have argued that it is the best alternative among the various efforts designed to provide essential drugs to developing countries, especially for treating HIV/AIDS. The authors of one article argue that 'making use of the . . . TRIPS provision or even breaking international trade agreements might be a given developing country's most effective means of providing life-saving medication time-efficiently to its people' (Schüklenk and Ashcroft 2002: 191). In an article discussing the moral responsibility of drug companies, Dan Brock concurs. He argues that developing countries are justified in not respecting product patents when this is the only effective means of making available pharmaceuticals necessary to save lives and protect the health of their citizens. '[T]his may be a case', Brock says, 'where two wrongs make a right' (Brock 2001: 37). In a just world, of course countries would be morally required to respect product patents. However, given existing global injustices, the decision not to respect product patents is morally justified.

The Declaration on the TRIPS Agreement and Public Health, issued at the WTO Ministerial conference on 14 November 2001, was not the best that might have been achieved. Nevertheless, it was an improvement over the previous situation, which not only left much uncertainty, but also held a strong presumption against the right of developing countries to gain access to much-needed drugs. Paragraph 4 of the 2001 Declaration states:

We agree that the TRIPS Agreement does not and should not prevent Members from taking measures to protect public health. Accordingly, while reiterating our commitment to the TRIPS Agreement, we affirm that the Agreement can and should be interpreted and implemented in a manner supportive of WTO Members' right to protect public health and, in particular, to promote access to medicines for all.   (WTO 2001)

In light of the statement in paragraph 4, the document goes on to say in paragraph 5: 'Each Member has the right to grant compulsory licenses and the freedom to determine the grounds upon which such licenses are granted'; and 'Each Member has the right to determine what constitutes a national emergency or other circumstances of extreme urgency, it being understood that public health crises, including those relating to HIV/AIDS, tuberculosis, malaria and other epidemics, can represent a national emergency or other circumstances of extreme urgency.' These statements make it explicit that the developing countries themselves are the ones to make determinations regarding compulsory licensing and national emergencies, surely an improvement over the previous situation. What, then, are the shortcomings of the Declaration on the TRIPS agreement?

The Declaration still did not go far enough since it contained a prohibition against importing inexpensive, generic drugs from countries that have the capability of manufacturing them. Paragraph 6 states:

We recognize that WTO members with insufficient or no manufacturing capacities in the pharmaceutical sector could face difficulties in making effective use of compulsory licensing under the TRIPS Agreement. We instruct the Council for TRIPS to find an expeditious solution to this problem and to report to the General Council before the end of 2002. (WTO 2001)

In effect, the Ministerial Conference sent this important issue back to committee.

The net effect of paragraph 6 was that only a small group of developing countries would be able to manufacture affordable generic medications for their own populations. Argentina, China, India, Mexico, and South Korea are among the developing countries in which the level of development of their pharmaceutical industries is sufficiently high to have innovative capabilities. Countries at the next lower level (having pharmaceutical industries with reproductive capabilities—active ingredients and finished products) include Brazil, Cuba, Egypt, Indonesia, and Turkey. There is a long list of countries with no pharmaceutical industry, including many in Africa, with high rates of HIV/AIDS: Botswana, Burkina Faso, Burundi, Central African Republic, Congo, Rwanda, and Senegal (Correa 2002).

The end of 2002 marked the deadline for finding an expeditious solution to the problem posed by paragraph 6 of the TRIPS agreement. The year 2002 came and went without a solution. In late December of that year the United States led other industrialized nations in refusing to accept the draft accord because it covered more drugs and more diseases than the United States was willing to accept. As in the March 2002 meeting, the United States insisted on limiting the drugs for those needed to combat HIV/AIDS, tuberculosis, and malaria, 'or other infectious epidemics of comparable gravity and scale' (Becker 2002). The other countries joining the United States in its opposition were Canada, the European Union, Switzerland, and Japan. All were seeking to protect the patents of the pharmaceutical industry, while still making available medicines to treat HIV/AIDS, malaria, and tuberculosis.

These countries balked at broadening the scope of any exceptions to paragraph 6 of the TRIPS agreement to include diseases like cancer and asthma. The United States and its industrial allies argued that allowing countries like China, Brazil, and India to manufacture generic copies of patented drugs for export without the consent of the patent holders would 'open the door to copying Viagra as well as ointments for baldness' (Becker 2002). In addition, the United States continued to insist that only the poorest countries should be able to benefit, which rules out countries such as Peru and the Philippines. The United States and its industrial allies cared more about protecting the pharmaceutical companies from inroads into their profits from remedies for sexual dysfunction and baldness than they cared about the suffering of millions of inhabitants of developing countries who have diseases other than the big three: AIDS, malaria, and tuberculosis.

There is, however, a reasonably happy ending to this story of intransigence on the part of the pharmaceutical industry and the United States as industry's major champion. In August 2003 the deadlock was broken when the United States signed an implementation agreement that enabled individual governments to determine which health problems could justify compulsory licenses that would allow for the export of medications. The decision effectively waives the obligations countries had under the provision of the TRIPS agreement (Article 31(f)) that prohibits such exports. WTO member nations agreed that this waiver would remain in effect until the article is formally amended. An interesting feature of this 2003 agreement is the voluntary exclusion from the waiver of twenty-three developed countries, despite the eligibility of all WTO members to import under the decision (*WTO News* 2003).

In contrast to what appeared to be a concession by the United States in its stalwart protection of the patent rights of pharmaceutical companies, in other less noticeable actions the United States continued to wield power preventing poor countries from gaining access to generic drugs for their populations. One example is the US–Central American Free Trade Agreement (CAFTA), made public in February 2004. That agreement revealed that a level of intellectual property protection greater than that of the amended TRIPS agreement restricts access to medicines for countries in Central America.

According to a report by Médecins sans Frontières (MSF):

> Provisions related to marketing authorization are particularly worrisome. For instance, if an existing AIDS drug is not registered in one of the five CAFTA countries because the manufacturer has no interest in the market, under CAFTA, registration of generics would be prevented for five years, even if the drug is not patented, and until the end of the patent term if it is. Unlike with patents, which authorities can redress through compulsory licensing, there is no recourse to provisions restricting marketing authorization. (MSF 2004)

MSF observed that weak or small countries that negotiate with the United States in small groups tend to agree to provisions that are less favorable to them than the international standards for trade and intellectual property rights such as those established by the WTO. Negotiators from these Central American countries caved in to pressures from the United States, providing further evidence that when it comes to medications badly needed in poor countries, the benefits of globalization accrue to industry, backed by the most powerful nations.

GLOBAL HEALTH AND HUMAN RIGHTS

Scholars in human rights and public health have identified several different provisions in human rights instruments as a basis for the claim that there exists a right to health care, as well as the right to health. Although some people have ridiculed the very idea that there can be a 'right to health', that criticism reflects a confusion between the right to *health* and the right to *be healthy*. Properly understood, the right to health is understood in terms of the obligations that governments have to protect the health of their populations and to establish policies that promote health and eliminate or decrease causes of disease. Since human rights pertain to all people, wherever they may live on this earth, the connection between human rights and health is global in scope.

The relevant human rights provisions begin with Article 25 of the Universal Declaration of Human Rights, which explicitly recognizes a claim to health:

'Everyone has the right to a standard of living adequate for the health and well-being of himself and his family, including food, clothing, housing and medical care and necessary social services, and the right to security in the event of unemployment, sickness, disability, widowhood, old age or other lack of livelihood in circumstances beyond his control.' Article 27 of the UDHR identifies another pathway to a right to health: 'Everyone has the right freely . . . to share in scientific advancement and its benefits.' To share in the benefits of scientific advancement can be interpreted to mean that the fruits of biomedical research must be made available to everyone who needs information or products developed in such research.

Article 12 of the International Covenant on Economic, Social and Cultural Rights (ICESCR) addresses 'the right of everyone to the highest attainable standard of physical and mental health', requiring states to take certain defined steps, including 'the prevention, treatment and control of epidemic, endemic, occupational and other diseases' and 'the creation of conditions which would assure to all medical service and medical attention in the event of sickness'. The wording of Article 12 recalls the preamble of the 1946 constitution of WHO, a member of the United Nations family of organizations: 'The enjoyment of the highest attainable standard of health is one of the fundamental rights of every human being without distinction of race, religion, political belief, economic or social conditions.'

How can these fundamental human rights claims regarding health care and health be realized in the poorest countries in the world today, given the prevalence of diseases that are difficult to prevent and costly to treat? Which actors should play a role in the progressive realization of these rights? Do the governments of industrialized nations have any human rights obligations to protect and promote the health of people in developing countries? As explained below, wealthier countries do have such obligations, whether or not they contributed in any way to the poor health of people in developing countries, and even if that poor health is a consequence of decisions and actions by the leaders of those countries.

One of the tasks of the United Nations committees authorized to monitor the implementation of human rights treaties is to make ongoing reviews of progress in light of changing circumstances. This process results in the periodic issuing of General Comments. One pertinent example is a comment issued by the Committee on Economic, Social and Cultural Rights when it revisited Article 12 of the International Covenant on Economic, Social and Cultural Rights: the right to the highest attainable standard of health. The Committee observed that much has changed in the world health situation since the ICESCR was adopted in 1966, noting that more determinants of health are now recognized, such as resource distribution and gender differences (Committee on Economic, Social and Cultural Rights 2000).

The Comment identifies *accessibility* as one of the essential elements required for fulfilling the right to health. This includes accessibility to health facilities, goods, and services with four overlapping dimensions: nondiscrimination (accessibility to everyone), physical accessibility, economic accessibility, and information accessibility. In addition to enumerating various detailed actions that states parties must undertake in order to respect, protect, and fulfill their obligations regarding this right, the Comment includes a section on international obligations. It refers states parties to a declaration that 'proclaims that the existing gross inequality in the health status of the people, particularly between developed and developing countries . . . is politically, socially and economically unacceptable and is, therefore, of common concern to all countries' (Committee on Economic, Social and Cultural Rights 2000: 11). Compliance with their international obligations requires countries with available resources to 'facilitate access to essential health facilities, goods and services in other countries, wherever possible and provide the necessary aid when required' (Committee on Economic, Social and Cultural Rights 2000: 11–12).

It is clear from this detailed commentary on the right to the highest attainable standard of health that wealthier countries (among those that have ratified the ICESCR) have international obligations to assist in providing access to health facilities, goods, and services to resource-poor countries. Although only states parties are accountable to fulfill this and other human rights obligations, the Comment also addresses nonstate actors. It states that all members of societies have responsibilities regarding the right to health, including intergovernmental and nongovernmental organizations, civil society, and the private business sector. The Comment specifically identifies the WTO, which is a member of the United Nations system, as one of the organizations that should cooperate effectively with states parties regarding the implementation of the right to health. Although the WTO ministerial conference at Doha did not go far enough, the agreement reached in August 2003 goes a long way toward allowing member states to make policies for importing or exporting drugs that fulfill their responsibility as stipulated in Article 12 of the ICESCR—the right of everyone to the highest attainable standard of physical and mental health.

Obviously, it is not sufficient to issue and reissue ethical and human rights guidelines. Monitoring activities are needed to ensure that implementation of provisions in these guidelines is taking place. To that end, a guideline that stipulates human rights obligations with regard to HIV/AIDS specifies a large array of actions that governments must take. These actions include setting benchmarks and targets for measuring progress; consulting with people living with HIV/AIDS, nongovernmental organizations, and international health organizations; enacting laws to ensure that an adequate supply of medicines is available in a timely manner; allocating funds for research, development, and promotion of therapies; and working with the private sector to achieve these goals; among many others.

A key recommendation for implementation of this human rights guideline for HIV/AIDS explicitly acknowledges the obligations of wealthier nations toward poorer countries in a globalized world. This recommendation says:

States and the private sector should pay special attention to supporting research and development that address the health needs of developing countries. In recognition of the human right to share in scientific advancement and its benefits, States should adopt laws and policies, at the domestic and international levels, ensuring that the outcomes of research and development are of national and global benefit, with particular attention to the needs of people in developing countries and people who are poor or otherwise marginalized. (Office of the United Nations High Commissioner for Human Rights and the Joint United Nations Programme on HIV/AIDS 2002)

An array of conceptual, ethical, and policy questions regarding the interpretation of human rights provisions require further study and discussion. How can it be determined when the highest attainable standard of health has been reached? Against which measures is 'highest attainable' to be defined? How should priorities be set among the competing health-related needs in developing countries, and what role, if any, should donor nations and international organizations play in promoting some priorities over others in working with ministries of health in developing countries? Making drugs more affordable to the populations in developing countries is only a first step toward realization of the human right to health, but it is a giant step.

INTERNATIONAL OBLIGATIONS OF JUSTICE

The facts of globalization raise the fundamental question of what, if anything, rich countries owe to poor countries in the realm of health. Is health essentially different from other public goods, such as education and police protection, for which it is the responsibility solely of national, state, or local governments to provide for their people? And if rich countries ought to provide major assistance in helping resource-poor countries meet the health needs of their populations, is it because there is a moral obligation to do so? Or is it because the interests of rich and powerful countries are threatened by the destabilization that occurs in countries where the crisis produced by AIDS and other devastating diseases affects not only the health infrastructure but also the entire governmental structure and its ability to provide education and social services? Do obligations of distributive justice cross international boundaries? Or should industrialized nations assist in providing health benefits to poor countries because it is in their own national self-interest to do so?

Depending on one's political convictions and views about social justice, different answers to these questions will be forthcoming. People of varying political persuasions are likely to agree that a global response to infectious diseases like SARS and avian influenza is warranted, since failure to take timely and effective steps can have dire health consequences for populations in all countries, rich or poor, industrialized or least developed. This is a case in which national self-interest coincides with global health interests. A straightforward application of the utilitarian principle, aimed at health maximization, serves as a justification for assisting other nations in their efforts to contain transmissible diseases. Disagreements will inevitably arise, however, on the justification for specific decisions and actions where a tension occurs between health and civil liberties. Additional disagreements are also inevitable regarding the amount of resources that should be expended for this purpose. These disagreements are no different from ones that occur regarding domestic situations that are relevantly similar.

Principled disagreements are likely to arise over whether wealthy nations have a moral obligation to assist poor nations in providing access to health care and necessary medications for their populations. Adherents of the principle of justice that calls for providing assistance to the least advantaged or worst off will use that principle as a direct justification for providing financial, technical, or medical assistance to combat diseases in poor countries. Among those adherents, disagreements may arise with regard to the severity or scope of diseases that affect the populations in resource-poor countries. Does the principle justify providing assistance to treat all diseases equally? Should priority be given to the most devastating diseases, such as HIV/AIDS, malaria, and tuberculosis? What about diseases that affect smaller numbers of people but are nonetheless serious and endemic in tropical areas, such as parasitic infections that pose no threat to countries in the North? Here again, specific disagreements are inevitable in making choices and setting limits.

Those who reject the principle that calls for providing assistance to the least advantaged in the global arena might still endorse a more limited basis for help in circumstances where rampant or endemic disease leads to destabilization of a country and thus ultimately threatens countries in North America and Europe. This is the 'enlightened self-interest' rationale for helping poor countries with their health needs in an era of globalization. Whether it is fear of being overwhelmed by illegal and unhealthy immigrants, worries about providing a breeding ground for terrorists, some other perceived threat, or unalloyed beneficence, even the 'America first' administration of George W. Bush can justify providing billions of dollars for antiretroviral drugs to treat people living with AIDS in Africa.

Only under the most severe international pressure did the United States and other industrialized countries that support huge pharmaceutical companies give in to proposed reforms of the WTO's TRIPS agreement. Permitting poor countries to import affordable generic drugs from other developing countries that manufacture them seems like such an obvious remedy in confronting the disease burden in developing countries, it is hard to conceive of a moral argument that could prohibit it. In fact, there is no moral argument. It is, rather, the age-old principle of 'might makes right': the power and influence of the pharmaceutical industry that have prevailed for so many years in this domain.

When it comes to the various United Nations human rights treaties, the United States has an abysmal record. The only major treaty that the United States has signed and ratified is the International Covenant on Civil and Political Rights. The United States has not ratified (but has signed) the International Covenant on Economic,

Social and Cultural Rights, the Convention on the Elimination of All Forms of Discrimination Against Women, or the Convention on the Rights of the Child. Does this mean that the United States does not have any obligations imposed by those treaties? No, because human rights can be identified in international custom and treaties, as well as in the decisions of treaty bodies and organizations that contain human rights as a central aspect of their mandate. Treaty laws may become customary international law if widely enough observed. Moreover, when a country signs but does not ratify a treaty, it is still bound not to contravene the treaty's terms.

Although bioethicists have devoted relatively little attention to the relationship between ethical principles and human rights provisions, the latter are a source of obligations recognized in a wide variety of global contexts. For those bioethicists who find merit in the use of ethical principles, the principles of both beneficence and distributive justice can readily serve to justify public health policies that have a global and not merely intranational reach. If the principle that calls for policies that maximize health and minimize the burden of disease applies domestically, why should it not also apply globally? If the principle that mandates an equitable distribution of health-related benefits and burdens applies within a country, why should it not also apply across national boundaries?

In today's globalized world, public health is global health. Since public health is a public good, it requires contributions and commitments from all sectors—public, private, governmental, nongovernmental, and international. Although some may argue that it is justifiable for national interests to override the plight of those in faraway lands, it is hard to see how it is in the interest of any nation to ignore or dismiss the health needs of everyone in a globalized world.

REFERENCES

ATTAWELL, L., and MUNDY, J. (2003), *Scaling up the Provision of Antiretroviral Therapy in Resource-Poor Countries: A Review of Experience and Lessons Learned* (London: DFID Health Systems Resource Center for the UK Department for International Development in collaboration with WHO).

BECKER, E. (2002), 'Trade Talks Fail to Agree on Drugs for Poor Nations', *New York Times*, 21 Dec.; <http://select.nytimes.com/search/restricted/article?res=F40D15F634590C728ED DAB0994DA404482>.

BLOCH, M. G., and JUNGMAN, E. R. (2003), 'Health Policy and the WTO', *Journal of Law, Medicine and Ethics*, 31/4: 529–45.

BROCK, D. W. (2001), 'Some Questions About the Moral Responsibilities of Drug Companies', *Developing World Bioethics*, 1/1: 33–7.

COMMITTEE ON ECONOMIC, SOCIAL AND CULTURAL RIGHTS (2000), 'Substantive Issues Arising in the Implementation of the International Covenant on Economic, Social and Cultural Rights', General Comment no. 14, E/C.12/2000/4, 11 Aug.

CORREA, C. M. (2002), 'Implications of the Doha Declaration on the TRIPS Agreement and Public Health', *WHO, Essential Drugs and Medicines Policy*, EDM Series, no. 12 (Geneva: World Health Organization), Annex 2, 1 n. 5.

CROSSETTE, B. (2001*a*), 'Brazil's AIDS Chief Denounces Bush Position on Drug Patents', *New York Times*, 3 May, A5.

—— (2001*b*), 'U.S. Drops Case Over AIDS Drugs in Brazil', *New York Times*, 26 June.

DANIELS, N., and SABIN, J. E. (2002), *Setting Limits Fairly* (New York: Oxford University Press).

FEACHEM, R. G. A. (2001), 'Globalisation Is Good for Your Health, Mostly', *British Medical Journal*, 323: 504–6, <http://bmj.bmjjournals.com/cgi/content/full/323/7311/504>.

INSTITUTE OF MEDICINE (2003), *Microbial Threats to Health: Emergence, Detection, and Response* (Washington, DC: National Academies Press), <http://www.nap.edu/catalog/10636.html?, <http://books.nap.edu/execsumm_pdf/10 636.pdf>.

INSTITUTE FOR BIOETHICS, HEALTH POLICY AND LAW (2003), *Quarantine and Isolation: Lessons Learned from SARS*, <http://www.louisville.edu/medschool/ibhpl/publications /SARS%20REPORT.pdf>.

LABONTE, R. (2003), *Dying for Trade: Why Globalisation Can Be Bad for Our Health* (Toronto: CSJ Foundation for Research and Education).

MSF (MÉDECINS SANS FRONTIÈRES) (2004), 'CAFTA Provisions Restrict Access to Medicines', <http://www.doctorswithoutborders.org/news/2004/02-03-2004.cfm>.

OFFICE OF THE UNITED NATIONS HIGH COMMISSIONER FOR HUMAN RIGHTS AND THE JOINT UNITED NATIONS PROGRAMME ON HIV/AIDS (2002), *HIV/AIDS and Human Rights: International Guideline*, Revised Guideline 6 (New York: United Nations).

PAGE, A. K. (2002), 'Prior Agreements in International Clinical Trials: Ensuring the Benefits of Research to Developing Countries', *Yale Journal of Health Policy, Law, and Ethics*, 3/1: 35–64.

PAPPAS, G., HYDER, A. A., and AKHTER, M. (2003), 'Globalisation: Toward a New Framework for Public Health', *Social Theory and Health*, 1: 91–107.

RAM, E. (2001), *Global Future* (First Quarter), 22.

RAWLS, J. (1971), *A Theory of Justice* (Cambridge, Mass.: Belknap Press).

RICUPERO, R. (2001), 'The Poverty of Globalisation, the Globalisation of Poverty', *Global Future* (First Quarter), 3–5.

SCHÜKLENK, U., and ASHCROFT, R. E. (2002), 'Affordable Access to Essential Medication in Developing Countries: Conflicts Between Ethical and Economic Imperatives', *Journal of Medicine and Philosophy*, 27/2: 179–95.

SINGER, P. (2002), *One World: The Ethics of Globalisation* (New Haven: Yale University Press).

STIGLITZ, J. E. (2002), *Globalisation and Its Discontents* (New York: W. W. Norton).

STOLBERG, S. G., and STEVENSON, R. W. (2003), 'Bush AIDS Effort Surprises Many, But Advisers Call It Long Planned', *New York Times*, 30 Jan., A19.

SWARNS, R. L. (2001), 'Companies Begin Talks with South Africa on Drug Suit', *New York Times*, 18 Apr., A3.

UNAIDS (2001), 'Global AIDS and Health Fund', <http://www.aegis.com/news/unaids /2001/UN010625.html>.

UNITED NATIONS (1948), *Universal Declaration of Human Rights*, General Assembly Resolution 217A (III).

—— (1966), *International Covenant on Economic, Social and Cultural Rights*, General Assembly Resolution 2200A (XXI).

Watal, J. (2001), 'Background Note', prepared for WHO–WTO Workshop on Differential Pricing and Financing of Essential Drugs (8–11 Apr.), 7.

WHO (World Health Organization) (2003), '3 × 5 Initiative', <http://www.who.int/3by5/en>.

WHO–UNAIDS (2003), *Treating 3 Million by 2005: Making It Happen* (Geneva: World Health Organization).

WTO (World Trade Organization) (2001), *Declaration on the TRIPS Agreement and Public Health, Ministerial Conference*, WT/MIN(01)/DEC/W/2 (14 Nov).

WTO News (2003), WTO News Press/350/Rev.1, 30 Aug., <http://www.wto.org/english/news_e/pres03_e/pr350_e.htm>.

CHAPTER 30

BIOETHICS AND BIOTERRORISM

JONATHAN D. MORENO

UNTIL the terrorist attacks of 11 September 2001, and the subsequent anthrax scare, modern bioethics paid little attention to issues concerning preparation for and response to bioterrorism (Moreno 2002). Yet a number of foundational bioethical problems are engaged or given a new twist by this topic, including the rights of human research subjects, resource allocation, the appropriate balance of human rights and public health, and special responsibilities of emergency health care workers. Bioterrorism also takes bioethics into novel territory, such as the social obligations of private industry and the uses of genetics both in developing terror weapons and in defending against them.

Although the term 'bioterrorism' has only recently come into widespread use, the tactical notion of using biological or chemical agents to spread terror among enemy forces reaches back to the First World War. The psychological impact of waging terror campaigns against civilians using various destructive means was first evident in the American Civil War, especially during Union General William T. Sherman's infamous march through Georgia. In the Second World War both sides attempted to terrorize non-combatants, the Nazis by bombing the British mainland, and the Americans with firebombs in Germany and Japan and, of course, the first atomic weapons. Terror campaigns by radical political movements, rather than nation-states, took place in the 1960s in Europe and the United States, mainly in the form of attacks on financial institutions and the air transportation system. The novelty of twenty-first century bioterrorism lies in the prospect that it will combine political radicalism with techniques that were once largely the province of state military establishments.

The term 'bioterrorism' seems to have become a kind of shorthand for sowing terror through the use of other 'unconventional' weapons, especially chemical, nuclear, and radiological weapons, or 'dirty bombs'. The ethical problems associated with these other threats are closely associated with those raised by biological agents. Therefore, this chapter will necessarily refer to these related potential terrorist technologies, all of them made more available to militant organizations through the spread of knowledge and material in the post-cold war era.

Biological Weapons and the Ethics of Human Experiments

Following the anthrax attacks in the fall of 2001, the US government made efforts to expedite the restocking of smallpox vaccine supplies and to develop safer and more effective medical responses to biological weapons generally. The smallpox vaccine trials in particular demonstrated that the general public is enthusiastic about volunteering for clinical trials when fears of a bioterrorism attack are widespread. Although the initial phase of the clinical research on the viability of the vaccine had taken place well before 11 September 2001, the project generated little public interest until after the anthrax attacks.

The smallpox vaccine studies were conducted mainly to determine whether vaccine derived from dilutions of stocks 'on the shelf' since the 1970s could register a 'take' in a human being. It would have been unethical to expose a human being deliberately to smallpox in order to determine the efficacy of the vaccination. This ethical obstacle to efficacy studies in humans has been a matter of concern to governmental authorities for some years. An alternative to human efficacy testing was exemplified in July 2000, when the US Food and Drug Administration approved ciproflaxicin (Cipro) for use as post-exposure therapy for inhalational anthrax based on laboratory data, animal studies, clinical trials for other diseases, and experience with the drug in routine clinical use. This model essentially became law in 2002, when the FDA adopted the 'animal rule', which allows certain important therapies that could be used in the case of a terror attack to be approved based on animal rather than human efficacy testing (Moreno 2003).

Although bioethics has only recently discovered issues associated with bioterrorism (ACHRE 1996; Moreno 2003), the history of medicine and warfare is replete with examples of attempts to use disease as a weapon, even before the mechanism of bacterial infection was understood. In one famous example, blankets used by soldiers dying of smallpox during the French and Indian wars are said to have been given to Indians in the hopes of spurring an epidemic. In the twentieth century a number of governments tried to enlist medical science, including human experimentation, in an effort both to produce and to defend against biological weapons that could create terror. Discussions of medical ethics and policy concerning such experiments took place at high governmental levels, especially following the trials of Nazi experimenters at Nuremberg, West Germany, in 1946–7. The imperial Japanese military pursued a massive research and development program on biological and chemical weapons in occupied Manchuria. Though thousands died, none of the scientists involved was subjected to prosecution by the American administrative authority (Moreno 2001).

During the early 1950s, while the US Department of Defense was trying to assess the utility of biological and chemical weapons, Pentagon officials determined that there was no policy governing the use of human subjects in atomic, biological, and chemical (ABC) weapons research. At the time there was suspicion that both the Soviets and the Communist Chinese were surpassing the United States and its allies in developing these technologies. Reports from the Korean War suggested that psychoactive drugs were being used on American prisoners of war in an attempt to 'brainwash' them into providing sensitive information or even to program them to become Communist agents. Following a highly contentious secret internal debate, in 1953 the Secretary of Defense established the Nuremberg Code as the official policy of the Department for defensive ABC warfare research, including a requirement for written consent (Moreno 2001).

One specific issue that arose repeatedly in these discussions was who would be appropriate candidates for human experiments. Military personnel were an obvious possibility, for exposure to elevated risk is part of what it is to serve in the military. On the other hand, the use of service members as 'human guinea pigs' seemed to be both an affront to their dignity and a threat to morale. Both positions were taken before, during, and after the Second World War. Another option was the use of long-term prisoners. Their captivity made them attractive subjects in any case, and various inducements could be employed to obtain 'volunteers'. But the Nuremberg Nazi doctors' trial rendered this option potentially embarrassing. Hospitalized patients were another possibility, but studies with these individuals would mainly be limited to addenda to their regular treatment (as in the case of cancer patients undergoing radiation therapy); and sick patients were not necessarily the best model for a general population, let alone for healthy young military personnel. By the early 1950s there was no entirely satisfactory solution to this problem and instead a mix of subjects was utilized, sometimes with consequences that became scandals when publicly revealed years later (Moreno 2001).

There are at least two striking aspects of this concern about human experiment policies in the allied defense establishment in the early cold war era. First, these discussions presaged the academic debate about research ethics that began in the mid-1960s following several scandals; in fact, there was virtually no conversation on these issues in the early 1950s outside the military, and even the World Medical Association's Helsinki Declaration took until the mid-1960s to become final. Second, the effects of these early policies were, at best, modest. Although there is evidence that attempts were made to disseminate the conditions intended to govern human experiments funded or sponsored by national security agencies, in many instances the rules were not applied.

The US Army Inspector General reached this conclusion in 1975, following the revelations of LSD experiments on thousands of soldiers in the 1960s (Moreno 2001).

Other activities that possess characteristics of medical experiments have not been classified as such, and therefore have not been subject to informed consent requirements. One prominent example is the deployment of thousands of soldiers, sailors, and airmen to atomic bomb test shots from the late 1940s to the early 1960s. Another example, about which more was learned only in 2002, is a program of aerosolized nerve gas field tests over ships at sea and in proximity of soldiers on the ground in the late 1960s. The rationale for excluding some experimental activities from informed consent procedures is mainly the need to develop force protection methods as new threats become known. This problem has become especially salient in the war on terror, in which it is assumed that soldiers are among the most likely victims of biological or chemical attacks. In the civilian context there is an analogous justification in public health, a subject I will address in the next section.

Among the unsettled ethical issues concerning human experiments in an era of bioterrorism is whether special rules should apply to classified research studies undertaken by governments. Some would argue that there is no justification for classified human experiments, others that information must be denied to an adversary, such as which strains of a certain biological agent can and cannot be defeated by available therapy. In any event, if classified human experiments are to be undertaken as part of the war on terror, as was the case during the cold war, then ethical principles of respect for persons and beneficence appear to require both prior review by a research ethics board and informed consent on the part of potential subjects. In turn, all involved parties will require the appropriate level of security clearance so that they can receive relevant information. More difficult to implement under classified conditions will be an appeals procedure in which complaints about secret research can be reviewed.

Observational studies are another sort of human experiment that may follow a catastrophic event. These projects may be undertaken by life scientists, as in the case of the long-term study of survivors of the atomic bombs at Hiroshima and Nagasaki, or behavioral scientists, such as those who interviewed persons exposed to the collapse of the World Trade Center. Protection of potential human subjects is especially difficult because there is no confidentiality for those who have been affected by the event. They are easily identified, perhaps even named in newspaper stories or interviewed by the broadcast media. Traumatized survivors may welcome the opportunity to talk to authority figures like physicians and psychologists, but may not in the acute period appreciate the scientific rather than therapeutic purpose of the study (Fleischman and Wood 2003).

Besides the standard requirements of prior review by a research ethics committee and informed consent there are no well-established special protections for the survivors of a terrorist event. It is not clear that any further conditions are warranted, but at the very least the visibility of victims suggests that they may be subject to repeated contacts by multiple teams of well-meaning investigators, a problem that is largely unique to this population of potential subjects.

PUBLIC HEALTH AND CIVIL LIBERTIES

In the fall of 2001 the deliberate contamination of letters with anthrax and their subsequent distribution through the US mail system resulted in five deaths, thousands of exposures, and hundreds of persons treated. As no one could know the extent of the threat while it unfolded, the ensuing public health crisis called attention to what many regarded as weaknesses not only in bioterrorism preparedness but also in the legal framework that empowers public health authorities to act in an emergency.

In response to a request by the federal Centers for Disease Control and a number of national organizations, a group of public health law scholars developed the Model State Emergency Health Powers Act (MSEHPA). The MSEHPA is intended to provide a comprehensive set of legal standards for the response to catastrophe while also respecting civil liberties. At the time of writing more than twenty states have adopted versions of the model act (Center for Law and the Public's Health 2003). The ink had barely dried on the MSEHPA, however, when critics charged that its provisions represented infringements on freedoms that were unjustifiable on ethical or public health grounds.

State law is the traditional repository of public health authority, but the MSEHPA authors believed that they were inadequate, obsolete, and therefore sufficiently variable from one jurisdiction to another to hamper efficient emergency response, as such events do not respect state borders. At the time, many states did not require that a strategic plan be in place for a public health emergency or ensure that channels of communication among responsible officials in neighboring states can be kept open. As well, there was significant variation in state laws concerning surveillance for early detection of pathogens so that containment and treatment plans could be triggered. Reporting systems for dangerous potential bioterrorism agents were varied or altogether absent, nor was it legally possible in some states for public health agencies to monitor data acquired from the health system, which might provide signals of unusual disease patterns (Hodge and Gostin 2003).

These and other perceived deficiencies in the status quo were partly due to concerns about infringements on civil liberties. Adequate emergency planning and response may require such extreme actions as the seizure of property for decontamination and the imposition of medical treatment such as vaccination or quarantine. Individuals may be required to sacrifice some of their freedom for the common good. Yet the MSEHPA authors argued that such sacrifices both are justifiable and, with proper safeguards in place, present acceptable and temporary limits on individual rights.

The MSEHPA therefore authorizes the governor to declare a public health emergency that continues until the threat is eliminated or after thirty days, except when reinstated by the governor or annulled by the legislature or a court. An emergency is defined as an imminent threat caused by bioterrorism, or a fatal biological toxin, or a new or previously controlled infectious agent that presents a high probability of numerous deaths or disabilities. Thus action by a state's chief executive is authorized regardless of whether the public health emergency is the result of intentional human action, as in terrorism, or not (Hodge and Gostin 2003).

The model statute also requires, within twenty-four hours, reporting by doctors of cases of disease that may be caused by infectious agents, by coroners of deaths from such diseases, by pharmacists of unusual prescription patterns, and by veterinarians of deaths of animals that may have had diseases that present potential danger to humans. Besides the cooperation with government of these various professional groups, the MSEHPA encourages data-sharing among health agencies at all levels of government, with restricted access to medical records of quarantined persons in order to protect their privacy.

Under the Act property may be seized as needed to respond to a threat once the emergency has been declared. Assets needed to eliminate infectious waste, dispose of human remains safely, or otherwise to control the situation may be procured, with just compensation to any property owners who are deprived of their use. Measures may be taken to prevent or halt exploitive commercial practices like price gouging, for scarce public health services to be rationed, and for health care providers to be pressed into service.

During the emergency persons may be asked to submit to physical examinations and vaccinations, with the alternative their quarantine or isolation. These latter measures are thought to be rarely required and then are to be governed by a 'least restrictive' standard, consistent with the public health goal. Except for extreme cases, health officials must obtain a court order under the MSEHPA for the imposition of physical restrictions on individuals. If individuals are restricted without such an order, they are entitled to receive information and be represented by legal counsel if they wish to challenge the order or any of the conditions of isolation (Hodge and Gostin 2003).

The model statute's critics found it based on a post-11 September hysteria that neither improved existing public health protections nor squared with traditional civil liberties. It granted public health professionals the power to order citizens to undergo medical examinations and interventions and to force physicians and hospitals to do their bidding, all under the threat of prosecution. Such provisions, it was argued, are contrary to both constitutional law and medical ethics (Annas

2003*a*). They are also are said to be far too broad, applying not only to a smallpox outbreak but also to many kinds of non-emergency conditions such as the annual flu epidemic (Annas 2003*b*).

Critics of the MSEHPA objected particularly to its provisions for the use of force in public health emergencies. Not only has large-scale quarantine been of dubious efficacy as compared with less restrictive alternatives but it may also create difficulties with public compliance. Public trust, it is argued, is the most important factor in effective public health interventions and should not be jeopardized by overreaction. Indeed, the fall 2001 anthrax attacks resulted in demands for screening and treatment by those potentially exposed, though many believed that trust in the offered anthrax vaccine was compromised by the refusal of the Department of Health and Human Services to make a recommendation on vaccination, or on which groups should be vaccinated (Annas 2003*b*).

Besides objections to the model statute's details, a more general issue is the investment of public health resources in bioterrorism preparedness rather than those more familiar sources of morbidity and mortality—current infectious diseases, chemical accidents, food-borne illness, drug and alcohol abuse—for which prevention or treatment is available but under-utilized. The rationality of this critique runs afoul of the powerful symbolism of national security as somehow transformative of what might otherwise be a straightforward allocation question.

TRIAGE IN A BIOTERROR ATTACK

The Napoleonic armies were the first to practice a system of sorting casualties of war in order to maximize the good for the greatest number of injured combatants. This utilitarian approach is also thought to satisfy the formal requirement of justice: equity or the treatment of similar cases similarly. Equitable treatment will vary in its detail depending on the situation, but in any case should be guided by the greater likelihood that some individuals will benefit from treatment more than others, both in quality and duration, and in the urgency of treatment.

There are at least two senses of utility operative in triage for military and civilian disasters: the medical utility already described, and social utility. The latter refers to the value for the entire fighting force of returning wounded soldiers to duty. But it may also apply to a larger sense of common good that could justify an expanded form of triage in which egalitarian principles are modified to take into account the exceptional value of certain individuals to society, such as political leaders or those with rare technical expertise. A difficulty with a broad version of social utility is that it provides little guidance for specific judgments in the event of a terrorist attack or similar catastrophic event. A narrower version that provides more guidance is combined with medical utility, namely the multiplier effect of salvaging medical personnel so that they can in turn provide medical care to others (Childress 2003).

Although triage may justifiably compromise human equality, egalitarian approaches could be applied within sorted groups. Once those who offer exceptional services to society are identified, a weighted lottery could be employed so that they are exposed to some risk, albeit less than others. In this way the principle of equal human worth is honored while social utility is recognized.

Any triage arrangements that are part of planning for a terrorist attack should be publicly justifiable. Public confidence is a necessary condition for the social cooperation that will be critical in such an event, and in any case the nature of health care activities is such that they will be open to the scrutiny of many individuals. Individual physicians and other health care professionals should not be the only ones to bear the burden of developing triage criteria; the institutions of which they are a part, professional organizations, and government acting through appropriate agencies should all be partners in planning for allocating scarce resources. These entities must share in the accountability that should accompany decisions that will result in the death or suffering of some rather than others. Depending on the nature of the threat and the available resources, care may have to be provided in homes and civic institutions such as schools and houses of worship. To help ensure the trust and cooperation needed to execute plans that may bring the sick and dying into the heart of the community, some form of public participation should also be integrated into the planning process.

Community acceptability of triage arrangements will, as indicated, be especially important if an incident is of such magnitude that the infrastructure of health care institutions themselves are compromised by the scale of the attack and the subsequent number of injured, or by the infliction of massive casualties upon health care workers themselves, or by the nature of the attack that causes some patients to be a danger to many others. In catastrophic cases, illustrated by the atomic bombings of Hiroshima and Nagasaki in 1945 or widespread biological exposures that create a severe risk of further contamination if the victims are collected near those not exposed, medical care will have to be provided outside hospitals. Planning for this sort of emergency must be far-sighted as it entails decentralizing health resources in various community settings rather than in hospitals. These arrangements, too, involve allocation decisions that entail public participation and accountability (Kipnis 2003).

RESPONSIBILITIES OF EMERGENCY HEALTH CARE PROFESSIONALS

Emergency health workers implicitly accept a higher level of risk than other persons, and even other health care workers, in the course of their professional activities. Not only in terms of their commitment but also as a result of their training, they are better prepared than most to confront danger, as well as to know how to act in ways that may allow life and limb to be salvaged. But what sorts of responsibilities and risks must these individuals assume? And even the most skilled emergency worker cannot be effective without the cooperation of others. What sort of infrastructure should be in place to support the extraordinary efforts of a few?

Those who assume the responsibilities of emergency medical personnel are often supposed to be prepared to provide their services in an egalitarian fashion to all in need. Yet universal beneficence is never plausible as some distinctions must always be drawn. One basis for distinguishing between levels of obligation that is so common it is rarely questioned is that of geographic distance: it is generally thought to be acceptable to minister first to those nearby rather than those suffering far away. But virtually all of those who present themselves for emergency care are moral strangers. Yet there can be grievous social consequences to the failure to confront a distant crisis with the same degree of moral seriousness that one would a local one, even though practicalities may justify tragic choices.

After the determination of the commitment emergency workers must assess the nature of the threat following the initial incident. Security agencies in particular are in a position to support or hinder the free flow of information necessary to threat assessment. Their decision making must take into account not only the public health implications of withholding sensitive information but also the social implications if, for example, the incident has especially affected members of minority groups who may already harbor skepticism about government and health care institutions based on historic experience. Thus the broader implications of decisions by national security agencies can compromise not only threat assessment but also the public cooperation that makes emergency intervention more effective (Eckenwiler 2003).

Following threat assessment, the emergency response should follow from the advance planning, perhaps involving triage. As discussed above, in this phase the most effective response will be that which has included the broadest possible public participation, transparency, and accountability, relieving health care workers of any unfair burden of determining allocation criteria on their own.

When interventions are to be provided, health care personnel will often need to make rapid decisions on behalf of patients who are unable to consent to treatment. In these cases medical best interests can form a legitimate basis for intervening. If the injuries are such that there is no validated medical therapy, then emergency workers may find themselves in a state of equipoise, in which an innovative, albeit theoretically plausible, approach may be no less promising than the standard care. If such approaches are anticipated in the event of an emergency, they should arguably be presented to the public as part of the planning process, similar to the 'community consultation' requirement in advance of clinical trials in the emergency department (Eckenwiler 2003). Finally, health care workers may also be obligated to impose medical treatment or isolation on individuals who pose a threat to the public. Once again, appropriate legal and institutional structures should be in place so that emergency workers do not shoulder an unfair burden of responsibility for potentially controversial decisions.

We have seen that considerations of national security assume unique relevance in communicating information that has public health consequences when the source of the threat is thought to be a terrorist attack. Problems of information management arise not only in threat assessment at the outset, but also in the maintenance of conventions of privacy and confidentiality. Justifiable expectations about the privacy of health information records both honor respect for persons and also give individuals the confidence that presenting themselves for medical care will not expose them to stigmatization or other social risks. These expectations may be overridden when the implications of personal health information are relevant to actions that can preserve public health, as in the case of highly infectious disease. Arguably, considerations of national security may also justify the release of personal health information as needed, to help identify the source of an outbreak, for example. Conversely, national security authorities may determine that the health status of certain groups that would normally be available to health officials should be specially safeguarded, at least for some time (Eckenwiler 2003). Again, emergency health care personnel should not be solely responsible for interpreting the circumstances under which the release of information is desirable or not, nor should the rules under which these decisions are made be imposed upon the public without prior consultation.

Emergency physicians are accustomed to finding themselves implicitly in the position of agents of law enforcement, as when they care for individuals whose injuries may have been incurred in the course of a crime. Systematic ties to national security agencies in preparation for a terrorist attack may be viewed by some as likely to compromise the ideals of independence of medical practice and transparency of public health practice. Similarly, concentration on bioterrorism preparedness can take time away from other and arguably more pressing health initiatives in response to current rather than potential threats to public health. Particularly when contemplating extreme conditions, emergency health care personnel face unique conflicts of professional responsibility that should not be theirs to bear alone (Eckenwiler 2003).

An example of the way these conflicts can emerge is the decontamination of an individual who has been exposed to a dangerous chemical agent. Unlike bacterial or viral exposures, which generally require a longer-term response, there is a brief window of treatment for victims of a chemical attack. That window requires them to disrobe and be flushed with water. In the acute period victims may not feel terribly ill and may resist public nudity. Personal decontamination kits or even large trash bags can be slipped over the outer garments so that the individual can disrobe; in some cases underwear can be kept on. These measures require a degree of expertise and planning to avoid overt conflicts between patient autonomy and the emergency worker's beneficence-based duties in a crisis (Trotter 2004).

ORGANIZATION ETHICS

Organizations engaged in the delivery of services or production of goods for health care purposes incur special moral obligations. These moral obligations are sharpened in the event of a dire emergency. Yet non-governmental entities, whether technically 'for profit' or not, have a more tenuous relationship to the public good than government agencies. What is the relationship between their social obligations and their legitimate business interests? Under extreme conditions such as those that may be associated with a bioterror attack, privately held resources like pharmaceuticals or the time and skills of physicians that are normally strictly controlled by corporate interests could be needed for the public good (Mills and Werhane 2003).

A standard approach to the obligations of business entities is stakeholder theory, which states that corporate moral obligations are determined by the direct interests of shareholders. Yet a strict construal of stakeholder theory sanctions highly profitable products like child pornography that exploit the vulnerable and corrupt social life. Surely the narrow construction is unacceptable. Further, in the case of health care-related services and products, and especially in emergent circumstances, the stakeholders must be construed more broadly as including health care consumers. This broadened view of corporate stakeholders is incompatible with the notion that profit is the sole end of a business, but compatible with the view that profit is, and under ordinary conditions must be, an appropriate goal of business activity.

When extraordinary conditions prevail, then, private interests may be required to serve pressing social needs. Drug manufacturers, for example, should plan for special pricing strategies in the event of a widespread public health threat, a prudent step in any case as they risk losing control over a product if government chooses to assert its prerogatives for the greater good and withdraw patent protection. Similarly, although proprietary interests concerning sensitive product information should be protected, secrecy practices may extend beyond necessity and impinge on the public's need to know. Industry-wide secrecy standards could eliminate concerns about competitive advantage while preserving the free flow of socially valuable information (DeRenzo 2003).

Corporations engaged in the production and distribution of substances that could be turned to terrorist advantage also have an obligation to put adequate security measures in place and to provide educational programs for their employees. Cooperation with local, regional, and, depending on the nature of the business, even national authorities may be required, especially if the company's facilities could be directly exploited and toxic substances released (DeRenzo 2003).

GENETICS AND BIOTERRORISM

Finally, new scientific developments can become objects of interest for technically sophisticated groups bent on terror. In the late 1990s several government advisory groups warned that the conclusion of the human genome project and subsequent advances in genetics created risks for the United States concerning genetically modified bioterror organisms. In its extreme form, attempts might even be made to engineer bioweapons that target specific racial groups, though the scientific feasibility of such weapons is in grave doubt considering the genetic diversity within racial groups. More plausible are efforts to modify viruses so that they will elude currently available vaccines, or perhaps agents that could act on agriculture (Meslin 2003).

Fortunately, these worries are highly speculative. More immediate are the consequences of scientific security concerns for academic freedom and, in the long run, improved prevention and treatment of the ills that accompany bioterrorism. These improvements are most likely to occur rapidly in an atmosphere in which scientific cooperation flourishes, and the free flow of information is critical to that process. To help ensure that scientific progress for the public good is not stifled, the self-regulation of scientists with guidance from government seems preferable to heavy-handed restrictions on scientific exchange that, paradoxically, exacerbate the threat by preventing many groups of scientists from attempting to develop novel approaches.

In the era of bioterrorism a scientific event that would normally be a cause of unalloyed celebration, the publication on the World Wide Web of the 'map' of the human genome, raises concerns about the openness of science and the role of government in both utilizing and constraining scientific activity (Meslin 2003). This problem illustrates how far bioethics has traveled from its original concerns with the rights of patients and research subjects, the allocation of life-saving technology, and the implications of genetics for the future of humanity. Yet the bioethical issues stimulated by bioterrorism also revive each of these topics in a new light while they create new ones, challenging the creativity and resourcefulness of those interested in the life sciences and human values.

REFERENCES

ACHRE (ADVISORYCOMMITTEE ON HUMAN RADIATION EXPERIMENTS) (1996), *The Human Radiation Experiments* (New York: Oxford University Press).

ANNAS, G. J. (2003*a*), 'Terrorism and Human Rights', in Moreno (2003: 33–49).

—— (2003*b*), 'Blinded by Bioterrorism: Public Health and Liberty in the 21st Century', *Health Matrix*, 13: 33–50.

CHILDRESS, J. F. (2003), 'Triage in Response to a Bioterrorist Attack', in Moreno (2003: 77–93).

DeRenzo, E. G. (2003), 'The Rightful Goals of a Corporation and the Obligations of the Pharmaceutical Industry in a World with Bioterrorism', in Moreno (2003: 149–66).

Eckenwiler, L. A. (2003), 'Emergency Health Professionals and the Ethics of Crisis', in Moreno (2003: 111–31).

Fleischman, A. R., and Wood, E. B. (2003), 'Research Involving Victims of Terror: Ethical Considerations', in Moreno (2003: 185–97).

Gostin, L. O., et al. (2002), 'The Model State Emergency Health Powers Act: Planning for and Response to Bioterrorism and Naturally Occurring Infectious Diseases', *JAMA* 288: 622.

Hodge, J. G., and Gostin, L. O. (2003), 'Protecting the Public's Health in an Era of Bioterrorism: The Model State Emergency Health Powers Act', in Moreno (2003: 17–32).

Kipnis, K. (2003), 'Overwhelming Casualties: Medical Ethics in a Time of Terror', in Moreno (2003: 95–107).

Meslin, E. M. (2003), 'Genetics and Bioterrorism: Challenges for Science, Society and Bioethics', in Moreno (2003: 199–218).

Mills, A. E., and Werhane, P. H. (2003), 'After the Terror: Health Care Organizations, the Health Care System, and the Future of Organization Ethics', in Moreno (2003: 167–81).

Moreno, J. (2001), *Undue Risk: Secret State Experiments on Humans* (New York: Routledge).

—— (2002), 'Bioethics After the Terror', *American Journal of Bioethics*, 2: 60–4.

—— (2003), *In the Wake of Terror: Medicine and Morality in a Time of Crisis* (Boston: MIT Press).

Trotter, G. (2004), 'Chemical Terrorism and the Ethics of Decontamination', *Journal of Clinical Ethics*, 15: 149–60.

INDEX